General Surgery Board Review

Third Edition

Gallagher's steakhouse
245 5336
228 W. 52nd
(8th - BDWAY)

Maritime 354-1717
125/ 6th
(49th/6th
st/Ave)

Tupelo Grill
7602700
One Penn Plaza

General Surgery Board Review

Third Edition

Editors

Michael S. Gold, M.D., F.A.C.S.
Clinical Professor of Surgery
Columbia University
College of Physicians and Surgeons
Surgeon-in-Chief
The Mary Imogene Bassett Hospital
Department of Surgery
Cooperstown, New York

Larry A. Scher, M.D., F.A.C.S.
Chief, Division of Vascular Surgery
Associate Professor of Surgery
North Shore University Hospital/
New York University School of Medicine
Manhasset, New York

Gerard Weinberg, M.D., F.A.A.P., F.A.C.S.
Associate Professor
Department of Surgery and Pediatrics
Albert Einstein College of Medicine
Montefiore Medical Center
Bronx, New York

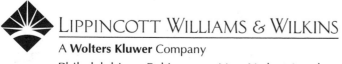

LIPPINCOTT WILLIAMS & WILKINS
A **Wolters Kluwer** Company
Philadelphia · Baltimore · New York · London
Buenos Aires · Hong Kong · Sydney · Tokyo

Acquisitions Editor: Lisa McAllister
Developmental Editor: Rebecca Irwin Diehl
Manufacturing Manager: Kevin Watt
Supervising Editor: Mary Ann McLaughlin
Production Service: Bermedica Production, Ltd.
Cover Designer: Patricia Gast
Indexer: Bermedica Production, Ltd.
Compositor: Compset
Printer: R. R. Donnelley

Printed in the United States of America

9 8 7 6 5 4 3 2

Library of Congress Cataloging-in-Publication Data

General surgery board review / editors, Michael S. Gold, Larry A.
   Scher, Gerard Weinberg. — 3rd ed.
      p.   cm.
      Includes bibliographical references and index.
      ISBN 0-397-51851-X
      1. Surgery—Examinations, questions, etc.   I. Gold, Michael S.
   II. Scher, Larry A.   III. Weinberg, Gerard.
      [DNLM: 1. Surgical Procedures, Operative examination questions.
   WO   18.2G326   1998]
   RD37.2G462   1998
   617'.0076—dc21
   DNLM/DLC
   for Library of Congress   98-29424
                                                                   CIP

Care has been taken to confirm the accuracy of the information presented and to describe generally accepted practices. However, the authors, editors, and publisher are not responsible for errors or omissions or for any consequences from application of the information in this book and make no warranty, expressed or implied, with respect to the contents of the publication.

The authors, editors, and publisher have exerted every effort to ensure that drug selection and dosage set forth in this text are in accordance with current recommendations and practice at the time of publication. However, in view of ongoing research, changes in government regulations, and the constant flow of information relating to drug therapy and drug reactions, the reader is urged to check the package insert for each drug for any change in indications and dosage and for added warnings and precautions. This is particularly important when the recommended agent is a new or infrequently employed drug.

Some drugs and medical devices presented in this publication have Food and Drug Administration (FDA) clearance for limited use in restricted research settings. It is the responsibility of the health care provider to ascertain the FDA status of each drug or device planned for use in their clinical practice.

Contents

Contributors

Mosses Bairamian, M.D. *Assistant Professor, Attending Anesthesiologist, Department of Anesthesiology, New York Medical College, Valhalla, New York 10595*

Robert Bibi, M.D., F.A.C.S. *Department of Plastic Surgery, Albert Einstein College of Medicine, 547 Gidney Avenue, Newburgh, New York 12550*

Lawrence S. Bizer, M.D., F.A.C.S. *Associate Professor of Surgery, Albert Einstein College of Medicine, 3424 Kossuth, Bronx, New York 10467*

Steven A. Blau, M.D., F.A.C.S. *Department of Surgery, Hackensack Medical Center, 30 Prospect Avenue, Hackensack, New Jersey 07601*

Neil J. Cobelli, M.D. *University Orthopedics Associates, 1180 Morris Park Avenue, Bronx, New York 10461*

Michael Coomaraswamy, M.D. *Assistant Professor of Surgery, Department of Surgery, Montefiore Medical Center, 1575 Blondell Avenue, Bronx, New York 10461*

Sanford Dubner, M.D. *Assistant Clinical Professor of Surgery, Department of Surgery, North Shore University Hospital, 200 Middle Neck Road, Great Neck, New York 11021*

Steven G. Friedman, M.D. *Department of Surgery, North Shore University Hospital, 300 Community Drive, Manhasset, New York 11030*

Elizabeth A. M. Frost, M.D. *Professor and Chair, Department of Anesthesiology, New York Medical College, Valhalla, New York 10595*

Brigid K. Glackin, M.D., F.A.C.S. *Clinical Instructor of Surgery, Tufts University School of Medicine, Department of Surgery, West Campus, Baystate Medical Center, Springfield, Massachusetts 01199*

Michael S. Gold, M.D., F.A.C.S. *Clinical Professor of Surgery, Columbia University College of Physicians and Surgeons; Surgeon-in-Chief, The Mary Imogene Bassett Hospital, Department of Surgery, Atwell Road, Cooperstown, New York 13326*

Robert D. Goldstein, M.D., F.A.C.S. *Associate Professor, Plastic and Reconstructive Surgery, Albert Einstein College of Medicine, 1625 Poplar Street, Bronx, New York 10461*

James T. Goodrich, M.D., Ph.D., F.R.C.M. (Lond.) *Professor of Clinical Neurological Surgery, Pediatrics, Plastic and Reconstructive Surgery, Leo Davidoff Department of Neurological Surgery, Albert Einstein College of Medicine, Montefiore Medical Center, 111 East 210th Street, Bronx, New York 10467*

Tito Gorski, M.D. *Fellow in Surgery, The Brooklyn Hospital Center, 121 DeKalb Avenue, Brooklyn, New York 11201*

Bruce Greenstein, M.D., F.A.C.S. *Department of Plastic Surgery, Albert Einstein College of Medicine, Montefiore Medical Center, 1825 Eastchester Road, Bronx, New York 10461*

Stuart Greenstein, M.D., F.A.C.S. *Associate Professor of Surgery, Department of Surgery, Albert Einstein College of Medicine, Montefiore Medical Center, 111 East 210th Street, Bronx, New York 10467*

Michael H. Hall, M.D. *Adjunct Associate Professor, Cardiothoracic Surgery, North Shore University Hospital, 300 Community Drive, Manhasset, New York 11030*

Keith S. Heller, M.D., F.A.C.S. *Clinical Professor of Surgery, Department of Surgery, North Shore University Hospital, 200 Middle Neck Road, Great Neck, New York 11021*

W. John B. Hodgson, M.D. *Professor of Surgery, Department of Surgery, Montefiore Medical Center, 1875 Blondell Avenue, Bronx, New York 10461*

David F. Jimenez, M.D. *Assistant Professor of Neurological Surgery, Division of Neurology, University of Missouri Hospital, N521 Health Science Center, 1 Hospital Drive, Columbia, Missouri 65212*

Ronald N. Kaleya, M.D. *Associate Professor of Surgery, Department of Surgery, Montefiore Medical Center, 111 East 210th Street, Bronx, New York 10461*

Dean Kim, M.D. *Resident in General Surgery, Department of Surgery, Montefiore Medical Center, 111 East 210th Street, Bronx, New York 10467*

Helen H. Kim, M.D. *Department of Otolaryngology, Montefiore Medical Center, Albert Einstein College of Medicine, 111 East 210th Street, Bronx, New York 10467*

Sylvain Kleinhaus, M.D. *Professor of Surgery and Pediatrics, Albert Einstein College of Medicine, Montefiore Medical Center, 111 East 210th Street, Bronx, New York 10467*

Sam Lan, M.D., Ph.D., *Clinical Associate Professor of Surgery, Montefiore Hospital and Medical Center, 1180 Morris Park Avenue, Bronx, New York 10461*

Stephen A. Michalski, M.D. *Assistant Professor of Surgery, Department of Surgery, The Jack D. Weiler Hospital of the Albert Einstein College of Medicine, 1825 Eastchester Road, Bronx, New York 10461*

Marek Rudnicki, M.D., Ph.D. *Head of Surgical Research and Attending Surgeon, The Mary Imogene Bassett Hospital, Atwell Road, Cooperstown, New York 13326*

Russell H. Samson, M.D., R.V.T., F.A.C.S. *Chief of Surgery, Sarasota Memorial Hospital, 5744 Bee Ridge Road, Sarasota, Florida 34233; Formerly, Associate Professor of Surgery, Albert Einstein College of Medicine, Bronx, New York 10461*

Gil Hauer Santos, M.D., F.A.C.S. *Professor of Thoracic Surgery, Albert Einstein College of Medicine, 1170 North Avenue, New Rochelle, New York 10804*

Richard S. Schechner, M.D. *Assistant Professor of Surgery, Department of Surgery, Albert Einstein College of Medicine, Montefiore Medical Center, 111 East 210th Street, Bronx, New York 10467*

Larry A. Scher, M.D., F.A.C.S.   *Associate Professor of Surgery, Chief, Division of Vascular Surgery, North Shore University Hospital/New York University School of Medicine, 300 Community Drive, Manhasset, New York 11030*

Vicki L. Seltzer, M.D., F.A.C.O., F.A.C.S.   *Professor of Obstetrics and Gynecology, Albert Einstein College of Medicine; Chairman, Obstetrics and Gynecology, Long Island Jewish Medical Center, Lakeville Road, New Hyde Park, New York 11040*

Carl E. Silver, M.D., F.A.C.S.   *Professor of Surgery, Albert Einstein College of Medicine, Chief, Head & Neck Surgery, Montefiore Medical Center, Bronx, New York 10467*

Ronald J. Simon, M.D., F.A.C.S.   *Assistant Professor of Surgery, Jacobi Medical Center, 1400 Pelham Parkway South, Bronx, New York 10461*

Andrew Stein, M.D.   *Department of Orthopedic Surgery, The Jack D. Weiler Hospital of the Albert Einstein College of Medicine, 1825 Eastchester Road, Bronx, New York 10461*

H. David Stein, M.D., F.A.C.A.   *Department of Surgery, Albert Einstein College of Medicine, Flushing Hospital Medical Center, 45th Avenue at Parsons Boulevard, Flushing, New York 11355*

Peter L. Stone, M.D.   *Department of Urology, Albert Einstein College of Medicine, 1578 Williamsbridge Road, Bronx, New York 10461*

Vivian A. Tellis, M.S., F.A.C.S.   *Professor of Surgery, Department of Surgery, Albert Einstein College of Medicine, Montefiore Medical Center, 111 East 210th Street, Bronx, New York 10467*

Sheel K. Vatsia, M.D.   *North Shore University Hospital, 300 Community Drive, Manhasset, New York 10030*

Francis J. Velez, M.D.   *Department of Surgery, Albert Einstein College of Medicine, Montefiore Medical Center, 111 East 210th Street, Bronx, New York 10467*

Gerard Weinberg, M.D., F.A.A.P., F.A.C.S.   *Associate Professor of Surgery and Pediatrics, Albert Einstein College of Medicine, Montefiore Medical Center, 1575 Blondell Avenue, Bronx, New York 10461*

Shelley Nan Weiner, M.D.   *Clinical Associate Professor, Department of Radiology, Albert Einstein College of Medicine, 175 Memorial Highway, New Rochelle, New York 10801*

Michael E. Zenilman, M.D., F.A.C.S.   *Associate Professor of Surgery, Chief, Surgical Services, Albert Einstein College of Medicine, Montefiore Medical Center, 1825 Eastchester Road, Bronx, New York 10461*

Preface

In the five years since publication of the second edition of *General Surgery Board Review,* significant advances have occurred in general surgery and many surgical specialties. The third edition of our book includes a new chapter on minimally invasive surgery and updated material covering all other aspects of general surgery. The format utilized for the previous two editions has been maintained. Factual material necessary to provide a framework for review has been updated and questions are again included for self-assessment. In addition, current references have been provided to facilitate further study in areas in which the reader feels deficient.

The favorable reception that the first two editions of this text received has been most gratifying and has encouraged us to present this revision. The editors hope that this edition will be as successful in continuing to help our readers succeed in the qualifying, certifying or recertifying examination.

Michael S. Gold
Larry A. Scher
Gerard Weinberg

Acknowledgments

The editors are indebted to the many individuals who were invaluable in making this text a reality. We start by thanking Dr. George W. Machiedo, Interim Chairman, Department of Surgery of Albert Einstein College of Medicine/Montefiore Medical Center for supporting and encouraging our efforts.

Most of the material in this book derives from The Annual Intensive Review in General Surgery, a course sponsored by the Montefiore Medical Center Office of Continuing Medical Education. The professionals who have organized this course for these past 32 years have made it into one of the premier courses of its kind in the country. We especially acknowledge the help of Mr. Jon Allen who had been so instrumental in organizing the vast amount of logistical detail necessary to have a successful course year after year.

A course or a book is only as good as the people who contribute to it. Thankfully, we are fortunate in having had an outstanding cadre of speakers and authors give of their time, knowledge, and specialized skills in making this project possible. Without them there would not have been this book.

Lippincott–Raven Publishers has been extremely supportive. We specifically wish to thank our developmental editor Rebecca Irwin Diehl for shepherding this project until it became a reality.

Finally, we especially acknowledge Joan Segall. Joan is able to administrate two busy academic departments, manage to run downtown to see to it that the course is running well, and still find time to help us organize and publish this book.

1

Diseases of the Esophagus

Gil Hauer Santos

ANATOMY

The esophagus is situated in three anatomic regions—cervical, thoracic, and abdominal—each with its specific blood supply. The cervical esophagus receives branches of the inferior thyroid artery. The upper thoracic esophagus blood supply is derived from bronchial arteries, and the inferior thoracic esophagus obtains blood from segmental branches of the aorta. The left gastric and splenic arteries supply blood to the abdominal segment of the esophagus. For descriptive purposes the esophagus can be divided in thirds: upper, middle, and lower, each measuring an average of 8 cm.

The esophagus is a muscular organ limited by an upper and a lower esophageal sphincter. The upper esophageal sphincter is comprised of the cricopharyngeus and is well defined. The lower esophageal sphincter is not well defined anatomically but physiologically is identified as a high-pressure zone. A sling of gastric muscle fiber known as the collar of Helvetius is occasionally found at the esophagogastric junction. The esophagus extends about 4 to 5 cm below the diaphragm before it blends into the stomach. Attached to the esophagus as it crosses the diaphragm is the phrenoesophageal ligament, which is a continuation of the transversalis fascia and peritoneum fused with the endothoracic fascia and pleura. The esophagus is lined by squamous epithelium throughout its length. It changes to columnar epithelium 1 to 2 cm proximal to the esophagogastric junction.

The upper esophageal muscularis externa is composed of striated longitudinal and circular layers. The striated muscle is replaced by smooth muscle at the distal three-fifths of the esophagus.

PHYSIOLOGY

The upper esophageal sphincter (UES) has a resting pressure that keeps it closed most of the time. The sphincter relaxes during swallowing, and the pressure falls to zero. When fluid is injected into the upper esophagus the pressure increases at the UES. The pressures measured at this sphincter are asymmetric, with posterior measurements being higher than those obtained anteriorly or laterally. The pressures measured are also different at different levels in the sphincter, which averages 4 cm in length. Swallowing relaxes this sphincter, making it possible for the contraction of the lower pharyngeal muscles together with the "pump" action of the tongue to push food into the upper esophagus. It is essential that relaxation of the UES precedes the rise in pressure in the lower pharynx produced by the contraction of the inferior constrictor of the pharynx. Once the bolus enters the upper esophagus, a propulsive wave, the primary peristaltic wave, brings it down to enter the stomach, which is made possible by the relaxation of the lower esophageal sphincter. In a different way secondary peristaltic waves originate from distension of the esophageal wall produced by contents inside the esophagus. It takes, on average, 6 seconds for a bolus to travel from the pharynx to the stomach. Cold food decreases peristaltic amplitude and frequency; warm food has the opposite effect.

Nonpropulsive contractions, when present, may have high amplitude and duration. On manometry they are identified as tertiary contractions.

The high-pressure zone (HPZ) found at the lower esophageal sphincter (LES) has a resting pressure that in normal individuals varies from as low as 6 mm Hg to as high as 24 mm Hg, and it is this continuous tone that prevents gastroesophageal reflux. When abnormal relaxation is present, gastric contents reflux into the lower esophagus, damaging the esophageal mucosa. In patients with duodenogastric reflux alkaline contents, represented by bile salts and pancreatic enzymes, can also be refluxed into the esophagus.

There is no consensus on a precise definition of normal esophageal pH. Most authors consider an esophageal pH below 4 to be indicative of reflux. It is proposed that normal individuals have an acidic pH in the lower esophagus no more than 6% of time, or 1.5 hours per 24 hours. Almost 90% of physiologic reflux occurs during and after meals. Alkaline reflux may interfere with evaluation of reflux based exclusively on pH monitoring and give a false idea of normalcy when there is frank alkaline reflux.

The length of the abdominal esophagus subjected to positive intraabdominal pressure is an important factor in the prevention of reflux. Reflux has been shown to occur when the total length of the LES is less than 2 cm or when the length of the intraabdominal LES is less than 1 cm. Reflux is certain to occur when the LES pressure is less than 6 mm Hg, the total length of the LES is less than 2 cm, and the intraabdominal LES measures less than 1 cm. Other, less important features in controlling reflux are the oblique angle of entry of the esophagus into the stomach, the mucosal folds at the LES, and the tightness of the diaphragmatic crura.

Acid regurgitated into the lower esophagus is cleared by the peristaltic activity of the esophagus. During waking time one peristaltic wave takes place each minute. This is different from sleeping time when the frequency of peristalsis decreases to four waves per hour. Esophageal emptying is also facilitated by gravity during daytime, and acid is neutralized by more abundant production of saliva. Regulation of LES pressure is under nervous control mainly through the vagus. Transection of the vagi below the atrial level does not affect the LES tone, as there is a rich network of intramural nerve plexi. α-Adrenergic receptors localized within the wall cause esophageal constriction, whereas β-receptors mediate relaxation. The LES is also under hormonal influence. Gastrin in vitro has been shown to double LES pressure, although the effect may not be physiologically important. Other substances that increase LES pressure are vasopressin, α-adrenergic drugs, cholinergic drugs, anticholinesterase, a protein meal, and gastric alkalinization. Some of the substances that decrease LES tone are secretin, vasoactive intestinal polypeptide, nitroglycerin, cholecystokinin, glucagon, progestational agents, α-adrenergic antagonists, β-adrenergic drugs, anticholinergics, prostaglandin E, nicotine, a fat meal, chocolate, and gastric acidification. The importance of these substances in the maintenance of LES competence is beginning to be clarified.

Several tests are used to test the functional integrity of the esophagus.

1. *Manometry:* The pressure of the sphincters and body of the esophagus, at rest and during deglutition, are measured via catheters placed at different levels and during withdrawal from the stomach as it passes through the HPZ.
2. *pH reflux:* A 300-ml dose of 0.1 N HCl is injected into the stomach after a pH electrode has been positioned 5 cm above the gastroesophageal (GE) junction. If the esophageal pH drops to 4 or less, GE reflux is assumed to be present.
3. *Acid clearing test:* This test measures the ability of the esophagus to clear regurgitated acid.
4. *Acid perfusion test (Bernstein):* Acid is introduced into the lower esophagus. The occurrence of symptoms is considered a positive result. This test has a high incidence of false positives and false negatives.
5. *pH monitoring (24 hours):* A pH probe is left in the lower esophagus. A continuous recording is made of the number of reflux episodes when the pH falls below 4, as is the amount of time it takes for the esophagus to clear the regurgitated acid. The value of the test may be obscured when duodenogastric reflux brings alkaline contents into the esophagus. In this situation a normal pH between 4 and 6 can be found even though significant reflux may be taking place. Daytime reflux in excess of 90 minutes is suggestive of gastroesophageal reflux disease. Nighttime reflux

is more damaging to the esophagus because of diminished protective mechanisms (gravity, saliva production, and peristaltic activity) when the patient is asleep. It should be mentioned that recognition of alkaline GE reflux initiated by duodenogastric reflux can make it difficult to interpret values obtained by esophageal pH monitoring.

MOTILITY DISORDERS OF THE ESOPHAGUS

Normal food progression from the lower pharynx to the stomach requires perfect coordination of the esophageal sphincters and the muscles of the esophageal body. When the inferior constrictor of the pharynx squeezes together with the "pump" action of the tongue, it pushes the food downward through an already relaxed cricopharyngeus. On entering the esophagus the food is then actively transported to the stomach by peristaltic activity. The LES relaxes in anticipation of the arrival of this peristaltic wave, permitting the food to enter the stomach. Passage of the bolus from the pharynx to the stomach takes an average of 6 seconds. When there is lack of coordination of this normal sequence at any level, dysphagia occurs. Depending on the level where the disturbance takes place, different symptoms are referred by the patient.

Transfer dysphagia is seen when the disturbance is at the level of the cricopharyngeus, interfering with transfer of food from the pharynx to the esophagus. Transport dysphagia relates to disturbances in the esophageal body that interfere with transport of food from the UES to the LES. Delivery dysphagia refers to disturbances at the LES that prevents food entry into the stomach.

Transfer Dysphagia

Cricopharyngeal Dysphagia

Cricopharyngeal dysphagia is characteristic of transfer dysphagia, where there is delayed and or incomplete relaxation of the UES. The peak pressure produced inside the lower pharynx by muscular contraction does not find a relaxed cricopharyngeus, and so the food has difficulty entering the esophagus. A high-pressure region is generated between the inferior constrictor and the cricopharyngeus. At this point an area with attenuated muscles, described by anatomists as Killian's triangle, is observed. In the past complaints of swallowing difficulties at this level were sometimes diagnosed as

"globus hystericus" and considered to be of psychogenic origin. Radiographic studies can demonstrate the delay of contrast getting through the UES into the esophagus. With this radiologic finding and in the presence of obvious symptoms, cricopharyngeal myotomy is indicated. Some authors believe that the simultaneous presence of gastroesophageal reflux is the triggering factor in some patients.

Zencker's Diverticulum

The basic motility disturbance of Zencker's diverticulum is the same as that of cricopharyngeal dysphagia. In these patients, however, the condition goes untreated for a long time, which makes it possible for the pressure generated between the oblique fibers of the inferior constrictor of the pharynx and the transverse fibers of the cricopharyngeus to push out the mucosa between the two muscles at or near Killian's triangle, producing a diverticulum. Its size depends on the length of time since the condition started as well as the degree of dysfunction. As food particles and liquid accumulate inside the diverticulum, symptoms are produced, including regurgitation, bad odor, and aspiration.

The disorder is seen more frequently in older patients. The provoking factor is not clear, and it is possible that spasm of the cricopharyngeus is the result of mucosal irritation secondary to gastroesophageal reflux, which is found in some patients.

Treatment includes myotomy associated with diverticulectomy. For minor diverticuli an alternative treatment is diverticulopexy in which the diverticulum is suspended posterior to the pharynx. The incidence of postoperative complications is more frequent in patients who had diverticulectomy.

Transport Dysphagia

Once thoracic pain of cardiac origin is ruled out, the next source of thoracic pain is the esophagus. High-amplitude peristaltic or nonperistaltic contractions are frequently the source of painful symptoms.

Diffuse Esophageal Spasm

Diffuse esophageal spasm (DES) is manifested by retrosternal pain that radiates to the neck and upper extremities, mimicking angina. Adding to the possibility of diagnostic confusion is the fact that this pain can be relieved by nitroglycerin. Manometry can detect the presence of a large number of high-amplitude tertiary (nonpropulsive) contractions. A contrast study during episodes of pain can demonstrate the presence of a typical "corkscrew" esophagus. Antispasmodics and calcium channel blockers comprise the first line of treatment. Surgery is rarely indicated.

High-Amplitude Peristaltic Contractions

High-amplitude peristaltic contractions (HAPCs), or hyperperistalsis, also known as "nutcracker esophagus," is produced by peristaltic contractions of high amplitude that in some cases reach 400 mm Hg (normal average 75 mm Hg). This condition manifests by painful swallowing. The treatment for both DES and HAPC is mostly conservative. Surgery is indicated only when symptoms do not respond to pharmacologic symptomatic and supportive treatment. Extended esophagomyotomy, sparing the upper and lower esophageal sphincters, is the procedure of choice. The results are not encouraging, however, with frequent recurrences having been reported.

Delivery Dysphagia

Achalasia

Achalasia, a clearly defined motility disturbance, is recognized by the presence of three main components.

1. Aperistalsis. High or low tertiary (nonpropulsive) contractions may be present.
2. Increased LES resting pressure. This pressure can increase to more than double the normal values.
3. Incomplete LES relaxation. Only about 30% of relaxation of the original resting pressure is achieved.

Histologically, there is a decrease in the number of ganglion cells in Auerbach's plexus at all esophageal levels. Some authors have suggested that possibly neurotropic viruses are responsible for their destruction, which would be similar to the destruction of these cells due to *Trypanosoma cruzi,* observed in Chagas' disease.

The symptoms of achalasia are progressive dysphagia associated with regurgitation of undigested food, particularly at night when the patient lies down. This food has been lying in the esophagus without being de-

livered into the stomach. Esophageal carcinoma develops in 2% to 4% of patients with untreated achalasia.

Achalasia is diagnosed by esophagography, which shows obstruction at the GE junction and a dilated esophageal body. These changes are more or less pronounced depending on the progression of the disease. Early in the course of the disease, before dilatation has occurred, the obstruction at the GE junction may be difficult to distinguish radiologically from a carcinoma. Manometry reveals the resting LES pressure to be two to three times the normal values associated with decreased or absent LES relaxation. Also noted is absent peristalsis, even though sporadic tertiary nonpropulsive waves can be identified. In the variant of achalasia known as vigorous achalasia, nonperistaltic high-amplitude contractions are present, sometimes in great numbers.

There are two well established options for the treatment of achalasia. The "conservative" treatment consists in dilating the LES with a pneumatic balloon until it ruptures the sphincter muscles. Frequently, more than one dilatation is necessary to obtain enough relaxation. The most serious complication of dilatation is rupture of all esophageal layers. When this occurs surgery is required to repair the ruptured esophagus, and a myotomy should be performed on the side opposite the rupture.

The surgical alternative to dilatation is a myotomy, described by Heller. Myotomy is the recommended treatment for children and for the rigorous form of the disease. A dreaded complication of myotomy is reflux. There is no consensus on whether an antireflux procedure should be added routinely to prevent such reflux. Even with proper, careful technique, reflux occurs in 3% of cases. The proponents of myotomy alone advocate minimal dissection of the GE junction. The muscle division should not advance more than 1 cm into the stomach. This operation can easily be done transthoracically. When properly done, the resting pressure of the sphincter decreases an average of 15 mm Hg. The proponents of more extensive myotomy recommend extending it as much as 2 cm into the stomach and adding an associated antireflux procedure. It should be noted that the barrier introduced by the antireflux procedure can interfere with proper emptying of an esophagus already impaired by decreased peristaltic activity. This operation has been done more recently through a laparoscopic approach.

Other treatments include botulinum toxin, which has been used as the primary treatment for achalasia. Injections are made above the Z zone in four quadrants for a total dose of 80 units. Botulinum toxin type A acts by preventing release of acetylcholine from peripheral nerve endings, thereby reducing the LES pressure. Trials using pharmacologic agents such as nifedipine are in progress, with initial results being reported as providing only short term relief to patients with mild symptoms.

Epiphrenic Diverticulum

Epiphrenic diverticula are better visualized by contrast studies than by endoscopy. They are situated just above the diaphragm and are often associated with motility disturbances such as achalasia or diffuse esophageal spasm. This frequent association requires a motility study prior to surgery.

The treatment is surgical and consists in excising the diverticulum. If achalasia is present, a Heller esophago-myotomy is added.

Some diverticula of different origin are located in the midesophagus and are produced by inflammatory changes in the mediastinum. These are the so-called traction diverticula, which in reality are not diverticula but localized esophageal retraction. They are produced by scars located outside the esophageal wall pulling the esophagus in that direction. They are asymptomatic, are often discovered incidentally, and need no treatment.

Gastroesophageal Reflux Disease

Gastroesophageal reflux is a normal event that occurs occasionally during the day, mostly associated with swallowing. When reflux of gastric contents occurs more frequently than can be tolerated by the esophageal mucosa, gastroesophageal reflux disease (GERD) is present.

It occurs in response to a hypotensive LES permitting excessive reflux of gastrointestinal contents into the esophagus. There is a close relation between esophageal injury and esophageal exposure to contents of pH below 4 or above 7. Even though reflux esophagitis was initially described by Winkelstein in *JAMA* as early as 1935, it was only in recent years that researchers arrived at a better understanding of this entity.

Presently there are two known mechanisms responsible for the production of esophageal mucosal damage (esophagitis), and both are based on the action of proteolytic enzymes on the esophageal mucosa. The better known, more extensively studied mechanism is that as-

sociated with acid pepsin. The less well known mechanism is related to alkaline pancreatic enzymes and bile salts. Initially, pepsinogen secreted by chief cells at the gastric fundus is activated to pepsin by gastric acid. It is significant that in animal experiments no injury to the esophageal mucosa occurs when the esophagus is perfused with HCl alone. The presence of pepsin is required for injury to occur. Similarly, acid is critical for damage to occur when the esophagus is exposed to bile salts. This explains the beneficial effects of reducing the acid content in patients with bile-associated reflux esophagitis. In adults a hiatus hernia is responsible for hypotensive LES in almost 90% of the cases.

Diagnosis

In patients with symptoms produced by reflux, the diagnosis is suspected by esophagography results and confirmed by esophagoscopy, which reveals inflammatory changes and mucosal erosion. Histologic examination is not universally recommended as it often does not add to the information seen by the endoscopist. It is useful, however, when fungal or viral esophagitis is suspected. Pain provocation techniques are also not always informative. In cases of duodenogastric reflux finding bile in the esophagus can help clarify the etiology of the injury. Presently, the only system capable of determining bile injury to the esophagus is the Bilitec 2000 fiberoptic system, which can detect bilirubin by its specific absorption peak (450 nm).

When the diagnosis is in doubt, a motility study can be a valuable diagnostic tool; and pH monitoring can provide additional information even though it may not detect reflux when alkaline reflux predominates. In uncomplicated situations 24-hour pH monitoring can demonstrate increased esophageal exposure to refluxed acid when the pH is at or below 4 for more than 6% of the time (1.5 hours).

Three stages of esophagitis are described. During the first stage the esophagus is inflamed and shows areas of superficial erosion. The second stage is heralded by ulcerations that are more frequently seen on the posterior esophageal wall. These ulcers can be complicated by bleeding and perforation. During the third stage of esophagitis the healing process supervenes, with local deposition of fibrin and collagen. Throughout the healing process the damaged esophagus undergoes scarring and contracture, which results in stricture of its lumen, evident on the esophagogram. Other, more detailed classifications of esophagitis exist (Savary, MUSE) but we use this one because of its simplicity and ease of clinical correlation.

Treatment

For patients with first-stage esophagitis, before complications take place, medical treatment is used with the objective of decreasing the acidity of gastric contents and optimizing the reflux-preventing function of the LES. Foods that decrease the LES resting pressure should be avoided. At nighttime, to help gravity clear the regurgitated acid, the head of the bed can be elevated.

A large number of medications are available, starting with simple antacids and progressing to H_2-blockers (cimetidine, famotidine, ranitidine). However, blocking acid production does not address the underlying motility disorder, as acid production is normal in GERD. Prokinetic agents exemplified by metoclopramide and cisapride are important in the treatment of esophagitis as they act by increasing the LES pressure, stimulating gastrointestinal smooth muscle, accelerating gastric emptying, and coordinating gastric pyloric duodenal motor activity. GERD is a lifelong disease in 90% of the patients, and cisapride appears at present to be the only prokinetic agent effective for maintenance treatment of esophagitis.

Other agents with demonstrated healing power for esophagitis belong to the group of proton pump inhibitors (omeprazole). Omeprazole is used as a first-line medication in several European countries. The role of sucralfate as a mucosal protectant to prevent esophagitis has not been defined. In most patients the above measures are enough to promote significant improvement.

When these measures fail, complications develop as esophagitis progresses to stage II (ulceration, bleeding, perforation, intractable pain). Surgical treatment is indicated for these patients. Several procedures have been developed to reposition the distal few centimeters of the esophagus inside the positive-pressure environment of the abdomen and at the same time reinforce the LES.

When the disease is detected at advanced stage III, when stricture had already occurred, dilatation of the stricture must precede antireflux surgery. Commonly used procedures include the Nissen procedure, represented by a 360-degree transabdominal fundoplication. A 240-degree anterior fundoplication, the Belsey Mark IV, is done transthoracically. The Hill procedure consists in a posterior gastropexy in which the LES is attached to the median arcuate ligament. According to some anatomists this "ligament" is in reality the lateral border of the right crus of the diaphragm. Some authors advocate a Toupet or Lind partial wrap instead of the more widely used Nissen procedure. Some surgeons claim success with a laparoscopic antireflux procedure.

The goal for all these antireflux procedures is to obtain a resting pressure in the LES enough to prevent reflux while preserving a pliable GE junction that does not prevent food from entering the stomach. The crura should be closed to ensure that a segment of esophagus stays under the diaphragm.

With all these procedures the esophagus is restored to an intraabdominal position. When this is not possible because the esophagus is short, it can be "elongated" by performing a gastric fundoplasty as described by Collis. Selected patients who had a failed surgical procedure or who have poor tissues have benefited from the prosthetic ring devised by Angelchick, which has been used with good results in some of these cases.

When the problem is duodenogastric reflux, whereby excessive amounts of bile and pancreatic and intestinal enzymes are responsible for producing esophagitis, surgery is directed to preventing the alkaline substances from entering the stomach and refluxing from there into the esophagus. This can be accomplished by performing a Roux-en-Y procedure.

Barrett's Esophagus

A different sequence of events in a response to reflux is seen in 7% to 33% of patients. Here the damaged squamous epithelium is replaced with a metaplastic columnar lining, resulting in a columnar-lined esophagus (CLE). It measures at least 3 cm and is known as Barrett's esophagus.

Barrett's esophagus is often associated with increased alkaline reflux, which exposes the esophagus to bile salts and other duodenal contents. It has been shown that this lining is not simple columnar epithelium but a specialized epithelium with a villous appearance composed of mucin-containing columnar gastric cells interspersed with intestinal goblet cells. Patients with Barrett's esophagus have more episodes of alkaline reflux than patients with simple esophagitis.

Complications associated with CLE are stricture, ulcers, and cancer, which has been found to occur in these patients 30 to 125 times more often than in the general population. Two types of ulcers are seen in this epithelium: Barrett's ulcers found at the columnar area and Savari ulcers located at the squamocolumnar junction. The presence of a CLE does not change the treatment for reflux.

Patients with CLE who underwent an antireflux operation have been reported not to show regression of the columnar epithelium in sufficient numbers to justify surgery for that reason alone. Among 249 cases collected in the literature, 6.4% had partial regression and 2% had complete regression. Considering the difficulties encountered by endoscopists when defining exactly what they saw before and after surgery it is not surprising that even these low numbers must be questioned.

The incidence of CLE-related carcinoma in the population is 1.5 per 100,000, or almost 4,000 per year in the United States. Among patients followed for 10 years the incidence of carcinoma in those with CLE was found to be 1% to 2%. The carcinoma occurs mostly when there are extensive segments of metaplastic epithelium. Current indications for resection of CLE are the presence of a nondilatable stricture, malignancy including high-grade metaplasia, severe symptoms not responsive to conservative treatment, bleeding, or perforated ulcers.

Secondary Motility Disorders

Several central nervous system diseases can produce dysphagia owing to interference with normal swallowing mechanisms. That is the case, for example, with patients who have suffered a stroke, those with cerebral palsy, and those with Parkinson's disease. Similarly, muscular diseases may cause swallowing difficulties, as with myasthenia gravis and myotonic dystrophy. With some multisystem diseases, such as scleroderma, the esophageal component requires specific treatment. Patients with scleroderma exhibit a decrease in the lower esophageal resting pressure associated with decreased or even totally absent esophageal peristalsis, which together create a situation difficult to treat: There is gastroesophageal reflux into an esophagus devoid of peristaltic activity, which is therefore unable to defend itself against refluxed acid; hence esophagitis promptly develops.

Chemical Burns of the Esophagus

Chemical burns of the esophagus result from the accidental or voluntary ingestion of strong acids or alkalis. The local caustic action on the esophageal mucosa, when severe, may result in a deep necrosis. Alkalis produce liquefaction necrosis, which predisposes to extensive penetration, whereas acids produce a type of coagulation necrosis with more limited penetration into the esophageal wall. When healing occurs and the burn is circumferential, a stricture may form. The alkali usually implicated is NaOH (lye), which is found in a variety of household products. Acids produce more damage to the stomach. Sulfuric acid, which was an easily obtainable component of the early car batteries, is frequently responsible.

Symptoms are variable, depending on the nature, amount, and concentration of the substance ingested. The oropharynx, esophagus, and stomach are injured by these substances. When large amounts have been ingested, esophageal or gastric perforation with shock can occur, requiring immediate surgery as a life-saving measure. When perforation does not occur early, esophagoscopic inspection during the initial 24 to 48 hours is indicated to evaluate the extent of the burn. This initial evaluation cannot change the subsequent course of events but is helpful for documenting the extent of the damage. A brief inspection of the oropharynx, observing how patients handle their saliva and how they breathe and phonate, is a reliable way to evaluate the extent of the oropharyngeal injury. The early insertion of a prosthetic stent inside the esophageal lumen, as advocated by Reyes, to avoid the stricture produced by contraction of the burn scar has not been successful in our cases. This failure may be because the stent is left in place for only 2 to 3 weeks, whereas scar contraction continues for several months. The use of steroids has not helped decrease scar formation. Antibiotics are indicated to prevent bacterial colonization of the injured mucosa, which would increase the extent and depth of the injury.

Once stricture develops, peroral dilatation programmed to start 2 to 3 weeks after the original injury is recommended as the initial treatment. In cases when protracted treatment is anticipated, a gastrostomy helps pass the dilators in a retrograde fashion. Weekly or even biweekly dilatation sessions for several months may be necessary. If results are good and the lumen stays open, this process should continue until a satisfactory lumen is obtained.

If after 3 to 4 months of dilatation there is no permanent lumen, surgery is indicated. A colonic bypass in a retrosternal position is preferred, with anastomosis of the proximal colon to the divided proximal cervical esophagus. The divided distal cervical esophagus is sutured and left in place. Esophagectomy is not necessary, but proper esophageal drainage should be maintained by preserving esophagogastric continuity. The risk of malignant transformation has been reported only in the functioning esophagus, not in the bypassed esophagus; and it reaches 4% to 6% after 40 years.

Benign chemical burns occur with ingestion of certain medications, such as potassium chloride, and some antibiotics, such as doxycycline and tetracycline. The mucosal injuries produced by these medications usually heal within 2 to 3 weeks without specific treatment after discontinuing the use of the noxious agent. Localized burns and even perforations have been reported after accidental ingestion of coin-sized batteries.

Rupture of the Esophagus

Spontaneous rupture of the esophagus after forceful vomiting was first described by Boerhaave, and the syndrome carries his name. The usual location of the rupture is at the distal esophagus just above the diaphragm. Symptoms consist of acute retrosternal pain after an episode of vomiting, soon followed by fever and later by circulatory collapse. The symptoms may be mistaken for a myocardial infarction if the clinical history does not reveal the vomiting episode preceding the pain.

Physical examination reveals the presence of Hamman's sign resulting from mediastinal emphysema. A chest radiograph confirms the presence of mediastinal air. If the mediastinal pleura has ruptured, pleural effusion and pneumothorax are also seen. A contrast swallow is necessary to clarify the location of the perforation. The high mortality associated with spontaneous rupture of the esophagus is a consequence of the high pressure required for esophageal rupture. When the esophagus ruptures with an intraluminal pressure of 5 psi (260 mm Hg) or more, a true explosion takes place within the chest in the posterior mediastinum.

Bacteria, enzymes, chemical substances, and food particles are introduced into the mediastinum under high pressure. Even though rarer mechanisms for spontaneous rupture have been described, the rupture usually occurs in the patient who vomits after eating. This situation is more damaging than an instrumental perforation in a patient who was prepared for endoscopy by fasting for several hours.

Treatment of an early diagnosed rupture requires prompt surgical repair after débridement of necrotic tissue and removal of all particulate and liquid material from the mediastinum. Wherever possible a pleural flap, as recommended by Grillo, is used to reinforce the closure. A chest tube is placed close to the rupture. Inspection of the area of rupture in the esophagus frequently indicates that the tear in the submucosal layer is more extensive than the tear at the muscular layer. Therefore the surgeon must identify the proximal and distal limits of the mucosal tear for thorough repair. Parenteral hydration and broad-spectrum antibiotics are given pre- and postoperatively.

Mortality from esophageal rupture approaches 50% when the diagnosis is made 18 to 24 hours after the event. It is close to 85% when more than 36 hours has elapsed.

The treatment for late diagnosed rupture is controversial. Attempts should be made to close it primarily whenever technically feasible. When there is dehiscence of the repair during the postoperative period, some authors recommend exclusion of the esophagus by performing a proximal diverting cervical esophagostomy and tying the esophagus distal to the tear at the GE junction to prevent gastric reflux. An operation of such magnitude on a very sick patient is apt to be associated with major complications and high mortality rates. If the patient survives, later reconstruction is also difficult.

Considering that the lethal factor in esophageal rupture is sepsis due to mediastinitis, we direct our efforts to the treatment of mediastinitis and take advantage of the opening in the esophagus for treatment. One catheter is positioned inside the esophagus proximal to the rupture through which mediastinal irrigation fluid can flow. A chest tube positioned in the mediastinum near the esophagus is used to constantly suction the mediastinal irrigant. Using this technique we have been able to obtain results superior to those obtained with more radical techniques.

Perforation of the Esophagus

Instrumental perforation is the most common type of esophageal perforation and occurs with both rigid and flexible esophagoscopes. The most frequent site of perforation is proximal to the cricopharyngeus, that is, proximal to the UES. The next most common sites are at the level of the aorta and proximal to the diaphragm. Perforations may also occur proximal to an area of pathology such as a stricture. In cases of suspected perforation a radiograph should be obtained, looking for free air in the mediastinum. A contrast study can demonstrate its exact location.

Some small cervical perforations can be treated by drainage and antibiotics alone. It is these perforations with which the contrast material used for esophagograms returns to the lumen of the esophagus on late films. Thoracic perforations where the contrast material does not return to the lumen of the esophagus in late films but stays outside the esophagus must be repaired surgically. Small perforations caused by foreign bodies such as bones or pins can, in selected cases, be treated with antibiotics alone, but the surgeon should be ready to perform surgery if the patient becomes febrile and has a suspicious, changed radiograph. In most cases a surgical repair is indicated.

Mallory-Weiss Syndrome

Mallory-Weiss syndrome occurs when there is bleeding from a mucosal tear in the fundus of the stomach or, more rarely, in the distal esophagus as a result of retching produced by nausea or vomiting. It represents about 5% to 17% of cases of upper gastrointestinal bleeding and is associated with alcohol ingestion in about 30% of cases. Most of the tears occur only in the region of the gastric cardia. Only 10% to 25% extend to the esophagus. Endoscopic evaluation is the most accurate method for establishing the diagnosis; and it provides access for hemostasis by cautery, heat probe, or sclerosing agents.

Most patients stop bleeding spontaneously. When bleeding persists, it frequently responds to intravenous administration of vasopressin. Balloon tamponade should be reserved for the rare patient who is not a candidate for surgery and does not respond to more conservative treatment. Transabdominal transgastric suture of the tears is occasionally necessary when bleeding persists.

ESOPHAGEAL TUMORS

Benign Tumors

Leiomyoma

Leiomyoma, the most common benign tumor of the esophagus, arises from the smooth muscle of the esophageal wall. Usually they are single and occur in the lower half of the esophagus. They can grow into the esophageal lumen in a polypoid-like manner, or they can embrace the lumen circumferentially, as a napkin. The most frequently referred symptoms are dysphagia and a sense of fullness. A contrast radiograph shows a filling defect with an intact mucosa. Endoscopy is useful for confirming the diagnosis.

Treatment is surgical in all cases. An attempt is made to remove the tumor without entering the esophageal lumen whenever possible. This precaution is not possible when the tumor grows inside the lumen of the esophagus.

Other, rarer benign tumors, such as lipomas and hemangiomas, are found occasionally.

Duplication Cysts

Duplication cysts are the second most common benign masses of the esophagus. Most of them occur near the tracheal bifurcation and are within the esophageal wall. Large cysts in infants can produce severe respiratory symptoms that require urgent surgery. The cyst wall contains smooth muscle, and the cyst lining is composed of columnar or, more rarely, squamous epithelium. These cysts may communicate with the lumen of the esophagus, or they may have no communication, simulating a simple cyst.

Treatment of most cysts consists in enucleation. It is accomplished by carefully spreading the muscle fibers while avoiding entering the esophageal lumen.

Malignant Tumors

The number of esophageal cancer deaths in the United States for 1996 was estimated to be 10,900. This cancer is more common in men than in women and is more common in Blacks than in Whites. There is a high correlation between excessive hard liquor ingestion and esophageal squamous cell cancer. Achalasia, chemical burns of the esophagus, and Barrett's esophagus are considered to be premalignant lesions.

The most common malignant epithelial tumor of the body of the esophagus is squamous cell carcinoma— different from cancers at the GE junction, which are adenocarcinomas. Adenocarcinomas may originate at the junctional epithelium normally found in this location, or they may be gastric cancers that are growing proximally into the esophagus. It is important to remember that adenocarcinomas develop on Barrett's columnar-lined esophagus.

Other malignant tumors of the esophagus are rare; they include fibrosarcomas, liposarcomas, myosarcomas, mucoepidermoid carcinomas, and adenoid cystic carcinomas. Rarely, small-cell carcinomas have also been found in the esophagus.

Esophageal cancer spreads via local invasion and regional lymphatic and hematogenous dissemination. It spreads to distant organs, such as the liver, lung, and bones.

Diagnosis

Symptoms appear late in the course of the disease, often only when distant metastasis and invasion of local structures have already taken place. Symptoms are anorexia, weight loss, and progressive dysphagia typically manifested initially as dysphagia for solids, which progresses slowly to dysphagia for liquids.

The diagnosis is made with contrast radiographic studies, esophagoscopy, and biopsies. When the tumor is at or above the carina, bronchoscopy is indicated to detect possible airway invasion. Computed tomography (CT) scans are informative but fail to provide definitive information regarding invasion of neighboring structures. They are even less accurate for evaluating tumors at the GE junction, where their accuracy is only 30%. Magnetic resonance imaging (MRI) was not found to be superior to CT scans. Endoscopic ultrasonography (EUS) has been utilized to determine the depth of invasion in the esophageal wall; it is more accurate than CT scans, but overstaging the lesion with this technique has been reported. EUS has also been found to be useful for detecting lymph node invasion and can differentiate N0 from N1 lesions. A major drawback to the use of EUS has been the impossibility of advancing the probe through the lumen of an esophagus obstructed by tumor.

Molecular biology studies have found a number of possible oncogenes and tumor-suppressor genes that influence tumor growth. The *p53* gene is a tumor-suppressor gene located in chromosome 17p. Loss of 17p or mutations on *p53* are the most frequent molecular changes in cancer. Overexpression of *p53* in the esophageal tumor or in the invaded lymph nodes is associated with a much worse prognosis and decreased survival rate. When this overexpression is identified in Barrett's esophagus, it indicates an increased possibility of malignant degeneration and may be used in the future to determine treatment.

Treatment

The best treatment for esophageal carcinoma in a given patient requires determining the resectability of the lesion based on a thorough evaluation of the tumor's characteristics as well as the patient's ability to undergo a proposed treatment. After this evaluation the surgeon can determine if the patient is a candidate for a treatment aiming at cure or palliation.

The tumor factors are its histopathology and its location, size, and invasiveness. At this point preoperative staging is based on the TNM classification, taking into consideration the depth of penetration in the esophageal wall, length, lymph node invasion, and presence of distant metastasis. A tumor is amenable to curative resection when it is limited to the esophageal wall without invasion of the neighboring structures and without distant metastasis. Most often these conditions are not present when the tumor reaches 6 cm in length, at which time the tumor is already outside the esophageal wall invading neighboring tissues.

A patient is a good candidate for curative surgery when weight loss was not more than 8% to 10% of the original weight and when there is no associated pathology that would increase the surgical risk, especially cardiac or pulmonary disease.

If the tumor is not resectable or if the patient cannot undergo surgery, a palliative treatment is proposed. The goal of palliation is to make it possible for the patient to recover the ability to eat and control his or her saliva. Such palliation can be obtained by inserting an intraluminal prosthetic tube after proper dilatation of the obstructed esophagus through a retrograde transgastric or prograde transoral route. An isolated gastrostomy is not enough palliation for the patient with an esophageal obstructing tumor, as such patients cannot eat or control their saliva.

Radiotherapy and chemotherapy have a role to play in the symptomatic treatment of patients with esophageal cancer. These modes of treatment have also proved beneficial for short-term palliation in patients who cannot undergo surgical treatment. Laser therapy for relief of obstruction has no major advantage over debulking using large-cusp biopsy forceps.

Several authors have described the use of photodynamic therapy (PDT) as palliation for unresectable carcinomas. The results are still being evaluated. A few patients with complete remission from early superficial carcinomas have been reported. PDT is a complex treatment that takes advantage of the property that a photosensitizing drug, Photofrin (PF), injected intravenously, achieves a higher concentration in cancer tissues. A laser light is used to activate the concentrated PF, which then transfers the applied energy to oxygen, thereby obtaining a tumor necrosis effect. Because the PF is also absorbed in lesser quantities by normal tissues, the patients undergoing this treatment must avoid sunlight for a couple of months, covering all exposed skin and using gloves and sunglasses to avoid skin burns.

For the patient who is a surgical candidate, the best option is surgical resection associated with visual lymph node dissection. Results after surgical resection depend on the histology and the location of the cancer. A curative procedure for the patient with squamous cell carcinoma requires right thoracotomy for dissection of the esophagus and lymph nodes. After this initial step the thoracotomy is closed, leaving the dissected esophagus *in situ* ready to be removed. The patient is then repositioned, and the abdomen is entered with the patient in the supine position. The cervical esophagus is exposed by an incision on the left neck following the anterior border of the sternocleidomastoid muscle. A decision is then made whether to use the stomach or the colon as the esophageal replacement. Technical factors determine which replacement is better suited for the individual patient. If the stomach is elected, the blood supply to this organ through the right gastric and right gastroepiploic arteries must be carefully preserved. The stomach can be positioned in the bed of the removed esophagus or in the anterior mediastinum posterior to the sternum. After mobilizing the stomach, the highest point of the greater curvature is anastomosed to the remaining cervical esophagus. It is important to suture the stomach to the fascia covering the vertebral bodies so there is no tension at the anastomosis, which is possibly the cause of many anastomotic leaks.

Some surgeons prefer to approach low and mid esophageal squamous cell carcinoma by initially isolating the stomach and its blood supply. After performing a right thoracotomy, the involved segment of esophagus is identified and resected. The procedure is then finished by anastomosing the upper thoracic esophagus to the stomach high inside the chest, as initially described by Ivor-Lewis.

A gastric tube made from the greater curvature can also be used by preserving the blood supply through the left gastroepiploic and splenic arteries. This should be done only by surgeons well experienced with the technical details of this procedure.

If the colon is selected, its vascular pedicle containing the artery and vein is dissected and positioned without tension or torsion alongside the colon. The colon can be positioned in the esophageal bed or in the retrosternal position. The left colon has a good blood supply through the left colic artery and can be easily positioned as a peristaltic conduit. The transverse colon can also be used with its blood supply based on the middle colic artery; the ascending colon can be used with its blood supply based on the right colic artery.

Extended survival after curative resection is obtained in 25% of cases. Obviously, this number is significant only if there is minimal operative mortality and morbidity. In Japan, where patients are treated at an earlier stage and where an exhaustive lymph node dissection is carried out, the 5-year survival is 50% when no positive lymph nodes are found.

A different approach is indicated for patients with adenocarcinoma of the GE junction. These patients can be treated with a low left thoracotomy through the seventh interspace, which can be easily converted to a thoracolaparotomy providing the best possible exposure of the tumor. After resecting the tumor, the gastrointestinal tract is reconstituted with an end-to-side anastomosis, being careful to add a fundoplasty to prevent reflux.

Patients with cancers at the cricopharyngeal level can benefit from a pharyngolaryngoesophagectomy associated with a gastric pull-up and a pharyngogastric anastomosis. Except on the rare occasions when the tumor is localized in the mucosa and submucosa, a "blind esophagectomy" without opening the chest can be performed by dissecting the esophagus through a combined cervical and abdominal approach. This is not a curative operation, as it leaves behind involved lymph nodes and extraesophageal invasion. It is indicated occasionally as a palliative procedure.

Strong predictors for survival are the TNM stage before and after (pTNM) treatment and the postoperative residual (R) classification as defined by the UICC. According to this classification R0 is obtained when there is no residual tumor at the proximal and distal margins and no tumor at the lateral mediastinal resection planes. The postoperative result is deemed R1 when microscopic residual tumor is found in the specimen and R2 when there is macroscopic local and regional residual tumor. The R2 evaluation is made by the surgeon at the operating table. After an R0 resection, 15% to 40% five-year survival can be expected. R1 and R2 resections give a 5-year survival not above 5%.

INTRAMURAL PSEUDODIVERTICULOSIS

Other than Zencker's diverticulum, epiphrenic diverticulum, and mid-esophageal diverticulum (traction diverticulum), the esophagus presents one rare form of diverticulosis: so-called intramural pseudodiverticulosis. This rare condition is seen in patients older than 50 years of age. Esophagography shows narrowing of the upper or mid esophagus as well as small diverticula measuring 2 to 3 mm throughout the esophagus, producing an image that resembles a centipede. These "diverticula" are dilated esophageal glands located deep in the muscularis mucosae. Food is retained in the areas of esophageal narrowing. The condition remains asymptomatic or, when symptomatic, responds well to dilatation.

CANDIDIASIS

Candidiasis is the most frequent inflammatory lesion of the esophagus and is found in patients who have been treated with antibiotics and immunosuppressants. The presenting symptom is odynophagia. Contrast esophagography demonstrates a typical cobblestone picture. Treatment consists of oral administration of nystatin and discontinuation of the offending agent whenever possible. Other inflammatory lesions of the esophagus are produced by herpes simplex virus and cytomegalovirus.

HIATAL HERNIAS

There are two main groups of hiatal hernia. They have different etiologies and different symptomatologies.

Sliding Hiatus Hernia

Normally the distal 3 to 4 cm of esophagus is inside the abdomen, where it is exposed to positive intraabdominal pressure. This pressure in conjunction with the HPZ at the GE junction is enough to prevent abnormal GE reflux. A loose esophageal hiatus and stretched phrenoesophageal ligament permits cephalad migration of the GE junction and, less frequently, migration of segments of the lesser and greater curvatures. It may result in gastroesophageal reflux disease, already described in the discussion on motility disturbances.

Paraesophageal Hiatal Hernia

With paraesophageal hiatal hernia there is an asymmetric defect in the muscles comprising the crus of the diaphragm, making it possible for the phrenoesophageal ligament together with the peritoneum to stretch upward into the chest between the esophagus and the diaphragmatic hiatus. Here it forms a true hernial sac into which the stomach can enter. The GE junction remains under the diaphragm. The consequences of this herniation are gastric torsion, gastric volvulus with obstruction, and strangulation.

Treatment for this type of hernia is surgical and consists of closing the patent hiatus after delivering the stomach back to the abdominal cavity. Occasionally a paraesophageal hiatal hernia has a sliding component as well. In this case the gastroesophageal junction is found to be above the diaphragm.

QUESTIONS

Select one answer.

1. The three findings in achalasia are:
   a. Increased LES resting pressure, decreased LES relaxation, increased esophageal peristaltic activity.
   b. Decreased LES resting pressure, increased LES relaxation, decreased esophageal peristaltic activity.

a. Increased LES resting pressure, decreased LES relaxation, decreased esophageal peristaltic activity.
d. Decreased LES resting pressure, increased LES relaxation, increased esophageal peristaltic activity.

2. Esophageal precancerous conditions are:
   a. Cricopharyngeal dysphagia, epiphrenic diverticulum, achalasia.
   b. Achalasia, hiatus hernia, Zencker's diverticulum.
   c. Chemical burns of the esophagus, achalasia, Barrett's esophagus.
   d. Barrett's esophagus, hiatus hernia, achalasia.

3. Acidic pH in the lower esophagus should not exceed:
   a. 1 hour daily.
   b. 2 hours daily.
   c. 1.5 hours daily.
   d. 2.5 hours daily.

4. An antireflux procedure may be unsuccessful because of:
   a. Gastric outlet obstruction not previously identified.
   b. Well dilated previous stricture.
   c. Decreased saliva production.
   d. Transthoracic fundoplasty.

5. The most common etiology of esophageal perforations is:
   a. Spontaneous rupture (Boerhaave's syndrome).
   b. Instrumental perforation.
   c. Foreign bodies in esophagus.
   d. Barrett's esophagus.

6. Esophageal carcinoma confined to the esophageal wall is best treated by:
   a. Laser debulking.
   b. Prosthetic tube insertion.
   c. Local resection.
   d. Subtotal resection.

7. Middle-third esophageal carcinoma confined to the esophageal wall is best approached sequentially through:
   a. Left chest and abdomen.
   b. Right chest, abdomen, and neck.
   c. Abdomen and right chest.
   d. Left and right chest.

8. Cricopharyngeal dysphagia is associated with all but:
   a. Lack of coordination between contraction of the inferior constrictor of the pharynx and relaxation of the cricopharyngeus.
   b. Gastroesophageal reflux.
   c. Development of Zencker's diverticulum.
   d. Decreased primary peristaltic waves.

9. Esophageal tertiary waves are prevalent in:
   a. Esophageal carcinoma.
   b. Hiatus hernia.
   c. Diffuse esophageal spasm.
   d. Scleroderma.

SELECTED REFERENCES

Castell DO. *The esophagus.* Boston: Little, Brown, and Company, 1992.

Giuli R. *Primary motility disorders of the esophagus: O.E.S.O. 450 questions 450 answers.* Montrouge: John Libbey, 1992.

Giuli R. *The esophageal mucosa: O.E.S.O. 300 questions 300 answers.* Amsterdam: Elsevier Science, 1994.

Glenn's Thoracic and Cardiovascular Surgery, vol 1, 6th ed. Stamford, CT: Appleton & Lange, 1996.

2

Stomach and Duodenum

Michael E. Zenilman

ANATOMY

The stomach is divided into four portions. The cardia and fundus are located proximally near the gastroesophageal (GE) junction, proximal to the main body, or corpus. Distally the antrum begins at the incisura angularis; and its muscular contractions, along with those of the pyloric sphincter, control emptying of the stomach. The motility of the antrum and pylorus are neurally linked with the duodenum, and all three are referred to the antropyloroduodenal complex. The fundus and corpus contain the parietal cells and oxyntic cells. The antrum contains the gastrin G-cells and pyloric glands, which secrete mucosa. The ligamentous attachments of the stomach include the gastrohepatic ligament (which includes the lesser omentum), the gastrocolic ligament (which includes the greater momentum), and the lienogastric ligament (which contains the short gastric vessels).

The duodenum is divided into four portions: superior, descending, transverse, and ascending. The duodenal bulb is anatomically important because (a) most duodenal ulcers and their sequelae occur in the bulb; and (b) the common bile duct runs behind this portion of the duodenum as it goes toward the pancreas, putting it at risk for injury during ulcer surgery. The ampulla of Vater enters in the second portion of the duodenum, and the superior mesenteric artery crosses over the third portion of the duodenum. The ligament of Treitz suspends the fourth portion of the duodenum, and taking down this ligament is critical when exposing the fourth portion and areas posterior to it, such as the abdominal aorta.

Five vessels supply blood to the stomach. The right and left gastric arteries arise off the celiac axis. The right gastroepiploic artery arises from the gastroduodenal artery and the left from the short gastrics. The short gastrics feed the corpus of the stomach. A replaced left hepatic artery may arise from the left gastric artery and be visualized and palpated in the lesser omentum.

The duodenum is supplied by the superior pancreaticoduodenal arteries from the gastroduodenal trunk and the inferior pancreaticoduodenal arteries from the superior mesenteric trunk. The supra- and retroduodenal arteries are collaterals of both pancreaticoduodenal arteries.

Nervous control of the stomach is principally from the vagus nerve. This nerve is parasympathetic in origin and gives off branches to the stomach, liver (via the hepatic branch), antropyloric complex, celiac plexus, and small bowel. Vagal stimulation induces acid secretion directly and pepsinogen secretion; and it can stimulate or inhibit gastrin hormonal release.

The cells of the stomach include the parietal cells, which secrete hydrochloric acid and intrinsic factor, and the chief cells, which secrete pepsinogen. Pepsinogen is secreted in the inactive form and is cleaved to the active form (pepsin) in the acidic milieu of the stomach. Goblet cells and epithelial cells secrete mucus and extracellular fluid, respectively. The mast cells, located in the fundus and corpus, secrete histamine (which can stimulate acid secretion via the H_2-receptor), heparan, and vasoactive substances. The antrum contains the enteroendocrine cells, with two predominant types: G-cells, which secrete gastrin, and delta cells, which secrete somatostatin.

GASTRIC MOTILITY

The motility of the stomach varies by location. The fundus and corpus are relatively inactive during the normal fasted and fed states. Both, however, maintain a constant muscular tone during the fasted state. After feeding, the fundus and corpus relax; *a receptive relaxation* that allows the stomach to expand and store the food. Transit of a food bolus through the stomach takes 1 to 2 hours and can be quantitated using gastric emptying scintigraphy.

The antropyloric complex is the muscular center of the stomach. Antral contractions churn and shear solid foods into smaller portions, which increases the surface area available for digestive enzymes, and facilitate delivery of the food bolus into the duodenum. Antropyloric motility, coordinated with receptive relaxation and pyloric contraction, causes churning and shearing of food boluses. Increased fundic tone coordinated with antropyloric relaxation allows ejection of liquid food. Coordinated antropyloric motility with increased fundic tone is essential for effective solid food expulsion and gastric emptying.

The motility of the stomach is based on electrical events and is well controlled intrinsically and extrinsically. Intrinsic control is based on cell-to-cell connections called gap junctions. Gastric myocytes are electrically polarized, and the cellular electrical events can be measured using intracellular electrodes. In the fundus, intracellular resting membrane potentials are between -40 and -50 mV, and frequent and spontaneous slow waves of depolarization (e.g., three per minute) are seen. By comparison, the antrum cells are relatively hyperpolarized (-60 to -70 mV) and do not spontaneously depolarize as frequently (zero to two per minute). Waves of depolarization are communicated distally by cellular gap junctions. The net result is that the proximal stomach, with its more frequent waves of depolarization, drives the

waves of the distal antrum and pylorus. Therefore the proximal stomach contains a pacemaker that drives the motility of the distal stomach. A pacemaker region has been identified along the greater curvature of the stomach near the vasa brevia.

When extracellular electrodes are embedded in the muscular layer of the stomach, the electrical activity of groups of cells can be monitored. In the antrum, slow-wave depolarizations are typically seen two to three times per minute; they are not associated with muscular contractions. The slow waves can be detected on the surface of the skin by electrogastrography. Occasionally, rapid depolarizations are noted superimposed on slow waves; they are called spike potentials. Spike potentials are associated with calcium influx into the cells and muscular contractions. The cells of the corpus and fundus of the stomach rarely exhibit spike potentials, which corresponds with the minimal contractions noted in this region. Cells of the terminal antrum, however, frequently have spike potentials with depolarizations and therefore have frequent, strong contractions.

The extracellular control of motility is by vagal innervation. This innervation serves to coordinate the activity of the fundus, antrum, pylorus, and duodenum; it also extrinsically controls the pacemaker of the stomach.

PEPTIC ULCER DISEASE

Acid formation in the stomach goes through three phases. The cephalic response is mediated by direct vagus stimulation and can be induced by sham feeding. The gastric response is induced by the presence of food in the stomach and is mediated by both hormonal and local receptors in the antrum. The intestinal response is induced by the delivery of food into the duodenum and is driven by hormones, classically gastrin and cholecystokinin.

The parietal cell can concentrate hydrochloric acid one million times, secrete it, and acidify the stomach. Three receptors on the parietal cell are involved in the control of acid secretions. The acetylcholine receptor is mediated by a cyclic adenosine monophosphate (cAMP) second messenger. The gastrin receptor is mediated by a G-protein second messenger, as is the histamine receptor. The effects of combinations of acetylcholine, gastrin, and histamine on acid secretion from the parietal cell are not cumulative but potentiated. Specifically, if one gives a unit dose of acetylcholine or a unit of gastrin, a specific acid response occurs. If the two are given together, the acid response is more than doubled; this is called *potentiation*. This is why single pharmacologic agents such as H_2 blockers can reduce the acidity of the stomach by 60% to 80%: Along with the histamine receptor the effects of acetylcholine and gastrin are inhibited as well.

The antral G-cell, which secretes gastrin, can be stimulated extrinsically by acetylcholine (vagus) or locally by gastric distension. It is also stimulated by small peptides and amino acids. The G-cell has a feedback inhibition of gastrin by the presence of luminal acid.

Cholecystokinin, a member of the gastrin family, also stimulates acid secretion. Calcium infusion alone can stimulate acid formation by a direct effect on the parietal cell and by inducing gastrin release.

Gastric acid can be inhibited by hormones secreted by the duodenum during the intestinal phase, namely glucagon, secretin, and gastric inhibitory polypeptide (GIP). GIP was originally thought only to inhibit gastric acid secretion and motility. It is now called a glucose-dependent insulinotrophic polypeptide because its main function has been found to be as an incretin; that is, it enhances the insulin response from pancreatic beta cells during hyperglycemia. Other hormones that can inhibit gastric secretion are somatostatin, vasoactive intestinal peptide (VIP), and glucagon-like polypeptide. The glucagon–secretin family of proteins (which include GIP and VIP) inhibit acid secretion and motility by competing for and blocking the gastrin receptor on the parietal cell.

Gastrin appears in many forms. The human gastrin gene has been sequenced, and a series of posttranslational modifications converts a pre-pro-protein to a pro-protein to big gastrin. Big gastrin (G-34), 34 amino acids in length, is the form predominantly found in the serum. G-17 is the second most common form in serum. The C-terminal first four amino acids of gastrin contain the active fragment. Pentagastrin is a commercially available five-amino-acid analog.

Interestingly, gastrin is also a hormone with a trophic effect on cells of the gastrointestinal (GI) tract. Gastric mucosal hyperplasia and pancreatic growth are seen in patients with hypergastrinemia. Gastrin has also been implicated in mediating colonic mucosal growth. Studies have shown that gastrin can promote the growth of colon cancer, and that the antigastrin molecule proglumide can inhibit the growth of some colorectal cancers.

The defense of the stomach against back-diffusion of acid is based on the mucosal barrier. The gastric mucosal barrier is thought to be the result of tight junctions between mucosal cells and a luminal layer of mucus secreted by cuboidal epithelium. Prostaglandin E_2 (PGE_2) is believed integral to an intact mucosal barrier; nonsteroidal antiinflammatory agents (NSAIDs) injure the barrier by destroying products of PGE_2. The drug misoprostol is an oral preparation of PGE_2 and has been shown to enhance the acid mucosal barrier.

The rich blood supply of the stomach has also been proposed to protect the stomach by nourishing the cuboidal layer and allowing it to secrete more mucus. Low blood supply to the stomach in times of hemorrhagic shock or stress therefore results in mucosal erosion. Acid neutralization by bircarbonate is another important mucosal defense. Defective production of bircarbonate by the duodenum or impaired directional vectors of the antropyloric motility complex have been shown to be associated with peptic ulcers.

Peptic ulcer disease (PUD) is an international problem. The incidence of PUD has been decreasing over the last 20 to 40 years, but is not related to the development of drugs such as H_2 blockers. At the same time, the incidence of hospital admissions for complications of acid-derived peptic disease—perforation, bleeding, obstruction, and intractability—has not changed. The basic nature of PUD is injury of the stomach or duodenal mucosa by acid and peptic enzyme digestion. The theory of no acid–no ulcer is true for both gastric and duodenal ulcers. The peptidase pepsin is active if the pH is lower than 5.0, so keeping the gastric pH higher than 5.0 protects the mucosa from both direct burning and enzymatic digestion.

Our understanding of the pathogenesis of peptic ulcer disease has undergone a major shift with the identification of *Helicobacter pylori* (previously known as *Campylobacter pylori*). *H. pylori* has been cultured from the antrum and the duodenum of 95% of patients with ulcers and is typically not found in those with NSAID-induced ulcers. It is believed that *H. pylori* inhibits the mucosal defense by destroying the mucosal barrier. *H. pylori* thrives in an acidic environment and contains urease. *H. pylori* infection can be documented by culture, histologic staining, antibody analysis [enzyme-linked immunosorbent assay (ELISA) or Western], urease staining, or the urea breath test.

Infection with *H. pylori* is typically treated by administration of an antacid plus an antibiotic. The addition of aggressive treatment of *H. pylori* has decreased the recurrence rate for simple ulcer disease from 30%–50% to 2%–5%, a remarkable accomplishment.

Peptic ulceration can be divided into duodenal and gastric ulcers. Gastric ulcers are not typically associated with hyperacidity; usually the acid level in the stomach is low or normal. With a gastric ulcer the gastric mucosal barrier is damaged; acid and pepsin cause the ulcer. Gastric stasis and bile reflux have also been implicated in the genesis of gastric ulcers. About 95% of gastric ulcers are found on a lesser curvature near the incisura, which is really the antrofundic border. This location contains a transition zone where the two cell types (parietal and antral) meet. As patients age, this border moves cephalad.

By contrast, duodenal ulcers are associated with hyperacidity. Some patients increase their parietal cell mass, thereby increasing the effect from each dose of acetylcholine and gastrin. Some patients have an increased serum gastrin level, and some have defective secretion of bicarbonate from the duodenal mucosa. Other theories include antropyloric dysmotility, where increased, rapid emptying of an acid load to the duodenum overwhelms the mucosal defense.

Treatment options for peptic ulcer disease are multifold. Oral antacids such as Maalox or Mylanta are magnesium and aluminum complexes that neutralize gastric acid. H_2 blockers block the H_2 receptors on the parietal cell and inhibit gastric acid secretion by potentiation. Cimetidine, ranitidine, and famotidine have increasing potencies, respectively. Sucralfate is a complex sugar that is not digested in the stomach, but in an acidic environment it binds to the ulcer crater. Sucralfate coats the ulcer and protects it from acid damage, promoting healing. It also combines with protein growth factors such as epidermal growth factor (EGF), and studies have shown that it can facilitate the delivery of EGF to the ulcer crater. Misoprostol, a PGE_2 agonist, has a cytoprotective effect on the gastric mucosal barrier. Unfortunately, it is expensive; and although it has been demonstrated to be effective experimentally, clinically its effectiveness is not yet documented.

Omeprazole has been recently approved for use for peptic ulcer disease. It promotes complete achlorhydria because it inhibits the hydrogen-proton pump in the parietal cell. Omeperazole therapy can result in hypergastrinemia, and there is some experimental evidence that carcinoid tumors can occur after long-term treatment. Hence it is not currently advisable to use omeperazol for continued suppression.

The U.S. National Institutes of Health (NIH) held a consensus conference in 1994 in which suggestions were made about treating patients for *H. pylori*. At that time it was thought that if patients were asymptomatic, had no ulcer, and were *H. pylori*-positive there was no indication to treat. For patients with dyspepsia, gastritis by endoscopy, and *H. pylori* positivity, there is still was no indication to treat. Only in patients with gastric or duodenal ulcers with positive *H. pylori* cultures was there reason to treat the patient for *H. pylori*. More liberal criteria are used today for those with dyspepsia.

The first operation for PUD was proposed in 1881 by Woelfer, who advocated a gastroenterostomy. That same year, Billroth presented gastric resection with Billroth I (BI) reconstruction. The BII reconstruction was introduced in 1885. The prevailing thought at that time was that gastric ulcers were the result of stasis, so any type of drainage or resection of the stomach was needed. Dragstedt changed the way we understood ulcer disease during the early 1940s by noting that experimentally vagotomy decreased acid production by 60% to 70%. He introduced truncal vagotomy and 6 to 7 years later added drainage procedures because of the development of functional gastric outlet obstruction in 15% to 20% of the patients. Golligher and Holumbuck during the early 1970s introduced parietal cell, or highly selective, vagotomy.

Gastric Ulcers

Gastric ulceration can be divided into four types: type I, a single gastric ulcer; type II, simultaneous gastric and duodenal ulcers; type III, pyloric channel ulcer; and type IV, a gastric ulcer near the GE junction. The type I and IV gastric ulcers are associated with low or normal gastric acid secretion, whereas type II and III ulcers are associated with increased gastric acid secretion.

Gastric ulcer has its peak incidence during the fifth decade of life. The male/female ratio is 2 : 1. It can be documented by gastroscopy or radiography. Gastroscopy is better because biopsy specimens of the ulcer can be obtained. At least six specimens per endoscopy are suggested to determine that a gastric ulcer is benign. About 95% of benign ulcers occur along the lesser curvature of the stomach near the incisura angularis. Treatment for gastric ulcer is antacids (or H_2 blockade) and elimination of *H. pylori* (if the appropriate assay is positive). In general, 50% of gastric ulcers heal in 4 to 6 weeks and 90% by 12 weeks. Gastric ulcers have higher recurrence rates than duodenal ulcers.

Surgery is indicated for hemorrhage, perforation, intractability, or obstruction and to rule out cancer. The operation preferred for gastric ulcer (type I) is 50% gastrectomy or a simple excision. Vagotomy is not generally needed, as acid secretion is not the etiology. High lesser-curve ulcers (type IV) should be excised by 50% gastrectomy with teeing off medially to include most of the lesser curvature. This procedure is called a Shoemaker gastrectomy. A true GE junction ulcer can be treated by excision with reconstruction with a loop of jejunum (Csendes reconstruction) or by biopsy and distal drainage (Kelling Madlener operation).

Duodenal Ulcers

Duodenal ulcers occur in 5% to 15% of the population. Historically, the male/female ratio was a little higher than that for gastric ulcers, 4 : 1, but today the ratio is almost equal, probably because of the advent of smoking in women. The peak incidence of duodenal ulcer occurs during the fourth decade. It is associated with smoking, hyperparathyroidism, hypercalcemia, chronic obstructive pulmonary disease, uremia, liver disease, and polycythemia vera. Duodenal ulcers typically present with epigastric pain that is relieved by food and can awaken the patient during the night. Other symptoms include early satiety, anorexia, and nausea. Ethanol use and spicy and fried foods exacerbate the symptoms. About 15% to 20% are silent. The diagnosis is made radiographically or by endoscopy.

Historically, treatment of duodenal ulcer was with antacids, with a 70% to 85% success rate. Unfortunately, the recurrence rate was high without some sort of maintenance therapy. As previously noted, recurrences have decreased recently with the addition of antibiotic therapy for *H. pylori*.

About 70% to 80% of bleeding ulcers stop spontaneously. Treatment for acutely bleeding ulcers includes endoscopy, heater probe application, electrocoagulation, or direct injection with a vasoconstrictor such as epinephrine. A heater probe can increase the local temperature to 250°C and cauterize the vessel. The stigmata of bleeding include a cherry red spot (bleeding with a clot) and an ulcer with a visible vessel. The reported rebleed rates for endoscopically visualized ulcers with no evidence of bleeding are low. These can be treated with medical therapy. If a red spot, visible clot, or vessels are visualized, the rebleed rate increases significantly, and patients should undergo invasive therapy and intensive care observation. Once the bleeding vessel is treated, repeat endoscopy should be planned prior to discharge. If operation is indicated, suture ligation of the ulcer is advocated in four quadrants in addition to vagotomy and drainage. Studies have shown that operative morbidity and mortality increase significantly in the presence of a large bleed (more than 5 units), a large ulcer (more than 1 cm), or a concomitant medical illness.

Duodenal ulcers usually perforate when the lesion is located anteriorly. Typically, perforation presents as board-like rigidity and free air under the diaphragm. Surgery is indicated, and studies have shown that the operative risk increases significantly with age over 60 years, preoperative shock, or history of more than 24 hours since the perforation occurred. Operations include the Graham patch, vagotomy and drainage, or a patch with highly selective vagotomy. The operation performed should be tailored to the patient's history and risk of recurrence. The procedure with the least number of recurrences is truncal vagotomy with antrectomy (V&A), as both the vagal cholinergic fibers and the source of gastrin from the antrum are removed. V&A has a higher complication rate than either truncal vagotomy and pyloroplasty or highly selective vagotomy because the bowel is entered.

Obstruction due to a duodenal ulcer is typical in patients with a long-standing history of ulcer disease. Patients with obstruction present with a large, dilated stomach and hypochloremic, hypokalemic metabolic alkalosis. This metabolic derangement is due to the hydrogen and potassium lost during emesis and from active kidney excretion of potassium to preserve fluid. Gastric outlet obstruction can be diagnosed by endoscopy, radiography, or the saline load test, in which a 500-ml bolus of saline is instilled into the stomach by a nasogastric tube. The test is positive if 50% or more of the fluid remains in the stomach 2 hours later. Obstructive ulcer disease is usually treated by antrectomy and truncal vagotomy. Because of the derangements in motility of a chronically obstructed, dilated, floppy stomach, there is a high incidence (35%) of postoperative gastric stasis and gastroparesis after these operations.

The final indication for surgery for duodenal ulcer disease is intractability due to failure of antacid therapy or noncompliance. The operation is aimed at reducing acid secretion via vagotomy.

Stress Ulcer

The last peptic ulceration for review is the acute mucosal erosion. These lesions follow damage to the mucosal barrier by hemorrhagic shock, malnutrition, or bile reflux from an adynamic ileus. Cushing's ulcers are associated with central nervous system injury and have been thought to result from increased vagal activity. Curling's ulcers are associated with burn injuries and have been reported to be due to vagal activity as well. Acute mucosal erosions can bleed and perforate.

The treatment is usually nonoperative. Antacid therapy and angiography with pitressin and gelfoam embolization of the left gastric artery should be considered. If surgery is indicated, there is an associated 35% to 80% mortality rate. Some advocate resection with a truncal vagotomy, whereas others prefer selective devascularization of the stomach. With this procedure the left and right gastric arteries and the right and left gastroepiploic arteries are ligated. The short gastrics are left to nourish the stomach. The procedure is done in conjunction with a gastrotomy to identify and ligate the ulcer(s) that is bleeding. A more definitive treatment option for acute mucosal erosions is total gastrectomy.

MALLORY-WEISS TEARS

Mallory-Weiss tears cause bleeding from the upper GI tract. Tears are the result of forceful vomiting, usually associated with ethanol ingestion. Most bleeds are self limited. Once Boorrhaeve syndrome (esophageal perforation) is ruled out by radiography and the diagnosis is confirmed by endoscopy, the treatment is expectant. Sengstaken-Blakemore tubes, for tamponade, are used rarely. If operation is indicated, a high gastrotomy is performed, oversewing the tear.

ACUTE GASTRIC DILATION

Acute gastric dilatation is associated with severe illness, ileus, and the gastroparesis of diabetes. Patients rarely bleed, but a significant percentage can aspirate. Acute gastric ileus with distension rarely causes rupture. The best treatment for this condition is urgent placement of a nasogastric tube.

VAGOTOMY AND DRAINAGE

When performing truncal vagotomy, one should clear 3 to 4 cm above the GE junction to transect fibers prior to their branching to the stomach. After truncal vagotomy, a drainage procedure is generally performed. Antrectomy is followed by a Billroth I or II gastroenterostomy. There are several types of pyloroplasty. With the standard Heineke-Mikulicz pyloroplasty a longitudinal incision is made and then closed transversely. If the longitudinal incision is too long and an adequate transverse repair cannot be performed, a Finney pyloroplasty is preferred, where the bowel is left *in situ* and one simply approximates the bowel leaflets posteriorly and anteriorly.

The Jaboulay gastroduodenostomy is performed after two incisions are made, one in the duodenum and one in the antrum. The two incisions are then connected, leaving the pylorus intact.

Selective vagotomy is performed below the GE junction to preserve the hepatic and celiac branches. This technique was introduced to avoid postoperative gallbladder and intestinal dysmotility. This purpose has not been served, however, and highly selective vagotomy has replaced it.

Highly selected vagotomy (HSV) selectively denervates the fundus and corpus of the stomach, leaving the vagal nerve supply to the antrum and the rest of the bowel uninjured. The procedure preserves the innervation to the antroduodenal complex. Studies have shown that HSV has a lower incidence of sequela than vagotomy, and because an enterostomy is not performed. There is reduced morbidity.

SEQUELAE OF VAGAL TRANSECTION AND DRAINAGE

The sequelae of truncal vagotomy and drainage are postvagotomy diarrhea, dumping syndrome, alkaline reflux gastritis, early satiety, and afferent and efferent loop syndrome. Postvagotomy *diarrhea* occurs in 30% to 40% of patients, but most resolve on their own. Studies suggest that it is most likely the result of changed motility patterns previously controlled by the vagus nerve. The antrum, pylorus and small intestine exhibit the migrating motor complex, which normally cycles every 90 minutes. After oral nutrients are given, the migrating motor complex is inhibited, which halts motility in the upper GI tract allowing the food to be churned, digested, and absorbed. If vagal electrical activity is inhibited, this postprandial inhibition of the migrating motor complex does not occur, causing rapid transit of foodstuffs from the antrum and pylorus down to the terminal ileum. Undigested food is then delivered into the colon, and diarrhea results.

Studies have shown that small bowel transit in normal patients without diarrhea is about 350 minutes. In patients with vagotomy who do not have diarrhea, small bowel transit is faster, 260 minutes. In patients with vagotomy and diarrhea the small bowel transit time is only 100 minutes. Therefore patients with postvagotomy diarrhea should be treated with antimotility agents such as loperamide (Imodium) or diphenoxylate–atropine (Lomotil) to inhibit small intestinal transit. For patients who require surgery, an interposition of a reverse segment of small bowel in the distal gut sometimes helps.

Postvagotomy *dumping* occurs in up to 20% of patients after truncal vagotomy but is persistent in fewer than 10%. Dumping syndrome be divided into two types: early and late. Early dumping presents as intestinal fullness, dizziness, nausea, and vomiting within 30 minutes of eating a meal. Late dumping occurs 2 to 3 hours after the meal and has different symptoms, usually diaphoresis and tachycardia. Early dumping is the result of dumping of nondigested, highly osmotic fluid into the GI tract, causing fluid shifts within the GI tract and intravascular space. Late dumping is thought to be a humorally mediated event, resulting from abnormal release of enteroglucagon, a hormone counterregulatory to insulin. Early release of enteroglucagon results in an abnormally high insulin release, resulting in delayed hypoglycemia and its subsequent symptoms.

Late dumping can be treated with the hormone somatostatin (octreotide). Studies have shown that somatostatin halts the early release of enteroglucagon and other counterregulatory hormones, leading to normal insulin secretion. If medical treatments fail to manage symptoms, surgical intervention includes reversal of pyloroplasty or, for patients with a BI or BII gastroenterostomy, conversion to a Roux-en-Y gastrojejunostomy. For markedly severe cases placement of an isolated reverse segment between the proximal jejunum and the stomach has been advocated.

Early satiety occurs because of the loss of receptive relaxation of muscle fibers of the stomach corpus after vagotomy. Normally, vagal tone to this area relaxes postprandially to accommodate the food bolus. After vagotomy, the tone remains, and the patient feels full. *Afferent loop syndrome*, which classically occurs after loop gastrojejunostomy, is due to obstruction of the proximal Billroth II limb. Patients present with severe abdominal pain after eating followed by forceful vomiting of bilious material (without food), which relieves the obstruction. Complete obstruction can cause a closed loop, with fever and elevated white blood cell (WBC) count and amylase level. Treatment of afferent loop syndrome is revision of the Billroth II to a Roux-en-Y gastroenterostomy. *Efferent loop syndrome* is the result of obstruction of the efferent loop from a Billroth II anastomosis, typically from adhesive bands. It is treated surgically.

Many of the above sequelae of truncal vagotomy can be avoided by initially performing a highly selective va-gotomy. Highly selective vagotomy has only a 2% incidence of associated dumping. Postvagotomy diarrhea after highly selective vagotomy is seen in only 5%. Bilious vomiting occurs in 10% to 15% of patients after pyloroplasty, vagotomy, and antrectomy but in only 3% of patients with highly selective vagotomy.

Bile acid reflux gastritis occurs particularly after a Billroth I gastroduodenostomy but sometimes after a loop Billroth II gastrojejunostomy. The symptom is typically epigastric pain, resembling that of ulcer disease. It is diagnosed by visualizing bile-induced gastritis via endoscopy. Initial therapy is with cholestyramine. If unsuccessful, a Roux-en-Y operation is indicated, which diverts the biliary flow downstream.

A Roux-en-Y diversion is not always benign. The *Roux syndrome* occurs when the limb does not empty well, resulting in upper GI distress, nausea, and pain. The etiology is dysmotility in the limb. The migrating motor complex, which is initiated in the duodenum and moves caudally, is disrupted when the Roux segment is separated from the proximal duodenum. The limb then develops its own aberrant motility pattern, based on ectopic pacemakers. External pacing using wires have not had long-term success. An operation advocated by Keith Kelly's group at the Mayo Clinic has been the "uncut Roux-en-Y," which leaves the electrical control of the

Roux limb intact along with that of the duodenum. A loop gastrojejunostomy is brought up to the stomach, and the limb is stapled proximally; a concomitant proximal jejunojunostomy is done so there is intestinal continuity. The long-term utility of this procedure is still under investigation.

A devastating complication of gastric surgery is *duodenal stump blowout*, which manifests a few days after surgery as fever, abdominal pain, and elevated WBC count. Sometimes it is impossible to diagnose radiographically. Treatment is laparotomy and tube drainage of the blown segment.

GASTROPARESIS AND ZE SYNDROME

Gastroparesis can occur in operated and nonoperated patients. Gastroparesis in nonoperated patients is typically the result of diabetes. Studies have shown that acute hyperglycemia alone can inhibit gastric motility. Other studies have shown that diabetic patients develop a vagal neuropathy. Gastroparesis in patients with surgical disease is seen typically after relief of an obstruction, benign (peptic ulcer disease) or malignant (pancreatic cancer).

There are a few modalities available to document gastroparesis. Electrogastrograms (EGGs), performed with surface electrodes, measure the slow waves of the stomach (two to three per minute). Patients with gastroparesis exhibit tachygastrias and bradygastrias. A simpler test is radionuclide scintigraphy, which can measure both solid and liquid emptying.

Gastroparesis is treated with patience and prokinetic agents, such as metaclopropamide, cisapride, and erythromycin. The latter macrolide antibiotic has a structure similar to the GI hormone motilin, which directly stimulates the contraction of myocytes.

Partial gastrectomy is indicated for intractable gastroparesis. Some advocate total gastrectomy, accepting the risk of sewing the jejunum to the esophagus, as even a small cuff of stomach left cannot function. I prefer an 80% gastrectomy as a first step and if it fails conversion to total gastrectomy.

Recurrent ulceration is typically the result of a failed vagotomy, retained antrum, G-cell hyperplasia, or the Zollinger-Ellison (ZE) syndrome. A failed vagotomy can be documented by the Hollander test, congo red test, or a sham feeding. The Hollander test is based on the fact that hypoglycemia induces vagal activity and

acid secretion. Insulin-induced hypoglycemia is potentially dangerous, however, so the test is no longer performed. Congo red can be applied topically to the gastric mucosa during endoscopy to determine if acid is being produced. Sham feeding is the most commonly used test of vagal integrity. First a nasogastric tube is placed. Acid output in the stomach is measured and the baseline acid secretion measured. The patient is shown and allowed to chew food, and if the vagus is intact acid production increases. If the vagus has been fully transected, no acid increase is observed. For the last part of the test a dose of intravenous pentagastrin is given to document that the stomach can produce acid. In clinical practice, all the above tests are difficult and can give equivocal results.

Hypergastrinemia after vagotomy and drainage results from retained antrum, G-cell hyperplasia, or ZE syndrome. Retained antrum can be determined by looking at the operative note and, more importantly, the pathology of the distal part of the resection. Typically, serum gastrin levels are elevated two to three times above normal, but no response to secretin stimulation is noted. Antral G-cell hyperplasia also exhibits gastrin levels two to three times normal. A high protein bolus in the stomach increases gastrin levels upward (three to four times higher), but here too there is no response to secretin stimulation.

Gastrinoma is diagnosed when basal gastrin levels are over 200 pg/mL and the secretin stimulation test is positive. Within 2 minutes after a secretin injection, absolute serum gastrin increases to more than 200 pg/mL. A baseline serum gastrin level over 500 to 800 pg/mL is diagnostic of gastrinoma.

Zollinger-Ellison syndrome manifests as recurrent ulceration and associated diarrhea and malnutrition. The diarrhea is the result of acid dumped into the small intestine and the motility that is induced. Normal basal acid secretion is 10 mEq/hr, whereas in patients with ZE it is well over 15 mEq/hr. ZE syndrome may occur sporadically, or it may be associated with endocinopathies, specifically multiple endocrine neoplasia type I (MEN-I). MEN-I includes parathyroid tumors, pituitary tumors, and pancreatic endocrine tumors. Patients with MEN-I typically have multiple gastrinomas at duodenal sites.

Once ZE syndrome is diagnosed, localizing the tumor is attempted with computed tomography (CT), magnetic resonance imaging (MRI), octreotide scans, angiography, or portal venous sampling. Intraoperative evaluation by ultrasonography or duodenal transillumination can help locate very small tumors. About 80% to

90% of gastrinomas are found in the gastrinoma triangle, defined as the junction of the cystic duct and common bile duct along with the second, third, and fourth portions of the duodenum plus the head and neck of the pancreas.

As many as 50% of patients with ZE have metastatic disease, and most should be explored if the tumors are resectable. Debulking has been shown to be beneficial. If operation is not indicated because of widespread metastatic disease, patients can be maintained on long-term omeprazole treatment. Interestingly, ZE syndrome is historically an important disease because total gastrectomy was initially advocated (resecting the end-organ to prevent severe ulceration) to improve long-term survival.

GASTRIC TUMORS

Benign tumors of the stomach include hyperplastic polyps, which are regenerative and have been associated with atrophic gastritis and hypoclorhydria. Ménétriere's disease is a hypertrophic gastropathy and is usually benign, although rarely there is some malignant degeneration. Adenomas are single tumors with atypical glands. Concerns about malignant transformation should be present in lesions more than 2 cm in size (25% incidence). Familial polyposis and Gardner syndrome can give rise to duodenal and gastric adenomas as well.

Hamartomas, typical of Peutz-Jeghers syndrome, can occur in the stomach. Islands of heterotopic pancreas are also sometimes found, as are Brunner's gland adenomas.

Gastric leiomyoma and **leiomyosarcomas** are smooth muscle tumors. Today they are considered part of the gastrointestinal stromal tumor (GIST) group, which includes tumors derived from smooth muscle and other stromal elements. GIST tumors are typically intramural and have some submucosal expansion. Gastric leiomyomas typically cause GI bleeding, pain, and a palpable mass. There is ulceration in 50%.

It is difficult to distinguish leiomyomas from leiomyosarcomas. Usually the larger tumors (more than 4–5 cm) are malignant, but the only way to diagnose the lesion is by looking at the number of mitotic figures per high-power field. If a tumor exhibits more than 5 to 10 mitotic figures per high-power field, it is considered malignant. Occasionally, these tumors grow to enor-mous size, pedunculate, and separate from the stomach wall. I have seen leiomyosarcomas present as an isolated mass behind the stomach and in front of the pancreas.

Malignant or not, resection for a GIST is the same. Leiomyomas and leiomyosarcomas should be resected with a 2- to 3-cm margin. A lymphadenectomy is not indicated, as no data show any improvement in survival with larger resections. If one encounters a small submucosal nodule that appears benign, local enucleation is usually adequate.

Gastric carcinoma is a disease of significance in both the United States and Japan. The U.S. death rate is 6.6/100,000, whereas the Japanese death rate is 59/100,000. In the United States the incidence has declined by 65% over the last 30 years. Gastric carcinoma has been associated with diet, specifically salted or pickled foods, nitrites, and nitrosamines. Smoking and familial, racial, and socioeconomic factors are also involved. There is an association with blood group A, and evidence has linked gastric adenocarcioma with previous infection with *H. pylori*.

Risks for carcinoma of the stomach include chronic atrophic gastritis, the hypochlorhydric or achlorhydric state, pernicious anemia, adenoma, polyps larger than 2 cm, and a history of gastric surgery. Patients 20 years after Billroth II reconstruction are considered to be at two to six times the normal risk.

Signs and symptoms include pain, anemia, weight loss, and fatigue. An epigastric mass can be palpated on physical examination. With advanced disease, Virchow's nodes can be palpated in the left neck, Sister Mary Joseph's nodes in the periumbilical region, and a Bloomer shelf on rectal examination. Krukenberg tumors are metastatic lesions to the ovary.

Gastric cancer is diagnosed typically by barium contrast study or endoscopy. On barium study the ulcers are typically seen to be more than 1 cm in diameter, and the folds do not radiate to the center as they do with benign lesions. The folds are usually elevated. An abdominal CT scan can help determine the extent of illness. Staging is usually by the TNM system, which is based on the extent of wall penetration and regional lymph node involvement. The 5-year survival for stage I (a small tumor limited to the mucosa) is more than 90%. The stage II 5-year survival is 50%; survival with stage IV is zero. Other classification systems include that of the World Health Organization, with different types signet ring, mucinous, and tubulous. Signet ring and undifferentiated lesions have the worst prognosis. Another system is based on the histologic appearance—intestinal or diffuse—with the former having a better survival.

The Japanese Gastroenterological Endoscopy Society developed a system based on invasion: submucosal versus more advanced. Early disease is isolated to the mucosa or superficial submucosa. Once the muscularis is involved, the tumor is considered advanced by these stages; if the tumor is confined to the mucosa, a 95% five-year survival rate can be predicted.

Studies have shown that the presentation of gastric cancer is changing in the older person, leading to the need for more aggressive surgery. Older patients present with a predominance of the intestinal type, which is less aggressive than the diffuse type; moreover, the location of the tumor is more often in proximal areas of the stomach. This has led to more patients requiring total gastrectomy for curative resection. The incidence of total gastrectomy being required in elderly patients is 13% to 34%. No difference between resectability or the rate of positive lymph nodes found at surgery has been noted between young and old patients (60% to 70%).

Japanese groups have reported endoscopic resections: local resection of very early gastric cancer. These data are the result of intense screening procedures. In the United States, we consider gastric cancer surgery more as a palliative procedure because most of the patients present with submucosal and serosal invasion and positive lymph nodes.

Surgical treatment of a typical distal stomach tumor includes greater omentectomy, and the lesser curve is resected towards the GE junction. A 3-cm distal margin by the duodenum and a 6-cm proximal margin are considered adequate, and one should try to resect the left gastric artery as well.

Total gastrectomy is advocated for large GE junction lesions. Proximal gastrectomy is associated with significant morbidity (acid or alkaline reflux). Esophagogastrectomy is indicated only for pure GE junction lesions, whereas total gastrectomy is reserved for lesions in the cardia. Prophylactic gastrectomy is only rarely indicated for patients with atrophic gastritis, Ménétriere's disease, or gastric polyposis.

The lymphatic spread of gastric cancers has been mapped carefully. They spread first to the R1 lymph node level, which is the perigastric or periantral region and the pancreatic lymph node. The R2 lymph nodes are next, which include some those near the proximal

hepatoduodenal ligament and the splenic artery near the stomach antrum. The R3 nodes are last, which include all those of the hepatoduodenal ligament, celiac axis, and splenic hilum. Data suggest that extensive lymphadenectomy (i.e., inclusive of the R2 and R3 nodes) results in improved survival. The results of clinical trials in the United States have been equivocal. It is probable that large resections show better survival stage per stage, but the course of the disease is not changed; it is just that the patient is more accurately staged. Specifically, patients with R3-negative nodes survive longer than those with positive nodes; but if no R3 resection was done, all would be averaged together for an overall poor survival rate.

With respect to adjuvant therapy, gastric cancer is one of the least sensitive gastrointestinal tumors. In general, 5-fluorouracil and radiation can increase survival in patients with metastatic disease from 6 months to 12 months. There is only a 50% response rate.

Our understanding of the etiology of **gastric lymphoma** has changed. Gastric lymphoma is now known to be highly associated with *H. pylori* infection. Its precursor is believed to be mucosal associated lymphoid tissue (MALT). MALT is currently the terminology for what was previously called pseudolymphoma: lymphoid infiltration of the gastric mucosa resulting from chronic infection with *H. pylori*. In general, there is no lymphoid tissue in the stomach, so when it is observed on biopsy MALT is diagnosed. Studies show that MALT is a prelude to malignant lymphoma. Remarkably, MALT tissue regresses with adequate antibiotic therapy directed at *H. pylori*.

Most primary GI tract lymphomas are located in the stomach. Eighty percent of patients with gastric lymphoma present with pain usually due to ulceration. Forty-two percent have a complication, either bleeding, perforation, or obstruction. The prognosis is determined by the size of the tumor, degree of invasion, and lymph node status. Stage I and II lymphoma (confined to the stomach and regional lymph nodes) can be treated by resection for cure followed by adjuvant chemotherapy and irradiation. This protocol is controversial, however, as some believe it should be treated first with chemotherapy, and others believe it should be treated surgically. Stage III and IV disease is treated with chemotherapy and irradiation; operative resection is indicated only for complications.

The overall survival for gastric lymphoma is 34% to 50% over 5 years. Those with stages I or II have a survival rate of 90%; survival of those with stage III or IV is lower: 20% to 30%.

SURGERY FOR MORBID OBESITY

Morbid obesity is defined as body weight more than 100 pounds over the ideal weight. A more scientific measurement is the body mass index (BMI), which is the weight divided by the body mass. Normal BMI is 25 kg/m^2; a BMI over 28 kg/m^2 is considered to reflect obesity. Persons with a BMI over 40 kg/m^2 are morbidly obese, and those whose BMI is over 60 kg/m^2 are considered superobese. Complications of obesity include high mortality rates, pulmonary insufficiency, cardiac disease, high blood pressure, stroke, diabetes, arthritis, infertility, gallstones, gout, and socioeconomic problems. The indications for surgery include failed diet (multiple times) and the development of complications of obesity.

Surgery for morbid obesity has undergone significant evolution over the last 20 years. One of the original operations was jejunoileal (JI) bypass, but it was associated with a 58% complication rate, including bypass enteritis with bacterial overgrowth, liver failure, and renal failure (the latter due to calcium oxalate stone disease). About 23% of patients who underwent JI bypass eventually needed the surgery to be reversed.

The two types of gastric operation currently being performed are vertical banded gastroplasty (VBG, Mason), a restrictive procedure, and Roux-en-Y gastric bypass procedure (RGB, Greenville), which is both restrictive and induces malabsorption by dumping food into the jejunum. The bypass procedure has been shown to be more successful in patients who eat large amounts of sweets.

Successful surgery results in loss of 40% to 60% of excess body weight. Complications of surgery include anastomotic leak, strictures, stomal ulcerations, erosion of the wraps, rapid weight loss with malnutrition, and development of gallstones after rapid weight loss.

DUODENUM

Common tumors arising primarily from the duodenum are villous adenomas and periampullary carcinomas. Survival after resection of the latter is much better than with other tumors of this region (pancreatic or bile duct tumors).

Annular pancreas causes gastric outlet obstruction, duodenal stenosis, or peptic ulceration in the pediatric population. It is treated by duodenogastrostomy.

Vascular compression of the duodenum is associated with loss of the fat pad near the superior mesenteric artery, causing compression of the third portion of the duodenum and resulting in an obstruction. This condition is rare and is usually treated by duodenojejunostomy.

Gastric and duodenal Crohn's disease occur infrequently. In a large series of patients with Crohn's disease, noting the bowel segments in which it appeared, showed that the stomach and duodenum were associated in about 9%, the duodenum in 8%, and the stomach 1%. Upper GI radiography of patients with duodenal Crohn's disease revealed frozen motility in the antropyloric complex and gradual tapering of the antrum to the bulb. Surgery is rarely required.

Trauma to the duodenum can result from blunt injury to the trunk and is usually associated with other life-threatening injuries. Intramural hematomas of the duodenum can cause obstruction and are usually managed conservatively; they rarely need to be bypassed. Pancreaticoduodenal trauma is highly lethal. Because of concomitant wounds and the insidious nature of pancreaticoduodenal injury, it is usually not diagnosed in a timely fashion. Pancreaticoduodenectomy should almost never be done for trauma because of the excessive associated morbidity.

Duodenal rupture must be handled operatively. One should initially attempt to close the rupture primarily and drain the region; if it is a large defect, a Roux-en-Y limb can be brought up and patched with a serosal patch. For duodenal injury some advocate performing a pyloric exclusion in which the pylorus is stapled and a gastrojejunostomy is created to divert gastric flow to this region; the region is then drained. The pyloric exclusion eventually opens in most patients.

QUESTIONS

Select one answer.

1. For the evaluation of a patient for the etiology of a recurrent ulcer after a vagotomy and antrectomy, the following tests are contributory except:
   a. Sham feeding test.
   b. Serum gastrin level.
   c. Pathology of previous operative specimen.

d. Technetium scan.

e. Gastric biopsy.

2. The operation(s) most appropriate for severe stress ulcer bleeding are:

a. Vagotomy and pyloroplasty.

b. Highly selective vagotomy.

c. Near-total or total gastrectomy.

d. Ligation only of the bleeding sites.

e. Antrectomy and Billroth I reconstruction.

3. What percentage of patients with perforated duodenal ulcer but without previous symptoms when treated by suture closure only of the perforation site remain asymptomatic postoperatively?

a. 90%.

b. 10%.

c. 50%.

d. 0%.

e. 70%.

4. In patients with Zollinger-Ellison syndrome with hyperparathyroidism in need of surgical intervention for severe peptic ulcer disease who are poorly responsive to H_2 blocker therapy, what is the preferred first procedure?

a. Gastric resection.

b. Neck exploration for hyperparathyroidism.

c. Both operations simultaneously.

d. Change in medical therapy.

5. For type I gastric ulcer disease, the elective operation(s) of choice are:

a. Pyloroplasty and vagotomy.

b. Subtotal gastrectomy.

c. Hemigastrectomy with Billroth I reconstruction.

d. Vagotomy and antrectomy.

e. Vagotomy and gastroenterostomy.

6. For management of significant duodenal trauma, all of the following procedures should be considered as options except:

a. Primary repair.

b. Pyloric exclusion and gastroenterostomy.

c. Duodenal diverticulization.

d. Choledochoduodenostomy.

e. Double-tube jejunostomy.

7. The overall 5-year survival rates for gastric carcinoma not resected and resected are, respectively:

a. 1% and 10%.

b. 10% and 21%.

c. 40% and 90%.

d. 20% and 60%.

8. Gastrin release is increased by which of the following?

a. Antral acidification.

b. Ischemia.

c. Histamine.

d. Antral distension.

e. Trauma.

9. Which of the following are risk factors for patients with perforated ulcer?

a. Blood pressure <100 mm Hg.

b. Perforation >24 hours.

c. Diabetes.

d. All of the above.

e. None of the above.

10. Giant gastric ulcers:

a. Are defined as >5 cm.

b. Respond to surgical therapy only.

c. Respond to medical therapy only.

d. Are all malignant.

e. Sometimes respond to medical therapy.

SELECTED REFERENCES

Barragry T, Blatch JW, O'Connor MO. Giant gastric ulcers: a review of 49 cases. *Ann Surg* 1986;203:255–259.

Berne CJ, Rosoff L. Peptic ulcer perforation of the gastroduodenal artery complex: clinical features and operative control. *Ann Surg* 1969;169:141–144.

Boey J, Choi SK, Poon A, Alagaratnam TT. Risk stratification in perforated duodenal ulcers: a prospective validation of predictive factors. *Ann Surg* 1987;205:22–26.

Boey J, Branicki FJ, Alagaratnam TT, et al. Proximal gastric vagotomy: the preferred operation for perforations in acute duodenal ulcer. *Ann Surg* 1988;208:169–174.

Cook AO, Levine BA, Sirinek KR, Gaskill HV. Evaluation of gastric adenocarcinoma: abdominal computed tomography does not replace celiotomy. *Arch Surg* 1986;121:603–606.

Crofts TJ, Park KGM, Steele RJ, Chung SS, La AK. A randomized trial of nonoperative treatment for perforated peptic ulcer. *N Engl J Med* 1989;320:970–973.

Csendes A, Braghetto I, Smok G. Type-IV gastric ulcer: a new hypothesis. *Surgery* 1987;101:363–365.

Deitel M, Jones BA. Petrov vertical banded gastroplasty: results in 233 patients. *Can J Surg* 1986;29:322.

Driks MR, Craven DE, Celli BR, et al. Nosocomial pneumonia in intubated patients given sucralfate as compared with antacids or histamine type 2 blockers: the role of gastric colonization. *N Engl J Med* 1987;317:1376–1382.

Duncombe VM, Bolin TD, David AE. Double-blind trial of cholestyramine in postvagotomy diarrhoea. *Gut* 1977;18: 531–535.

Feliciano DV, Martin TD, Cruse PA, et al. Management of

combined pancreatoduodenal injuries. *Ann Surg* 1987;205: 673–680.

Herrington JL, Davidson J. Bleeding gastroduodenal ulcers: choice of operations. *World J Surg* 1987;11:304–314.

Herrington JL. The afferent loop syndrome: additional experience with its surgical management. *Am Surg* 1968;34: 321–329.

Hogan RB, Hamilton JK, Polter DE. Preliminary experience with hydrostatic balloon dilation of gastric outlet obstruction. *Gastrointest Endosc* 1986;32:71–72.

Howard TJ, Passaro E. Gastrinoma: new medical and surgical approaches. *Surg Clin North Am* 1989;69:667–681.

Hubert JP, Kiernan PD, Welch JS, Remine WH, Beahrs OH. The surgical management of bleeding stress ulcers. *Ann Surg* 1980;191:672–679.

Hunt P. Bleeding gastroduodenal ulcers: selection of patients for surgery. *World J Surg* 1984;11:32–36.

Ingvar C, Adami HO, Enander LK, Enskog L, Rydberg B. Clinical results of reoperation after failed highly selective vagotomy. *Am J Surg* 1986;152:308–312.

Irvin TT. Mortality and perforated peptic ulcer: a case for risk stratification in elderly patients. *Br J Surg* 1989;76:215–218.

Jensen HE, Hoffman J, Wille-Jorgensen P. High gastric ulcer. *World J Surg* 1987;11:325–332.

Johnson HD. Gastric ulcer: classification, blood group characteristics, secretion pattern and pathogenesis. *Ann Surg* 1965;162:996–1004.

Kozarek RA. Hydrostatic balloon dilation of gastrointestinal stenoses: a national survey. *Gastrointest Endosc* 1986;32: 15–18.

Kurata JH, Corboy ED. Current peptic ulcer time trends: an epidemiological profile. *J Clin Gastroenterol* 1988;10:259–268.

Larson G, Schmidt T, Gott J, Bond S, O'Conner C, Richardson D. Upper gastrointestinal bleeding, predictors of outcome. *Surgery* 1986;100:765–773.

Lowe RJ, Saletta JD, Moss GS. Pancreatoduodenectomy for penetrating pancreatic trauma. *J Trauma* 1977;17:732–741.

Lundegardh G, Adamik H-O, Helmick C, Zack M, Meirik O. Stomach cancer after partial gastrectomy for benign ulcer disease. *N Engl J Med* 1988;319:195–200.

Maruyama K, Okabayashi K, Kinoshita T. Progress in gastric cancer surgery in Japan and its limits of radicality. *World J Surg* 1987;11:418–425.

Mason EE, Ito C. Gastric bypass. *Ann Surg* 1969;170:329.

McGee GS, Sawyers JL. Perforated gastric ulcers: a plea for management by primary gastric resection. *Arch Surg* 1987;122:555–561.

Mimpriss TW, Birt JMC. Results of partial gastrectomy for peptic ulcer. *BMJ* 1948;2:1095.

Mulholland MW, Debas HT. Chronic duodenal and gastric ulcer. *Surg Clin North Am* 1987;67:489–507.

Pories WJ. The surgical approach to morbid obesity. In: Sabiston, DC Jr. ed. *Textbook of surgery,* 14th ed. Philadelphia: WB Saunders, 1991;851–866.

Rosen CB, van Heerden JA, Martin JK Jr, Wold LE, Ilstrup DM. Is an aggressive surgical approach to the patient with gastric lymphoma warranted. *Ann Surg* 1987;205:634–640.

Shiu MH, Karas M, Nisce L, Lee BJ, Filippa DA, Lieberman PH. Management of primary gastric lymphoma. *Ann Surg* 1982;195:196–202.

Shiu MH, Moore E, Sanders M, et al. Influence of the extent of resection on survival after curative treatment of gastric carcinoma: a retrospective multivariate analysis. *Arch Surg* 1987;122:1347–1351.

Sugerman HJ, Starkey JV, Birkenhauer R. A randomized prospective trial of gastric bypass versus banded gastroplasty for morbid obesity and their effects on sweets versus nonsweets eaters. *Ann Surg* 1987;205:613.

Taylor TV, Gunn AA, MacLeod DA, et al. Mortality and morbidity after anterior lesser curve seromyotomy with posterior truncal vagotomy for duodenal ulcer. *Br J Surg* 1985;72:950–951.

Turner WW, Thompson WM, Thal ER. Perforated ulcers: a plea for management by simple closures. *Arch Surg* 1988;123:960–964.

Weiland D, Dunn DH, Humphrey EW, Schwartz ML. Gastric outlet obstruction in peptic ulcer disease: an indication for surgery. *Am J Surg* 1982;143:90–93.

Yamada E, Miyaishi S, Nakazato H, et al. *The surgical treatment of cancer of the stomach.* Int Surg *1980;65:387.*

Yajko RD, Seydel F, Trimble C. Rupture of the stomach from blunt abdominal trauma. *J Trauma* 1975;15:177–183.

3

Diseases of the Small Bowel

Stephen A. Michalski and Gerard Weinberg

ANATOMY

The small intestine, a tubular viscus about 13 ft long *in vivo,* is divided into three segments: duodenum, jejunum, and ileum. The duodenum is 10 in. long and largely retroperitoneal. This portion and operations on it are described in another chapter. The jejunoileal segment begins at the ligament of Treitz and ends at the ileocecal valve. It is intraperitoneal and is suspended in coils by a dorsal mesentery. The proximal half of the mesenteric small bowel is arbitrarily designated the jejunum and the distal half the ileum. There are no anatomic features that allow clear distinction between these two segments.

The wall of the small intestine is made up of four concentric layers: serosa, muscularis, submucosa, mucosa. Circular folds of mucosa and submucosa called valvulae conniventes are present throughout but decrease in number and prominence distally in the ileum. They are useful for radiographic identification of small bowel.

At the mesenteric aspect of the small bowel the leaves of the mesentery split and encircle the bowel to form the visceral peritoneum. Blood vessels, nerves, and lymphatics run within the two peritoneal layers of the mesentery to enter and exit the intestine. The arterial supply arises from the superior mesenteric artery. Venous drainage is through the superior mesenteric vein into the portal vein. Lymphatic channels accompany the mesenteric arteries and drain into the cisterna chyli, which empties into the thoracic duct. Both divisions of the autonomic nervous system innervate the small bowel. The parasympathetics are carried by the celiac division of the posterior trunk of the vagus nerve. The sympathetics reach the bowel through the celiac and superior mesenteric ganglia. Sympathetic afferent fibers detect luminal distention, which is perceived as pain in the periumbilical region.

PHYSIOLOGY

The principal functions of the small intestine are to propel the gastric chyme it receives forward, continue its digestion, and absorb into the blood and lymphatics the water, electrolytes, minerals, and nutrients released by digestion.

Gastric effluent is hypertonic and acidic. It is neutralized in the duodenum with bicarbonate and rendered isotonic with secretions. Although daily oral ingestion amounts to only 1.0 to 1.5 liters of fluid, the salivary, gastric, pancreatic, biliary, and intestinal secretions add another 7 to 8 liters. Most of this fluid is absorbed by the time it reaches the ileocecal valve, which leaves approximately 1.0 to 1.5 liters for colonic absorption. The maximum daily capacity for small bowel fluid absorption is estimated to be 12 liters.

Carbohydrate digestion occurs in the mouth, stomach, duodenal lumen, and brush border of the small intestine. Salivary and pancreatic amylase begin starch digestion, and brush border disaccharidases complete the process. Carbohydrate absorption begins in the duodenum and is completed in the jejunum.

Protein digestion begins in the stomach with pepsin, but the gastric contribution is small and nonessential under normal circumstances. Most protein digestion occurs in the proximal small bowel lumen, the brush border, and the enterocyte cytoplasm. Pancreatic enzymes hydrolyze proteins to small peptides and free amino acids in the lumen. Brush border and cytoplasmic peptides complete the digestion of oligopeptides. Peptide absorption occurs in the jejunum and accounts for most of the protein assimilation. Amino acid absorption occurs in the ileum.

Fat digestion occurs rapidly in the duodenum by pancreatic lipases. Absorption begins there and is completed in the proximal 100 cm of jejunum. Bile salts are required to solubilize the products of fat digestion in the form of mixed micelles before absorption can occur. Medium-chain triglycerides contain fatty acids with 6 to 12 carbon atoms that are water-soluble and are processed differently than the more common long-chain triglycerides, which make up 90% of dietary fat. Medium-chain triglycerides can be absorbed intact without pancreatic lipase or micellar transport. Hydrolysis of these triglycerides within the enterocyte releases the medium-chain fatty acids, which can enter the portal circulation directly and thereby bypass the lymphatic channels. Clinical applications include the use of medium-chain triglycerides in patients with pancreatic insufficiency (fat maldigestion), chylous effusions from lymphatic leaks (chylous ascites, chylothorax), and short bowel syndrome (deficient bile salt pool and fat malabsorption).

After participating in lipid absorption, 95% of the bile salts are actively absorbed in the distal ileum. They then return to the liver to be recycled into bile to complete the enterohepatic circulation of these substances.

Most water-soluble vitamins are absorbed in the jejunum with the exception of vitamin B_{12}, which binds the gastric intrinsic factor to facilitate absorption in the distal ileum. The fat-soluble vitamins (A, D, E, K) are solubilized by the mixed micelles and are absorbed with fat in the proximal jejunum. Calcium and magnesium absorption occurs throughout the small bowel, although most takes place in the ileum. Iron absorption occurs in the duodenum and proximal jejunum.

DISEASES OF THE SMALL INTESTINE

Crohn's Disease

Crohn's disease is a chronic transmural inflammatory disease that affects any part of the gastrointestinal tract from the mouth to the anus. Most commonly the disease affects the terminal ileum with or without colonic involvement. In some patients the disease is limited to the colon and rectum. Ileitis afflicts approximately 30% of the patients, ileocolitis 40%, and colitis 20% to 30%. Crohn's disease limited to the colon is considered in a subsequent chapter.

Crohn's disease is characterized by progression and frequent recurrence. Its cause is unknown. Medical and surgical therapy is palliative not curative. Both sexes are affected equally. The disease tends to run in families, but no clear mode of transmission has been established. In the United States Crohn's disease occurs two to three times more often among Jews than non-Jews. Onset is typically during the second or third decade, but later onset during the sixth, seventh, or eighth decades is not unusual.

The bowel wall is thickened by fibrosis and edema, which ultimately narrows the lumen in advanced cases and converts the involved segment to a rigid stenotic tube. Although the disease is transmural, the submucosa shows some of the most striking changes in terms of fibrosis and edema. Noncaseating granulomas with Langerhans giant cells are found in 60% of the diseased intestines, primarily in the submucosal layer. The intestinal wall is infiltrated transmurally with inflammatory cells, but lymphoid aggregates tend to concentrate in the submucosa. The mucosa is usually ulcerated. Early aphthous ulcers are small, superficial, and discontinuous. They are thought to arise from a microabscess in an underlying lymphoid follicle. With more advanced disease, deep longitudinal ulcers and transverse fissures give the mucosa a cobblestone appearance with edematous mucosal islands situated between the ulcers.

Involvement of the small bowel is occasionally (25%) discontinuous, with skip areas of disease separated by regions of normal-appearing intestine. The mesentery is inflamed, thickened, and shortened; it contains enlarged lymph nodes, some with noncaseating granulomas. The mesenteric fat tends to creep onto the serosal aspect of the involved small bowel. Burrowing fissures can traverse the wall of the bowel and penetrate adjacent adherent noninvolved loops of bowel or other structures such as the bladder, with the development of fistulas. Penetration into the mesentery or retroperitoneum can lead to abscess formation.

Perianal manifestations of the disease include fistulas, fissures, ulcers, and abscesses. They are encountered in up to 30% of the patients with small bowel Crohn disease and in up to 50% of those with colonic involvement.

Clinical presentation can be that of an acutely developing disorder that mimics appendicitis. More frequently the early symptoms are vague and nonspecific. They include episodic mild abdominal discomfort and diarrhea. Patients are often diagnosed as having irritable bowel syndrome until an acute exacerbation delineates the true nature of the disorder. During this interval of misdiagnosis, which lasts on average 2 to 3 years, the patient may experience malaise, weight loss, and periods of unexplained fever.

The abdominal pain is intermittent and crampy when caused by partial obstruction. It is persistent when caused by an abscess or tender mass of inflamed intestine encountered during an acute exacerbation of the disease.

The diarrhea is usually nonbloody and worse at night. Causes include partial small bowel obstruction, impaired bile salt absorption from extensive ileal disease, bacterial proliferation proximal to a partial obstruction, ileosigmoid fistula formation, and extension of the disease to the colon. Steatorrhea may complicate the picture when extensive segments of small bowel are involved.

Rectal bleeding is uncommon in small bowel Crohn's disease, occurring in 10% of these patients. This symptom occurs more frequently in those with colonic involvement. Massive bleeding is rare.

With progression of the disease, increasing fibrosis may result in signs and symptoms of small bowel obstruction. The ureters may become encased by retroperitoneal inflammation that results in hydroureter and hydronephrosis.

Free perforation is rare, occurring in 1% to 2% of the patients. More common is the development of fistulas and intraabdominal abscesses. Most fistulas are associated with sepsis to a variable extent. Enteroenteral fistulas may be asymptomatic unless associated with an abscess. Enterovesical fistulas cause dysuria, pyuria, hematuria, and occasionally pneumaturia and fecaluria. Ileosigmoid fistulas may present as sepsis or an exacerbation of the diarrhea. Enterocutaneous fistulas usually occur through old abdominal scars from an appendectomy or bowel resection. The source of the fistula is frequently recurrent disease at an ileocolic anastomosis following bowel resection. The source of the fistula is frequently recurrent disease at an ileocolic anastomosis following bowel resection. External drainage of an intraabdominal abscess may result in a residual enterocutaneous fistula. Spontaneous fistulas are uncommon and result from the discharge of purulent material from an underlying abscess. Intraabdominal abscesses occur in 20% of the patients and develop when a perforation is walled off by surrounding loops of bowel, omentum, mesentery, and parietal peritoneum.

There is an increased incidence (60- to 300-fold increased risk) of small bowel adenocarcinoma in patients with Crohn's disease of the small intestine. The adenocarcinomas tend to occur in the ileum. The symptoms of carcinoma are similar to those of Crohn's ileitis. As a result, delayed recognition has led to a poor prognosis with cure rates less than 10% (versus 20% to 30% in those with small bowel adenocarcinoma unassociated with Crohn's disease). Crohn's colitis is associated with a 4- to 20-fold increased risk of colon cancer. However, many patients require resection before a carcinoma can develop.

Extraintestinal manifestations may precede overt bowel disease, including polyarthritis, ankylosing spondylitis, iritis, uveitis, erythema nodosum, and pyoderma gangrenosum. Patients with ileal involvement have an increased incidence of gallstone formation due to failure to reabsorb bile salts.

Inadequate protein-calorie intake is primarily responsible for the nutritional complications of this disease. Patients are reluctant to eat because food aggravates the abdominal pain. In addition, bacterial proliferation proximal to partially obstructed bowel (blind loop syndrome) or as a consequence of small to large bowel fistula formation can result in fat, protein, carbohydrate, and vitamin malabsorption. A variety of anemias are encountered, including iron deficiency anemia secondary to occult blood loss and megaloblastic anemia secondary to vitamin B_{12} malabsorption from the diseased or resected terminal ileum.

The diagnostic evaluation of a patient with suspected Crohn's disease should begin with a complete history and physical examination, which includes a careful rectal examination. Perianal disease can appear before symptomatic intestinal disease. The perianal lesions are relatively painless except for an abscess. Fissures are often wide, multiple, painless, and in atypical locations. Anal canal ulcers can also occur, which may give rise to pain on defecation. Fistulas may be single and simple or multiple and complex. They tend to be asymptomatic.

The colon should be evaluated with either colonoscopy or double-contrast barium enema. Colonoscopy has the advantage of obtaining material for histologic examination, and the presence of noncaseating granulomas in a rectal or colonic biopsy is helpful for diagnosing Crohn's disease. Studies have questioned the value of a routine rectal valve biopsy in the absence of proctocolitis. Barium enema has the advantage of demonstrating transmural disease, where extravasation of barium into an abscess cavity or into a neighboring viscus would differentiate Crohn's disease from ulcerative colitis.

An upper gastrointestinal series with small bowel follow-through should be performed in all patients after the colorectal evaluation. The presence of small bowel lesions in a patient with colitis supports the diagnosis of Crohn's disease. Small bowel lesions seen on contrast evaluation include thickened blunted valvulae conniventes, cobblestoned mucosa, strictures, skip areas, and fistulas.

A computed tomography (CT) scan or ultrasonography is helpful for identifying abscess formation and directing percutaneous drainage.

Treatment of Crohn's disease includes medical management to achieve temporary remission of an acute exacerbation and to modify a complication. Antiinflammatory corticosteroids are effective in active ileitis or ileocolitis and can settle an acute exacerbation over the course of days to weeks. Their role in disease isolated to the colon is less certain. Steroids should be withdrawn once remission is achieved, as they do not prevent recurrent disease. Patients whose disease relapses as steroids are tapered may benefit from maintenance steroids to control their disease. Sulfasalazine, which contains the antiinflammatory salicylate moiety, can be effective in patients with Crohn's colitis or ileocolitis but has little effect on isolated ileitis. As with steroids, sulfasalazine as a prophylactic agent has not been shown to prevent recurrent disease. The immunosuppressant azathioprine or its metabolite mercaptopurine can be combined with steroids or sulfasalazine to control active disease. These immunosuppressants have an unusual ability to cause fistulas to close. They have also permitted the decrease or elimination of steroid therapy in many instances. The antibiotic metronidazole, which

is bactericidal to intestinal anaerobes, has shown some benefit in colonic and perianal Crohn's disease.

Antidiarrheals, cholestyramine, and a low-fat diet may be required to provide satisfactory bowel function. Antibiotics effective against enteric aerobes and anaerobes are used to combat septic complications. Nutritional support with elemental diets and total parenteral nutrition (TPN) may help bring active disease into remission when combined with other existing medical therapy; TPN has been used for operative preparation of nutritionally depleted patients in an attempt to reduce postoperative morbidity and mortality.

Although a well planned nonoperative approach can successfully treat most acute exacerbations and complications as they develop, most patients (75% or more) eventually require an intestinal operation. As with medical management, surgical intervention cannot cure Crohn's disease, but a remission can be achieved for a variable length of time. Postoperative recurrence rates are 40% at 5 years, 60% at 10 years and 75% at 15 years. Most recurrences occur in the region of the anastomosis at the neoterminal ileum. Neither the amount of grossly normal bowel removed proximal and distal to the lesion, the presence or absence of microscopic disease at the resection margins, nor any combination of drugs can prevent a recurrence after resection. Therefore the surgeon should be conservative: the goal is to treat a specific complication, and every attempt is made to preserve bowel.

For the most part, surgery is performed for complications of the disease. However, not all complications are absolute indications for surgery, with the exception of undrained intraabdominal abscesses, free perforation of the intestine (rare), and uncontrolled intestinal hemorrhage (rare).

Acute small bowel obstruction can usually be managed successfully without surgical intervention, as the obstruction is usually partial and responds to intravenous fluids, bowel rest, nasogastric suction, and steroids. Mural fibrosis occurs with chronic disease, and the bowel has a diminished capacity to recover. The patient experiences recurrent attacks, persistent obstructive symptoms, or both, which are best managed with an operation. Intestinal obstruction is the most common indication for surgery in small bowel Crohn's disease.

When the obstructing lesion is in the terminal ileum, resection of the involved ileum and cecum with anastomosis of the neoterminal ileum to the ascending colon is the operation of choice. The proximal margin should be free of gross disease. Because the mucosa of the ileocecal valve is almost always involved, the distal margin should be placed in the ascending colon just above the cecum or distal to any colonic disease in cases of ileocolitis. Stricturoplasty is useful for proximal skip areas and cases of diffuse jejunoileitis with multiple strictures. This procedure preserves bowel length and prevents short bowel syndrome, especially if there have been previous resections. The Heineke-Mickulicz technique can be used for short-segment strictures and the Finney technique for long-segment strictures.

Bypass of diseased segments is avoided. Future problems with the bypassed segment include closed loop obstruction, blind loop syndrome, free perforation, and carcinoma.

The distinction between an inflammatory mass or phlegmon and an abscess is difficult but has important clinical implications. Both present as a right lower quadrant tender mass (in ileitis or ileocolitis) with associated fever and leukocytosis indicative of a suppurative process caused by transmural penetration of fissures. A phlegmon is treated conservatively with bowel rest, intravenous fluids, and systemic antibiotics. This suppurative process has a capacity for resolution without surgical intervention. However, if the suppurative process extends and pus loculates, an abscess forms; drainage then frequently becomes necessary if the patient does not respond promptly to antibiotic therapy. Steroids may increase the morbidity of these suppurative processes. A CT scan may define the pathology. If a frank abscess is present, CT-guided percutaneous drainage may be effective for resolving the sepsis. A residual enterocutaneous fistula may occur. This approach would then necessitate subsequent resection to treat the fistula. Clinical deterioration from an undrained abscess or persistent phlegmon and signs of spreading peritonitis from abscess rupture or free perforation are indications for immediate operation. Primary resection plus drainage is effective. Surgical judgment must be used to determine if an anastomosis can be safely performed. Otherwise an end-ileostomy and mucous fistula can be constructed, as most perforations and abscesses originate from the ileum rather than the jejunum.

Because many fistulas are associated with sepsis to a variable extent, antibiotics are generally indicated; steroids are generally contraindicated. Enterovesical fistulas should be treated surgically to prevent repeated urinary tract infections. At operation the fistula is disconnected, the diseased bowel is resected, and the bladder is closed. Catheter drainage of the bladder is maintained for 7 to 10 days to ensure healing.

An enteroenteral fistula is not an absolute indication for surgery unless other surgical problems such as obstruction or abscess are present. Ileosigmoid fistulas can lead to severe diarrhea and are managed surgically in that instance. Fistulas are common between adjacent loops of ileum or between the ileum and cecum or ascending colon and have no physiologic consequence in the absence of sepsis. Many remain clinically unrecognized until a contrast evaluation demonstrates their presence. In fact the process of fistulization may have resolved a remote episode of sepsis as an abscess decompressed into an adjacent loop of bowel. When such a fistula is associated with sepsis, surgery is indicated to drain the abscess and resect the fistulous intestine. The extent of Crohn's disease in both segments of intestine involved in the fistulization should be assessed. If both are diseased, two resections are performed. With ileosigmoid fistulization, in most instances the sigmoid is passively involved, as Crohn's disease does not spread into that viscus. Therefore the treatment is takedown of the fistula and ileocecal resection with débridement and closure of the sigmoid.

Enterocutaneous fistulas are managed operatively for the most part. Although a regimen of TPN, bowel rest, and immunosuppressants can close these fistulas, they usually reopen with resumption of oral intake. The fistula is taken down and the diseased bowel resected. Patients with early postoperative enterocutaneous fistulas arising from apparently normal bowel after resection of diseased bowel have been successfully managed with TPN provided there has been no distal obstruction or undrained septic focus.

If acute ileitis is encountered on exploration for appendicitis, the terminal ileum should not be resected because many of these patients recover spontaneously and do not have other attacks. Specific etiologic agents (e.g., *Yersinia* sp.) have been identified in some of these cases. Even if the patient was known or suspected to have Crohn's disease prior to laparotomy, resection of uncomplicated ileitis is not indicated. If the cecum is soft, pliable, and otherwise normal, appendectomy is performed to prevent future diagnostic dilemmas. Excision of the appendix if the cecum is involved may lead to a postoperative colocutaneous fistula. When enterocutaneous fistulas occur after appendectomy and the cecum is uninvolved, the origin of the fistula is almost always the diseased ileum, not the appendiceal stump.

Operations for growth retardation are being performed less frequently with modern nutritional support. Provision of adequate protein and calories (with TPN if necessary) restores growth in many children.

Most patients with Crohn's disease require only one or two operations over the entire course of their disease and are able to lead normal productive lives.

SMALL BOWEL OBSTRUCTION

Mechanical small bowel obstruction (SBO) is a common problem confronting surgeons. The usual cause in adults is adhesions following surgery. Congenital and postinflammatory adhesions are occasionally responsible. Hernias are the second most common cause. Abdominal wall hernias, including inguinal, femoral, umbilical, and incisional, account for most cases of obstruction from hernias. Rarer forms exist. Internal hernias are related to abnormalities of intestinal rotation and fixation or are caused by mesenteric defects or internal traps created following bowel resection. Primary benign and malignant or metastatic malignant neoplasms are the third most common cause. Adhesions, hernias, and neoplasms account for 90% of the cases of SBO. Gallstones, Crohn's disease, and many other etiologies account for the rest.

Simple obstruction implies an adequate blood supply to the obstructed segment. Strangulation obstruction implies vascular compromise. Closed loop obstruction indicates occlusion at both ends of an obstructed segment with no possibility of antegrade or retrograde decompression. Partial obstruction indicates a residual narrowed lumen through which intestinal contents can pass. Complete obstruction indicates total occlusion of the lumen.

When the bowel lumen becomes occluded the proximal bowel distends with fluid and swallowed air. The fluid is initially derived from the normal daily 8-liter output of salivary, gastric, pancreatic, and biliary secretions. As the luminal pressure rises proximally, intestinal absorption decreases followed by an increase in intestinal secretion. Because intestinal fluid has a tonicity and electrolyte composition similar to that of extracellular fluid, electrolyte and acid–base abnormalities are not remarkable initially unless there is a high small bowel obstruction (duodenum, proximal jejunum) with

copious vomiting. Here gastric losses of H^+, Cl^-, and K^+ lead to a hypochloremic, hypokalemic metabolic alkalosis. As the extracellular fluid compartment shrinks from losses into the bowel (third space) or externally (vomiting), oliguria follows. Attempts by the kidneys to conserve Na^+ (elevated aldosterone) aggravate the tendency toward hypokalemia in the setting of copious vomiting. With distal obstructions and little vomiting the tendency is toward a metabolic acidosis because of starvation, ketosis, and loss of pancreatic secretions in the intestinal lumen.

With closed loop obstructions there is no possibility for antegrade or retrograde decompression. The bowel becomes markedly distended. A vicious circle is established: distension increases secretion, which further increases distension. Intraluminal pressures rise to 40 mm Hg or more, and intestinal blood flow diminishes. At first there is venous obstruction with vascular engorgement and bowel wall edema, followed by arterial vasospasm and local tissue anoxia. Capillary integrity is lost, and intramural hemorrhage can occur. A strangulation obstruction has occurred and, if unrelieved, results in necrosis of tissue and proliferation of bacteria in the affected segment. Eventually bacteria and endotoxin escape transmurally into the free peritoneal cavity even before free perforation has occurred. A dark blood-tinged peritoneal fluid is produced. Sepsis, cardiovascular collapse, and death follow if the infarcted segment is not resected.

Patients classically present with crampy abdominal pain, nausea and vomiting, abdominal distension, and obstipation. One or more of these characteristics may be missing depending on the anatomic level of obstruction (proximal or distal), degree of occlusion (partial or complete), and presence or absence of strangulation. Patients with proximal obstruction present with pain and vomiting on the first day and are less likely to experience distension and obstipation. Patients with distal obstruction present with pain for a couple of days followed by distension, vomiting, and obstipation once the distal unobstructed segment empties. With late established obstructions, as bacteria proliferate in the stagnant contents of the obstructed loops the vomitus turns feculent. On physical examination borborygmi correlate with abdominal cramps. In neglected cases bowel motility diminishes, and the abdomen becomes distended, silent, and tender. Patients with partial obstruction may continue to pass flatus and have explosive bouts of diarrhea with sudden relief of the pain. Patients with strangulation obstruction ultimately develop continuous pain and peritoneal signs.

Unfortunately, the clinical picture does not allow one to distinguish reliably between simple and strangulation obstruction. The distinction is important, as mortality rates for simple obstruction range from 0% to 6%, whereas for strangulation obstruction the rates range from 15% to 30%. Patients with simple obstruction may have a low-grade fever, mild tachycardia, and mild generalized tenderness related to compression of distended loops of bowel. Patients in extremis with diffuse peritonitis and septic shock obviously have advanced gangrene of the bowel. The goal that has been so elusive is to recognize the early reversible ischemia of strangulation. No combination of clinical criteria or laboratory data has reliably met that goal. In this era of nasogastric (NG) intubation and intestinal decompression as initial primary therapy, there is always the possibility of delaying treatment of potentially reversible ischemia.

Recognizing the above limitations, many authorities recommend immediate operation after resuscitation for patients with feculent vomiting or NG aspirate, marked leukocytosis (more than 18,000/mm^3), peritoneal signs, absent bowel sounds, high fever, and marked tachycardia. Some patients with simple obstruction have one or more of the above, and some patients with strangulation obstruction have none. A more aggressive approach is taken in elderly patients in whom the physical findings accompanying peritonitis may be unimpressive.

Abdominal radiographs confirm the diagnosis 85% of the time and allow differentiation of small bowel and large bowel obstruction. False-negative abdominal films occur when there is no intestinal dilatation, as is occasionally seen with early or very proximal small bowel obstruction. False-negative films also occur when the bowel loops are filled with fluid rather than air.

Contrast studies with barium (small bowel series or enteroclysis study) can be helpful if the diagnosis of SBO is unclear from the plain films or if an attempt at nonoperative therapy is chosen.

The management of all cases of SBO begins with fluid resuscitation, electrolyte replacement, and NG decompression. A Foley catheter is required, and central venous pressure monitoring should be considered. Patients with complete SBO (i.e., whose abdominal films show dilated proximal loops with empty distal small bowel, colon, and rectum) and those with suspected strangulation should be given prophylactic antibiotics and taken promptly to surgery once resuscitation is com-

plete. Patients with prior abdominal surgery and partial SBO (i.e., whose abdominal films show some colonic gas and feces or in whom intermittent episodes of diarrhea persist) thought to be secondary to adhesions may benefit from continued nonoperative management if they show improvement over the initial 24 hours. Unfortunately, abdominal films cannot reliably differentiate partial from complete SBO. Patients with early complete SBO have residual colon gas and feces until it is expelled and obstipation becomes complete. Nonoperative therapy is successful in only a few patients with complete SBO (15% to 25%) but helps in most patients with partial SBO (65%) caused by adhesions. Contrast studies differentiate between the two entities.

Other circumstances in which nonoperative therapy is a reasonable alternative to immediate operation include early postoperative obstruction, carcinomatosis, multiple recurrent adhesive obstruction, radiation enteritis, and Crohn's disease. Failure to resolve any obstruction nonoperatively makes operative therapy mandatory.

Incarcerated abdominal wall hernias frequently represent a closed loop obstruction of bowel with the potential for strangulation. Therefore all such hernias should be considered surgical emergencies. Patients without prior abdominal surgery or an incarcerated abdominal wall hernia should also be promptly operated once resuscitation is complete, as the obstruction requires surgical relief in most instances. Operative treatment involves lysis of adhesions, reduction of hernias with obliteration of the defect, repair of intestinal injuries, and resection of nonviable bowel.

NEOPLASMS OF THE SMALL INTESTINE

Neoplasms of the small intestine occur frequently. Although the small bowel contains 90% of the mucosal surface area of the alimentary tract, only 5% of all gastrointestinal neoplasms and 2% of all gastrointestinal malignancies arise from the small bowel.

Benign tumors of the small bowel are frequently asymptomatic and are found incidentally at the time of laparotomy or autopsy. The most common benign tumors include adenoma (adenomatous polyp and villous adenoma), leiomyoma, lipoma, and hemangioma. These tumors occur 20% of the time in the duodenum, 30% in the jejunum, and 50% in the ileum. When symptomatic it is because the lesions have caused bleeding or obstruction. Evidence suggests an adenoma-to-adenocarcinoma sequence, as has been proposed for the colon: large sessile villous adenomas are particularly worrisome in this regard.

When found incidentally at the time of laparotomy, a small bowel tumor should be assessed for evidence of malignancy (i.e., hard consistency, invasion, or lymphatic metastasis). If none of these features is present and the tumor is small, intraluminal, and presumably epithelial in origin (i.e., adenoma), an enterotomy, submucosal excision, frozen section examination if doubt remains, and transverse closure should be performed. Wide resection would be appropriate for intermediate-size benign lesions and those involving the submucosa (i.e., hemangioma). Large benign lesions involving much of the bowel circumference, especially leiomyomas, should be managed with segmental resection of the bowel with an end-to-end anastomosis.

When a benign small bowel tumor causes an obstruction, the preoperative evaluation frequently identifies only the obstruction, not the etiology, although it is easily discernible at laparotomy. Adult patients without prior abdominal surgery, incarcerated abdominal wall hernias, or evidence of gallstone ileus who present with small bowel obstruction have an increased incidence of obstructing small bowel tumors. This obstruction can result from intussusception or rarely a mass effect. Unlike childhood intussusception, adult intussusception in most instances has some obvious etiologic factor, which is usually a benign small bowel tumor acting as the lead point. Adult intussusception is frequently relapsing and intermittent with spontaneous reduction and pain relief until incarceration occurs. A patient who gives a history of intermittent postprandial crampy abdominal pain with a variable degree of bloating and occasional vomiting should be evaluated for a small bowel obstruction. Small bowel series and especially enteroclysis studies are helpful for demonstrating small bowel tumors.

At laparotomy an intussusception is reduced by milking the intussusceptum backward. Traction is never used on intussuscepted bowel. After manual reduction, resection of the small bowel lesion is performed. If the bowel is necrotic or the intussusception cannot be reduced, *en bloc* resection of the intussusceptum and intussuscipiens is performed.

Benign small bowel tumors can cause chronic slow blood loss with iron deficiency anemia and intermittent melena or, rarely, acute brisk blood loss with blood expelled per rectum. Leiomyomas and hemangiomas are more apt to bleed. The diagnostic workup for occult gastrointestinal bleeding after gastroduodenal and colonic sources are ruled out includes a bleeding scan, angiography, enteroclysis, and small bowel enteroscopy. Surgical exploration, combined with intraoperative enteroscopy if necessary, can be both diagnostic and therapeutic. Small, soft polyps should not be missed when using this approach.

The tumors of the Peutz-Jeghers syndrome are hamartomas that are found throughout the gastrointestinal tract but tend to concentrate in the jejunum and ileum, where they can cause intussusception and bleeding. This syndrome is inherited as an autosomal dominant trait and has the additional feature of mucocutaneous melanotic pigmentation. Because there is widespread involvement, extensive resections are not indicated and treatment should be limited to the segment responsible for the complication.

Malignant tumors of the small bowel include adenocarcinoma (the most common), carcinoid tumor, leiomyosarcoma, and lymphoma. Adenocarcinomas have been found alone, within villous adenomas, and in association with Crohn's disease. Most of these tumors occur in the duodenum, especially in the periampullary region, and in the proximal 100 cm of jejunum. Duodenal tumors are discussed elsewhere in this text and are not considered here further. Ileal lesions are less frequent except when associated with Crohn's disease. These lesions infiltrate the intestinal wall, metastasize to regional lymph nodes, and spread to the liver and peritoneal surfaces.

There is no specific symptom complex. Patients may experience abdominal pain, anemia, weight loss, obstruction, bleeding, and perforation (rarely). A palpable mass is present one-third of the time. Barium studies may identify an apple-core defect with mucosal ulceration, but a correct preoperative diagnosis is made only one-third of the time. Most cases are diagnosed at laparotomy for intestinal obstruction.

Jejunoileal carcinomas are removed by segmental resection with an approximately 10-cm margin on either side and a wedge of continuous mesentery. The proximal extent of the lymphadenectomy is limited by the superior mesenteric artery. Tumors of the terminal ileum require right colectomy. Five-year survival rates are poor (20%) because of the late clinical presentation of advanced disease.

Carcinoid tumors develop from the enterochromaffin cells situated in the crypts of Lieberkühn. They are slow-growing yellow-gray submucosal neoplasms that have the capacity to invade locally and to metastasize. Malignant potential depends on the location of the tumor and its size. The appendix is the most common site of a carcinoid tumor, but the malignant potential here is low. The small bowel is the next most common site, and most of these tumors are located in the ileum within 2 ft of the ileocecal valve. The malignant potential for small bowel carcinoids is high. Lesions less than 1 cm in diameter rarely metastasize. Lesions between 1 and 2 cm have a 50% incidence of metastasis, and lesions larger than 2 cm have an 80% incidence of metastasis. Altogether 75% of the lesions are less than 1 cm in diameter, 20% are 1 to 2 cm, and 5% are larger than 2 cm. Carcinoids of the small bowel are multiple in 30% of cases. They frequently (20% to 30% of the time) coexist with a second malignant neoplasm of a different histologic type.

Most small bowel carcinoids are asymptomatic and are found incidentally at laparotomy or autopsy. When symptomatic a carcinoid frequently has metastasized. Symptoms are usually obstructive in nature secondary to an extensive desmoplastic reaction around the tumor or its mesenteric metastases, which leads to kinking and matting of intestinal loops with constriction and partial obstruction. Intussusception and bleeding are unusual. Additional symptoms of metastatic disease in general (anorexia, weight loss, fatigue) may be present. Small bowel series may show partial obstruction with thickening of the bowel wall, tethering of its folds, and kinking of loops. This picture can resemble Crohn's disease or other inflammatory conditions. Unlike the carcinoid syndrome, urinary levels of 5-hydroxyindoleacetic acid (5-HIAA) are normal.

Local excision is adequate for small lesions less than 1 cm in diameter with no evidence of metastatic disease encountered incidentally at laparotomy. For lesions more than 1 cm in diameter, a standard cancer operation is indicated. When the tumors are in the distal ileum, right colectomy is indicated to include the node-bearing tissue in the resection. Otherwise a segmental resection with *en bloc* removal of adjacent mesentery suffices. With advanced disease and hepatic metastases the primary tumor should be resected if possible to avoid future complications (e.g., obstruction). Nonanatomic resection of liver metastases (tumorectomy) is performed whenever feasible. Five-year survival rates following curative resection approach 70%. Twenty percent of those with liver metastases live 5 years.

The carcinoid syndrome is usually caused by metastatic liver disease and is related to a variety of vasoactive substances produced by the tumor: serotonin, histamine, bradykinin, and others. About 5% to 10% of the patients with small bowel carcinoids develop this syndrome. For the syndrome to occur, sufficient disease must be present in the liver to overwhelm the normal detoxifying mechanisms. The symptoms include episodic cutaneous flushing of the head and upper trunk, watery diarrhea, and bronchospasm. Symptoms can occur spontaneously or can be precipitated by foods, alcohol, emotional stress, or defecation.

A life-threatening carcinoid crisis consisting of intense flushing, severe diarrhea, tachycardia, arrhythmias, and vascular collapse has been described. Permanent manifestations include endocardial fibrosis (carcinoid plaques), which most commonly affects the right side of the heart and leads to tricuspid insufficiency and pulmonary stenosis with subsequent right-side heart failure. The cutaneous lesions of pellagra may appear, as functioning tumors divert most of the essential amino acid tryptophan into the serotonin path way, leaving less available for niacin production.

Diagnosis is made by finding increased 24-hour urinary excretion of 5-HIAA, which is the major metabolite of serotonin. Rare patients have normal 5-HIAA levels. A CT scan can demonstrate metastatic liver disease, which is usually massive once the syndrome manifests.

Treatment of carcinoid syndrome is palliative. Surgical debulking and hepatic artery embolization have been tried with some success, but the responses are frequently short-lived. A somatostatin analog has been most effective in controlling the diarrhea and flushing. Chemotherapy with streptozotocin, 5-fluorouracil, and doxorubicin has yielded some palliation as well.

Jejunoileal leiomyosarcomas arise from smooth muscle cells in the muscularis propria and grow extrinsically away from the bowel lumen to reach a large size before causing symptoms. Most tumors are larger than 5 cm in diameter when discovered. Spread is by direct extension to adjacent structures and hematogenous dissemination. Intermittent abdominal pain with weight loss and a palpable abdominal mass is a common clinical presentation. There is a high incidence (50% in some series) of bleeding because these tumors have a tendency to outgrow their blood supplies and develop central necrosis and mucosal ulceration. Perforation occurs in 10% of patients. Obstruction can occur and is often caused by external compression rather than intrinsic circumferential growth or intussusception.

Small bowel series demonstrate a large extraluminal mass effect causing obstruction with pooling of barium in the necrotic center of a cavitating lesion. A CT scan frequently shows a large mass with a central lucent area that represents necrosis. In patients who present with gastrointestinal bleeding, mesenteric angiography shows irregular tumor vessels, a tumor blush, or pooling of contrast in the mass.

Surgical treatment consists in wide resection with associated mesentery. Lymphatic involvement with leiomyosarcomas is not common, and the mesenteric resection is performed more or less to achieve clear margins. Leiomyosarcomas are radioresistant, but combination chemotherapy using doxorubicin, cyclophosphamide, and vincristine has shown some activity against advanced disease.

INTESTINAL ISCHEMIA

The small intestine is susceptible to interruption of its normal circulation resulting in ischemia, which if left untreated can result in catastrophic consequences to the patient. Four types of mesenteric ischemic syndromes have been recognized, each having a different etiology, clinical picture, and treatment.

1. Acute mesenteric arterial embolism. Most emboli to the superior mesenteric artery (SMA) originate from thrombi in the left atrium or the left ventricle. Often these thrombi have been there for some time and are suddenly dislodged by an arrhythmia, such as sudden onset of atrial fibrillation, or an episode of hypokinesia of the heart following an acute myocardial infarction. Twenty percent of emboli to the SMA are associated with emboli to other arterial beds. Most of the emboli lodge in the SMA just beyond the origin of the middle colic artery; about 15% lodge in the proximal SMA.

2. Acute mesenteric arterial thrombosis. Thrombosis of the SMA occurs in a vessel that has become progressively more diseased, often over a period of time. The vessel is usually narrowed or filled with plaque. A sudden episode of low flow, as can occur during an intercurrent illness or a bout of sepsis, can aggravate a critical stenosis resulting in complete thrombosis. Often these patients have had symptoms of chronic mesenteric ischemia for years. The symptoms include post-prandial abdominal pain, early satiety, or weight loss. Unlike emboli, most thromboses of the SMA occur in its proximal portion just beyond its takeoff.

3. Nonocclusive mesenteric ischemia (NOMI). This condition is less well understood than the first two and has a different set of symptoms, making the diagnosis much more difficult. Patients with NOMI have decreased mesenteric perfusion without specific vessel blockage. The poor blood flow is often associated with cardiac failure or sepsis or is found in patients taking digitalis. Digitalis has been found sometimes to cause contraction of the smooth muscle in both the mesenteric arterial and venous mesenteric vessels resulting in poor flow and symptoms of ischemia.

4. Acute mesenteric venous thrombosis. These patients often have a hypercoagulable state such as portal hypertension, protein S or C, or antithrombin III deficiency: or they are on oral contraceptives. Other conditions predisposing patients to venous thrombosis include trauma to the abdomen and malignancies.

Clinical Presentation

Acute mesenteric ischemia usually presents with sudden, severe abdominal pain. Ischemia due to arterial embolization tends to be the most precipitous with exquisite abdominal pain accompanied by nausea and vomiting. Often a cardiac arrhythmia is present as well.

Mesenteric ischemia due to thrombosis, nonocclusive ischemia, or mesenteric venous thrombosis presents in a less dramatic fashion, with pain increasing in nature over several days. The pain is associated with nausea, vomiting, and progressive abdominal distension. Most patients have guaiac-positive stools. As the ischemia progresses, the entire thickness of the bowel wall necroses, and the abdominal examination reveals classic signs of peritonitis, with rebound and guarding. Laboratory findings include nonspecific elevation and the white blood cell count; elevated levels of amylase, lactate dehydrogenase, and creatine phosphokinase, and an increasing base deficit.

Radiographs are often nonspecific, with 25% of them reported as normal. Some specific findings in patients with intestinal ischemia include adynamic ileus with bowel wall thickening. Duplex ultrasonography can detect poor or absent blood flow in the celiac axis or SMA, but these tests are highly operator-dependent.

Large air-filled loops of overlying bowel may make accurate ultrasonography difficult.

The CT scan has proved somewhat helpful in diagnosing embolic occlusion to the SMA, but the definitive study is still the mesenteric angiogram, obtaining both anteroposterior and lateral views of the SMA and, if needed, of the celiac axis. As mentioned above, most SMA emboli are lodged 3 to 10 cm from the origin of the SMA, whereas most thrombi are found near the origin of the SMA.

Nonocclusive mesenteric ischemia usually is associated with narrowed, irregular branches of the SMA, whereas the vessel itself is patent. With mesenteric venous thrombosis, the arterial phase is prolonged. The venous phase shows filling defects within the superior mesenteric view or in the protal vein itself.

Treatment

Initial treatment of patients suspected of having acute mesenteric ischemia is fluid resuscitation, correction of acidosis, and administration of antibiotics. Anticoagulation with intravenous heparin should be part of the regimen. A Foley catheter is placed to monitor urine output, and a nasogastric tube is placed on suction to decompress the stomach.

The key to treatment is obtaining the appropriate imaging studies. Emergency angiography must be done in an expedient fashion. In selected patients in whom the angiogram shows an SMA embolus and in whom there are no signs of peritonitis and symptoms have been present for 8 hours or less, thrombolytic therapy through the SMA catheter can be instituted. If there is no response within 4 hours of beginning therapy or if peritonitis appears, surgical exploration is warranted. The abdomen is opened and the SMA is exposed by elevating the root of the transverse mesocolon and mobilizing the duodenum all the way to the ligament of Treitz. A transverse arteriotomy is made over the SMA, a Foley catheter is inserted and the embolus is extracted. Care is needed to make sure that no fragments of clot are passed into the distal vessel. Once blood flow is restored, the bowel is examined; and any obviously necrotic bowel is resected. Marginally viable areas should be resected unless they are extensive, in which case they can be left in place and a second-look operation planned for 24 hours later.

Patients with an SMA thrombosis have a more complex problem. Thrombectomy is unlikely to maintain long-term patency in the circulation, and most of these patients require some sort of aortomesenteric artery bypass surgery.

The treatment of NOMI is usually nonoperative, involving the use of intraarterial vasodilators, such as papaverine, in conjunction with anticoagulation with heparin. Patients who develop signs of peritonitis must undergo surgical exploration while continuing the intraarterial infusion of papaverine. Any obviously necrotic bowel is resected. Marginally viable bowel is left in place, and a second-look operation is planned for 24 hours later.

The treatment of patients with mesenteric venous thrombosis is surgical. The long-term results of venous thrombectomy have been poor, with recurrent thrombus appearing more often than not. These patients should be explored and all nonviable bowel resected. The bowel that is marginally viable can be resected if the segment removed is not too long or left in place and then reexamined 24 hours later at a second-look operation.

Patients with mesenteric ischemia comprise a group of high-risk patients. Their ultimate prognosis depends on the speed with which the diagnosis is made and how quickly and appropriately the treatment can be started.

QUESTIONS

Select one answer.

1. Which of the following does not contribute to the digestion of the fats in the small intestine?
   a. Brush border enzymes.
   b. Pancreatic lipases.
   c. Bile salts.
   d. Lacteals.
2. Which of the following is not characteristic of Crohn's disease?
   a. Perianal disease.
   b. Rectal bleeding.
   c. Diarrhea.
   d. Abdominal pain.
3. Which of the following complications of Crohn's disease is least common?
   a. Enteroenteral fistulas.
   b. Enterocutaneous fistulas.
   c. Free perforation.
   d. Strictures.

4. What percentage of patients with Crohn's disease eventually need surgery:
   a. 20%
   b. 50%
   c. 75%
   d. 90%

5. A patient is taken to the operating room for appendicitis and is found to have ileitis. What is the correct management?
   a. Biopsy of ileum.
   b. Ileal resection with ileocolic anastomosis.
   c. Appendectomy.
   d. Ileostomy.

6. Which of the following can most reliably distinguish simple from strangulation small intestinal obstruction?
   a. High nasogastric output.
   b. Fever over 101°F.
   c. Tachycardia.
   d. None of the above.

7. Which of the following is true of nonoperative management of patients with small bowel obstruction (SBO)?
   a. It is most likely to be successful in patients who have SBO from adhesions.
   b. Long-tube decompression is superior to nasogastric tube decompression.
   c. It is most useful for the younger patient.
   d. It is successful in cases of complete SBO.

8. Which is the most likely cause of intussusception in a 20-year-old man?
   a. Idiopathic.
   b. Lymphoma of the small bowel.
   c. Carcinoid.
   d. Adhesions.

9. Which is true of the lesions responsible for the symptoms in patients with Peutz-Jeghers syndrome?
   a. They are sessile adenomas.
   b. They tend to cluster in the duodenum.
   c. They are hamartomas.
   d. The syndrome is inherited as an autosomal recessive trait.

10. A patient is found to have a small bowel carcinoma 2 cm in diameter in the distal ileum. Which of the following is the operation of choice:
    a. Wedge resection with 2-cm margins.
    b. Biopsy and chemotherapy.
    c. Right hemicolectomy.
    d. Wedge resection with 5-cm margins.

SELECTED REFERENCES

Bizer LS, Liebling RW, Delany HM, Gliedman ML. Small bowel obstruction. *Surgery* 1981;89:407–413.

Cameron JL. *Current surgical therapy,* 4th ed. St. Louis: Mosby Year Book, 1992.

Moody FG. *Surgical treatment of digestive disease,* 2nd ed. Chicago: Year Book Medical Publishers, 1990.

Scott HW, Sawyers JL. *Surgery of the stomach, duodenum and small intestine.* Boston: Blackwell Science, 1987.

Ziudema GD. *Shackelford's surgery of the alimentary tract,* 3rd ed. Philadelphia: WB Saunders, 1991.

4

Diseases of the Colon, Rectum, and Anus

Lawrence S. Bizer

The physiologic and pathophysiologic problems of the lower bowel are presented and briefly discussed in this chapter. No attempt is made to be encyclopedic in this effort, and the focus is on information likely to be asked on the written or oral examinations of the American Board of Surgery. A small number of references have been appended that appear to be of value to the reader.

GENERAL CONSIDERATIONS

The colon, rectum, and anus are approximately 1.5 m (5 ft) in length, with the distal anorectum (anal canal) comprising the last 4.0 to 4.5 cm. The diameter is greatest in the cecum (8 cm) and narrowest at the distal descending colon (2.5 cm). In the presence of distal obstruction the colon is most likely to perforate in the cecum because tension is greatest where the radius of the lumen is largest, intraluminal pressures being approximately equal (LaPlace's law).

The colonic wall has the same layers (mucosa, submucosa, muscularis, serosa) as the small intestine. However, the outer longitudinal layer of smooth muscle is incomplete and converges in three teniae coli that are confluent at the base of the appendix. The teniae are no longer recognizable in the extraperitoneal rectum. Partial outpouching of the colon wall (haustra) and partial mucosal infoldings (plicae semilunares) are probably produced by the short length of the bowel wall (compared to the entire bowel wall length) under the taeniae coli. The serosa is incomplete posteriorly in the fused ascending and descending colon and completely absent in the lower one-third of the rectum.

The colonic arterial blood supply is via the superior and inferior mesenteric arteries, and their branches occasionally form a continuous vessel along the mesenteric border of the colon wall (marginal artery of Drummond). Gaps in this vessel most frequently occur in the splenic flexure area (Griffith's point) or between the last sigmoid branch and the superior rectal artery (Sudek's point). The upper rectum receives its arterial blood supply from the superior hemorrhoidal (rectal) artery (a distal branch of the inferior mesenteric artery); and the lower rectum and anorectum receive arterial blood from the middle and inferior hemorrhoidal arteries, respectively, both of which are derived from the internal iliac artery. Venous drainage follows the superior and inferior mesenteric veins to the portal system and is the usual venous drainage route for the rectum and colon except in the presence of portal hypertension, when collateralization to the internal iliac veins is important.

Most of the lymphatics follow the regional arteries to preaortic nodes and then to the cisterna chyli, but some lymphatics parallel the venous drainage of the colorectum. Except for the anus, nervous innervation is via sympathetic (thoracolumbar) and parasympathetic (vagal and sacral) nerve fibers. Parasympathetic activity is mainly stimulatory, with internal sphincter relaxation, and sympathetic activity is the opposite. Much of this bowel activity is merely reflexic and occurs even with severance of the spinal cord or vagotomy; it is mediated through the intramural nerve plexuses of Meissner and Auerbach.

Active absorption of sodium and chloride (up to 200 mEq/day), potassium, carbohydrates, and short-chain fatty acids occurs in the colon; and water is passively absorbed with sodium. Potassium is also secreted by the mucosa. The maximum amount of water absorption may exceed 2 liters per day. The colon converts 20% of daily urea production to ammonia, which is either excreted or reabsorbed depending on the pH in the colon lumen. Conjugated bile acids are absorbed through the ileal and colon walls, but deconjugation by colonic bacteria interferes with sodium and water absorption and may be responsible for diarrhea. This process becomes a significant factor in the development of diarrhea if the distal ileum is absent or diseased. Fiber (nonabsorbable carbohydrate) is fermented by colonic bacteria, producing short-chain fatty acids (butyrate) that are trophic for colonic mucosal cells.

Giant migrating contractions in the left colon produce mass movement of fecal content toward the rectum. Continence at the distal end of the rectum is maintained by tonic contraction of the internal sphincter (involuntary control) and the external sphincter and puborectalis muscle (voluntary control). If large amounts of stool enter the rectum, there is reflex relaxation of the internal sphincter and conscious contraction of the external sphincter and puborectalis muscle. This rectal–anal inhibitory reflex in the internal sphincter is mediated by nitric acid. When satisfactory conditions are met for defecation, there is voluntary relaxation of the external sphincter along with a voluntary increase in intraabdominal pressure, allowing stool evacuation.

TRAUMA

Blunt and penetrating abdominal or pelvic trauma may injure the colorectum. Injuries are far more frequent after penetrating trauma, and in 80% of patients at least one other organ is injured as well (only 5% of injuries are due to blunt trauma).

Initial supportive therapy (intravenous fluids, blood, nasogastric suction, and antibiotics) is important for all patients preoperatively. When resuscitation is satisfactory (normal blood pressure, pulse, urine output, and central venous pressure), exploratory celiotomy through a vertical midline abdominal incision is commenced.

Concomitant injuries affect the definitive treatment of the colonic injury. Prolonged hypovolemia, delayed celiotomy (more than 6 hours), and massive peritoneal contamination with blood, bile, gastric contents, formed stool, and small bowel content probably make intraperitoneal closure of a colonic wound or resection and a colonic anastomosis more likely to fail. The type and extent of the colonic injury itself is also important. One-layer closures of colonic wounds are as effective as two-layer closures. If there is any doubt about the safety of a colonic closure, it is safer to exteriorize the injury as a colostomy, close the injury and exteriorize the closure, resect the injured bowel and form a proximal colostomy and distal mucus fistula or Hartmann-type closure, or protect a suture closure with a proximal colostomy. Colostomies should completely divert the fecal stream and be matured if possible. Following treatment of the colon injury the peritoneal cavity should probably be copiously irrigated with saline and suctioned dry. Abdominal closure should leave the skin and fat open for either delayed primary closure (4 to 7 days) or healing by secondary intention. Primary closure or resection-anastomosis of colonic injuries is frequently satisfactory unless multiple adverse factors (see above) are present at the time of operation. It is now usually the treatment of choice for civilian injuries and avoids the morbidity of a colostomy closure.

Rectal injuries frequently produce massive bacterial contamination of the pelvic soft tissues. After initial resuscitation, as with intraperitoneal colon injuries, the abdomen is explored after confirmation of the injury by anoscopy or sigmoidoscopy, and a completely diverting sigmoid colostomy is fashioned. Small rectal lacerations, if seen early, can be sutured; but usually the injury and early pelvic cellulitis mitigate against suture closure. Instead, the rectal injury and pelvic soft tissues are débrided, and wide, dependent drainage is established through the perineum. Finally, the distal rectum is irrigated to remove all residual fecal content, preventing continuing pelvic soft tissue contamination, although this last maneuver is of unproved efficacy, as is suture closure of the rectal laceration itself.

IATROGENIC TRAUMA

A second group of traumatic injuries of the colorectum are iatrogenic and frequently follow diagnostic or therapeutic maneuvers. Reports of these injuries do not commonly appear in the medical literature. They follow the use of cleansing enemas, barium enemas, sigmoidoscopy, colonoscopy, and the use of rectal tubes. A few are associated with sexual acts or pranks. If the lower bowel is diseased or fixed by adhesion, perforation is more likely especially in the sigmoid colon.

On recognition of the injury, treatment is much the same as for external blunt or penetrating colorectal trauma except that some of these injuries occur in patients who have had mechanical cleansing of the lower intestine and, occasionally, intraluminal antibiotics. For most of these injuries, simple operative closure of a perforation is possible. If barium spill into the peritoneal cavity has occurred, it rapidly becomes adherent. Attempts to remove it are futile and only increase the inflammatory reaction and the subsequent appearance of adhesions. Barium attached to omentum, however, can often be resected.

A more controversial approach is to treat the patient with supportive measures (bowel rest, antibiotics, observation) and avoid operation. This approach may be recommended for patients in whom formal operation presents a prohibitive risk or for a small perforation after colonoscopy in a well prepared colon with minimal or no symptoms.

APPENDIX

The appendix, at the base of the cecum, is about 0.8 cm wide and 4 to 12 cm in length. It is part of the gut-associated lymphoid tissue and secretes immunoglobulins. Appendicitis occurs most frequently between ages 15 and 30. Only 10% of cases occur under age 10 or over age 50. The history and physical findings and their variability should be known to all surgeons, and laboratory tests play a minor role in the diagnosis of appendicitis. Fever and elevated white blood cell (WBC) counts are common, but most useful is the differential of the WBC count, where mature and immature granulocytes are seen to be increased. The diagnosis is more difficult in female patients than male patients. Among the former about 50% have gynecologic pathology when appendicitis is *not* found at operation (salpingitis, tuboovarian abscess, mittelschmerz, ovarian torsion, ruptured ovarian follicle, endometriosis, or ectopic pregnancy). Ultrasound examination in questionable cases of appendicitis has poor sensitivity but high (80% to 90%) specificity.

The patient who presents several days after the onset of symptoms with a palpable mass in the right lower quadrant of the abdomen may be treated medically or by immediate operation. If an abscess is present on ultrasound examination, percutaneous drainage is appropriate. With resolution of the inflammatory process, recurrent appendicitis occurs in 10% to 30% of patients. Open or laparoscopic appendectomy is acceptable; randomized studies thus far have not substantiated the overall superiority of either approach.

Tumors of the appendix are uncommon. Carcinoids generally have a benign clinical course, and appendectomy is adequate therapy. Tumors that are larger than 2 cm, involve the base of the appendix or extend to the mesoappendix, or involve regional lymph nodes should be treated by right colectomy. Adenocarcinoma is treated like other right colon cancer. Mucoceles result from obstruction of the appendiceal lumen without sufficient distal bacterial flora to produce appendicitis and are treated by appendectomy, carefully avoiding perforation at operation to reduce the threat of subsequent pseudomyxoma peritonei.

INFLAMMATORY DISEASE

Granulomatous colitis (Crohn's colitis) and ulcerative colitis are the commonest generalized chronic inflammatory diseases of the colorectum. Both are of unknown etiology, but the prevalent concept now is that both are related to hyperactivity of the gut immune system with increased lymphocyte activation, increased tumor necrosis factor, interleukin-1 levels, increased tissue macrophages, and circulating antibodies to colonic mucosal cells. Rectal bleeding and diarrhea occur in both diseases but tend to be of greater severity in ulcerative colitis. Pathologically, ulcerative colitis involves the mucosa and submucosa, whereas the disease is characteristically transmural in granulomatous colitis. Granulomas are common (50%) in patients with granulomatous colitis but are not seen in those with ulcerative colitis. Serositis with segmental involvement, thickened mesentery, and enlarged regional nodes are all common features of granulomatous colitis and are not features of ulcerative colitis. Initial involvement of the rectum is present in almost all cases (90% to 95%) of ulcerative colitis, but rectal involvement is present in only 15% to 25% of cases of granulomatous colitis. Despite this fact, perineal disease (abscesses, fissures, fistulas) commonly occurs with granulomatous disease (25% incidence in colonic Crohn's disease and about 10% in small intestinal Crohn's disease) but uncommonly with ulcerative colitis; and it may be the first sign of Crohn's colitis (10% of cases) or its *only* manifestation for as long as 5 years. It is not improved by resection of proximally involved small bowel or colon. Furthermore, abdominal wall or internal fistulas are rare with ulcerative colitis but common with granulomatous colitis.

Systemic diseases (iritis, uveitis, arthritis, erythema nodosum, vasculitis, sclerosing cholangitis, retroperitonitis, hepatic cirrhosis, pyoderma gangrenosum) are associated with both diseases but more commonly occur with ulcerative colitis (one-third of patients), and their response to colectomy is not entirely predictable. Sclerosing cholangitis and axial arthritis are least likely to improve after colectomy. Reports suggest that patients with granulomatous colitis have a somewhat increased risk of colonic cancer, but malignancy assumes much greater importance in patients with universal colorectal involvement with ulcerative colitis, particularly when the disease has been present for 7 to 10 or more years (the incidence of malignancy averages about 0.5% per year beyond the first 7 years). It also is common in patients with schistosomal colitis. Furthermore, a malignancy is difficult to detect when it occurs, and some authors believe that colonic mucosal high-grade dysplasia or DNA aneuploidy (random biopsies) should be an indication for colectomy to treat idiopathic ulcerative colitis. A stricture in the colon of a patient with ulcerative colitis is a malignancy until proved benign. Gallstones occur with increased frequency in Crohn's disease but not ulcerative colitis.

Ulcerative colitis is "cured" by removing the entire colorectum, but this operation leaves the patient with a permanent ileostomy. Ileal endorectal pull-through is the procedure of choice in most patients (young, nonmorbidly obese, and without perianal disease or incontinence). Subtotal colectomy is still an option, however, in some patients with this disease. Generally conceded

indications for operation are stricture, carcinoma, perforation, massive hemorrhage, fulminant disease with or without toxic megacolon, and rarely, a Coombs'-positive hemolytic anemia or complications of long-term steroid use. Relative indications for operation include growth retardation in children, failure to respond to medical management (5-aminosalicylic acid, steroids, or immunosuppressives), high-grade dysplasia, high DNA aneuploidy, and chronic debility.

Operation is generally reserved for complications of granulomatous disease. Any operation here should be conservative because recurrence in the remaining colon and subsequent small bowel involvement are common (more than 80% incidence at 25 years). Segmental resection should be done whenever possible, and anastomoses for microscopic disease do no harm and do not affect recurrence rates. Strictureplasty is frequently used in the small intestine to avoid a short bowel syndrome, but experience with this operation in the colon is too limited to discuss. Chronic obstruction, fistulas (enterocolonic, enterourinary, enterogastric, enteroenteric, or enterocutaneous), abscess, and rarely, hemorrhage, perforation, and questionable malignancy usually constitute indications for operation.

Interestingly, the distinction between these two diseases cannot be discerned in about 10% of the patients despite adequate microscopic examination of colonic tissue.

TOXIC MEGACOLON

Toxic megacolon (smooth muscle paralysis without nerve plexus destruction) occasionally (2%) occurs with ulcerative colitis and rarely with granulomatous colitis. It may also occur with *Salmonella, Shigella,* and cholera infections, Chagas' disease, and ischemic and pseudomembranous colitis. The patient presents with fever, tachycardia, high WBC counts, abdominal pain, distension, bloody diarrhea, and localized or generalized abdominal tenderness. The etiology is unknown, but the disorder may be precipitated by opiates, antidiarrheal agents or barium enema.

Management remains controversial. Initial management includes sigmoidoscopy; stool cultures and biopsy; nasogastric suction; fluid, electrolyte, and blood replacement; broad-spectrum antibiotics; parenteral corticosteroids; nutritional support; and avoidance of anticholinergic or narcotic medications. Barium enema should not be done.

Early operation (within 24 hours) is advocated by some surgeons, and controversy exists as to whether the optimal operation is subtotal colectomy or the less traumatic Turnbull procedure (loop ileostomy and blowhole transverse or sigmoid colostomy, or both). Total proctocolectomy should be avoided. Others believe that nonoperative therapy should continue unless the patient's condition deteriorates (peritonitis, massive bleeding, free intraperitoneal air or subserosal air in the colon wall) or fails to improve. No controlled studies of the therapy for toxic megacolon have ever been done. It seems reasonable that early operation (at 24 to 48 hours) should be performed unless improvement occurs during this period of nonoperative therapy. The ultimate value of the Turnbull procedure (when free colonic perforation is not present), remains to be determined. The overall mortality of toxic megacolon is 10% to 40%.

DIVERTICULAR DISEASE

True diverticula of the colon are rare, congenital, and usually solitary. They occur more frequently on the right side of the colon and, when inflamed, are confused with appendicitis. Most right colon diverticula are false (pseudodiverticula). False diverticula (mucosal outpouchings covered by serosa) are common, increase in number with increasing age (two-thirds of patients 80 years of age have them), and are most frequent in the left colon. False diverticula tend to occur in two or three rows between the teniae coli and are etiologically related to increased intraluminal colonic pressure, perhaps abetted by low-residue diets and stressful lives. There is evidence that patients with so-called irritable colon syndrome are at high risk for the development of false diverticula and frequently have areas of high intraluminal pressure in their colons.

Classifications designating this disease diverticulosis or diverticulitis may overlap. Diverticulosis may be associated with localized pain (spasm?) and diverticulitis with microscopic or macroscopic perforation and signs of infection. Treatment of diverticulosis usually includes a high-residue diet with or without stool softeners to decrease the transit time of stool in the colon and decrease intraluminal pressures. A giant diverticulum may rarely result from recurrent inflammation with fi-

brosis at a diverticular base resulting in a ball-valve phenomenon with increasing gaseous distension of the diverticulum. If present the colonic segment should be resected to prevent abscess or perforation.

Acute diverticulitis (peridiverticulitis) usually signifies that entrapped fecaliths have obstructed and eroded the mucosa and that infection has spread intramurally or into the pericolic tissues. The patient develops lower abdominal pain with fever and elevated WBC counts; and frequently a tender mass is felt in the left lower quadrant or on rectal or pelvic examination. Sigmoidoscopy shows only mucosal edema at the rectosigmoid area but is helpful for ruling out a distal carcinoma or colitis (ischemic or infectious). Barium enema may be the diagnostic procedure of choice and can be safely done in the absence of generalized peritonitis. The radiologist requires visualization of extraluminal barium (intra- or extramural) to assign a diagnosis of diverticulitis. This requirement tends to underdiagnose the disease radiographically, and the error may be reduced by computed tomography (CT) scanning with bowel contrast. This technique is more accurate than barium enema for diagnosing complications of diverticulitis but less accurate for diagnosing an associated carcinoma or other diseases in the differential diagnosis of diverticulitis (Crohn's disease, ischemia, cancer, radiation colitis). Treatment with bowel rest, intravenous fluids, and antibiotics (ampicillin, an aminoglycoside, and clindamycin or Flagyl) frequently results in resolution of the peridiverticular inflammation (60% to 70% of patients). A distal cancer may have incited the attack of diverticulitis and should be excluded during the diagnostic evaluation.

Occasionally, a large abscess develops and can be drained through the rectum or vagina or transabdominally (surgically or radiologically), resulting in resolution of the inflammatory process. Even if a fecal fistula ensues subsequent to abscess drainage, it often closes spontaneously or can be resected at a subsequent elective sigmoid resection after the inflammatory process has resolved.

Peridiverticulitis that resolves without operative drainage can be further treated with a high-residue diet and stool softener if there is no question of the sigmoid disease being carcinoma. A second episode (30% to 35% incidence) of diverticulitis suggests that elective sigmoid resection is needed. If the septic picture remains unresolved on antibiotic treatment or spreading peritonitis develops, the patient should be operated. The procedure of choice is resection of the diseased sigmoid colon with proximal and distal colostomy or, more frequently, proximal sigmoid colostomy and distal rectosigmoid closure. This protocol rids the patient of continuing contamination from the diseased colonic segment. A poor second choice is to drain the sigmoid colon abscess and create a proximal diverting colostomy. Rarely, it is the safe alternative if the left ureter cannot be found in the inflamed pelvic mass. Some surgeons have recommended sigmoid resection and primary anastomosis as an emergency procedure, but it is not generally recommended in a contaminated abdomen and an unprepared colon. Partial or complete obstruction due to chronic diverticulitis results from edema, fibrosis, muscular thickening, and spasm. Lack of resolution on conservative therapy indicates the need for colonic resection with proximal colostomy and distal mucous fistula or rectosigmoid closure. If this procedure cannot be safely done, an initial transverse colostomy (or descending colon colostomy) is constructed and sigmoid resection undertaken as a second-stage procedure 2 to 3 weeks later, particularly if there is worry about an associated carcinoma. The transverse colostomy is later closed when the patient is well, but it should be preceded by a barium enema that shows normal healing of the sigmoid colon anastomosis.

Massive hemorrhage (1500 ml of blood or transfusions required; definition variable) may result from a diverticulum. It is likely that some degree of diverticulitis accompanies the hemorrhage, although clinically the patients rarely have symptoms or signs of infection (presumably stool erodes from a diverticulum into an adjacent peridiverticular arteriole). Although false diverticula are less common in the right colon, at least 50% of diverticular bleeding originates at that site. Many of these right-sided colonic bleeders are caused by arteriovenous anomalies (angiodysplasia) that are not diagnosed. They are frequently multiple and may be the source of hemorrhage particularly in patients older than 60 years of age. Recurrent small hemorrhages appear to be more frequent if angiodysplasia is the cause of the bleeding, rather than a diverticulum. The remaining 10% to 20% of massive colonic bleeds are due to cancer (primary lesion or metastases), ulcers, renal failure, chemotherapy, hematologic disease, inflammatory bowel disease, acquired immunodeficiency syndrome (AIDS) or related infections or neoplasms, hemorrhoids, or unknown causes. As many as 25% of patients

with bleeding angiodysplastic lesions have aortic stenosis, but the cause of this association is unknown. In children and adolescents the most frequent cause of lower gastrointestinal (GI) bleeding is a Meckel's diverticulum.

Initially, a rectal examination and sigmoidoscopy should be done to exclude a lower rectal source of bleeding and a nasogastric tube passed to exclude a gastroduodenal bleeding source. If these studies are normal, isotope scanning with intravenously tagged red blood cells is done. Emergency colonoscopy is difficult during active hemorrhage, but it is the best diagnostic procedure if bleeding is slight or has ceased. If isotope scanning is positive it may be followed by arteriography, and in poor-risk operative patients a bleeding vessel may be embolized or intraarterial pitressin used. Otherwise, emergency or, preferably, elective segmental resection of the colonic bleeding site is the treatment of choice. Rarely, subtotal colectomy is needed when no specific bleeding site in the colon can be identified, and a primary ileoproctostomy is done for most patients. *Remember:* knowing the exact site of bleeding is more important than knowing the cause if an emergency operation is necessary.

POLYPS AND CANCER OF THE COLORECTUM

Colorectal Polyps

Polyps of the colorectum are in many cases associated with carcinoma, or carcinoma may arise from the polyp itself. This transition from polyp to cancer probably develops over 5 to 10 years or longer. It frequently involves loss or mutation of the tumor-suppressor genes on chromosomes 5, 17, or 18; activation of an oncogene (K-*ras, myc* or *src*); or mutations on chromosomes 2, 3, or 7 that interfere with maintenance of DNA fidelity during replication. This is generally true with large adenomatous (tubular) polyps (> 1 cm), villous adenomas, mixed villoadenomatous (villoglandular) polyps, and adenomatous polyps associated with genetically determined syndromes (familial polyposis, Gardner syndrome, Turcot syndrome, and Lynch syndromes I and II (hereditary nonpolyposis colorectal cancer syndromes).

Adenomatous (tubular) polyps occur most frequently in the rectum and sigmoid but are common throughout the colon. They are frequently multiple. Malignant change is uncommon (1% to 2%) in polyps less than 1 cm and most commonly manifest as rectal bleeding (gross or occult). The larger the polyp and the wider its base, the higher the incidence of malignant change. Invasion of malignant cells deep to the muscular mucosa is associated with the possibility of metastatic spread (5% to 20% incidence of lymph node metastases). Polyps should be completely excised, if possible, during sigmoidoscopy or colonoscopy. The polyps should be treated as an invasive carcinoma of the colon if invasion is deep to the muscularis mucosa, invasive cancer exists at the margin of polyp excision, or lymphovascular invasion is demonstrated microscopically.

Villous adenomas occur most frequently in the rectum, sigmoid, and cecum (15%) and infrequently in other areas of the colon. They tend to be single. Induration and large size (> 2 cm) raise suspicion of invasive malignancy, which occurs in 20% to 30% of cases. They should be completely excised if possible at endoscopy or by transanal excision if they lie below the peritoneal reflection. Villous adenomas are frequently large, and endoscopic biopsies sample only a portion of the polyp. If the polyp is incompletely excised or biopsied and lies above the peritoneal reflection, celiotomy and excision of the entire lesion (segmental resection) is necessary. Villoglandular polyps have a malignant potential between that of adenomatous polyps and the more frequently malignant villous adenomas.

Adenomatous polyps associated with the genetically determined syndromes begin to populate the colorectum after the age of puberty and number in the hundreds or thousands by adulthood. They are associated with congenital hypertrophic retinal pigmentation, increased levels of mucosal ornithine decarboxylase, and allelic deletions or mutations on chromosomes 5, 12, 17, or 18. The patient, generally aged 20 to 40 years, subsequently develops diarrhea, anemia, bloody stools, and abdominal cramping. The diagnosis is confirmed by sigmoidoscopy and air-contrast barium enema or colonoscopy. In addition to the proband, all family members should be investigated for the disease.

Treatment may include total colectomy, ileoproctostomy, and fulguration if the patient can be reliably followed at frequent intervals, the rectal segment can be easily endoscoped, no rectal carcinoma is present, and the rectal polyps are amenable to fulguration. (Most mortality after this procedure results from operative complications or the later development of desmoids or upper GI malignancies, *not* from rectal cancer.) If these criteria cannot be met, it is safer to perform a coloproc-

tectomy because virtually all these patients develop carcinoma of the colorectum by age 50. A superior alternative is total colectomy, mucosal proctectomy, and an ileoanal anastomosis. A few investigators have reported long-term regression of the rectal polyps after abdominal colectomy alone by feeding the patient vitamin C or a prostaglandin inhibitor (sulindac). Subsequently, these patients are at increased risk of developing desmoid tumors and periampullary neoplasms, as noted above.

Polyps that usually are *not* associated with the risk of invasive malignancy include the pseudopolyps of ulcerative colitis and granulomatous colitis, inflammatory or lymphoid polyps, the hamartomatous polyps of children (juvenile polyps), Cronkhite-Canada and Puetz-Jehgers syndromes, and hyperplastic polyps of the colorectum (usually less than 0.5 cm in size). Fecal occult blood testing remains the screening test of choice among patients at low risk for colorectal polyps or cancer, but sensitivity is low and specificity is poor (the patient should avoid raw meat, beets, radishes, iron, vitamin C, and aspirin prior to testing). Cumulative mortality reduction from colon cancer has been demonstrated with the use of yearly fecal occult blood testing in patients age 50 or older.

Colorectal Carcinoma

Colorectal carcinoma is diagnosed in about 150,000 patients per year in the United States with 60,000 deaths per year and equal distribution for the two genders. Carcinoma of the colorectum is conveniently divided into: (1) right-side lesions (supplied by the superior mesenteric artery), including lesions close to the splenic flexure; (b) left-side lesions (supplied by the inferior mesenteric artery), including the descending colon, sigmoid colon, and upper rectum; and (c) rectal lesions, with no serosal covering. Duke's pathologic classification for prognosis is improved by adding the Astler-Coller C1 and C2 designations. The TNM classification is used now more frequently for prognostic evaluation of this disease and should be adopted.

Surgical removal is generally the accepted treatment for carcinoma of the colorectum. It generally includes removal of bowel at least 5 cm proximal and distal to the carcinoma and encompasses a wide band of mesentery back to the origin of the arterial supply to include the primary lymphatic drainage of the tumor. Although direct adherence of the tumor to an adjacent organ (stomach, spleen, small intestine, abdominal wall, female genital organs, bladder) may be from inflammatory adhesion (50%) or direct microscopic tumor extension (50%), cure is still possible with *en bloc* resection of the adjacent organ. The Turnbull "no-touch" technique of resection for intraabdominal colonic malignancy produced excellent results in his hands but was not definitely superior to standard wide resection of intraabdominal colonic malignancy in a prospective randomized trial. Coles' suggestion of isolating the bowel tumor between umbilical tapes to prevent intraluminal spread of tumor is of confirmed value in experimental animals and is recommended. Subtotal colectomy should be considered in patients with two or more malignancies or one malignancy and multiple premalignant polyps.

Synchronous carcinoma occurs in about 5% of patients and synchronous polyps in 25% to 30%. Hence preoperative colonoscopy alters the surgical procedure to be performed in about 20% of patients.

Perioperative blood transfusion (plasma or whole blood) is avoided if possible, although its role as a negative prognostic factor is controversial. The role of extensive resection for colorectal cancer remains unproved. The place of laparoscopic resection of these tumors is unclear at this time, but it appears to be equivalent to open resection with equal removal of bowel length and lymph nodes but with an increased possibility of seeding cancer into operative ports.

Mechanical cleansing (polyethylene glycol solutions) and intraluminal antibiotics preoperatively is of proved benefit for reducing wound and intraabdominal infectious complications postoperatively. In addition, perioperative use of a broad-spectrum systemic antibiotic can further decrease the incidence of infectious complications. These results are not improved by the addition of an elemental diet, which is expensive and fails to improve mechanical cleansing of the colon. Surgical procedures exceeding 2 hours and operations in the rectum benefit most from the addition of a perioperative systemic antibiotic. Postoperative nasogastric tubes are unnecessary.

Blood samples for a carcinoembryonic antigen (CEA) assay should be obtained preoperatively. If the CEA is elevated preoperatively with a subsequent fall to normal postoperatively (about 6 weeks), elevation at a later date *may* be the first sign of recurrent disease that *may* be amenable to a second "curative" resection. Several reports have confirmed the value of the CEA assay for detecting early recurrent disease, and some of these lesions

can be resected. Whether increased long-term disease-free survival (> 5 years) results is still unclear. Patients with CEA elevations at follow-up after resection may have a negative workup (e.g., CT scans, colonoscopy). In these instances radioimmune localization of a neoplasm using radiolabeled monoclonal antibodies may detect residual tumor. Markedly high CEA levels prior to the initial tumor resection are associated with poor long term survival, as are high tumor DNA content, advanced TNM stage, and microscopic venous invasion (particularly extramural venous invasion). Patients who present with complete colonic obstruction or perforation (at the tumor site or proximal to it) have a poor long-term prognosis and increased operative mortality. Staged resection with an initial colostomy remains an option for obstruction except in the right colon, where immediate right colectomy and ileocolic anastomosis can usually be done safety and perhaps in the left colon as well in selected cases. Otherwise a resection with colostomy may be done; or resection, anastomosis, and a proximal protective colostomy are possible for lesions in the left colon. Reports suggest that primary resection (subtotal colectomy and ileoproctostomy) is appropriate for an obstructive left colonic lesion above the peritoneal reflection.

If the patient presents with a perforated colon, treatment of the perforation and resulting peritonitis take precedence over treatment of the neoplasm because they pose the immediate threat to life. In the left colon the perforated colonic segment and tumor should be resected and a proximal colostomy and distal mucous fistula or Hartmann-type colonic closure established. If a tumor in the right colon has perforated, it can frequently be resected and a primary anastomosis done. If the right colon perforation is proximal to an obstruction in the left colon, no anastomosis is usually safe. Here subtotal colectomy is the treatment of choice. Any patient who presents with *Streptococcus bovis* septicemia should be investigated for colorectal cancer as its source.

Carcinoma of the rectum is generally treated by abdominal perineal resection if the lower border of the tumor is in the lower one-third of the rectum (0 to 5 cm from the anal verge) and by anterior resection if the tumor is in the upper third (above 10 to 11 cm). Surgical treatment in the middle third of the rectum is controversial. In general, these tumors are now treated with an abdominal sacral resection or low anterior resection and anastomosis with an EEA stapler. Operations other than abdominal perineal resection may not allow 5-cm clearance distal to the tumor, but this point may not be important (distal intramural spread seldom exceeds 2.5 cm). Five-year survival is claimed to be as good as with abdominoperineal resection, and it is; but local pelvic recurrence may be increased. This local recurrence is usually from lateral tumor growth and increases as the tumor comes closer to the anus; local recurrence is also increased by anastomotic leaks or rectal perforation during resection. Neither preoperative CT scans nor intrarectal ultrasonography can accurately determine lymph node involvement, but the latter fairly accurately determines depth of invasion by rectal lesions (70% to 80% sensitivity and specificity).

Electrocoagulation or local excision has a role as definitive therapy for rectal lesions below the 10-cm level, especially with a small (less than 4 cm), well differentiated, nonmucinous, exophytic, freely movable lesion or in patients who are poor operative risks, refuse a major surgical procedure, or have distant metastatic disease. Obviously, nodal disease is not treated, and patients with stage III lesions in this area have less than a 20% five-year disease-free survival, although external radiotherapy and systemic chemotherapy may be added to the local procedure. High-dose radiotherapy with an intraluminal tube, insertion of radon seeds, or both has also been used successfully for these lesions by Papillon and other radiotherapists. In the future, the use of local excisional therapy may be extended with improvements in adjuvant chemotherapy and radiotherapy.

Preoperative radiotherapy (40 to 50 Gy) appears to be useful for converting some large, fixed rectal tumors to resectable lesions. No strong evidence exists that its routine preoperative (or postoperative) use (20 to 40 Gy) increases 5-year disease-free survival of patients with carcinoma of the rectum, but radiotherapy does decrease the local recurrence rate. The combination of adjuvant radiotherapy and chemotherapy of rectal cancer (stages II and III) increases disease-free survival; and postoperative adjuvant therapy with 5-fluorouracil, leukovorin, and levamisole in Duke C (stage III) colon cancer patients increases disease-free survival if begun within 6 weeks of operation. Overall 5-year *disease-free* survival (operations with curative intent) in the United States averages 60% for those with colon cancer and about 50% for those with rectal cancer. Direct portal vein chemotherapy infusion as adjuvant therapy for Duke C disease does not demonstrate a survival advantage over systemic chemotherapy.

Bilateral oophorectomy is a reasonable addition to colorectal resection for carcinoma in women (especially when perimenopausal or postmenopausal). The ovaries are involved with microscopic metastases in about 3% to 5% of cases, and oophorectomy obviates the development of primary ovarian carcinoma or large colonic metastases that may require resection at a later date. Unfortunately, oophorectomy does not increase the 5-year disease-free survival of those with colorectal cancer.

Liver metastases from colorectal cancer may be surgically resectable, which results in long-term survival if there is no extrahepatic recurrence, the metastases can be resected with a free margin of 1 cm or more, and generally they number three or fewer. The disease-free interval between resection of the primary lesion and documentation of hepatic metastases seems to be unimportant, unlike for other neoplasms. Of course, only a small number of patients with liver metastases meet the above criteria for surgical resection, but 5-year survivals of 25% to 30% are possible in this highly selected group of patients. Equal results occur with the use of cryotherapy in these patients. Intraoperative ultrasonography improves the detection of additional liver metastases, as may immunoscintigraphy using labeled monoclonal antibodies that demonstrate undiagnosed extrahepatic metastasis. Patients with unresectable liver metastases are reported to benefit (increased mean survival) from hepatic intraarterial chemotherapy with fluorouracil derivatives, in contrast to those who receive systemic chemotherapy, although this treatment is controversial.

ISCHEMIC COLITIS

Ischemic colitis, increasingly identified in elderly patients, usually results from small-vessel vascular disease in or near the colonic wall. A contributing factor is the "low flow" state (e.g., shock, vasopressor use), and the splenic flexure of the colon is most frequently involved. The severity correlates with the degree of ischemia and extent of colon involved; the disease may vary from mild mucosal edema (with or without mucosal sloughing) with healing, to circumferential mucosal sloughing and subsequent stricture, to full-thickness bowel wall necrosis and perforation. The presenting clinical signs and symptoms are frequently mistaken for diverticulitis or inflammatory bowel disease. It occurs most frequently in the left colon but may involve any portion of the intraabdominal colon. Barium enema

shows typical thumb-printing due to areas of edematous, hemorrhagic submucosa and mucosa. Colonoscopy is the most accurate diagnostic test.

Treatment is generally with bowel rest, intravenous
fluids, and broad-spectrum antibiotics. Operation is undertaken for signs of colonic gangrene or perforation,
obstruction, or lack of resolution.

COLONIC PSEUDOOBSTRUCTION

Acute obstruction in the absence of any identifiable
mechanical cause, ischemia, or infection is called
pseudoobstruction. Colonic pseudoobstruction typically occurs in elderly, bedridden, hospitalized patients.
They frequently are on narcotics or anticholinergic
medications or have pneumonia, renal failure, sepsis,
pancreatitis, or spinal or pelvic trauma.

Classically, the patient is noted to have painless abdominal distension and obstipation. Abdominal radiographs show massive colonic distension that is usually
worse in the right colon. The major risk for the patient
is cecal perforation. Colonoscopy is both diagnostic
and therapeutic and should be combined with nasogastric suction, bowel rest, intravenous fluids, and correction of abnormalities that contribute to the problem
(hypokalemia, hypomagnesemia, hypoalbuminemia,
hypothyroidism, or primary hyperparathyroidism). Cecostomy or colostomy is occasionally necessary if
colonoscopy is unsuccessful or unavailable. If the colon
is ischemic or perforated, resection is required. Mortality exceeds 50%.

VOLVULUS

Volvulus of the colon is an entity in which a mobile
portion of the colon twists on itself, producing a closed-
loop obstruction. The disease occurs most frequently in
the sigmoid colon (75% to 85%), occasionally in the cecum or ascending colon (10% to 15%), and rarely in the
transverse colon or the splenic flexure.

Sigmoid volvulus (counterclockwise rotation) tends
to occur in patients with a long, redundant sigmoid loop
with or without a narrow attachment at the base of the
sigmoid mesentery. Interestingly, if the patient's ileocecal valve is competent, a sigmoid volvulus results in
two closed-loop obstructions within the colon. In the
United States the disease tends to occur in older patients with chronic constipation, neglected bowel

habits, or neurologic disease. They frequently are taking medications that further decrease colonic motility.

The clinical picture is that of a colonic obstruction
with abdominal pain, distension, and obstipation. Vomiting occurs late or not at all. There may be a history of
episodes with spontaneous resolution. If the loop becomes gangrenous, signs of peritoneal irritation with
fever appear and the WBC count is elevated, although
in some elderly patients the WBC count remains normal
or low with a "left shift."

Supine and upright abdominal films show a large,
distended colonic loop with its apex frequently in the
right upper abdomen (bent inner tube or omega sign). If
there are no signs of peritonitis, sigmoidoscopy or
colonoscopy may be diagnostic and therapeutic with release of the obstruction by the sigmoidoscope or a rectal tube gently passed beyond the end of the scope. Barium enema may be necessary to establish the diagnosis
of sigmoidoscopy is not diagnostic. A "bird's beak" deformity is seen on barium enema and points to the site
of obstruction.

If there are no signs of gangrene (strangulation) of
the sigmoid loop, a rectal tube is left in place for several
days. The bowel is then prepared and elective sigmoid
resection is performed to avoid the high incidence (50%
to 90%) of recurrence. Signs of strangulation demand
emergency celiotomy, resection of the sigmoid loop
with proximal sigmoid colostomy (without detorsion of
the counterclockwise rotated sigmoid loop), and either
creation of a distal mucous fistula or oversewing of the
distal sigmoid, which usually cannot easily be brought
to the abdominal wall skin.

If volvulus occurs in the cecum or ascending colon
(clockwise rotation), it is usually because of a congenital lack of fixation or failure of the right colon to descend into the right lower quadrant of the abdomen.
This variety frequently occurs in a younger age group
than sigmoid volvulus.

Adhesions developing to the right colon from previous operations may be important in the development of
a volvulus. Sometimes a true volvulus does not develop; rather, a mobile cecum flops upward and lies on
the ascending colon (cecal bascule). The clinical picture
suggests a distal small intestinal obstruction, and previous episodes with spontaneous resolution are common.
Abdominal films are frequently diagnostic, with a large
distended cecum seen along with numerous loops of dilated small intestine. If necessary, the diagnosis is confirmed with a barium enema. Rarely, reduction is ac-

complished at colonoscopy if there are no signs of gangrene, with elective cecopexy or resection at a later date. With nonresolution or signs of gangrene, celiotomy is undertaken. Right colectomy with ileocolostomy is performed for a necrotic colon. If the colon is viable, cecopexy, right colectomy, or a lateral cecostomy may be done (colectomy preferred). Infectious postoperative complications increase if the colon is entered despite the use of perioperative antibiotics.

RECTAL PROLAPSE

Rectal prolapse is a disease in which some or all of the layers of the rectal wall prolapse externally. It occurs six times more commonly in women than men. Historically, this entity has been divided into three categories. Type I is prolapse only of the rectal mucosa through the anus and is frequently associated with internal hemorrhoids that enlarge and push the mucosa ahead of them in radial folds. Type II denotes a protrusion of all layers of the rectal wall through the anus (rectal intussusception) without an associated hernia of the pelvic cul-de-sac. Type III is a full-thickness prolapse with a perineal sliding hernia of the pelvic cul-de-sac. There is a large defect in the pelvic diaphragm, and the cul-de-sac hernia invaginates the anterior rectal wall, producing the intussusception. The development of a type II or III prolapse is associated with loss of adherence of the rectum to the sacral curve, with elongation, straightening, and eventually a lax, dilated external sphincter and loss of continence and mucous discharge. These symptoms are often preceded by a long history of severe constipation and frequently tenesmus or anterior rectal ulceration. As time passes, the rectal mucosa (concentric folds) constantly prolapses outside the anal canal with persistent soilage, odor, and mucosal excoriation with bleeding from minor trauma. Many patients with type II or III prolapse are elderly and have multiple chronic medical diseases. Incontinence is common (50%) and apparently results from pressure and stretching of the pudendal or perineal nerve denervating the internal anal sphincter and puborectalis muscles as well as stretching of the internal and external anal sphincters. A solitary rectal ulcer may develop from a prolapse that does not present externally. The etiology of complete prolapse is unclear.

Numerous operative procedures have been devised for the disease. Type I mucosal prolapse is well handled by hemorrhoidectomy or sleeve resection of the rectal mucosa to establish the distal extent of the mucosa at the pectinate line. Type II and III prolapses are most frequently managed by a transabdominal operation that mobilizes the rectum and fixes it to the presacral fascia. The operation may include repair of the hernia at the pelvic diaphragm, if present, and resection of the sigmoid colon if it is redundant. These procedures may be combined with a posterior repair of the puborectalis muscle. A perirectal circular suture may be used alone to palliate the problem in poor-risk patients but frequently results in fecal impaction. Alternatively, perineal rectosigmoidectomy (Altemeier) may be performed, particularly if the bowel is prolapsed and gangrenous. The medical literature describes numerous other procedures and modifications of the operations described here.

RADIATION PROCTITIS

The deleterious effects of radiation on the rectum and other areas of the intestinal tract are roughly dose-dependent (rarely occurs if the tissue dose is less than 40 Gy). The effect is also determined by the method of fractionation and the rapidity with which the total dosage is delivered. Rapidly proliferating intestinal epithelium is highly sensitive to the effects of ionizing radiation. When used long term, progressive vasculitis with subintimal foam cells leads to arteriolar occlusion and thrombosis that is worsened in patients who are elderly, diabetic, or severely atherosclerotic or who have fixed bowel.

The rectum is most frequently injured when radiotherapy is used to treat malignancies of the uterus, bladder, or prostate (true incidence unknown). Early proctitis is frequently treated successfully with a low-residue diet and steroid or 5-aminosalicylic acid enemas. Late symptoms (months to years after radiotherapy) include chronic proctitis, rectal ulcers, a rectovaginal fistula, strictures, or perforation. The lesions are usually 4 to 8 cm above the pectinate line and are worse on the anterior rectal wall.

Initial management must include rectal or vaginal biopsies to exclude the possibility of residual cancer. The conservative measures mentioned above should be used if they are effective. If not, an end-sigmoid colostomy is usually safe and effective. Localized lesions in the rectum may be resected but should be protected by a proximal colostomy until satisfactory healing is ensured. Nonirradiated colon is used to replace the re-sected radiation-damaged rectum.

ANORECTAL DISEASES

Basic knowledge of the anatomy of the anorectum is presumed in the following brief discussion of anorectal diseases. The discussion concerns an area about 4.0 to 4.5 cm in length where the entoderm of the lower rectum (2 cm) meets the ectoderm of the anus (2.0 to 2.5 cm) and their junction at the pectinate or mucocutaneous line. This area is frequently referred to as the anal canal, and the area distal to the pectinate line is called the anal margin.

Hemorrhoids

Hemorrhoids are varicosities of the submucosal veins with or without arteriovenous communications of the area. Like varicosities of the lower extremities, they have a strong hereditary predisposition. Their development is abetted by straining to pass hard stools, pregnancy, and increased resting anal pressure (internal sphincter). Internal and external hemorrhoids are separated from one another at the intersphincteric line (distal to the pectinate line) but are connected by small anastomosing venous channels.

Internal Hemorrhoids

Internal hemorrhoids may bleed but are otherwise asymptomatic except when they prolapse and become thrombosed. Bleeding may be severe enough to produce anemia. It is important to exclude other sources of bleeding from the colorectum by sigmoidoscopy and barium enema or colonoscopy.

Bleeding internal hemorrhoids may be treated by sclerotherapy, laser, or rubber band ligation; these methods are appropriate if the hemorrhoids are not prolapsed. Following treatment the patient is best managed with a high-residue diet and stool softeners to produce soft bowel movements that do not require excessive straining for evacuation. Injection sclerotherapy is contraindicated in the presence of concomitant fissure, abscess, or fistula in ano.

Large internal hemorrhoids that prolapse with defecation or exertion may not retract because of sphincter spasm. They then thrombose and develop perivenous

edema, and the overlying mucosa becomes gangrenous. If the patient is seen early (less than 24 hours) an emergency closed hemorrhoidectomy is beneficial, but usually the patient presents at a later time when associated edema, gangrene, and infection are more appropriately treated with bed rest, stool softener, and analgesia. Surgical hemorrhoidectomy is frequently desirable after resolution of the above symptoms (results are not improved by adding anal dilatation to hemorrhoidectomy).

External Hemorrhoids

External hemorrhoids may rupture or thrombose from straining, and the initial pain is produced by separation of the anal skin from the underlying soft tissues. If the patient is seen during the first 24 to 48 hours, evacuation of the clot (using local anesthesia) is helpful. Later the overlying anal skin frequently becomes inflamed and necrotic, and it sloughs. The conservative treatment described for strangulated internal hemorrhoids is then appropriate.

Anorectal Abscess and Fistula In Ano

Anorectal abscess and fistula in ano usually are due to infection in anal glands in the space between the muscle layers (external and internal sphincters) of the rectal wall. Delay in recognition and drainage of the abscess results in further tissue destruction. In patients with poor resistance to infection (diabetics, immunosuppressed individuals, corticosteroid users) it may be lethal. The infected anal glands rupture, and the infection may spread in multiple directions (perianal, ischiorectal, intersphincteric). Occasionally pus tracts up the rectal wall to rupture back into the rectal lumen or into the supralevator space. When satisfactory external drainage is performed without fistulotomy, the patient frequently (50% to 60%) develops a fistula in ano or a recurrent abscess; anal function disturbances are infrequent. With added fistulotomy at the time of abscess drainage, fistula in ano development is less common (5%) but anal function disturbances are increased. When healing occurs without the development of a fistula in ano, it is probably because the involved anal crypt and its glands have been destroyed by the intense inflammation or because of a concomitant fistulotomy at the time the perirectal abscess is drained.

Fistulas in ano usually represent sequelae of a perirectal abscess and are more common in men than women. They are frequently intersphincteric but may be transsphincteric or suprasphincteric. Goodsall's rule generally predicts the path between the external and internal openings: curved with a posterior external opening and straight with an anterior external opening. Multiple tracts are sometimes present and should raise a suspicion of Crohn's disease. The tracts should be opened (fistulotomy) and chronic granulations in the tract curetted or cauterized along with the anal crypt of origin. The tissue is biopsied to rule out Crohn's disease or carcinoma. Setons should be used in suprasphincteric fistulas to avoid the certain incontinence resulting from division of the puborectalis muscle.

Fissure In Ano

Fissure in ano most frequently occurs in the posterior midline where the anal skin is overstretched owing to passage of a hard stool and where the least striated muscular support is present, although as many as 10% occur in the anterior midline in women. The disease is also associated with inflammatory bowel disease with diarrhea and cryptitis. In this situation the fissure may occur laterally or be multiple. Once the anal skin is torn there is associated edema, inflammation, and spasm of the underlying internal and external sphincters. Rarely a subcutaneous abscess also forms in the area. The patient then avoids having bowel movements, which produces severe pain and a small amount of blood on the stool or toilet paper or in the toilet bowl. The diagnosis is easily made by spreading the buttocks. The fissure extends from the anal skin to within a millimeter of the dentate line. Conservative treatment of the acute fissure with high-residue diet, stool softener, nitic oxide, and topical anesthetic ointments is successful in about one-half to three-fourths of the patients. For those whose fissures do not heal or that recur should undergo lateral internal sphincterotomy with close attention to bowel habits subsequent to the operation. Operation should be avoided for fissures associated with inflammatory bowel disease, as they usually respond to conservative medical treatment, as does fissure in ano in infants.

Anal Cancer

For the purpose of discussing anal cancer and because the clinical courses and responses to therapy are similar, the pathologic variants of squamous carcinoma are considered together (cloacogenic, basaloid, mucopidermoid, transitional cell). These tumors tend to invade sphincteric muscles early and, like esophageal epidermoid carcinoma, may extend submucosally upward into the rectal wall. They are frequently related to human papilloma virus infection. The closer the primary lesion is to the dentate line, the more likely it is that lymphatic spread will occur superiorly into mesenteric or internal iliac lymph nodes. Pain and bleeding in small amounts are the most common symptoms. The symptoms mimic those of benign anorectal disease and so frequently the diagnosis is delayed.

Unlike that for colorectal adenocarcinoma, the prognosis is related to the size of the primary lesion. Tumors of the perianal skin (anal margin) can be widely excised similar to squamous cell carcinoma elsewhere. Inguinal node dissection is reserved for nodes proved to be pathologically involved with neoplasm (prophylactic inguinal node dissection has not been beneficial). Lesions at the anal margin or in the anal canal, if larger than 2×2 cm, were usually treated by abdominoperineal resection in the past.

These tumors are radiosensitive, but full-dose irradiation (4500 to 7000 rad) is likely to produce such complications as stricture, necrosis, hemorrhage, and postirradiation pain. Some radiotherapists have avoided this problem by highly fractionating the dosage and supplementing the external irradiation with interstitial implants.

In recent years numerous papers have described the use of radiotherapy (30 Gy) plus 5-fluorouracil and mitomycin C (both radiosensitizers) followed by local excision or abdominoperineal resection if there is residual cancer. Many of these patients (30% to 50%) have been found to have no residual disease in the surgical specimen after radiotherapy-chemotherapy. Overall, patients with small lesions that are not in the anal canal and are locally excised have a 5-year disease-free survival of 60% to 80%: for those with larger lesions treated by abdominoperineal resection the 5-year disease-free survival rate is 40% to 50%.

Treatment of these lesions with chemotherapy-radiotherapy as described improves the disease-free survival obtained by local excision, radiotherapy, or abdominoperineal resection and is now the preferred therapy. One exception is the Buschke-Lowenstein tumor (large squamous cell cancer frequently mistaken for condyloma acuminata), which appears to be best treated by radical surgical excision.

Anorectal melanoma is infrequent. It is amelanotic in 50% or more of patients, and the anorectal area is the third most common site of this neoplasm (after skin and eyes). Long-term survival after surgical treatment is uncommon and as poor after abdominoperineal resection as with wide local excision, although local recurrence is more frequent with the latter. Local excision is also the treatment of choice for basal cell carcinoma, Bowen's disease, and Paget's disease of the perianal region. Patients with the latter two diseases should be investigated for other solid internal malignancies.

Human Immunodeficiency Virus

Anorectal disease is common in patients with human immunodeficiency virus (HIV) disease (especially homosexuals). The spectrum includes condylomas (papilloma virus), fissures, abscesses, fistulas, Kaposi's sarcoma, squamous cell cancer, herpes simplex, and cytomegalovirus ulcerations, and even B cell lymphomas. Standard treatments are generally applicable, but those with advanced AIDS and low CD4+ lymphocytes counts should have conservative surgical procedures when possible, as wound healing may be impaired. This group of AIDS patients are usually starving and immunosuppressed, and surgical wounds heal poorly in them or not at all.

QUESTIONS

Which of the following statements (*one or more*) are correct:

1. Rectal cancer, compared with cancer of the intraperitoneal colon, has a:
   a. Higher local recurrence rate.
   b. Higher CEA levels.
   c. Lower survival rate.
2. Pouchitis can frequently complicate the ileal pouch–anastomosis procedure. With regard to this procedure, which of the following is/are true?
   a. It occurs with equal frequency in patients with familial polyposis and ulcerative colitis.
   b. Most patients are treated successfully with oral metronidazole.
   c. The responsible pathogen is *Bacteroides*.
   d. Recurrent pouchitis invariably necessitates pouch excision.

3. The safest procedure for radiation proctitis with rectal-vaginal fistula is:
   a. Low anterior resection and fistula closure.
   b. Sigmoid colostomy.
   c. Abdominosacral resection of the rectum and low anastomosis.
4. With regard to colonic fluid and electrolytes absorption, which of the following statements is/are correct?
   a. The colon protects against hyponatremia by actively absorbing sodium against both concentration and electrical gradients.
   b. The colon is not involved in urea metabolism.
   c. Chloride is actively absorbed from the colon lumen in exchange for bicarbonate.
   d. The maximum absorptive capacity of the colon is about 5 liters per day.
5. Biopsy of an ovoid-shaped villous lesion beginning at 4 cm shows cellular atypia. Which is the most appropriate treatment?
   a. Abdominoperineal resection.
   b. Intracavitary radiotherapy.
   c. Transanal excision.
   d. Fulguration.
6. With regard to colorectal polyps, which of the following is/are considered precancerous?
   a. Hyperplastic polyp.
   b. Villous adenoma.
   c. Colitis cystica profunda.
   d. Tubulovillous adenoma.
7. Which of the following is the *most* important determinant of survival after treatment of colorectal cancer?
   a. Lymph node involvement.
   b. Transmural extension.
   c. Tumor size.
   d. Histologic differentiation.
   e. DNA content.
8. Which of the following is the most frequent cause of massive (> 1500 ml in 24 hours) colonic bleeding in a 45-year-old patient?
   a. Ulcerative colitis.
   b. Diverticulosis.
   c. Cancer.
   d. Diverticulitis.
   e. Angiodysplastic lesions.
9. CEA is:
   a. An accurate screening test for colon cancer.
   b. An independent prognostic factor in colon cancer if elevated.

c. Useless for long-term follow-up of patients with resected colorectal cancers.

d. Elevated in some nonmalignant diseases.

10. Mandatory treatment of penetrating injuries of the rectum includes:

a. Diverting sigmoid colostomy.

b. Suture closure of the rectal laceration.

c. Washout of fecal material in the rectum.

d. Pelvic drainage.

11. The extraintestinal manifestation of idiopathic ulcerative colitis *least* likely to improve after total proctocolectomy is:

a. Uveitis.

b. Sclerosing cholangitis.

c. Pyoderma gangrenosum.

d. Erythema nodosum.

12. An absolute contraindication to primary repair of penetrating trauma of the intraabdominal colon is:

a. Hypotension.

b. Concomitant small bowel laceration.

c. Celiotomy delayed 4 hours after injury.

d. None of the above.

13. Initial treatment of a 4-cm squamous cell cancer at the pectinate line (after biopsy) should be:

a. Abdominoperineal resection.

b. External radiotherapy with 60 Gy.

c. 5-Fluorouracil, mitomycin C, and radiotherapy.

d. Abdominoperineal resection and bilateral prophylactic groin lymph node dissections.

14. Bilateral oophorectomy should probably be performed when a postmenopausal woman undergoes curative resection for colon cancer because:

a. Five-year survival is improved.

b. It may prevent the subsequent need for ovarian resection of Krukenberg metastases.

c. It prevents the subsequent development of primary ovarian cancer.

d. Restricts world population growth.

15. Sigmoid colon volvulus with a competent ileocecal valve results in:

a. Decompression of proximal colon gas and fluid into the ileum.

b. Two closed loop intestinal obstructions.

c. Early vomiting.

d. Massive abdominal distension.

SELECTED REFERENCES

Abulaf AM, Williams NS: Local recurrence of colorectal cancer: the problem, mechanisms, management and adjuvant therapy. *Br J Surg* 1994;81:7–19.

Baum ML, Anish DS, Chalmers TC, Sacks HS, Smith H Jr, Fagerstram RM. A survey of clinical trials of antibiotic prophylaxis in colon surgery: evidence against further use of no-treatment controls. *N Engl J Med* 1981;305:795–798.

Becker JM. Ileal pouch-anal anastomosis: current status and controversies. *Surgery* 1993;113:599–602.

Berry AR, Campbell WB, Kettlewell MGW. Management of major colonic hemorrhage. *Br J Surg* 1988;75:637–640.

Birnkrant A, Sampson J, Sugarbaker PH. Ovarian metastasis from colorectal cancer. *Dis Colon Rectum* 1986;29:767–771.

Burch JM, Martin RR, Richardson RJ, Muldowny DS, Mattox KL, Jordon GL Jr. Evolution of the treatment of the injured colon in the 1980's. *Arch Surg* 1991;126:979–984.

Burke EC, Orloff SL, Freise CE, et al. Wound healing after anorectal surgery in human immunodeficiency virus-infected patients. *Arch Surg* 1991;126:1267–1271.

Deans GT, McAleer JJA, Spence RAJ. Malignant anal tumors. *Br J Surg* 1994;811:500–508.

Deans GT, Parks TG, Rowlands BJ, Spence RAJ. Prognostic factors in colorectal cancer. *Br J Surg* 1992;79:608–613.

Heppel J, Farouk E, Dube S, Peloquin A, Morgan S, Bernard D. Toxic megacolon: an analysis of 70 cases. *Dis Colon Rectum* 1986;29:789–792.

Longo WE, Ballantyne GH, Cahow CE. Treatment of Crohn's colitis. *Arch Surg* 1988;123:588–590.

McKee RF, Deighan RW, Krukowski ZH. Radiologic investigation in acute diverticulitis. *Br J Surg* 1993;80:560–565.

Moertel CG. Chemotherapy for colorectal cancer. *N Engl J Med* 1994;330:1136–1142.

Moertel CG, Fleming TR, MacDonald JS, et al. Levamisole and fluorouracil for adjuvant therapy of resected colon carcinoma. *N Engl J Med* 1990;332:352–358.

Moran BJ, Jackson AA. Function of the human colon. *Br J Surg* 1992;79:1132–1137.

Mortesen PE, Olson J, Pedersen IK, Christiansen JA. A randomized study on hemorrhoidectomy combined with anal dilatation. *Dis Colon Rectum* 1987;3:755–757.

Playforth MJ, Smith GMR, Evans M, Pollack AV. Antimicrobial bowel preparation: oral, parenteral or both. *Dis Colon Rectum* 1988;31:90–93.

Podolsky DK. Inflammatory bowel disease. *N Engl J Med* 1991;928–937:1008–1016.

Rustgi AK. Hereditary gastrointestinal polyposis and nonpolysis syndromes. *N Engl J Med* 1994;331:1694–1702.

Saadia R, Schein M. Local treatment of carcinoma of the rectum. *Surg Gynecol Obstet* 1988;166:481–486.

Toribara NW, Sleisinger MH. Screening for colorectal cancer. *N Engl J Med* 1995;332:861–867.

Wiggers T, Jeekel J, Arends JW, et al. No touch isolation technique in colon cancer: a controlled prospective trial. *Br J Surg* 1988;75:409–415.

5

Diseases of the Biliary Tract

Michael S. Gold and Marek Rudnicki

ANATOMY

Biliary tract anatomy is perhaps the most variable in the abdominal cavity. Questions on the Board examinations regarding the blood supply to the liver and pancreas, the anatomic variability, and the relations and anomalies of the gallbladder and bile ducts can be expected.

Within the liver the proximal bile ducts drain into one main channel. The final common pathway for the left lobe is always a single trunk. The right lobe drains in one of two ways: In 75% of patients the right anterior and right posterior ducts join to form a single right hepatic duct; in 25% there are two right segmental ducts, each of which joins with the left hepatic duct. About 2 to 4 mm of the left and right hepatic ducts is almost always external to the liver. The length of the common hepatic duct is dictated by the entrance point of the cystic duct. The average diameter of the common hepatic and common bile duct is 8 mm with a normal range of 4 to 15 mm. The size increases slowly with age and does so slightly following a cholecystectomy.

Ducts that in the past were termed "accessory ducts" are now thought to represent a nonjoined right hepatic duct. Thus three ducts drain from the liver. When they are recognized, caution must be taken not to assume that these ducts are aberrant or accessory ducts and subsequently divide or ligate them.

In 0.5% of a large series of autopsies, the cystic duct entered the right hepatic duct, presenting a potential for right hepatic duct injury during cholecystectomy. Cholecystohepatic ducts are probably not congenital but acquired, resulting from large stones eroding through the gallbladder wall into the hepatic parenchyma. Subvesical ducts are slender (1 to 2 mm) ducts that occasionally emerge from the liver in the gallbladder fossa, pass toward the hilum, and join with the right hepatic or common hepatic duct. Ligation of these small ducts presents no problem, although division without ligation may result in short-term bile leak.

The gallbladder lies in a fossa in a line with the vena cava, separating the anatomic right and left hepatic lobes. The infundibulum is located at the point where the gallbladder leaves the fossa. The cystic duct exits from the infundibular segment of the gallbladder and has an average diameter of 2 to 3 mm. In 80% of patients the cystic duct joins the common hepatic duct on the right lateral side of the hepatoduodenal ligament. The triangle bounded by the cystic duct, common hepatic duct, and inferior border of the liver forms the triangle of Calot. An absent cystic duct probably represents effacement by a stone in Hartman's pouch and is rarely congenital. In 80% of patients the cystic artery is single and arises from the right hepatic artery posterior to the cystic duct; 20% originate from the left or common hepatic artery, and a small number originate directly from the superior mesenteric artery. Venous drainage of the gallbladder is directly to the liver via small venous plexuses.

The common bile duct lies to the right of the hepatic artery and anterior to the portal vein. The arterial supply is via small vessels from the surrounding arteries, and venous drainage is via small tributaries to the portal vein. Lymphatics drain toward lymph ducts around the celiac axis. The common bile duct runs behind the duodenum and enters a groove in the dorsal portion of the head of the pancreas. A symmetric narrowing at the distal intrapancreatic bile duct is normal. The bile duct then joins the main pancreatic duct (Wirsung) in a short common channel and enters the ampulla of Vater. The bile duct is posterior and to the right of the pancreatic duct in 80% of patients. The ampulla of Vater is on the medial or postcromedial side of the duodenum, usually in the mid or distal half of the descending duodenum. The most common error when performing a duodenotomy for surgical access to the ampulla is making the incision too proximal on the duodenum.

Anomalies of the gallbladder are common, with some variation occurring as frequently as 50% in autopsy series. Rarely, gallbladder is absent (0.02%), and when this occurs it is often associated with other congenital anomalies. Double or, rarely, triple gallbladders have been reported as well. Left-sided gallbladders have been reported with and without situs inversus. A partially intrahepatic gallbladder is common, but one that is totally intrahepatic is rare.

PHYSIOLOGY

About 500 to 1,000 ml of bile is secreted continuously by the liver each day; it enters the gallbladder, where it is concentrated six to ten times. Major constituents of bile include water, bile acids, cholesterol, phospholipids, and bile pigments. Bile acids are synthesized from cholesterol and consist mainly of cholic and chenodeoxycholic acids. Cholesterol is maintained in a solution by forming a mixed micelle and aggregates with lecithin. When secreted, these substances are activated by pancreatic lipase in the duodenum.

Bilirubin is a waste product of hemoglobin, and conjugated bilirubin is actively secreted into the bile. The daily hepatic excretion of bilirubin is approximately 300 mg, most of which is excreted in the feces. Bile acids are reabsorbed, primarily in the terminal ileum, returning to the liver via the portal vein. Therefore the liver secretes 20 to 30 g of bile per day from a total bile acid pool of 3 to 5 g recycled 4 to 12 times a day. Hepatic bile acid synthesis is controlled via a negative feedback mechanism. Serum levels of bile acids are low. Less than 5% of total bile acids are excreted in the feces, approximately 500 to 600 mg per day. The process of reabsorption of bile acids from the intestine and their secretion from the liver is known as the enterohepatic circulation.

Biliary tract pain is related to distension. The rapidity of the distension directly correlates with the degree of pain. The nerve supply consists of splanchnic nerves via the celiac ganglion from T7 to T10, branches of the right phrenic nerve from C3 to C5, and the intercostal nerves from T8 to T10. Biliary colic is probably not true colic but is caused by sudden stretching or distension. Gradual distension is usually painless.

The gallbladder functions to concentrate bile by reabsorption of water and electrolytes. The release of cholecystokinin is stimulated within 10 minutes of the appearance of food in the duodenum, resulting in contraction of the gallbladder and relaxation of the sphincter of Oddi. The duodenal muscle contracts and relaxes with the sphincter, and contraction generally concludes in 30 minutes. Truncal vagotomy doubles the resting volume of the gallbladder, but the significance of this in the etiology of stone formation is unclear. Normal resting pressure in the sphincter of Oddi is 8 to 15 cm H_2O.

The incidence and significance of biliary pancreatic reflux in normal subjects are not clearly known. Using intraoperative and postoperative cholangiography, the incidence has been variously reported as 7% to 46%. However, reflux is probably rare at normal physiologic pressure.

DIAGNOSTIC PROCEDURES

Abdominal Radiography

A plain abdominal film may reveal significant diagnostic information. Approximately 15% of gallstones contain sufficient calcium to be radiopaque and are visualized on a plain film. Other helpful information, such as the presence of air in the biliary tree or a calcified gallbladder, may also be apparent. Air in the biliary tree is present in 75% of patients with a cholecysten-teric fistula in conjunction with a gallstone ileus, rarely with a choledochoduodenal fistula from stones, or more commonly with a duodenal ulcer.

Ultrasonography

Ultrasonography is 95% accurate for demonstrating the presence of biliary tract stones. It should be the pri-mary screening test for initial evaluation of the patient presumed to have biliary tract disease, gallbladder disease, or obstructive jaundice. Choledocholithiasis, when present, is demonstrated in 50% of patients. Al-though less accurate than computed tomography (CT), masses in the head of the pancreas larger than 3 cm in diameter may be visualized with ultrasonography.

Ultrasonography is now generally accepted as the initial diagnostic test to confirm the presence of gall-stones, biliary tract dilatation, and pancreatic pathol-ogy. Ultrasonography occasionally shows tiny stones or sludge after an oral study has produced normal results. Because ultrasonography only rarely gives false-positive results (less than 1%), there seems to be little reason to follow a positive sonogram routinely with an oral cholecystogram (OCG).

One important indication for obtaining an OCG fol-lowing a normal sonogram is unexplained biliary tract pain secondary to cholesterolosis or dysfunctional emp-tying. In these patients the delayed emptying, seen as opacification of the gallbladder beyond 36 hours, is highly suggestive of biliary dyskinesia, and improve-ment with cholecystectomy can be expected in 75% to 90% of cases.

Oral Cholecystography

The incidence of false-positive and false-negative re-sults on OCGs is each less than 5%. Contraindications for an OCG include significant hepatic or renal failure, vomiting, a bilirubin level of 2 mg/dl, or a known sensi-tivity (rare) to iopanoic acid. Reasons for nonvisualiza-tion include significant gallbladder disease due to an in-ability to concentrate the dye or cystic duct obstruction. Vomiting or failure to take pills, gastric outlet obstruc-tion, unnoticed jaundice, previous cholecystectomy, or acute pancreatitis also results in nonvisualization. This test is rarely used because of the availability and accu-racy of ultrasonography as an initial diagnostic tool.

HIDA Scanning

Scanning with hepatoiminodiacetic acid (HIDA) is the procedure of choice for the diagnosis of acute chole-cystitis. It is also useful for documenting the patency of any biliary–enteric anastomosis or for demonstrating the presence of a biliary fistula or emptying of the afferent limb in a gastroenterostomy. Nonvisualization of the gallbladder at 2 hours after injection is reliable evidence of cystic duct obstruction, although in about 5% of pa-tients gallbladders not visualized at this point may be vi-sualized at 4 hours. Delayed visualization is indicative of chronic cholelithiasis and cholecystitis in 80% of pa-tients. There are virtually no contraindications, and side effects are almost unknown. A HIDA scan followed by cholecystokinin (CCK) administration is helpful for documenting biliary dyskinesia when gallbladder con-traction accompanies typical biliary tract pain in patients without evidence of stones. Following infusion of CCK, measurements of the gallbladder ejection fraction (GBEF) (normal is more than 35%), gallbladder ejection period (GBEP) (normal is 8 to 12 minutes), gallbladder latent period (GBLP) (normal is under 3.0 minutes), and gallbladder ejection rate (GBER) (normal is 3.5% per minute) are performed. Abnormal values in association with reproduced pain suggest a high likelihood of symp-tomatic relief from cholecystectomy.

Cholangiography: Endoscopic Retrograde Cholangiopancreatography and Percutaneous Transhepatic Cholangiography

Cholangiography has remained the gold standard for diagnosis of biliary tree obstructive diseases. Endo-scopic retrograde cholangiography and pancreatogra-phy (ERCP) is indicated for suspected obstructing le-sions of the distal bile duct or the head of the pancreas. Many endoscopists believe that ERCP is the preferred procedure following ultrasonography when dilated ducts have been demonstrated. Others think that ERCP should follow ultrasonography regardless of ductal di-latation. When choledocholithiasis is suspected, ERCP followed by endoscopic papillotomy may be indicated. Contraindications include sensitivity to oral contrast and pyloric obstruction. Data suggest that Billroth II gastrectomy, acute pancreatitis, pancreatic pseudocyst, or known hepatitis antigen do not represent contraindi-cations for ERCP.

Although it is safe in experienced hands, the incidence of complications with ERCP, especially when combined with papillotomy, is still significant. Hyperamylasemia follows ERCP in 25% of patients, although it is usually of no clinical significance.

Percutaneous transhepatic cholangiography (PTC) is indicated in patients when endoscopic retrograde cholangiography (ERC) is not successful or the biliary tree proximal to a stricture was not adequately filled. In addition to its diagnostic value, PTC can be followed by placement of transhepatic catheters to assist in therapy (decompress the biliary system, guidance during surgical reconstruction, provide access for nonoperative dilation).

GALLSTONE DISEASE AND MANAGEMENT

At least 16 million Americans have gallstones, and 800,000 new cases occur each year. Generally, a combination of pure cholesterol, mixed cholesterol, phospholipids, or pigment stones is found. Most patients with cholesterol stones can be shown to have supersaturated bile. The relative proportion of cholesterol, phospholipids, and bile acids determines whether cholesterol is maintained in micellar solution or precipitates and forms the nidus for stones.

Asymptomatic Gallstones

It is now generally accepted that asymptomatic gallstones do not require treatment. Older data suggested that 50% of asymptomatic patients would develop symptoms within 10 years; and that significant complications would develop in 25%. More recent studies, however, refute this suggestion, noting that fewer than 10% of asymptomatic patients develop symptoms within 10 years. No significantly increased mortality or morbidity was noted when treatment was delayed until the onset of symptoms. In the past, diabetics and patients on steroids or immunosuppressants were thought to require cholecystectomy for asymptomatic gallstones due to the high complication rate with acute cholecystitis. Again, recent data have refuted this concept, and cholecystectomy is no longer suggested in any asymptomatic patient. Transplant surgeons often recommend cholecystectomy for asymptomatic gallbladders prior to transplantation procedures.

Laparoscopic Cholecystectomy

Laparoscopic cholecystectomy is a method of removing the gallbladder using laparoscopic techniques. In 1987 Phillip Mouret in France removed a diseased gallbladder during a laparoscopic gynecologic procedure. Indications are the same as for the open technique, including symptomatic gallstones, gallstone pancreatitis, symptomatic gallbladder polyps, acute cholecystitis, and a calcified gallbladder wall.

Two 1.0-cm ports and two 0.5-cm ports are used. A nasogastric tube is mandatory. The basic principles are the same as for the open procedure. Limitations are a two-dimensional view, a field of vision limited to the view of the endoscope, and an abdomen that cannot be explored manually. Equipment includes a high-resolution camera, two video monitors, a high-intensity light source, a high-flow insufflator (6 L/min), and a cautery or laser device. Techniques of dissection utilize an electrosurgical hook, scissors, a spatula, a suction irrigator, and a cautery device or an Nd-YAG laser.

Absolute contraindications are portal hypertension and cirrhosis, major bleeding disorders, and sepsis with diffuse peritonitis. Relative contraindications are significant bowel distension, previous major upper abdominal surgery, obesity, and acute pancreatitis. Pregnancy was previously thought to be a contraindication, but recent reports have refuted it. Emphysematous cholecystitis and suspected gangrenous cholecystitis are considered indications for open cholecystectomy.

A 5% to 10% conversion rate to open cholecystectomy reflects good judgment. Reasons for conversion include bleeding, bile leak or bile duct injury, rupture of an empyema, instrument failure, a thick-walled gallbladder, and an inability to correctly identify the anatomy. Pressure to complete a laparoscopic procedure can lead to technical misadventures. The safety net is an open cholecystectomy.

The major postoperative complications reported to require laparotomy are bleeding, common bile duct injury, biliary peritonitis, bowel perforation, sepsis, and subcapsular hematoma. Early large series have reported major complication rates well below 1%. The incidence of complications seems to be related to the experience of the surgeon. The true incidence of bile duct injuries is not known. Initially, numerous authorities in referral centers suggested a bile duct injury rate 5 to 10 times higher than with the open technique. Newer data report an injury rate equivalent to that with open cholecystectomy.

Laparoscopic management of common duct stones is still evolving. Indications for cholangiography are identical to those for the open technique. The controversy over routine cholangiography or with specific indications is also present with laparoscopic cholecystectomy. Patients with no history of pancreatitis, jaundice, or recent acute cholecystitis, normal liver function tests (LFTs), and a common bile duct (CBD) less than 5 mm on ultrasonography are considered at low risk and do not require a cholangiogram. Medium-risk patients with mildly abnormal LFTs, an enlarged CBD (5 to 9 mm), a history of pancreatitis, or recent acute cholecystitis should undergo intraoperative cholangiography. High-risk patients with clinical jaundice, a CBD larger than 9 mm, acute cholangitis or CD stones on ultrasound examination should undergo preoperative ERCP and papillotomy.

Options for management of common duct (CD) stones when found on the cholangiogram include (a) conversion to open CD exploration; (b) laparoscopic CD exploration via the cystic duct; (c) laparoscopic T-tube insertion, followed by closure and postoperative ERCP; and (d) close observation of small stones (less than 5 mm) in a nondilated duct. The appropriate choice depends on the operator's skill and experience.

Acute cholecystitis can be managed laparoscopically. The gallbladder is decompressed with a needle for easier manipulation, and if possible a cholangiogram is obtained. Approximately one-third of patients require conversion to open cholecystectomy.

The main benefits of laparoscopic cholecystectomy are a short hospital stay (often ambulatory, less than 24 hours) and a short recovery. Most patients can return to normal activity by 1 week. Cosmesis is also significantly improved.

Several series comparing laser cautery have failed to show any advantage for laser dissection. In fact, operating time, costs, and perhaps rates of injury are higher with laser; certainly the potential for technical misadventures is higher.

We are entering an exciting new era of minimal access general surgery. It is important to remember that the access may be minimal, but the operations and potential for complications are major.

Medical Dissolution of Stones

Because cholecystectomy is a safe, effective, remarkably well tolerated procedure, the role of medical disso-

lution of gallstones must be defined. Chenodeoxycholic acid and ursodeoxycholic acid have been approved for general use. The basic mechanism is to increase the bile acid pool and allow dissolution of gallstones. Criteria for treatment include (a) a functioning gallbladder, determined on an oral cholecystogram; (b) nonradiopaque stones (mainly cholesterol); (c) no stones larger than 2 cm diameter; (d) no evidence of significant liver disease; (e) infrequent pain; and (f) no risk or anticipation of pregnancy during treatment.

Most patients require treatment for at least 1 year and many for 2 years. An oral cholecystogram or ultrasound scan is obtained every 3 to 6 months. Lack of reduction in the size of the stones is considered treatment failure. About 8% to 10% of patients develop acute cholecystitis or other complications and require cholecystectomy while on treatment. By 5 years after treatment is terminated, 50% have been reported to re-form stones. Currently, oral dissolution is recommended for patients who fulfill the above criteria and have a strong medical contraindication for cholecystectomy.

Extracorporeal Shock Wave Therapy

Acoustic energy properly focused may fragment biliary stones. Lithotripters generate longitudinal waves that are able to pass through the body and concentrate on stones. The goal is to fragment the stones into pieces small enough to proceed through the cystic duct and papilla of Vater. Oral dissoluting agents should be used as adjuvant therapy after the procedure. Repeated extracorporeal shock wave therapy (ESWL) is necessary 4 to 6 weeks later if there are residual stones larger than 5 mm.

The cost of the equipment, the need for repeated procedures, the use of dissolution agents, and specific clinical indications with a large body of contraindications have limited the use of ESWL after laparoscopic techniques were developed.

Acute Cholecystitis

In 95% of patients acute cholecystitis results from a stone obstructing the cystic duct. Acalculous cholecystitis most often accompanies conditions that result in significant inactivity of the gastrointestinal (GI) tract with biliary stasis. Bacterial contamination in cholecystitis is secondary and probably occurs via lymphatics. *Escherichia coli* is the most commonly found organism, followed by other enteric organisms, such as *Klebsiella, Proteus, Pseudomonas,* and *Streptococcus faecalis.* Anaerobes are uncommon and are usually mixed with aerobes; *Clostridium* is most common, and *Bacteroides* is rare.

Clinical resolution of acute cholecystitis can be accomplished in 85% of patients by GI rest, antibiotics, and intravenous fluid replacement. Acute free perforation occurs in 2%, most commonly diabetics. The HIDA scan is 95% accurate for demonstrating cystic duct obstruction. Ultrasonography may show ductal dilatation, stones, or thickening of the gallbladder wall, but it is not specific for cystic duct obstruction. Some degree of jaundice is noted in 25% of patients with acute cholecystitis. Bilirubin elevation as high as 8 mg without the presence of stones in the CBD may be due to pericholedochal edema and ampullary stasis.

Prompt cholecystectomy, within 24 to 48 hours, is generally accepted as the preferred treatment for acute cholecystitis. Diabetics should undergo surgery with more urgency. Significant sepsis with high fevers and shaking chills is rare and more suggestive of cholangitis; but if a rapid response to fluids and antibiotics is not seen, surgery is performed without delay.

Choledocholithiasis

The overall incidence of CD stones varies from 8% to 15%, increasing with age to as high as 40% at age 80. Primary CBDs account for 5% to 40% of stones in the CBD depending on the criteria used. Usually soft, ovoid, crumbling, and heavily pigmented, they are often associated with ampullary dysfunction.

Indications for CBD exploration include a palpable stone, ductal dilatation over 17 mm, a positive cholangiogram, and clinical cholangitis. Other indications are multiple small calculi, elevation of bilirubin and alkaline phosphatase, and a history of jaundice. Using the above criteria, a palpable stone yields a positive exploration in 95%, a positive cholangiogram in 70%, clinical cholangitis in 70%, and dilatation of more than 17 mm in 50%. The generally reported incidence of postexploration retained stones is 5% to 10%. Several reports suggest that combining cholangiography with choledochoscopy for all duct explorations reduces this incidence to near zero.

Choledochoduodenostomy

A common duct with a diameter larger than 1.4 cm containing multiple stones is an indication for choledo-

choduodenostomy (CDD). Providing the duct is at least this size and that a bypass of 2.5 cm is constructed, CDD is safer statistically than T-tube drainage and is associated with almost no long-term sequelae. Other indications for CDD include a benign distal stricture or a periampullary diverticulum. The morbidity and mortality of cholecystectomy are roughly doubled when common duct exploration with T-tube insertion is added. Late cholangitis following CDD when the criteria for duct and stoma size are met is less than 5%. Postoperative evaluation of a CDD should be done when needed with HIDA scanning or an upper GI series.

Surgical sphincteroplasty should be reserved for an impacted distal stone in a duct smaller than 1.4 cm diameter. The complication rate is reported to be substantially higher for a sphincteroplasty than for CDD. Postoperative pancreatitis has been reported to occur in as many as 5% of cases. Failure to remove an impacted distal stone has not been shown to result in any long-term sequelae and should not be considered a contraindication for CDD.

The management of retained stones has now progressed to a point where few patients require reoperation. Flushing of T-tubes with materials ranging from chloroform to heparin solution have been tried and discarded. Relaxation of the sphincter by local anesthetics and glucagon followed by vigorous flushing with saline may allow passage of stones up to 1 cm in size. Infusion with monoctanoin, a normal metabolic product of short-chain triglycerides, may be successful; and reports indicate successful dissolution of cholesterol stones in up to 60% of cases. Infusion may be started as early as 1 week postoperatively and continued for up to 4 weeks. Side effects are minimal and can generally be controlled by reducing the rate of infusion.

After waiting a minimum of 4 weeks, mechanical extraction via the T-tube tract can be accomplished successfully via fluoroscopically controlled basket retrieval or under direct visualization with a flexible choledochoscope in 90% of patients. If unsuccessful, endoscopic papillotomy usually allows retrieval or passage. Fewer than 5% of patients with retained CD stones ultimately require surgical removal.

Endoscopic Papillotomy

Endoscopic papillotomy is indicated in patients with postcholecystectomy choledocholithiasis or benign ampullary stenosis. Patients with symptomatic CD stones or cholangitis and an intact gallbladder who are poor risks for surgery have been treated with endoscopic papillotomy alone, with satisfactory results. Contraindications include hematologic disorders, stones larger than 2.5 cm in diameter, inability to locate the papilla, or the papilla located in a duodenal diverticulum. Biliary pancreatitis is not a contraindication. Although technically more difficult, patients have undergone successful papillotomy after a Billroth II gastrectomy. An international survey of a large number of patients undergoing papillotomy reported a 95% success rate, with an overall complication rate of 9%. The most frequent complication was hemorrhage, which generally is self-limited; 2% required laparotomy. An overall mortality rate of approximately 1% was reported. Retroperitoneal air occurs in 10% of patients but usually does not require laparotomy. Cholangitis, especially if the papillotomy is unsuccessful, mild pancreatitis, and free perforation are other reported complications.

OTHER BILIARY TRACT PROBLEMS AND MANAGEMENT

Benign Biliary Strictures

Benign strictures most commonly result from operative bile duct injuries. The reported frequency of duct injuries varies from 1 : 300 to 1 : 500 cholecystectomies. The rate of injury during laparoscopic cholecystectomy was initially higher but is now thought to be equivalent to that seen with open surgery. Injuries most commonly result from inadequate demonstration of ductal anatomy or hazardous attempts to control bleeding, often when the cystic artery has "escaped." Bile duct anomalies are a far less common cause.

When recognized initially, management varies depending on whether the injury is circumferential or partial. Partial injuries are repaired and stented with a T-tube inserted via a separate choledochotomy using a limb of the tube as a splint. Most authors recommend leaving the tube in place for a minimum of 1 month. A circumferential injury may be managed by primary anastomosis with fine interrupted absorbable sutures, provided an adequate length can be obtained for a tension-free anastomosis. A T-tube stent through a separate choledochotomy is used and left in place for at least 4 to 6 weeks. If any doubt exists about the adequacy of a primary reanastomosis, a biliary intestinal anastomosis to a Roux-en-Y jejunal limb is undertaken. In fact, there is mounting evidence that initial management of bile duct injuries with Roux-Y jejunal anastomosis yields superior results. The incidence of late stricture formation varies between 30% and 50% and usually occurs within 3 years.

Cholangitis

Cholangitis is an acute bacterial infection within the biliary tree. Malignant strictures are considered to be the main cause of cholangitis, followed by choledocholithiasis, benign duct strictures, and sclerosing cholangitis. Biliary duct obstruction with bacterial contamination of the bile may lead to a clinical presentation known as *Charcot's triad* (fever with chills, jaundice, abdominal pain). The entire *triad* is found in 19% of patients. The diagnosis is based on clinical findings, an elevated WBC count and LFTs, and ultrasonography and CT results. Endoscopic or percutaneous transhepatic cholangiography is required in most patients to define the biliary pathology. The results of blood cultures are positive in 30% of patients with cholangitis, helping to identify the causative organism and guiding antibiotic treatment.

Traditionally, aminoglycosides can provide adequate coverage of gram-negative bacteria, with addition of ampicillin for *Enterococcus* and metronidazole or clindamycin for anaerobic pathogens such as *Bacteroides fragilis*. Endoscopic biliary decompression or transhepatic external drainage is indicated for approximately 30% of patients not responding to initial supportive therapy. Both procedures are preferable to surgical decompression.

Primary Sclerosing Cholangitis

Most commonly associated with ulcerative colitis, sclerosing cholangitis may occur alone or, rarely, with other inflammatory bowel diseases. Although unproved, various bacterial or viral agents have been implicated. A characteristic pattern of diffuse ductal thickening, usually with intra- and extrahepatic involvement, is evident. Surgical decompression is rarely possible. A course of steroids is of limited value, and antibiotics only help to control secondary bacterial cholangitis. There is some evidence that colectomy may result in alleviation of sclerosing cholangitis in patients with ulcerative colitis, but the overall prognosis is poor, with 90% undergoing progressive liver failure and death within 5 years. Liver transplant may be necessary.

Papillary Stenosis

Benign ampullary dysfunction and stenosis are associated with a dilated, often thickened common duct. Typically, the patient has undergone cholecystectomy with a pain-free interval followed by the onset of right upper quadrant abdominal pain and abnormal liver chemistries. HIDA scan, ERCP, and transhepatic cholangiography are useful diagnostic tools.

Endoscopic papillotomy is the primary treatment of benign papillary stenosis. If surgery is needed, CDD is performed.

Biliary Tumors

Benign biliary tumors include adenomyomatosis (also called Rokitansky-Aschoff sinuses, adenomyoma, or cholecystitis cystica), polyps, and sessile mucosal tumors (adenomas and papillomas). They are most commonly diagnosed on an ultrasound scan or by oral cholecystography. Cholecystectomy is indicated if the tumors produce biliary symptoms or are associated with gallstones.

At cholecystectomy, 1% to 2% of patients, usually 65 years of age or older, are found to have carcinoma of the gallbladder. About 70% to 80% of gallbladder carcinomas occur in older patients with a long history of gallstone disease (usually more than 10 years). It is the most common biliary tract neoplasm and the fifth most common malignancy in the digestive tract. Porcelain gallbladder (calcification of the gallbladder wall), when seen on a plain abdominal film, should be considered a premalignant state and is an indication for cholecystectomy. In patients over age 50 with symptomatic gallstones for 10 years or more, the risk of carcinoma is as high as 6%. The female/male ratio is 3 : 1.

No diagnostic modality can reliably distinguish symptomatic chronic cholelithiasis from gallbladder carcinoma. Sonography and CT may suggest malignancy, but their accuracy is still questionable. Radical surgery, including wedge resection of adjacent liver and hepatic lobectomy, has been suggested but has not been shown to provide significant cures. The prognosis is poor: 80% of patients die within 1 year, and the 5-year survival is 2% to 5%.

Bile Duct Carcinoma

Bile duct carcinoma, a relatively rare tumor, is occasionally polypoid but more often scirrhous, infiltrating, and generally hypocellular. There is a slightly increased incidence of bile duct carcinoma in association with gallstones. The proximal common hepatic duct, including the hilum and hepatic ducts (Klatskin's tumor), accounts for 40% to 50% of these tumors. *En bloc* resection with liver resection is occasionally possible. Palliation with some form of stenting, usually a T-tube, is generally undertaken. Although these tumors are usually fatal by 12 to 24 months, distant metastases are rare; and prolonged benefit may be obtained by intubation.

Tumors of the mid and distal bile ducts are less common. Mid-duct tumors can occasionally be resected with reconstruction via Roux-en-Y hepatojejunostomy. Distal bile duct tumors require pancreaticoduodenectomy (Whipple resection), after which a 20% to 30% five-year survival can be attained.

Biliary Cysts

Choledochal cysts are usually seen in children, although they do appear in adults. The symptom complex consists of abdominal pain, jaundice, and a palpable abdominal mass. Ultrasonography used as the primary diagnostic modality can outline the cyst in most cases. Additional helpful data are obtained from CT, transhepatic cholangiography, and ERCP. Complications include infection, rupture (rare), and malignant degeneration.

Bile duct malignancy in association with choledochal cysts is 20 times more common than malignancy in the general population and is almost uniformly fatal. Traditionally, Roux-en-Y bypass was the preferred treatment because resection was considered too risky, but an awareness of the increased risk of malignancy combined with better surgical techniques has led most recent authors to recommend resection of the cyst with Roux-en-Y reconstruction.

Biliary Fistulas

External biliary fistulas most commonly occur after biliary tract surgery. They are easily documented with

HIDA scanning. Anatomic delineation should be accomplished with either ERCP, transhepatic cholangiography, or fistulography. These procedures determine the presence or absence of distal obstruction. If no distal obstruction is seen, the fistulas close with local control and adequate nutrition. Uncontrollable sepsis or distal obstruction (e.g., stone, stricture) require surgical intervention.

An internal bile leak following laparoscopic cholecystectomy is suspected when patients develop fever, pain, and abnormal liver chemistries, usually within 24 hours of surgery. Initial confirmation with a HIDA scan should be followed by ERCP with stenting. If a leaking cystic duct is the cause, no further intervention may be needed. Additional surgery is usually not needed. Cholecystenteric fistulas from gallstones occur to the duodenum and less commonly to the stomach, colon, or small intestine. Gallstone ileus may result from obstruction at the ligament of Treitz, terminal ileum (most common), or sigmoid colon. Most patients with cholecystenteric fistulas have air in the biliary tree. Obstructing stones are at least 2.5 cm in diameter. In the United States gallstone ileus comprises 2% of mechanical intestinal obstruction.

It is still controversial as to whether a cholecystectomy should be undertaken at the time of laparotomy for stone extraction in the presence of gallstone ileus. There is general agreement, however, that if another large stone is present in the gallbladder, the stone must at least be removed.

Hemobilia

Hemorrhage through the biliary tract is most commonly due to blunt or penetrating trauma. Ascarides is common in the Orient but rare in the West. Gallstone disease, primary biliary tract malignancies, true or false intrahepatic aneurysms, or iatrogenic causes (percutaneous transhepatic cholangiography or removal of stones high in the biliary tree) are reported causes of hemobilia. The most common presenting symptom is melena followed by colicky pain, anemia, hematemesis, jaundice, shock, and fever, in that order. The diagnosis is established by endoscopic visualization of blood from the ampulla, and the site is best confirmed by angiography.

Treatment consists of embolization by arteriographic techniques or suture of false aneurysms or traumatic

tears. Cholecystectomy should be performed when the gallbladder is found to be the source of bleeding. In most instances, hepatic artery ligation with intrahepatic suture, if needed, can control the bleeding. Hepatic resection is rarely needed.

QUESTIONS

1. Which of the following is true?
   a. The cystic duct, common hepatic duct, and cystic artery form the triangle of Calot.
   b. The venous drainage of the gallbladder is directly to the portal vein via small venous plexuses.
   c. In most cases the hepatic artery passes cephalad within the hepatoduodenal ligament to the right of the bile duct and anterior to the portal vein.
   d. In 20% of patients the cystic artery originates from the left or common hepatic artery.
   e. The falciform ligament defines the anatomic right and left hepatic lobes.
2. Acute cholecystitis secondary to cystic duct obstruction is best diagnosed by:
   a. Ultrasonography.
   b. Oral cholecystography.
   c. Intravenous cholangiography.
   d. HIDA scanning.
   e. Elevated direct plasma bilirubin.
3. The disease most often associated with primary sclerosing cholangitis is:
   a. Crohn's disease
   b. Diabetes mellitus
   c. Rheumatoid arthritis
   d. Ulcerative colitis
   e. Chronic pancreatitis
4. The most common site of biliary tract malignancy is the:
   a. Confluence of hepatic ducts.
   b. Common hepatic duct.
   c. Gallbladder.
   d. Common bile duct.
   e. Retroduodenal portion of the common bile duct.
5. Patency of external and internal biliary fistulas is preferably documented by:
   a. Fistulography.
   b. ERCP.
   c. Intravenous cholangiography.
   d. ^{99m}Tc Iminodiacetic acid scan.
   e. Percutaneous transhepatic cholangiography.

6. All of these stimulate bile flow, *except:*
   a. Secretin.
   b. Cholecystokinin.
   c. Bile salts.
   d. Vagal stimulation.
   e. Splanchnic stimulation.

7. Elimination of retained common duct stones via T-tubes has been successful using all of these, *except:*
   a. Bile acids.
   b. Ureteral basket.
   c. Glucagon infusion.
   d. Heparin infusion.
   e. Monooctanoin infusion.

8. The primary screening test for the initial evaluation of obstructive jaundice is:
   a. ERCP.
   b. CT scan.
   c. HIDA.
   d. Ultrasonography.
   e. Intravenous cholangiography.

9. An increased incidence of cholelithiasis may be associated with which of the following:
   a. Sickle cell anemia.
   b. Chemotherapy.
   c. Prosthetic valve replacement.
   d. Hereditary spherocytosis.
   e. All of the above.

10. A 65-year-old patient presents with jaundice of 2 weeks' duration, with no history of significant abdominal pain. Ultrasonography revealed a markedly distended gallbladder. The most likely diagnosis is:
    a. Acute cholecystitis.
    b. Common bile duct obstruction from a stone.
    c. Cancer of the head of the pancreas.
    d. Common bile duct obstruction from pancreatitis.
    e. Peptic ulcer penetrating to the retroduodenal portion of the CBD.

SELECTED REFERENCES

Adamek HE, Sorg S, Bachor OA, Riemann JF. Symptoms of post-extracorporeal shock wave lithotripsy: long-term analysis of gallstone patients before and after successful shock wave lithotripsy. *Am J Gastroenterol* 1995;90:1125–1129.

Andrews RT, Bova DA. Visualization of a postoperative bile leak during cholescintigraphy: morphine augmentation prevents a false-negative study. *Clin Nucl Med* 1995;20:642–643.

Bass EB, Pitt HA, Lillemoe KD. Cost-effectiveness of laparoscopic cholecystectomy versus open cholecystectomy. *Am J Surg* 1993;165:466–471.

Carey MC. Pathogenesis of gallstones. *Am J Surg* 1993;165:410.

Dawson SL, Mueller PR. Interventional radiology in the management of bile duct injuries. *Surg Clin North Am* 1994;74:865–874.

Farges O, Malassagne B, Sebagh M, Bismuth H. Primary sclerosing cholangitis: liver transplantation or biliary surgery. *Surgery* 1995;117:146–155.

Go PM, Stolk MF, Obertop H, et al. Symptomatic gallbladder stones: cost-effectiveness of treatment with extracorporeal shock-wave lithotripsy, conventional and laparoscopic cholecystectomy. *Surg Endosc* 1995;9:37–41.

Graham SM, Flowers JL, Schweitzer E, Bartlett ST, Imbembo AL. The utility of prophylactic cholecystectomy in transplant candidates. *Am J Surg* 1995;169:44–49.

Joseph VT. Surgical techniques and long-term results in the treatment of choledochal cyst. *J Pediatr Surg* 1990;25:782–787.

Lee YM, Kaplan MM. Primary sclerosing cholangitis. *N Engl J Med* 1995;332:924–933.

Lipsett PA, Pitt HA. Acute cholangitis. *Surg Clin North Am* 1990;70:1297.

Liu CL, Lo CM, Fan ST. Acute biliary pancreatitis: diagnosis and management. *World J Surg* 1997;21:149–154.

McDonald ML, Farnell MB, Nagorney DM, Ilstrup DM, Kutch JM. Benign biliary strictures: repair and outcome with a contemporary approach. *Surgery* 1995;118:582–590.

Meyers WC. What's new in gastrointestinal and hepatobiliary surgery. *J Am Coll Surg* 1996;182:100–106.

Moser AJ, Abedin MZ, Cates JA, Giurgiu DI, Karam JA, Roslyn JJ. Converting gallbladder absorption to secretin: the role of intracellular calcium. *Surgery* 1996;119:410–416.

NIH consensus conference statement of gallstones and laparoscopic cholecystectomy. *Am J Surg* 1993;165:390.

Pereira SP, Hussaini SH, Kennedy C, Dowling RH. Gallbladder stone recurrence after medical treatment: do gallstones recur true to type? *Diagn Dis Sci* 1995;40:2568–2575.

Reding R, Buard J-L, Lebeau G, Launois B. Surgical management of 552 carcinomas of the extrahepatic bile ducts (gallbladder and periampullary tumors excluded). *Ann Surg* 1991;213:21–25.

Ribeiro LC, Correia AP, Contente LF, de Moura MC. An aggressive protocol of ESWL and dissolution therapy of gallbladder stones. *Hepatogastroenterology* 1995;42:259–264.

Rossi RL, Tsao JI. Biliary reconstruction. *Surg Clin North Am* 1994;74:825–841.

Russell JC, Walsh SJ, Mattie AS, Lynch JT. Bile duct injuries, 1989–1993: a statewide experience; Connecticut Cholecystectomy Registry. *Arch Surg* 1996;131:382–388.

Scheeres DE, Simon I, Ponsky JL. Endoscopic retrograde cholangiopancreatography in a general surgery practice. *Am Surg* 1990;56:185–191.

Tang E, Stain SC, Tang G, Fores E, Berne TV. Timing of laparoscopic surgery in gallstone pancreatitis. *Arch Surg* 1995;130:496–499.

Terblanche J, Worthley CS, Krige JEK. High or low hepatico-jejunostomy for bile duct strictures? *Surgery* 1990;108:828–834.

Tompkins RK, Saunders K, Roslyn JJ, Longmire WP. Changing patterns in diagnosis and management of bile duct cancer. *Ann Surg* 1990;211:614–621.

Tudyka J, Wechsler JG, Kratzer W, et al. Gallstone recurrence after successful dissolution therapy. *Dig Dis Sci* 1996;41:235–241.

Van Erpecum KJ, Portincasa P, Eckardt E, Go PM, VanBerge-Henegouwen GP, Groen AK. Ursodeoxycholic acid reduces protein levels and nucleation-promoting activity in human gallbladder bile. *Gastroenterology* 1996;110:1225–1237.

6

Aspects of Liver Surgery

W. John B. Hodgson and Tito Gorski

SURGICAL MILESTONES

As early as 600 AD Aeginata is said to have cauterized injured protruding liver. More than 1,000 years later Beata in 1716 excised a portion of protruding liver in a madman. More than 100 years after that, in 1846, McPherson excised traumatically eviscerated chunks of liver, and some of his patients lived. The next step forward was an approach to control a pedicle containing the vessels, usually by a mass ligature or large clamp, left in place until thrombosis occurred. The offending portion of liver could then be cut off. This idea of developing a pedicle was used by Luis unsuccessfully, by Langenbuch successfully, and by Keen at the end of the nineteenth century in more than 100 cases. It is the basis of segmental resection today, which involves careful control of vessels.

At the beginning of the twentieth century various sutures were developed for mass ligation of liver tissue, which did not require any anatomic knowledge and were useful only to a point. They certainly helped delay the development of controlled liver surgery, and I do not advise their use.

The anatomic approach was used by Pringle, who controlled inflow to the liver by clamping the porta hepatis. Understanding of the bilaterality of the liver began during the 1930s and culminated in the description of surgical segmental anatomy in 1957 by Couinaud.

Methods of getting through the liver parenchyma to find the intrahepatic vessels have included the thumb nail, scalpel handle, finger and scalpel handle, finger and thumb, Bovie, Cavitron ultrasonic surgical aspirator (CUSA), Nd-Yag laser, and water jet. According to Little, the CUSA appears to be the most effective, safest, and least bloody. Methods of identifying intrahepatic anatomy, used particularly by the European and Japanese, involve intraoperative ultrasonography and sometimes needle-stick and dye injection directly into portal venous branches.

Honjo and Araki from Japan reported preliminary hilar dissection in 1955 but probably operated on their patient before Quattlebaum, who reported the same technique in 1953. In 1957 Goldsmith and Woodburne described the left medial lobe, and in 1975 Starzl reported on right trisegmentectomy and capped it in 1982 with a description of left trisegmentectomy.

Increasingly, Couinaud's "segmental anatomy" has dominated liver surgery, and liver-sparing surgery has gained in importance. On the other hand, liver surgery training programs in transplantation units emphasize control of hepatic vascular inflow and outflow. Complete vascular occlusion, at a physiologic cost, sets the stage for liver resection without blood transfusion, and there is some evidence that this protocol enhances patient survival after tumor resection.

ANATOMY

Hepatic Ligaments

The superior surface of the liver can be seen through a bilateral subcostal incision. It is supported by the falciform ligament, which separates the left medial and lateral lobes. It is also supported by the right and left coronary ligaments. A line can be drawn across the smooth surface of the liver from the fundus of the gallbladder back to the point at which the falciform ligament splits into right and left coronary ligaments: this line separates the right and left lobes of the liver.

The first step during liver surgery is to divide the falciform ligament all the way back to the suprahepatic cava, which drops the liver away from the diaphragm. Next, the appropriate coronary ligament is divided to mobilize the liver further. On the left, the gastrohepatic ligament (lesser omentum) must also be divided. Care must be taken dividing the left superior coronary ligament, as it is easy to enter the left hepatic vein. On the right, the coronary ligament is extremely posterior, and the liver sometimes must be pulled hard to the left to expose it. I usually start division at the falciform ligament and proceed laterally. Note that the posterior hepatocaval veins may be encountered dividing the inferior right coronary leaf.

Hepatic Veins

After dividing the ligaments, the liver can be rotated forward to expose the cava and hepatic veins. These hepatic veins are major anatomic landmarks. For example, the middle hepatic vein runs from the fundus of the gallbladder obliquely back to the cava, marking the separation of liver into right and left lobes.

Blood Supply

The next step is to identify the foramen of Winslow and pass the index finger through to the lesser sac. This sac is opened, and a 0.5 in. Penrose drain is passed from left to right. This drain can be tightened as necessary to perform a Pringle maneuver. Stripping peritoneum from the porta hepatis reveals, from right to left, in their most common configuration, the common bile duct, hepatic artery, and portal vein. If the decision has been made to perform a formal lobectomy (right or left) at this stage, it is often helpful to first take down the gallbladder to act as

an anatomic marker. It is also helpful in order to apply traction to demonstrate the portal vein bifurcation, which is posterior to the artery. The right hepatic artery is usually posterior to the common hepatic duct. Incidentally, the right portal vein branch is often horizontal, peeking out from behind Hartman's pouch, whereas the left portal vein branch is often vertical. Individual branches should always be identified before ligation and division.

Inside the liver parenchyma the hepatic arterial branches, portal venous branches, and bile ducts are deep and closely applied to each other. On the other hand, during division of the parenchyma many of the vessels initially encountered are branches of the hepatic vein. Only as the main trunks are approached do these vessels become posterior.

Arterial Supply

It is a myth that hepatic arteries are end-arteries. Bengmark and Rosengren demonstrated as long ago as 1970 that intrahepatic collaterals open up to maintain perfusion of the whole liver if the right or left hepatic artery is occluded. However, there is some evidence that floxuridine infusion via these collaterals is not as effective as direct arterial infusion, perhaps indicating inadequate flow via collaterals. It must be remembered that when death occurs after hepatic artery ligation it is always associated with hypotension and hypovolemia, and there is minimal mortality associated with hepatic artery ligation alone.

The common hepatic artery usually originates from the celiac axis; and after giving rise to the gastroduodenal artery it becomes the hepatic artery proper, which then divides into right and left branches in the hepaticoduodenal ligament. This situation is seen in 50% to 60% of cases. In 12% to 25% of cases the right hepatic artery originates from the superior mesenteric artery; in 17% there is an anomalous right hepatic artery; and in 10% the left hepatic artery originates from the left gastric artery. An accessory left hepatic artery rises from the left gastric artery in 8%. Patient may therefore vary depending on whether the blood supply is dominated by the celiac axis, the superior mesentery artery, or both.

Segmental Anatomy

Diagrammatically, the liver can be divided vertically by the hepatic veins into the right, middle, and left scissura. It is divided at the transverse plane by branches of the portal vein. This division allows a useful surgical separation into segments. Because the caudate lobe is excluded by this system, it is called segment I. The left hepatic vein splits the left lateral segment into II and III. The left medial lobe lies between the left hepatic and middle hepatic veins and is segment IV. The part above the left portal vein is IV(a) and the part below IV(b). The remaining 60% of the hepatic volume is divided by the transversely lying right portal vein and right hepatic vein into segment V inferomedially; VI inferolaterally; VII, the posterosuperolateral part of the dome of the right lobe; and VIII, the supramedial portion. This anatomic division assumes increasing importance as liver-sparing procedures are done.

Hepatic Resection

After mobilizing the liver for a *formal right lobectomy,* the right hepatic duct, artery, and right portal vein branch are ligated and divided, resulting in an avascular zone from the right of the gallbladder fossa. This surface of the liver is then scored about 1 in. to the right of this zone with the Bovie on high power, and the liver parenchyma is entered. Standing on the patient's right side with the left hand supporting the right lobe, and using the CUSA with the right hand, the parenchyma is aspirated off the intrahepatic vessels. The assistant, on the patient's left, uses a right-angle clamp to secure the exposed vessels, which are then tied or clipped (or both) and divided. Progress is rapid and relatively bloodless, with only about 600 ml of blood lost per case. The open surface of the liver is left open, as it is only necessary to place one or two Jackson-Pratt drains.

Right trisegmentectomy is similar to formal right lobectomy except that the plane of division is moved toward the left of the liver, next to the falciform ligament. The right hepatic duct is divided, which opens the way to the umbilical fissure, which is not as thick as the liver itself. At its base, the right portal vein and right hepatic artery are secured and divided. The caudate may or may not be removed at this point. Finally, the right hepatic vein and middle hepatic vein are removed; a vascular stapler may be of use here.

Left trisegmentectomy involves removing segments V and VIII in addition to the entire left lobe. The plane is developed anterior to the point of transection of the left hepatic vein, through the middle hepatic vein, and

anterior to the right hepatic vein. This plane emerges near the base and at right angles to the gallbladder bed.

Inferior transverse hepatectomy is an *en bloc* resection of segments IVB, V, and VI. Segment III can also be included. Ultrasonic fragmentation greatly facilitates this procedure, allowing dissection in the transverse plane. Care is taken to preserve the posterior and superior portal vein branches so as not to compromise the remaining segments.

Isolated resection of the caudate lobe remains a challenge. Left, right, and central approaches can be used. The approach through "bloody gulch" is essentially direct removal of the caudate from the cava, finishing with parenchymal division to separate it from the right hepatic lobe. It may be safer to use cryotherapy in these cases.

Direct approaches are used for *segmental resection* and sometimes *lobectomy.* So long as the liver is mobilized and fully controlled, this approach saves time. Careful dissection with an ultrasonic scalpel allows accurate delineation of surgical anatomy, but prior anatomic knowledge is important. Use of intraoperative ultrasonography not only helps define anatomy, it also may change the clinical management of patients undergoing hepatic resection for malignancy.

Hepatic Physiology

The liver is the only organ in the body with a double blood supply. The hepatic artery carries oxygenated blood and accounts for 25% of the hepatic blood flow. The portal vein accounts for 75% of hepatic blood flow and carries hepatic regeneration factors from the splenic bed. These factors include glucagon and insulin and are thought to enhance the effects of other nitogens. Epidermal growth factor (EGF) is heavily taken up by the periportal areas in the lobule where regeneration is pronounced. DNA synthesis is started within 18 hours of resection but appears to require the presence of transforming growth factor alpha (TGFα), which is generated in the liver. Hepatocyte growth factor (HGF) is similar to hepatopoietin A and is probably generated in nonparenchymal cells. When regeneration is complete, the process is shut down by a combination of chalones, locally produced inhibitors of growth. TGFβ1 may stimulate or inhibit proliferation depending on the circumstances and is normally present at low levels, exerting an inhibitory effect; it appears to require being overcome by heparin-binding growth factor I for regeneration to occur. Cytokines released from endothelial cells or macrophages also appear capable of inhibiting hepatocyte proliferation.

Nonparenchymal cells include the reticular endothelial system. The latter consists of the phagocytic Kupffer cells and endothelial cells.

Coagulation Factors

Coagulopathy may occur immediately after hepatic resection secondary to the inability of the liver to synthesize prothrombin. Decreases in growth factor V (proaccelerin, Christmas factor, factor VII), proconvertin, fibrinogen, and platelets have been noted in hepatic disease. Postsurgical management with fibrinogen for 2 to 4 days is sometimes required. A platelet count of less than 100,000/mm³ is a bad prognostic sign, and a falling platelet count may require correction by platelet transfusion. With obstructive jaundice, reduction of bile results in decreased absorption of vitamin K.

Liver Function Tests

Liver function tests give an overall idea of hepatic function and some indication of liver pathology. Other tests are required, however, to make diagnoses.

Serum albumin may fall rapidly after extensive liver resection, which may lead to anasarca. I have found that intravenous albumin given in sufficient quantities to maintain the serum albumin close to 3 g/dL helps obviate these effects. Serum protein is also correlated to the extent of liver failure but not as closely as albumin. Decreased serum cholesterol levels reflect parenchymal disease or hepatic failure, as synthesis, esterification, and excretion of cholesterol is turned off. The liver is also responsible for glyconeogenesis, glucagon storage, glycogenolysis, and conversion of galactose to glucose. I have not generally found that hypoglycemia has been a problem after liver surgery.

Liver enzymes rise in response to acute cellular damage, such as after a prolonged warm ischemia time following the Pringle maneuver during resection. Alkaline phosphatase measures the patency of bile channels and is highest with distal obstruction. These tests are poor indicators of tumor growth, as they generally become abnormal only when the tumor is large or extensive.

Measurement of dye excretion is particularly useful for evaluating severely cirrhotic livers for suitability of resection. Sulfobromophthalein is only 80% cleared by the liver (the rest is cleared extrahepatically), but indocyanine green and rose bengal are more completely cleared and hence more accurate.

EVALUATION OF LIVER MASS

Liver chemistries are generally not helpful unless the mass is large or the liver diseased. Tumor markers such as α-fetoprotein (AFP) and carcinoembryonic antigen (CEA) can be helpful for suggesting primary or metastatic disease if positive and if their levels rise on repeated testing. CA 19-9 may have a place in detecting pancreatic or ovarian metastases.

Imaging techniques vary depending on the information required. Generally, nucleotide scanning is performed using technetium sulfur colloid and has a 65% accuracy for detecting focal defects. In good hands ultrasonography can detect 95% of tumors. CT scanning is too expensive to be used as a screening technique, but when the index of suspicion is high it can detect tumors as small as 8 mm. Magnetic resonance imaging (MRI) is more expensive and as accurate as CT scanning. It can be particularly helpful for detailing hepatic anatomy when questionable results are obtained on CT scans. Angiography can diagnose various tumors, such as follicular nodular hyperplasia, adenoma, and cavernous hemangioma. Used in combination with CT, during the portal phase after superior mesenteric artery injection (CTAP) tumors as small as 5 mm can be detected. Spiral CT is less cumbersome and is achieving similar results.

Fine-needle aspiration biopsy (FNAB) can give close to 100% accuracy for posthepatic and postnecrotic cirrhosis but may miss small, nodular lesions. It is particularly useful during laparoscopic examination of the liver.

TRAUMA

As a rule, most general surgeons are first presented with liver surgery because of trauma. The liver is the most frequently injured organ with abdominal trauma, but hepatic injuries are often associated with other injuries and therefore careful initial evaluation of the patient is important. An airway must be established, the cervical spine checked, central lines set up, and blood given if required.

Management of the liver injury is expectant or invasive, depending on the degree of liver injury. The latter has been classified in various ways. I believe that the simpler the classification, the better it is. For example, Moore in 1988 defined *class I* injury as capsular avulsion or parenchymal fracture less than 1 cm deep with no active bleeding. *Class II* includes parenchymal fractures 1 to 3 cm deep, peripheral penetrating wounds, or subcapsular hematomas less than 10 cm in diameter. *Class III* injuries include deep penetrating wounds and stellate parenchymal tears, both with active bleeding. This class also includes nonexpanding subcapsular hematomas larger than 10 cm. With *class IV* injuries the parenchymal destruction is severe enough to involve major vascular inflow, and with *class V* it is worse because there is major venous outflow involvement.

Knudson, in 1990, refined this classification. *Class I* was the same. In *class II* the subcapsular hematoma covers 10% to 50% of the surface area, and there may be active bleeding of a laceration. In *class III* the subcapsular hematoma covers more than 50% of the surface area or is expanding or ruptured. The stellate injury is larger than 2 cm or expanding. *Class IV* involves parenchymal rupture. *Class V* also includes major outflow injury as massive parenchymal disruption. Note that there is also a *class VI,* which indicates hepatic avulsion and is invariably fatal.

For a patient to be stable, there must be stable blood pressure, pulse, and respiration. There should be no peritoneal signs. Blood replacement should be minimal and not recurrent. An immediate CT scan should not show free fluid; but if a small amount is seen, selective arterial embolization may effectively stop bleeding. Laparoscopy can be used to ascertain whether the bleeding has stopped. The patient should be kept on bed rest for 7 to 10 days and a repeat CT scan done (which probably looks the same if there is extensive subcapsular hemorrhage). In fact, it can appear the same for weeks.

To reach the liver in the unstable patient, a bilateral subcostal incision is used—if necessary as an adjunct to a midline incision—and the liver is mobilized as quickly as possible by an experienced team to expose the injured area. Note that even if there is a concurrent injury elsewhere, other than perhaps a severe neurologic injury, the liver takes precedence: The liver produces coagulation factors and if severely injured ceases to do so. In such cases irreversible disseminated intravascular coagulation results, leading to the death of the patient.

With the abdomen opened and the liver fully exposed, sutures can be used to close the injured area completely, leaving no deadspace, in class II patients.

For class II, III, IV, and sometimes class V patients packing can be lifesaving, but bleeding should be expected to recur with class IV and V injuries. It is therefore advisable to transfer patients to a liver center for subsequent definitive management. In Japan, good results have been obtained with hepatectomy, either as a completion procedure in unstable patients or as a formal lobectomy in stabilized patients.

Nonetheless, certain steps can be taken as a routine. (a) Packs are placed in both upper quadrants and the liver firmly grasped or squeezed posteriorly. (b) After aspirating the blood and confirming the liver injury, a Pringle maneuver is done using a 0.5-in. Penrose drain. (c) The falciform ligament is divided backward until it splits over the cava. (d) The coronary ligament is divided, usually on the right, so the surgeon can hold the liver firmly in two hands. The situation can then be assessed.

For class III injuries débridement of devitalized tissue is the main focus. For class IV injuries the hepatic artery can be embolized or ligated as distally as possible but as proximal as necessary. The portal vein is controlled and repaired if possible. The major right or left portal vein branch can be ligated without resecting the appropriate lobe of the liver in a difficult situation. It is preferable, however, to ligate more distal branches. Nonetheless, major portal venous injury is associated with a mortality as high as 70%. For class V injuries, full mobilization of the liver can expose the cava in minutes and it can be clamped above and below the liver as repairs are carried out. Right and left hepatic veins can be sutured if they can be seen, but mortality varies from 50% to 100%. Packing is probably more likely to save a life than is caval shunting because it gives the trauma team time to stabilize the patient for 24 hours or so before another attempt is made to control bleeding.

LIVER METASTASIS

In the United States metastases from colon cancer are the most frequently seen liver tumors, with about 50,000 new cases annually. To identify the resectable cases (estimated to be about 12,000 annually) careful follow-up using markers and imaging techniques is required. A rising CEA level is the most useful marker. By the time liver chemistries, such as alkaline phosphatase, become abnormal, it is usually too late. Although nucleotide scanning and ultrasound scanning can give useful information, currently with a rising CEA titer a CT scan is normally done. A spiral CT scan gives the most information, with good views of the portal and hepatic veins and their relation to the tumor; it may determine whether the tumor is resectable. This scan rivals CTAP (in which CT is performed in combination with arteriography—the scan performed during the portal phase of a superior mesenteric artery dye injection) for detecting small tumors. MRI is also increasingly accurate but is not as readily available.

If at the time of colonic resection a peripherally placed synchronous metastasis is seen, it should be removed immediately. However, if there is evidence of a large or deep-seated lesion, resection is delayed 6 weeks or so for the workup to be completed. Cady and his colleagues were particularly concerned with the biology of the tumor and believed that a rapidly growing tumor will rapidly recur even after successful resection. Conversely, a slowly growing tumor is more likely to have a successful outcome after resection. Patients with a CEA level of less than 200 ng/mL, 1-cm surgical margins, and less than 1,000 g of liver tissue removed have an estimated 5-year survival of more than 50%. In other words, patients with small tumors that are detected early do best, so it is incumbent on us to remain vigilant, even after resecting all other known tumors. Less certain, because of the small number of patients reported, are the effects of resecting metastatic disease from other primaries. There are increasing number of anecdotal cases of successful results after resecting metastases from other areas of the GI tract and, for example, the breast, or after resecting sarcomas, endocrine tumors, and even melanomas.

Major resection is now being done routinely with less than 1 liter of blood loss, particularly when the CUSA is used. Decreased blood use seems to have a direct association with increased survival. Furthermore, few patients develop abscesses or bile leaks with the CUSA technique, so the overall morbidity is about 5% to 10%. Almost no patients die on the operating table. The 30-day mortality is less than 4%, and the deaths are usually due to extrahepatic causes or irreversible liver failure after massive resection. In the days when thoracoabdominal incisions were used, morbidity was 100%, blood loss was on the order of 5 liters per case, postoperative infection rates were 22%, and respiratory complications occurred in 15%. We have come a long way.

Long-term follow-up indicates that survival of patients with four or fewer metastases, even if bilateral, is the same as for patients with one metastasis. Some authors, including ourselves, did not find any statistical difference in survival between patients where the original colon cancer was Dukes' B or C. Other authors found that Dukes' B patients did better. The median survival in our patients was 56 months, and the actuarial survival rate was 35% at 5 years.

When resection is not possible, other methods can be considered, such as embolization, portal vein branch ligation, intraarterial chemotherapy, cryotherapy, brachytherapy, and various combinations of systemic chemotherapy. Cryotherapy, in particular, seems to be gaining ground. Performed with intraoperative ultrasonography to ascertain if the ice ball is encircling the tumor, 5-year survival rates of 20% are possible. To render the patient disease-free with cryosurgery, temperatures must be below ⁻20°C throughout the tumor. Problems remain, with the inability to freeze tumors completely in close proximity to major vessels such as the portal vein and hepatic veins. Care must be taken with tumors near the portal vein because the larger branches of the biliary tree may be destroyed in the process.

HEPATOCELLULAR CARCINOMA

Primary carcinoma of the liver is not a common disease in America, with only about 16,000 new cases annually; equal numbers of men and women are affected. Risk factors include hepatitis B infection, which is so important to the surgeon that vaccination is recommended. Those with hepatitis B infection who also have chronic active hepatitis are at greatest risk. In the United States alcoholic cirrhosis is an important factor as well. Less important in the American experience is kwashiorkor, *Clonorchis sinensis* infection, and aflatoxins from grains spoiled by *Aspergillus flavus*.

The clinical presentation is often heralded by a sudden deterioration in the patient's usual state of health, the result of a rapid decline of liver function. The median time from diagnosis to death is only about 2 months. Noncirrhotic patients (36% to 46%) have a more subtle presentation; for example, right upper quadrant pain, Budd-Chiari syndrome, jaundice, or distal metastases to the lungs or bones may be the first presentation.

Hepatocellular carcinoma (HCC) is one of the tumors most commonly associated with remote hormonal and hematologic syndromes. HCC may be multicentric in cirrhotic patients and impossible to identify except by microscopy. Patients in high-risk groups can be monitored with serum AFP levels. There is about a 2-year window from the time of first detection of a rise in AFP to over 500 ng/mL before these tumors become unresectable, which tends to occur when they are more than 5 cm in diameter. The diagnosis is strongly suspected if there is portal vein or hepatic vein invasion; neovascularity is common, and a pronounced tumor stain is seen 70% of the time during angiography. The lesion can be hypodense on CT scans without contrast. Technetium scanning shows a photopenic lesion.

Chemotherapy with doxorubicin (Adriamycin) has a response rate of 25%, but the survival rate in this group is only about 7 to 9 months. Resection is the treatment of choice usually done as segmentectomies. Survival appears to depend on the tumor margin and varies from Japan to America, perhaps because different patient groups were being compared. Of all factors, however, vascular invasion, whether lymphatic, arterial, or portal, seems to be the most important predictor of survival. Mortality, which varies between 2% and 15%, rises as more liver is resected. The 3-year survival varies between 26% and 52%. American patients are highly selected. The 5-year survival for tumors up to 5 cm has been reported to be as high as 75%, but it drops to 35% if the tumor is larger than 5 cm. When the tumor size is less than 3 cm, transplantation results in a 3-year survival of 83%, equal to that of patients with no tumors. Other treatment options include percutaneous alcohol injection for small tumors, with results equivalent to those seen with resection. Arterial chemoembolization for unresectable HCC appears to provide some extension of survival, but this is difficult to gauge as some patients who did not undergo resection or other treatment can survive for as long as 3 years. Using iodized oil (selectively retained by HCC) as a carrying agent for chemotherapy may hold some promise.

The fibrolamellar variant is important. It occurs in young people, and risky procedures are justified for resecting these large tumors. The female/male incidence ratio is 4 : 3. The presentation is usually dull right upper quadrant pain, and persistent fatigue often leads to a full workup. The tumor appears to be somewhat nodular and may have a central stellate scar. Biopsy may falsely appear to be benign. Although the CEA level is only sometimes elevated, the presence of neurotensin in the serum is diagnostic. There is also a high vitamin B_{12}-

binding capacity. The resectability rate of these tumors is 49%, with a median survival of 50 months; the 5-year survival is 45%. In the absence of lymph node metastases, for solitary tumors the 5-year survival can be as high as 66.7%. Results after transplantation are similar to those in patients with common HCC.

BENIGN TUMORS

Follicular nodular hyperplasia (FNH) is a rare non-neoplastic epithelial tumor often found incidentally during surgical exploration. It is often nodular, and about 20% are pedunculated. Another 20% are multiple. They are usually 4 to 7 cm in diameter but can be as large as 18 cm. On CT scans there may be a central stellate scar (but this is a common finding with many liver tumors). Blood vessels are large at the periphery and radiate like spokes of a wheel. About 35% of FNH tumors take up technetium and so give a normal radionucleotide scan. Biopsy shows mixed hepatocytes, Kupffer cells, and biliary radicals. Resection is rarely necessary.

On the other hand, there is a 10% chance that adenomas may rupture, and they can be difficult to differentiate from HCC. They may be associated with use of steroids or birth control pills or with pregnancy; they are commonest in women. Although they may have a central stellate scar on the CT scan, they show up on radionucleotide scanning as a cold area.

If the adenoma ruptures, the patient may present in shock. The appropriate hepatic arterial branch is then ligated. If invasive angiography is available, occlusion coils can be placed selectively using the Seldinger percutaneous puncture technique. Six weeks later the tumor can be resected. A nonruptured adenoma should always be resected because of the danger of HCC foci. The tumor appears as a soft, pink mass and can be removed using a liver-sparing technique.

Multiple adenomas (more than eight) cannot be resected. They are usually associated with taking oral contraception which should be withdrawn. Spontaneous regression may then occur.

Regenerative nodules should not be resected but biopsied, if necessary, under direct vision. On radionucleotide scanning these tumors show disordered uptake; but the rest of the liver is usually severely cirrhotic, which also would show disordered uptake. HCC appears as a cold area.

Hemangiomas are frequently found incidentally on ultrasound scanning. They are usually asymptomatic and hence do not need treatment. Their size is variable. A regular or amorphous calcification is sometimes seen on scanning. Dynamic CT scanning shows a centripetally enhancing lesion that appears to shrink and finally becomes isodense with the hepatic parenchyma. Blood lakes, slow to clear, may be seen on angiography.

Giant hemangiomas can cause thrombocytopenia and pain due to necrosis when eddies are set up so ischemic areas result. These tumors also cause pressure symptoms. They can be resected, which is difficult, or they can be devascularized by ligation of the hepatic arterial branch and sometimes the portal vein branch. Enucleation done with inflow exclusion has been shown to be a safe and technically sound procedure especially with the ultrasonic dissector (CUSA). Transplant surgeons find it technically easier to first perform total exclusion, cross-clamping the inflow and inferior van cava below and then the suprahepatic vena cava in the fully mobilized liver.

A special variety occurs in children less than 6 months of age. In this Kasabach-Merritt syndrome there is hepatomegaly, cutaneous hemangiomas, and high-output cardiac failure. These symptomatic hepatic hemangiomas may involve both lobes and are actually large arteriovenous malformations.

CYSTS

Simple cysts are left alone unless they cause pressure symptoms. They may be single or multiple, in which case they are associated with polycystic kidneys 51% of the time. There have been several reports of laparoscopic marsupialization of hepatic cysts with no recurrence. Unroofing is inadequate, as the cyst usually recurs. If possible, the entire cyst lining should be removed; or if it is close to major vessels, such as the cava, that portion of the cyst wall may be sclerosed by absolute alcohol on a peanut. Percutaneous drainage and sclerosis may be successful with small cysts. However, some patients with multiple cysts have pressure symptoms, and they may be severe enough to compromise liver function. We have laparoscopically excised more then 24 cysts in one patient to good effect.

Biliary cystadenomas connect to the biliary tree, and the connection must be severed, or else bile leaks occur. Alternatively, the cyst can be drained via Roux-en-Y.

Preferably the cyst is completely excised and the differential diagnosis made between this entity and biliary cystadenocarcinoma.

Echinococcal (hydatid) cysts may be unilocular when caused by *Echinococcus granulosis* or alveolar when caused by *Echinococcus multilocularis*. This disease is endemic in farming areas of the world where sheep, pigs, and cattle are raised. The unilocular type is found in the liver 70% of the time, and 85% of cases are in the right lobe. The cysts have an inner germinative layer and an outer laminated or adventitial layer. Outside that is the pericyst, a dense, fibrous host-produced reaction to the parasite. This cyst may be under a pressure as high as 300 mm H_2O. Cysts contain clear fluid and live daughter scolices. The alveolar hydatid has no capsule and may present as multiple metastases.

The complications of hydatid cysts are intrabiliary rupture, which occurs 5% to 25% of the time; but intraperitoneal rupture is much worse, as further parasitic infection can then occur. Secondary bacterial infection kills the daughter cysts.

It is diagnosed by a positive Casoni skin test, indirect hemagglutination tests, or complement fixation tests. It is suggested by the presence of eosinophilia, which is seen in up to 58% of cases. Confirmation is obtained by CT and sometimes by endoscopic retrograde cholangiopencreatography (ERCP).

Surgical treatment is in a state of flux. Europeans have the most experience and have preferred hepatic resection or pericystectomy using the CUSA. However, 14% morbidity and 7% mortality with pericystectomy is driving surgery back to more conservative methods, such as omentoplasty where the morbidity is 7% and mortality 1%. Even more radical is the use of laparoscopic decompression, using a 10- to 12-mm port, through which hypertonic saline can be injected for irrigation and the cysts and contents aspirated. At the end, the cyst can be closely inspected using the end-viewing scope. Capitonnage and cyst jejunostomy are also available. ERCP with papillotomy is necessary to drain cysts from the biliary tree, and cholecystectomy may be required to remove the parasitic reservoir after intrabiliary rupture.

HEPATIC ABSCESS

About 24% of hepatic abscesses are due to amebic infestation and are usually solitary in the right lobe of the liver. Cysts are ingested, and the cyst wall is digested in the cecum or pelvic colon by trypsin. Large trophozoites (20 to 60 μm in diameter) live on erythrocytes, penetrate the gut wall, and pass to the liver via the portal vein. The amebic nature of the abscess is usually not appreciated until fine-needle aspiration produces "anchovy sauce"-like pus. A slightly elevated white blood cell (WBC) count and low hematocrit suggest amebic infestation in a patient with a travel history. The diagnosis is confirmed by specific complement fixation tests. CT shows a single lesion with a necrotic center, a zone of parenchymal destruction, and an outer layer that may contain live amebae.

Treatment with metronidazole is effective, although percutaneous catheter drainage or open surgical drainage, which are equally effective, may be required. Nonetheless, even after the patient becomes asymptomatic, resolution may take months or years. Hence some authorities continue treatment with metronidazole for as long as a year.

Pyogenic liver abscesses usually present with fever, right upper quadrant pain, and weight loss. The patient has a high WBC count, and blood cultures may be positive 30% to 50% of the time. The infecting organism is commonly *Escherichia coli*, *Staphylococcus aureus,* or *Bacteroides fragilis.* One study found unilocular abscesses in 57% of the cases and multiple abscesses in the other 43%. Both lobes were involved in 26%, the left lobe in 15%, and the right lobe in 59%.

The infectious origin of these abscesses is variable. In our experience the biliary tract is the commonest site of origin, but some authors note that any previous infection can be the culprit, arriving at the liver via hematogenous spread. Portal pyemia, however, cannot be denied.

Treatment has traditionally been surgical drainage because 50 years ago it was found that mortality in the undrained cases was 100%. We give the patient a trial with intravenous broad-spectrum antibiotics; if that does not work, we percutaneously drain the obvious or large abscess. Smaller abscesses often then resolve spontaneously. Sometimes this treatment must be repeated. When it fails, surgical drainage is done, preferably extraperitoneally. Finally, resection remains an option.

Patients with diabetes are at particular risk for the development of gas-forming cryogenic liver abscess. These abscesses are large, cause severe liver dysfunction, and run a fulminating course. Surgery must not be delayed if the patient does not improve after medical treatment and percuteaneous drainage. Diabetic patients are also at risk for rupture of the abscess, in which case surgical intervention is the only means of saving the patient's life.

PORTAL HYPERTENSION

Portal hypertension is clinically significant when the portal pressure is higher than 12 mm Hg, as measured by the hepatic vein wedge pressure gradient. Clinically, it manifests as ascites, portosystemic encephalopathy, and variceal hemorrhage.

Increased portal pressure has been attributed to a combination of increased portal venous inflow (forward flow theory) and increased vascular resistance offered by the portal circulation (backward flow theory). Deposition of fibrous tissue around the terminal hepatic venules and sinusoids is observed in cirrhotic livers and may account for the increased vascular resistance. Transient enlargement of hepatocytes may occur as a consequence of infectious or toxic insults to the liver and by compression of the sinusoids; it may be responsible for the reversible portal hypertension observed with alcoholic hepatitis. Increased splanchnic blood flow has been a consistent finding in patients with chronic liver disease and portal hypertension. Although it may be related in part to portosystemic shunting, its mechanisms and relation to portal hypertension are not fully understood.

Etiology

More than 90% of cases of portal hypertension worldwide are caused by intrahepatic obstruction of the portal circulation, as observed with alcoholic cirrhosis, postnecrotic cirrhosis, schistosomiasis, biliary cirrhosis, hemochromatosis, congenital hepatic fibrosis, and Wilson's disease. The major resistance to portal blood flow in these lesions is postsinusoidal, with the exception of congenital hepatic fibrosis and schistosomiasis, where the obstruction is presinusoidal. In this case parasite eggs are deposited in Disse's space, and reactive fibrosis occurs, with remarkable sparing of the liver parenchymal architecture and function.

Alcoholic cirrhosis is the most common cause of portal hypertension worldwide and results in portal obstruction at the sinusoidal level (secondary to deposition of collagen at Disse's space) and at the postsinusoidal level (secondary to compression of hepatic veins by regenerating nodules).

Postnecrotic cirrhosis results from progression of acute viral hepatitis or less frequently from toxic hepatic injury. It is the most common cause of portal hypertension in the Orient. It also causes mainly sinusoidal obstruction.

Prehepatic portal hypertension is most frequently caused by portal vein thrombosis and accounts for 50% of pediatric cases of portal hypertension. Posthepatic portal hypertension is uncommon and includes hepatic vein thrombosis (Budd-Chiari syndrome) and right ventricular heart failure. Rarely, portal hypertension is caused by massive splenomegaly and associated increased portal venous flow, in which case splenectomy alone may be therapeutic.

Anatomy

As portal pressure increases, collateral vessels develop in an attempt to decompress the portal system. These collaterals result in portosystemic shunting of blood. They are divided into two groups.

1. *Hepatopetal circulation* occurs when there is obstruction of the portal vein in the presence of a normal intrahepatic vasculature. It results in shunting of blood from the portal vein toward the liver. It includes the accessory vein of Sappey, deep cystic veins, epiploic veins, hepatocolic and hepatorenal veins, and diaphragmatic veins.

2. *Hepatofugal circulation* diverts the blood flow away from the liver when there is obstruction of the intrahepatic vasculature. It consists of the coronary vein, superior hemorrhoidal veins, umbilical and paraumbilical veins, and the retroperitoneal veins of Retzius. The coronary vein anastomoses with the esophageal veins, which drain into the azygos vein and is implicated in the development of esophageal varices in the presence of portal hypertension.

Esophageal Varices

Hemorrhage from esophageal varices is the most serious complication of portal hypertension, accounting for one-third of all deaths in patients with cirrhosis. Several factors are implicated in the development and rupture of esophageal varices, such as portal pressure above 12 mm Hg, inflammation of the distal esophagus secondary to gastroesophageal reflux, size of the varices, variceal wall tension, and thickness of the epithelium overlying the varix.

Hemorrhage occurs in approximately 30% of cirrhotic patients with demonstrable varices, usually within 2 years of the initial diagnosis. About 60% of these patients rebleed massively within 1 year after the initial episode of bleeding, with an overall mortality of 70%.

The diagnosis of variceal bleeding is established by endoscopy, which should be performed on an emergency basis in any cirrhotic patient who presents with upper gastrointestinal bleeding. Varices are the source of bleeding in 50% of the cases, followed by gastritis in 30%. Massive bleeding is usually caused by varices, and mild hemorrhage is more commonly related to gastritis or peptic ulcer disease.

Treatment of variceal bleeding is initially nonoperative, as these patients are at poor risk for emergency surgery. The initial aim is to obtain rapid control of the bleeding. Endoscopic sclerotherapy controls bleeding in more than 85% of patients and is the standard initial treatment for bleeding esophageal varices. Drug therapy is directed at reducing portal hypertension by vasoconstricting the splanchnic arterial circulation, thereby reducing the likelihood of further bleeding. The most frequently employed drugs are vasopressin and somatostatin. Balloon tamponade, which may be used in the case of sclerotherapy failure, requires placement and insufflation of an esophageal and gastric balloon (Sengstaken-Blakemore tube) to compress the varices directly. The esophageal balloon is inflated to 24 to 45 mm Hg and controls the hemorrhage in more than 85% of cases. Several complications have been reported with its use, however, including esophageal perforation, ischemic necrosis of the esophagus, and aspiration. Moreover, there is a high rate of recurrent hemorrhage after balloon deflation, further limiting its use during the initial treatment of variceal hemorrhage. Patients with tense ascites should undergo paracentesis, which promptly decreases portal pressure. Emergency surgical treatment of bleeding varices is usually reserved for the rare cases that do not respond to nonoperative measures.

Once the acute bleeding episode is controlled, therapy is directed at preventing recurrent hemorrhage. Repeated sclerotherapy is highly effective for long-term control of variceal bleeding, eradicating the varices in most patients. When the varices recur, they are easily managed by another course of sclerotherapy. There is a significant reduction in the number of rebleeding episodes but no improvement in survival.

Ascites

Patients with portal hypertension develop ascites as a consequence of alterations in the production and reabsorption of hepatic and splanchnic lymph; and it is secondary to impaired metabolism of salt and water by the kidneys. Obstruction of hepatic venous outflow causes congestion of the liver and increases the size of the lymphatic vessels, resulting in increased production of hepatic lymph, which extravasates through the liver capsule into the peritoneal cavity. Impaired renal excretion of water and salt, which contributes significantly to the formation and maintenance of ascites, is secondary to hyperaldosteronism, increased levels of antidiuretic hormone, and increased sympathetic activity.

Treatment of ascites in the patient with portal hypertension consists of fluid and sodium restriction associated with the use of diuretics such as furosemide and spironolactone when necessary. Approximately 10% of ascitic patients do not respond to medical treatment and should be considered for placement of a peritoneovenous shunt. Ascitic fluid is returned, via a one-way valve, into the systemic circulation, causing an increase in total blood volume, an increase in cardiac output, and a decrease in systemic vascular resistance. The renal blood flow also improves, causing a decrease in renin and aldosterone levels. Complications associated with the shunt include infection, shunt blockage, superior vena cava thrombosis, pulmonary edema, cardiac arrhythmia, variceal hemorrhage, and liver failure. Functioning shunts are always associated with an element of disseminated intravascular coagulation.

Encephalopathy

Hepatic encephalopathy occurs in patients with portosystemic shunts and advanced hepatocellular dysfunction. Initially there is mental confusion and hyperreflexia, which progress to muscular rigidity as the disease advances, and finally to flaccidity and coma. Hepatic encephalopathy seems to correlate with the degree of hyperammonemia. Other factors also play a role in the pathogenesis of encephalopathy, as some patients do not develop mental status changes even in the presence of high levels of ammonia, whereas others progress to coma when the levels are only moderately elevated.

Ammonia is formed from the metabolization of dietary protein by intestinal bacteria, and in the liver it is converted to urea. Cirrhotic patients cannot adequately metabolize ammonia. In addition, part of the portal flow delivers blood with high ammonia concentration directly into the systemic circulation. For this reason, many of the surgical portosystemic shunts cause worsening of encephalopathy postoperatively. This complication is observed mainly with portocaval and mesocaval shunts and less frequently with distal splenorenal shunts.

Treatment of encephalopathy consists of restriction of dietary protein and oral administration of lactulose and nonabsorbable antibiotics neomycin. Lactulose acts as a cathartic and decreases the colonic mucosal pH, interfering with the absorption of ammonia from the bowel lumen. Nonabsorbable antibiotics cause a reduction in the bacterial count in the bowel and consequently a decrease in the production of ammonia.

Surgical Therapy

The preoperative assessment includes measurement of the portal and inferior vena caval pressures because the presence of caval hypertension interferes with portal decompression. The anatomy of the major veins should be determined angiographically. Portal vein thrombosis is present in up to 2% of cirrhotic individuals and can be diagnosed by nonvisualization of the portal vein angiographically, by CT scan, or by Doppler ultrasonography.

Operative risk is related mainly to hepatic function. Child's classification of perioperative risk divides patients into three groups, taking in consideration the bilirubin and albumin levels, the presence of ascites and neurologic disorders, and nutrition. Patients in group A have a serum bilirubin level under 2 mg/dL, albumin level above 3.5 g/dL, no ascites, no neurologic impairment, and good nutritional status; they have a mortality risk of zero. In group B patients have a bilirubin level of 2 to 3 mg/dL, albumin of 3.0 to 3.5 g/dL, controlled ascites, mild neurologic problems, and fair nutrition; their postoperative mortality rate is 9%. Group C comprises patients with a bilirubin level above 3 mg/dL, albumin level below 3 g/dL, poorly controlled ascites, coma, and malnutrition; this state is associated with a postoperative mortality rate of 53%.

End-to-side portocaval shunt was the first decompressive operation to be used. It is technically the easiest and has the lowest incidence of postoperative thrombosis. The shunt diverts the portal flow completely away from the liver, resulting in total decompression of the portal system. However, this procedure is associated with a postoperative incidence of encephalopathy as high as 50%.

Side-to-side portacaval shunts have not been proved to be significantly different from end-to-end shunts in terms of function. They also cause total decompression of the portal vein, with marked reduction in the hepatic portal flow, resulting in the same survival and postoperative incidence of encephalopathy. Similar results have been observed with large-diameter mesocaval and central splenorenal shunts.

Selective shunts have been developed in an attempt to decompress the portal system while preserving some portal flow to the liver, thereby reducing the incidence of encephalopathy. Warren introduced the distal splenorenal shunt in 1967; it consists of an end-to-side anastomosis of the splenic vein to the left renal vein and gastric devascularization (excluding the right gastric artery and the short gastric veins). Theoretically, this operation should preserve the portal flow to the liver, decreasing the incidence of encephalopathy; but the development of new collaterals diverts the portal flow from the liver toward the caval circulation, resulting in significant reduction of liver portal flow within 1 year postoperatively.

A small-diameter portocaval H-graft shunt has been proposed as an alternative to the distal splenorenal shunt as a way of selectively decompressing the portal system. The current technique utilizes 8-mm polytetrafluoroethylene (PTFE) grafts to create a shunt between the portal vein and the inferior vena cava. These grafts do not dilate with time, as venovenous anastomoses do; and they are able to decompress the portal system selectively while maintaining prograde portal flow to the liver. Graft thrombosis is rare, being observed in fewer than 5% of cases. Recurrent variceal bleeding occurs in 5% of patients, and the incidence of encephalopathy is 15%.

In an attempt to reduce the high incidence of postoperative encephalopathy associated with portosystemic shunts, nonshunting operations were designed. These procedures aim to disconnect or interrupt the dilated venous collaterals from the esophagus without decreasing hepatic perfusion. Simple esophageal transection utilizes an EEA stapler to transect and simultaneously reanastomose the distal esophagus 2 cm above the esophagogastric junction. It may be performed using a transthoracic or transabdominal approach. The coronary vein is ligated, and the extrinsic veins of the esophagus are preserved. This technique is advocated for patients whose surgical risk does not allow a shunting operation, such as Child's class C patients, and in the presence of acute, uncontrollable bleeding. The hemorrhage is arrested in most cases, but postoperative mortality can be high. Also, although new encephalopathy is negligible, there is a high rate of variceal recurrence.

In 1973 Sugiura introduced a procedure consisting of transthoracic esophageal transection, paraesophageal devascularization, splenectomy, vagotomy, and pyloroplasty. The operation is associated with 7% mortality when it is done electively and 25% mortality in emergency situations. The incidence of postoperative encephalopathy is zero. Variceal recurrence was observed in 5% of cases, with a rebleeding rate of 1.5%.

Liver transplantation is currently the optimal therapy for patients with chronic liver disease complicated by portal hypertension. It is the only treatment that improves the survival for these patients. It reestablishes normal portal hemodynamics and restores liver function, resolving not only the gastroesophageal varices but also the encephalopathy. Because the availability of donor livers is limited, transplant candidates must be selected based on the severity and nature of their liver disease. Absolute contraindications for liver transplantation include malignancy not confined to the liver, sepsis, thrombosis of the portal venous system, active alcohol or drug abuse, acquired immunodeficiency syndrome, and the presence of other life-threatening conditions. The survival rate for Child's class C patients with transplants is 70% at 5 years compared to 13% to 35% for patients treated with portosystemic shunts or sclerotherapy. No improvement in survival has been observed in Child's A and B patients who undergo transplantation.

Transjugular intrahepatic portosystemic shunt (TIPS) has been used to treat patients with variceal hemorrhage refractory to sclerotherapy. To create the shunt, a catheter is placed in the hepatic vein by the transjugular route. A needle is then passed through the liver parenchyma toward the portal vein under fluoroscopic or sonographic guidance. Once a portal branch is entered, a guidewire is passed, the track is dilated with a balloon, and it is subsequently stented. TIPS is highly efficient in controlling refractory variceal bleeding, with a lower mortality rate than that with emergency surgery. Encephalopathy develops in approximately 25% of patients and recurrent variceal bleeding in 20%. Shunt patency is 66% at 1 year after the procedure and 42% at 2 years. The survival rate is not significantly improved. TIPS is the preferred temporizing measure in candidates for liver transplantation who present with variceal hemorrhage because it preserves the anatomy of the portal system, making the transplant operation technically easier.

QUESTIONS

Indicate whether each statement is true or false.

1. Postsinusoidal portal hypertension ensues because of obstruction of the hepatic veins in the Budd-Chiari syndrome.

2. A normal hepatic venous wedge pressure (HVWP) is obtained in patients with portal vein obstruction that causes esophageal varices.

3. Portal venous pressure may fall an average of 50% within 5 minutes after a continuous intravenous infusion of Pitressin (0.6 units/min) is begun.

4. Sclerotherapy should not be utilized to control an acute variceal hemorrhage because of its propensity for venous laceration.

5. Percutaneous transhepatic coronary vein occlusion (PTCVO) appears to be an effective method for permanent control of hemorrhage from esophageal varices.

6. The Suguira method of gastroesophageal devascularization is performed through separate thoracic and abdominal incisions.

7. A distal splenorenal shunt is the best method to achieve portal decompression when ascites has become a difficult clinical problem.

8. When the portal pressure is higher on the hepatic side of an occluding clamp on the portal vein, there is theoretically no flow or retrograde flow in the portal vein.

9. Increased amounts of ammonia effect an imbalance of plasma amino acids that leads to hepatic encephalopathy.

10. Levodopa and bromocriptine are highly effective drugs for the management of hepatic encephalopathy.

SELECTED REFERENCES

Liver Surgery

Bhattacharya S, Novell JR, Winslet MC, Hobbs KEF. Iodized oil in the treatment of hepatocellular carcinoma. *Br J Surg* 1994;81:1563–1571.

Cady B, Stone MD, McDermott WV, et al. Technical and biological factors in disease-free survival after hepatic resection for colorectal cancer metastases. *Arch Surg* 1992;127:561–569.

Chou FF, Sheen-Chen SM, Chen Y-S, et al. Prognostic factors for pyrogenic abscess of the liver. *J Am Coll Surg* 1994;178:727–732.

Federico JA, Horner WR, Clark DE, Isler RJ. Blunt hepatic trauma: non-operative management in adults. *Arch Surg* 1990;125:905–909.

Ger R. Surgical anatomy of hepatic venous system. *Clin Anat* 1988;1:15–22.

Goksoy E, Ulvalp KM, Kaner G, Gokdogan C. Hepatic echinococcosis: treatment without pericystectomy. *Contemp Surg* 1995;47:83–87.

Gibney EJ. Amoebic liver abscess. *Br J Surg* 1990;77:843–844.

Gozzetti G, Mazziotti GL, Grazi E, et al. Liver resection without blood transfusion. *Br J Surg* 1994;82:1105–1110.

Hodgson WJB. *Liver tumors: multidisciplinary management.* St. Louis: Warren H. Green, 1988.

Hodgson WJB, Morgan J, Bryne D, DelGuercio LRM. Hepatic resection for primary and metastatic tumors using the ultrasonic surgical dissector. *Am J Surg* 1992;163;246–250.

Hughes KS, Simon R, Songhorabodi S, et al. Resection of the liver for colorectal carcinoma metastases: a multi-institutional study of indications for resection; registry for hepatic metastases. *Surgery* 1988; 103:278–288.

Kasai T, Kobayashi K. Searching for the best operative modality for severe hepatic injuries. *Surg Gynecol Obstet* 1993; 177:551–555.

Knudson MM, Lim RC, Oakes DD, Jeffrey RB. Non operative management of blunt liver injuries in adults: the need for continued surveillance. *J Trauma* 1990;30:1494–1500.

Kotoh K, Sakai H, Sakamoto S, et al. The effect of percutaneous ethanol injection therapy on small solitary hepatocellular carcinoma is comparable to that of hepatectomy. *Am J Gastroenterol* 1994;89:194–198.

Magistrelli P, Masetti R, Coppola R, et al. Surgical treatment of hydatid diseases of the liver: a twenty year experience. *Arch Surg* 1991;126;518–523.

McDermott WV, Cady B, Georgi B, et al. Primary cancer of the liver, evaluation, treatment and prognosis. *Arch Surg* 1989;124:552–555.

Moore EE. Critical decisions in the management of hepatic trauma. *Am J Surg* 1984;148:712–716.

Pain JA, Gimson AES, Williams R, Howard ER. Focal nodular hyperplasia of the liver: results of treatment and options in management. *Gut* 1991;32:524–527.

Ravikumar TS, Kane R, Cady B, et al. A five year study of cryosurgery in the treatment of liver tumors. *Arch Surg* 1991;126:1520–1524.

Ringe B, Wittekind C, Weimann A, et al. Results of hepatic re-section and transplantation for fibrolamellar carcinoma. *Surg Gynecol Obstet* 1992;175:299–305.

Rogiers X, Bloechle C, Bloechle CE. Safe decompression of hepatic hydrated cyst with a laparoscopic surgiport. *Br J Surg* 1995;82:111.

Saifi J, Fortune JB, Graca L, Shah DM. Benefits of intra-abdominal pack placement for the management of nonme-chanical hemorrhage. *Arch Surg* 1990;125:119–122.

Schwartz ME, Sung M, Mor E, et al. A multidisciplinary ap-proach to hepatocellular carcinoma in patients with cirrho-sis. *J Am Coll Surg* 1995;180:596–603.

Schwartz SI, Henderson JM, Jones RS, Nagorney DM, Sitz-mann JV. Symposium: management of benign liver tumors. *Contemp Surg* 1995;46:269–282.

Stain SC, Yellin AE, Donovan AJ, Brien HW. Pyogenic liver abscess: modern treatment. *Arch Surg* 1991;126:991–996.

Steele G, Bleday R, Mayer RJ, et al. A prospective evaluation of hepatic resection for colorectal carcinoma metastases to the liver: Gastrointestinal Tumor Study Group protocol 6584. *J Clin Oncol* 1991;9:1105–1112.

Vauthey JN, Klimstra D, Fanchschi D. Factors affecting long-term outcome after hepatic resection for hepatocellular car-cinoma. *Am J Surg* 1995;169:28–35.

Portal Hypertension

Collini F, Brener B. Portal hypertension. *Surg Gynecol Obstet* 1990;170:177–189.

Forster J, Delcore R, Payne M, Siegel E. The role of transjugu-lar intrahepatic portosystemic shunts in the management of patients with end stage liver disease. *Am J Surg* 1994;168: 592–596.

Henderson M. The distal splenorenal shunt. *Surg Clin North Am* 1990;70:405–423.

Hoefs JH, Jonas GM, Sarfeh J. Diagnosis and hemodynamic assessment of portal hypertension. *Surg Clin North Am* 1990;70:267–289.

LaBerge J, Somberg KA, Lake JR, et al. Two year outcome following transjugular intrahepatic portosystemic shunt for variceal bleeding: results in 90 patients. *Gastroenterology* 1995;108:1143–1151.

Levine B, Sirinek KR. The portocaval shunt. *Surg Clin North Am* 1990;70:361–378.

Lillemoe KD, Cameron JL. The interposition mesocaval shunt. *Surg Clin North Am* 1990;70:379–394.

Mahl TC, Groszmann RJ. Pathophysiology of portal hyperten-sion and variceal bleeding. *Surg Clin North Am* 1990;70: 251–255.

McCormick PA, Dick R, Panagou EB, et al. Emergency transj-ugular intrahepatic portasystemic stent shunting as salvage treatment for uncontrolled variceal bleeding. *Br J Surg* 1994; 81:1324–1327.

Rypins EB, Sarfeh IJ. Small diameter portacaval H-graft for variceal hemorrhage. *Surg Clin North Am* 1990;70:395–404.

Terblanche J, Krige JE, Bornman PC. Endoscopic sclerother-apy. *Surg Clin North Am* 1990;70:341–359.

Wexler MJ, Stein BL. Nonshunting operations for variceal hemorrhage. *Surg Clin North Am* 1990;70:425–448.

Wood RP, Shaw BW, Rokkers LF. Liver transplantation for variceal hemorrhage. *Surg Clin North Am* 1990;70:449–461.

7

Surgical Diseases of the Pancreas

Michael S. Gold and Marek Rudnicki

Hidden in the posterior recesses of the abdominal cavity, the pancreas has been approached surgically with great trepidation. More accurate and informative diagnostic modalities, greater knowledge of the physiologic implication of surgical procedures, and a better understanding of the complex anatomy have increased the confidence with which surgical approaches to this organ can be made.

ANATOMY

The main arterial supply to the pancreas is via branches of the celiac and superior mesenteric arteries. The gastroduodenal artery, arising from the common hepatic artery in 75% of patients, provides the major blood supply to the head of the pancreas. The neck, body, and tail receive their primary blood supply from the splenic artery. In 5% of patients the entire hepatic blood supply arises from the superior mesenteric artery, and in at least 15% a portion of it does so. Resection of the pancreatic head may interrupt the superior mesenteric-to-celiac artery connections and interfere with all, or a portion of, the hepatic blood supply. Similarly, with congenital or acquired celiac occlusion, resection of the pancreatic head may result in ischemia of the liver, stomach, spleen, or remaining pancreas.

The superior mesenteric and splenic veins join to form the portal vein posterior to the neck of the pancreas. Venous drainage of the pancreatic head is via the anterosuperior pancreaticoduodenal vein. Usually the neck and body drain via the transverse or the inferior pancreatic vein. Venous drainage of the body and tail is by numerous small tributaries that enter the splenic vein directly. The most important surgical implication of pancreatic venous drainage is that no pancreatic tributary enters the portal vein or superior mesenteric vein on its anterior aspect.

PHYSIOLOGY OF THE EXOCRINE PANCREAS

One liter of pancreatic secretion, consisting mostly of water, electrolytes, and digestive enzymes, is produced daily. In general, the acinar cells secrete enzymes and the ductal cells secrete electrolytes, which are mostly bicarbonate. Enzymes, secreted as inactive proenzymes, are primarily lipolytic and proteolytic. Pancreatic fluid is alkaline and isosmotic. A low concentration of trypsin inhibitor prevents autodigestion.

There are three phases of pancreatic response to a meal. The cephalic phase, mediated through the vagus nerves, is partially abolished by vagotomy. The gastric phase, responding to gastric distension with secretion of gastrin, stimulates the pancreas slightly. By far the most important stimulant to pancreatic secretion is the intestinal phase, because the presence of acid in the duodenum and jejunum produces secretin, stimulating pancreatic water and bicarbonate secretion. Cholecystokinin (CCK) is the most potent endogenous intestinal hormone known to stimulate pancreatic enzymes.

Inhibition of pancreatic secretion may be mediated through glucagon, somatostatin, pancreatic polypeptide, and peptide YY secondary to enteropancreatic reflexes induced by distal intestinal stimulation from products of food digestion. Neural mechanisms, still poorly understood, also have an inhibitory effect on pancreatic secretion.

PANCREATITIS

Etiology

Acute pancreatitis is a process of autodigestion caused by the premature activation of pancreatic zymogens to active proteolytic enzymes within the pancreas. It is believed that the earliest events of acute pancreatitis most likely involve acinar cells themselves. This process can be triggered by a variety of mechanisms. In 90% of cases the cause is related to biliary duct obstruction or excessive alcohol intake. With gallstone pancreatitis, evidence for the impaction or, more importantly, passage of stones is overwhelming. Transient pancreatic duct obstruction, rather than bile reflux, is likely to be the precipitating factor for pancreatic injury. Progression of the disease continues with sequential alteration of the ductal-mucosal barrier and disruption of ductal membranes, which sets the stage for intrapancreatic trypsinogen activation. Reflux of bile into the pancreatic duct, once thought to be abnormal, is now believed to be present normally in many instances.

Alcohol probably augments resistance to the sphincter of Oddi at the ampulla of Vater. It also stimulates gastrin and acid output, increasing pancreatic exocrine secretion. Elevated intrapancreatic pressure, facilitated by an increase in pancreatic ductal permeability, may result in acute parenchymal injury.

Miscellaneous causes of pancreatitis include sequelae of some metabolic diseases (hyperparathyroidism, hyperlipidemia, porphyria), mumps, scorpion bites, and drugs (diuretics, immunosuppressives, cytotoxins, contraceptives, steroids). Chronic pancreatitis results mainly

from ongoing pancreatic hypersecretion with precipitation of protein in the small ducts resulting in intraductal plugs.

Diagnosis

Supraumbilical abdominal pain radiating through to the back is the clinical hallmark of pancreatitis. Serum amylase is the most useful laboratory test in the diagnosis of acute pancreatitis; levels higher than 100 IU/L are considered diagnostic in patients who do not have a reduction in pancreatic function from previous bouts of pancreatitis. Serum amylase levels of 200 to 600 IU/L are commonly seen during recurrent bouts of chronic pancreatitis. Serum amylase elevation occurs within 2 to 12 hours of the onset of pancreatitis, and amylase may remain elevated for up to 4 weeks. The rapidity, degree, and duration of elevation are not necessarily related to the severity of the attack.

Other causes of hyperamylasemia include any of the following: parotitis, ectopic pregnancy, perforated duodenal ulcer, small bowel obstruction or infarction, ruptured or dissecting aneurysm, acute cholecystitis, mesenteric ischemia, and almost any diffuse peritonitis. Measurement of amylase components may help differentiate between acute pancreatitis (elevated P-type isoamylase from the pancreas) and extrapancreatic amylase (increased S-type isoamylase, derived from salivary glands, breast, lung, prostate, ovaries, fallopian tubes, endometrium, and possibly liver). The presence of more than two small bowel fluid levels on an abdominal radiograph should suggest intestinal obstruction, not pancreatitis. Acute cholecystitis accompanied by hyperamylasemia can often be differentiated from pancreatitis of biliary tract origin by the degree of amylase elevation, the clinical presentation, and often nuclear biliary imaging [hepatoiminodiacetic acid (HIDA) scan].

The amylase/creatinine clearance ratio was initially thought to be highly specific for pancreatitis, but reports now suggest that it is no more useful than a spot urinary amylase test. A spot urinary amylase level above 750 IU/L is considered diagnostic of acute pancreatitis. A 24-hour collection of urine for amylase assay is helpful because persistent elevation signifies continued disease activity. Renal clearance of amylase has been shown to be increased during pancreatitis.

The white blood cell (WBC) count, hematocrit, and blood glucose and calcium assays are not diagnostic but indicate the severity of the disease. Serum lipase rises at a rate parallel to but somewhat slower than serum amylase, and it remains elevated. A difficult assay to perform, with no real advantages over serum amylase, the serum lipase assay has fallen into disuse by many laboratories. Hyperglycemia is seen in 50% of patients with acute pancreatitis and hypocalcemia in 25%.

A plain abdominal radiograph may show a diffuse ileus, a sentinel loop of dilated jejunum, or a colon cutoff sign. Pancreatic calcifications occur in 50% of patients with chronic pancreatitis but rarely before 10 years of active disease has been experienced. Ultrasonography should be performed on all patients with known or suspected acute pancreatitis because a swollen, edematous pancreas is often confirmatory of a diagnosis. Neither ultrasonography nor computed tomography (CT) scans distinguish a pancreatic mass as being inflammatory or neoplastic. Dynamic CT is useful for determining severity and assessing the necrotic devitalized pancreas. Gallstones, when present, are visualized in 95% of patients. Evidence suggests that endoscopic papillotomy is of benefit to patients with gallstone pancreatitis if performed within 24 to 48 hours of the onset.

Eighty-five percent of acute attacks of pancreatitis are uncomplicated, with recovery occurring in 3 to 7 days. Rapid deterioration with death within 48 hours occurs in 2% to 3% of patients, and another 6% to 8% have a downhill, fluctuating course lasting 2 to 6 weeks. The mortality of any bout significant enough to require hospitalization is 11%, and major complications can occur at any stage. Severe pancreatitis may be associated with the Grey Turner sign or Cullen's sign and the presence of methemalbumin and blood on peritoneal or pleural aspiration. The overall mortality for hemorrhagic pancreatitis is 30% to 50%. Cardiovascular involvement manifested by shock, persistent tachycardia, and arrhythmias is also present. Renal and pulmonary failure may be seen, as may dyspnea, low PO_2, and capillary leak with edema and rales. Cytokines have been suggested to participate in multiple organ failure following severe acute pancreatitis.

Treatment

Fluid replacement, gastrointestinal (GI) rest, and nasogastric suction remain the mainstays of therapy.

Meticulous monitoring is essential, as sophisticated critical care is the single most important factor in reducing the mortality due to pancreatitis.

Numerous drugs have been used to treat acute pancreatitis with little success. Controlled data show no advantage of anticholinergics. Early administration of antibiotics has been shown to reduce the incidence of septic complications. Cimetidine may be helpful. Somatostatin has shown promise but as yet is not approved for general use for pancreatitis. Peritoneal lavage has been shown to decrease the early mortality of hemorrhagic pancreatitis, but the effects on late mortality and prevention of sequelae are controversial. Total or near-total pancreatectomy for fulminant hemorrhagic pancreatitis has been recommended in several recent papers. Although some increase in survival is reported in small series, acceptance of this approach is by no means universal, and its current application must be viewed with caution.

Indications for surgery in patients with acute pancreatitis include uncertainty in the diagnosis of pancreatitis or continued deterioration despite all other therapeutic efforts. If a laparotomy is performed, it should include drainage of the pancreatic bed and biliary decompression. If gallstones are present, a cholecystectomy is indicated if technically possible; if not, cholecystostomy should be done. An operative cholangiogram is desirable, if possible; and common duct exploration is performed if the duct can be safely exposed and approached. Most authors recommend a jejunostomy for feeding, and many include a gastrostomy.

In deteriorating patients with severe pancreatitis and areas of necrosis confirmed by dynamic CT, needle aspiration should be performed to detect the presence of bacteria. If no bacteria are present, surgery may be of little benefit. If bacteria are present, prompt surgery with débridement and drainage is recommended.

Cholecystectomy for biliary tract pancreatitis should be performed during the patient's hospitalization but after resolution of the acute attack of pancreatitis. It can usually be done laparoscopically. Cholangiography is recommended and endoscopic retrograde cholangiopancreatography (ERCP) may be helpful preoperatively. Patients discharged before cholecystectomy have a 40% chance of a recurrent bout before readmission. If two attacks of "idiopathic" pancreatitis occur without identifiable etiology, cholecystectomy should be strongly considered.

PSEUDOCYSTS

Pseudocysts result from encapsulation of extravasated blood, pancreatic fluid, and debris in peripancreatic tissue following pancreatitis. Pseudocysts were originally thought to occur in 10% of patients with pancreatitis, but routine use of ultrasonography and CT has shown the incidence to be much higher, probably 40%. Through the use of ultrasonography, it is now known that at least 85% of these cases resolve spontaneously.

The diagnosis is suspected when persistent or recurrent symptoms of pain, vomiting, or fever follow pancreatitis. A mass is palpable with 50% of large pseudocysts, and persistent pain is present in 80% to 90%. In 50% the serum and urinary amylase levels remain elevated for a month or longer. Once a pseudocyst is suspected, ultrasonography should be undertaken. Abdominal CT is indicated when ultrasonography is not definitive or if an abscess is suspected. Angiography is performed if there is any question of bleeding into the cyst, and some authors consider angiography to be indicated for all pseudocysts prior to surgery due to the significant incidence of pseudoaneurysm and the potential for postoperative hemorrhage.

Complications include infection, free perforation, involvement of adjacent vessels with hemorrhage into the cyst, compression of adjacent viscera resulting in gastric outlet obstruction or common bile duct obstruction, and jaundice (10% of cysts). Spontaneous perforation into adjacent viscera may be associated with GI bleeding or may be asymptomatic with the disappearance of the cyst. Immediate free rupture can be catastrophic and is associated with high mortality. Surgery is indicated for any of the above complications or if the cyst suddenly enlarges. A slow leak results in pancreatic ascites or a pancreatic pleural effusion.

Data suggest that asymptomatic, nonenlarging pseudocysts can be treated nonoperatively without increased risk to the patient. Several series have now reported no increase in morbidity or mortality with nonoperative management. Early surgery (before 6 weeks) or for infected cysts should utilize external rather than internal drainage. Radiologic percutaneous drainage has been effective for a significant percentage of cysts and may eliminate the need for surgery. Endoscopic, transgastric, or transduodenal drainage of adherent cysts is also reported, but statistical confirmation is incomplete.

When surgery is required electively for enlarging or symptomatic cysts, internal drainage is undertaken via Roux-en-Y jejunal limb or into adherent stomach or duodenum via cyst–gastrostomy or cyst–duodenostomy. Large cysts (more than 10 cm diameter) have a lower recurrence rate with Roux-en-Y drainage than with cyst–gastrostomy or cyst–duodenostomy. The overall recurrence rates are 15% to 20% for internally drained cysts and as high as 50% for externally drained cysts.

PANCREATIC ABSCESS

Pancreatic abscess occurs in 5% to 10% of patients with pancreatitis. It is most commonly seen following a severe bout of hemorrhagic pancreatitis. The abscess consists of collections of infected, necrotic pancreas or peripancreatic fat in the lesser sac extending into the transverse mesocolon, small bowel mesentery, and retroperitoneum. About 48% of abscesses involve the head only, 28% the body and tail, and 24% the entire pancreas.

The more severe the pancreatitis, the more likely the formation of an abscess, which usually becomes apparent 10 to 14 days after the onset. Approximately 30% to 60% of patients have a rise in serum amylase, 60% have impaired liver function, and most are hypoalbuminemic. Although 30% to 50% of the abscess cultures reveal a polymicrobial population, the most common infecting organisms are, in order of frequency: *Escherichia coli, Proteus, Aerobacter, Staphylococcus, Klebsiella,* and *Pseudomonas.*

The diagnosis is made in 30% of patients by abdominal radiographs showing loculated retrogastric air. Ultrasonography is 50% accurate and CT 80% to 90% accurate. Dynamic CT should be requested to determine the amount of devitalized pancreatic tissue. When a pancreatic abscess is diagnosed, prompt surgical drainage is mandatory. The lesser sac must be opened, débrided of necrotic tissue, and drained or marsupialized. There is no statistical difference in survival with drains or marsupialization.

Mortality without surgery is nearly 100% and averages 30% to 50% with drainage. Initial CT-guided aspiration and drainage may be attempted if the fluid appears primarily liquid; if organisms are present, surgical drainage is advisable. Delay in diagnosis or in prompt drainage following diagnosis significantly increases the mortality.

PANCREATIC ASCITES AND PLEURAL EFFUSION

Pancreatic ascites follows ductal disruption that results in leakage of pancreatic fluid. If the leak is anterior, pancreatic ascites results; if it is posterior, fluid enters the retroperitoneal space, the mediastinum, and then the pleural space (usually the left). The most common presentation is painless distension and increasing abdominal girth often accompanied by weight loss. The diagnosis is based on a high ascitic or pleural fluid amylase level. Albumin levels in the ascitic fluid exceed 3 g/L. Serum amylase is usually mildly elevated but relatively less than its rise in the ascitic fluid.

Initial treatment is nonoperative, as more than 50% resolve with bowel rest, hyperalimentation, and somatostatin. If ascites or pleural effusion is still present at 2 to 3 weeks, surgery is indicated. ERCP is done prior to surgery to identify the location of the ductal disruption. If endoscopic cannulation is unsuccessful, a ductogram via the tail of the pancreas or ampulla must be obtained at surgery. Surgical management consists of Roux-en-Y drainage if the leak is central or in the pancreatic head. If the leak is distal, the tail is resected.

CHRONIC PANCREATITIS

Alcohol abuse is the etiology in 90% of patients with chronic pancreatitis, with the remainder of cases usually of idiopathic origin. Chronic gallstone pancreatitis is rare. Calcifications are usually seen radiographically 8 to 10 years after the initial attack, and the onset of diabetes appears approximately 10 years after the first bout of pancreatitis. Steatorrhea is almost always present when glucose intolerance occurs. Attacks of varying severity occur at 3- to 12-month intervals and last 3 to 7 days. The frequency of bouts of chronic pain following meals increases slowly with time and results in significant weight loss as patients avoid food.

Surgery is indicated for disabling pain in patients who have stopped drinking. Any procedure performed in a patient who continues to drink alcohol is doomed to failure. The choice of surgical procedure depends on the pattern of ductal obstruction. More commonly, the duct has intermittent areas of stricture and dilatation, the so-called chain of lakes. With this type of ductal obstruction, a filleting of the duct and pancreas with Roux-en-Y jejunal onlay (Puestow procedure) gives good to excellent results in 80% of patients. With a dis-

tal stricture, distal resection is occasionally possible. Near-total pancreatectomy with 90% to 95% resection is indicated if the entire duct is fibrotic or if a lesser procedure has failed. Satisfactory results can be expected 90% of the time with resection.

PANCREATIC TUMORS

Cystic Neoplasms

Cystadenoma represents 10% of all neoplastic pancreatic cysts. These lesions are most commonly seen during the fourth or fifth decade of life and have a female/male ratio as high as 6 : 1. They are slow-growing, and symptoms are usually vague. About 65% of patients present with abdominal pain and a mass, 25% with weight loss, and 10% with jaundice. Complications include GI bleeding, erosion into adjacent viscera, and intraperitoneal hemorrhage from free rupture. Calcifications are seen on a plain abdominal radiograph in 10% of patients. Ultrasonography, CT, and ERCP are useful diagnostic procedures; and preoperative angiography is helpful for determining the vascular anatomy. The differentiation between cystadenoma or cystadenocarcinoma must often be made at surgery. Generally, benign lesions can be enucleated from the surrounding pancreas. Serous microcystic lesions are always benign, whereas mucinous lesions, especially if multiloculated, are more commonly malignant. If the lesion cannot be easily enucleated, it is considered malignant and an appropriate resection is done. Cysts in the tail may be safely managed by resecting the distal pancreas, and central or head lesions may require a Whipple resection.

Cystadenocarcinoma presents in an identical manner but generally in an older population, most commonly during the sixth decade. Most patients present with pain and an abdominal mass. Management depends on the location of the tumor. A Whipple resection, distal pancreatectomy, and occasionally total pancreatectomy for large lesions are the required procedures. The overall 5-year survival for malignant lesions is 25% to 30%, with 50% of the patients who have undergone resection for cure surviving 5 years.

Carcinoma of the Ampulla

Other than carcinoma of the head of the pancreas, ampullary carcinoma represents the most common periampullary neoplasm. About 70% to 90% present with obstructive jaundice, and mild anemia is common. Occult blood in the stool in a jaundiced patient is considered highly suggestive. Ultrasonography can demonstrate 50% of lesions in the head of the pancreas but less than 30% of ampullary lesions. CT identifies 80% to 90% of head of pancreas lesions but less than 50% of ampullary lesions. Endoscopic visualization is easily done, and a positive biopsy is obtained for more than 80% of ampullary carcinomas. Angiography prior to resection is useful for demonstrating the celiac, superior mesenteric, and hepatic arterial anatomy.

Despite their relative accessibility to endoscopic biopsy, as many as one-third of ampullary lesions are thought to be head of pancreas lesions at surgery. Two-thirds of ampullary carcinomas are resectable, with many series reporting a 5-year survival of 25% or more. Operative mortality should be less than 5%.

Pancreatic Adenocarcinoma

Pancreatic adenocarcinoma is currently the fourth leading cause of cancer-related death in the United States. The incidence is increasing 15% per year and currently stands at 10 cases per 100,000 population. There are 25,000 new patients reported in the United States annually, of whom more than 90% die within 1 year of diagnosis.

As many as 50% to 60% of pancreatic carcinomas occur in the head of the pancreas. Most of these head lesions present with jaundice. Body lesions present with pain, weight loss, and abdominal mass. Back pain usually represents splanchnic nerve involvement and must be considered ominous. Ultrasonography is 60% to 70% accurate for demonstrating a lesion and 85% accurate for showing dilatation of the extrahepatic biliary tree. CT followed by ERCP is the mainstay of the diagnostic evaluation. If the pancreatic duct is cannulated, fluid for cytology and a carcinoembryonic antigen (CEA) assay is obtained. An angiogram is useful prior to surgery for definition of vascular anatomy and determination of resectability due to entrapment of vessels at the invasion point of the superior mesenteric or portal vein. Spiral or three-dimensional CT reconstruction has improved the usefulness of radiologic imaging and seems to make angiography unnecessary.

The 5-year survival of patients with pancreatic adenocarcinoma is still believed to be less than 5%, although it may be improving slowly up to 20% in experienced hands. Only 10% of head lesions are resectable at operation. Biopsy may be transduodenal, through a choledochotomy with a curette or choledochoscope or via a direct pancreatic biopsy. Often lesions are resected without obtaining a positive biopsy. Most authors agree that with a surgically resectable lesion and positive confirmatory studies resection should be undertaken even if a positive biopsy is not obtained. Laparoscopy is most reasonably used only if a positive finding results in avoidance of open exploration. Serologic tumor markers such as CA 19-9, α-fetoprotein (AFP), pancreatic oncofetal antigen, and CEA seem to be helpful for monitoring pancreatic carcinoma, but their accuracy needs to be improved, and they are of little value as screening tests.

For palliation, the benefits and type of biliary bypass are controversial. Bypass may relieve jaundice and pruritus, but longevity is not increased. Methods of bypass include cholecystojejunostomy, loop choledochojejunostomy, and choledochojejunostomy to a Roux-en-Y limb. Stents placed via ERCP or transhepatic approaches should be considered in patients with evidence of advanced disease. Choledochoduodenostomy is considered by many to be contraindicated for bypass in patients with pancreatic malignancy. Cholecystojejunostomy should not be used if there is evidence of gallstones. The overall surgical mortality for bypass is 15% to 30%. Gastrojejunostomy is employed for infiltration and obstruction of the duodenum by pancreatic tumor.

There is some evidence that external radiotherapy prolongs survival especially if combined with chemotherapy. Intraoperative radiotherapy or seeds have been tried, and some preliminary benefit is reported. Multidrug chemotherapy with 5-fluorouracil, doxorubicin (Adriamycin), and mitomycin (FAM) has been reported to have an initial response rate as high as 40%.

Pancreatic Endocrine Tumors

Endocrine tumors of the pancreas consist of cells that are capable of amine precursor uptake and decarboxylation (APUD) and are called APUDomas. The cells are believed to originate from neural crest or neural ectoderm.

Insulinoma

Insulinoma produces symptoms of hypoglycemia relieved by intake of sugar. About 65% of insulinomas are single, and 90% are benign. About 10% are associated with multiple endocrine neoplasia (MEN). About 10% of insulinomas are malignant. They are diagnosed by a blood glucose level below 60 mg/mL following an overnight fast or below 35 mg/dL after a 72-hour fast. Concomitant insulin levels should be higher than 24 U/mL. C-peptide levels are abnormally elevated. Various studies indicate that 30% to 80% of insulinomas can be seen on selective angiography; 80% are seen on careful CT scans. Ultrasonography is of little value. Selective portal and splenic vein catheterization with serial venous sampling should be done if localization fails. Diazoxide inhibits release of insulin and provides temporary control prior to surgery.

Unresectable malignant insulinomas are treated with streptozotocin. In 50% of the cases there is some improvement and in 20% complete remission. Enucleation of small, benign lesions is usually possible, whereas malignant lesions require appropriate pancreatic resection. If metastatic disease is found, removal of as much tumor as possible aids in subsequent control of hypoglycemia. With current methods of preoperative localization, the site of an insulinoma is identified in at least 85% of patients; in another 10% or more the lesion can be located at exploration. Intraoperative ultrasonography is useful in experienced hands. For those few remaining patients in whom no tumor is located preoperatively or found at surgery, "blind" resection of all pancreas to the left of the superior mesenteric vessels is recommended. If no tumor is found pathologically or if histologic evidence of diffuse hyperplasia is found, a 90% to 95% pancreatectomy should be done at a second procedure.

Gastrinoma

Zollinger-Ellison syndrome produced by a gastrinoma is characterized by a virulent ulcerous diathesis, often with ulcerations in atypical locations and diarrhea present in 30% to 60% of patients. Although slow-growing, at least 60% of gastrinomas are malignant; and often the only indication of malignancy is the presence of metastatic disease. Patients with metastatic disease often survive many years after detection. The pancreas is the most common site of gastrinoma. About 50% of tumors are multiple, and at least 37% are found in the duodenum. The syndrome has been diagnosed in patients 7 to 90 years of age, although it appears most commonly during the fifth and sixth decades.

Gastrinoma is suggested initially on an upper GI series, which shows gastric distension with a visible fluid level, prominent rugae, and multiple or atypical location of ulcers. Stimulated gastric secretion with augmented histamine or pentagastrin results in a basal/maximal acid output ratio of at least 0.6. A significantly elevated serum gastrin level in a patient who has increased gastric acid output is diagnostic. Serum gastrin is elevated in patients with pernicious anemia, but they are also achlorhydric. Intravenous secretin infusion produces a paradoxical elevation of serum gastrin in patients with gastrinomas, whereas in normal subjects and duodenal ulcer patients the serum gastrin levels remain unchanged. Localization techniques are identical to those described for insulinoma. Octreotide scanning uses a radioactive iodine-labeled somatostatin analog to image islet cells tumors based on the density of somatostatin receptors. This study determines the exact location of up to 80% of islet cell tumors. Intraoperative endoscopic transillumination of the duodenum with or without duodenotomy may localize small duodenal gastrinomas not detected by the other methods.

Management of gastrinomas (Fig. 7.1) initially begins with H_2 blocking agents. Most patients can be controlled with omeprazole. Diarrhea responds quickly, and in patients who have an initial response the recurrence of diarrhea may be an indicator of tumor recurrence or of treatment failure. Nonresponders are managed by complete tumor resection when possible; only when it is not possible is total gastrectomy indicated. Because of the high incidence of malignancy, medical responders should also undergo tumor resection when possible (about 25% of patients); if complete tumor resection is not feasible, continued medical control is recommended. A total gastrectomy is performed only if the disorder becomes refractory. The long-term effects of medical management and the number of patients who subsequently require total gastrectomy is still unknown but with the use of advanced drugs should be rare.

Other Islet Cell Tumors

Two other functioning islet cell tumors are vasoactive intestinal polypeptide-related tumor (VIPoma; so-called Verner-Morrison syndrome or pancreatic cholera) and the glucagonoma syndrome. VIPoma is characterized by secretory diarrhea, hypokalemia, hypochlorhy-

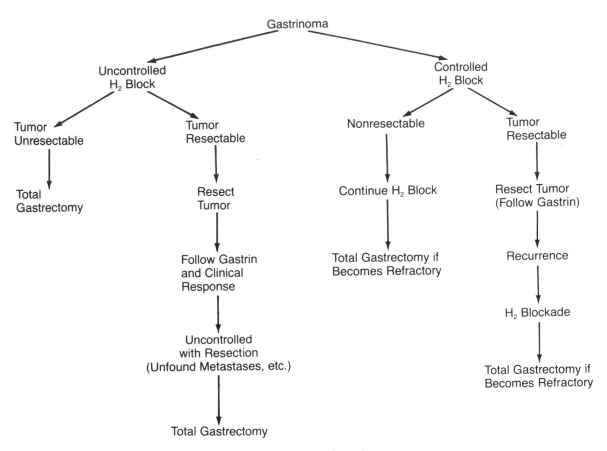

FIG. 7.1. Management of gastrinoma.

dria (WDHHA syndrome), and increased plasma VIP. Fifty percent of these lesions are malignant. Localization and management are similar to that for the above tumors, with resection done whenever possible. In contrast to gastrinoma, diarrhea is not controlled by H_2 blockade.

The glucagonoma syndrome is distinguished by a necrolytic migratory erythematous rash, which is characteristic; the lesion is often associated with diabetes. Many of these tumors can be cured by resection, but when they are not resectable debulking is usually helpful. Patients with incurable or recurrent disease have been treated with streptozotocin and dacarbazine with some success.

8/10

QUESTIONS

1. Which of the following statements is true?
   a. The gastroduodenal artery divides into the superior pancreaticoduodenal artery and the splenic artery.
   b. The splenic artery courses along the inferior border of the pancreas, supplying the body and tail.
   c. Similar to other adjacent organs, such as the kidneys and adrenals, the pancreas drains directly into the vena cava.
   d. The superior mesenteric vessel runs anterior to the uncinate process of the pancreas.
   e. The pancreas is anterior to the confluence of the

superior and inferior mesenteric veins forming the portal vein.

2. Which of the following is true regarding exocrine pancreatic physiology?
   a. Cholecystokinin is a strong stimulant of pancreatic water and bicarbonate secretion. *F*
   b. Vagal stimulation results in water and bicarbonate secretion. *T*
   c. Pancreatic polypeptide inhibits exocrine secretion. *?*
   d. Secretin is a strong stimulant of pancreatic enzyme secretion. *T*
   e. Pancreatic digestive enzymes are all secreted as inactive precursors. *F*

3. All of the following are indicative of poor prognosis in acute pancreatitis *except:*
   a. Serum calcium level less than 8.0 mg/dL.
   b. Hyperglycemia.
   c. Serum amylase level more than five times normal on admission.
   d. Arterial oxygen tension less than 60 mm Hg.
   e. Serum lactic dehydrogenase more than three times normal.

4. Which of the following is the best monitor of acute necrotizing pancreatitis:
   a. CT scan.
   b. MRI.
   c. Dynamic CT scan.
   d. Ultrasonography.
   e. Serum lipase.

5. Diagnostic tests for gastrinoma include all of the following *except:*
   a. Secretin test.
   b. Intravenous calcium.
   c. Octreotide test.
   d. Cholecystokinin–pancreozymin-stimulated gastrin secretion.
   e. Duodenal transillumination.

6. Which of the following tumors has the lowest malignancy rate:
   a. Gastrinoma.
   b. VIPoma.
   c. Insulinoma.
   d. Glucagonoma.
   e. Somatostatinoma.

7. Prior to operation for chronic alcoholic pancreatitis, the most helpful imaging modality is:
   a. Plain abdominal roentgenogram.
   b. Ultrasonography.
   c. Angiography.
   d. ERCP.
   e. Spiral CT scan.

8. A 50-year-old patient 6 months after a motor vehicle accident presents with occasional abdominal pain and a 5-cm cyst in the body of pancreas. The initial evaluation and treatment should include:
   a. Initial workup followed by surgical drainage using Roux-en-Y jejunostomy.
   b. Follow-up with regular CT scans.
   c. Complete excision of the tumor.
   d. Percutaneous CT-guided drainage.
   e. ERCP followed by a course of intravenous somatostatin.

9. Surgery for chronic pancreatitis should be mainly advised for the patient with:
   a. Exocrine insufficiency and steatorrhea.
   b. Progression of endocrine insufficiency.
   c. Decreased weight.
   d. Persistent pain.
   e. Pancreatic duct dilatation with "chain of lakes."

10. Regarding pancreatic carcinoma:
    a. Serologic marker CA 19-9 is accurate for diagnosis.
    b. Migratory thrombophlebitis is a common finding.
    c. It is usually associated with perineural invasion.
    d. It occurs less frequently in diabetic patients.
    e. Pancreatic fistula after pancreaticoduodenectomy is the most common fatal complication.

SELECTED REFERENCES

Barens SA, Lillemoe KD, Kaufman HS, et al. Pancreaticoduodenectomy for benign disease. *Am J Surg* 1996;171:131–134.

Barie PS. A critical review of antibiotic prophylaxis in severe acute pancreatitis. *Am J Surg* 1996;172(suppl 6A):38S–43S.

Bartz C, Ziske C, Wiedenmann B, Moelling K. p53 Tumour suppressor gene expression in pancreatic neuroendocrine tumour cells. *Gut* 1996;38:403–409.

Bieligk S, Jaffe BM. Islet cell tumors of the pancreas. *Surg Clin North Am* 1995;75:1025–1040.

Bluemke DA, Cameron JL, Hruban RH, et al. Potentially resectable pancreatic adenocarcinoma: spiral CT assessment with surgical and pathologic correlation. *Radiology* 1995;197:381–385.

Bradley EL III. A clinically-based classification system for acute pancreatitis: summary of the International Symposium on Acute Pancreatitis, Atlanta, GA, September 11 through 13, 1992. *Arch Surg* 1993;128:586–590.

Brenin DR, Talamonti MS, Yang EY, et al. Cystic neoplasms of the pancreas: a clinicopathologic study, including DNA flow cytometry. *Arch Surg* 1995;130:1048–1054.

Brennan MF, Moccia RD, Klimstra D. Management of adenocarcinoma of the body and tail of the pancreas. *Ann Surg* 1996;223:506–511.

Buchler MW, Friess H, Muller MW, Wheatley AM, Beger HG. Randomized trial of duodenum-preserving pancreatic head resection versus pylorus-preserving Whipple in chronic pancreatitis. *Am J Surg* 1995;169:65–70.

Cameron JL. Long-term survival following pancreaticoduodenectomy for adenocarcinoma of the head of the pancreas. *Surg Clin North Am* 1995;75:939–951.

Fernandez-del Castillo C, Warshaw AL. Cystic tumors of the pancreas. *Surg Clin North Am* 1995;75:1001–1010.

Geoghegan JG, Jackson JE, Lewis MP, et al. Localization and surgical management of insulinoma. *Br J Surg* 1994;81:1025–1028.

Gerkin TM, Eckhauser FE, Raper SE, Mulholland MW, Knol JA, Schork MA. Are traditional prognostic criteria useful in pancreatic abscess? *Pancreas* 1995;10:331–337.

John TG, Greig JD, Carter DC, Garden OJ. Carcinoma of the pancreatic head and periampullary region: tumor staging with laparoscopy and laparoscopic ultrasonography. *Ann Surg* 1995;221:156–164.

Kaiser MA, Saluja AK, Sengupta A, Saluja M, Steer ML. Relationship between severity, necrosis, and apoptosis in five models of experimental acute pancreatitis. *Am J Physiol* 1995;269:C1295–C1304.

Lerch MM, Weidenbach H, Hernandez CA, Preclik G, Adler G. Pancreatic outflow obstruction as the critical event for human gallstone induced pancreatitis. *Gut* 1994;35:1501–1503.

Lichtenstein DR, Carr-Locke DL. Endoscopic palliation for unresectable pancreatic carcinoma. *Surg Clin North Am* 1995;75:969–988.

MacFarlane MP, Fraker DL, Alexander HR, Norton JA, Lubensky I, Jensen RT. Prospective study of surgical resection of duodenal and pancreatic gastrinomas in multiple endocrine neoplasia type 1. *Surgery* 1995;118:973–979.

Machi J, Sigel B. Operative ultrasound in general surgery. *Am J Surg* 1996;172:15–20.

McArthur KE, Richardson CT, Barnett CC, et al. Laparotomy and proximal gastric vagotomy in Zollinger-Ellison syndrome: results of a 16-year prospective study. *Am J Gastroenterol* 1996;91:1104–1111.

Nitecki SS, Sarr MG, Colby TV, van Heerden JA. Long-term survival after resection for ductal adenocarcinoma of the pancreas: is it really improving? *Ann Surg* 1995;221:59–66.

O'Shea D, Rohrer-Theurs AW, Lynn JA, Jackson JE, Bloom SR. Localization of insulinomas by selective intraarterial calcium injection. *J Clin Endocrinol Metab* 1996;81:1623–1627.

Perry RR, Vinik AI. Endocrine tumors of the gastrointestinal tract. *Annu Rev Med* 1996;47:57–68.

Ranson JHC. Diagnostic standards for acute pancreatitis. *World J Surg* 1997;21:136–142.

Ruszniewski P, Amouyal P, Amouyal G, et al. Localization of gastrinomas by endoscopic ultrasonography in patients with Zollinger-Ellison syndrome. *Surgery* 1995;117:629–635.

Soper NJ, Brunt LM, Callery MP, Edmundowicz SA, Aliperti G. Role of laparoscopic cholecystectomy in the management of acute gallstone pancreatitis. *Am J Surg* 1994;167:42–50.

Sperti C, Guolo P, Polverosi R, Liessi G, Pedrazzoli S. Serum tumor markers and cyst fluid analysis are useful for the diagnosis of pancreatic cystic tumors. *Cancer* 1996;78:237–243.

Steer ML, Waxman I, Freedman S. Chronic pancreatitis. *N Engl J Med* 1995;332:1482–1490.

Tenner S, Banks PA. Acute pancreatitis: nonsurgical management. *World J Surg* 1997;21:143–148.

Thompson JS, Murayama KM, Edney JA, Rikkers LF. Pancreaticoduodenectomy for suspected but unproven malignancy. *Am J Surg* 1994;168:571–573.

Van Eijck CH, Lamberts SW, Lemaire LC, et al. The use of somatostatin receptor scintigraphy in the differential diagnosis of pancreatic duct cancers and islet cell tumors. *Ann Surg* 1996;224:119–124.

Yeo CJ, Bastidas JA, Lynch-Nyhan A, Fishman EK, Zinner MJ, Cameron JL. The natural history of pancreatic pseudocysts documented by computed tomography. *Surg Gynecol Obstet* 1990;170:411–417.

Yeo CJ, Cameron JL, Lillemoe KD, et al. Pancreaticoduodenectomy for cancer of the head of the pancreas: 201 patients. *Ann Surg* 1995;221:721–731.

8

Peripheral Arterial Disease

Larry A. Scher, Steven G. Friedman, and Russell H. Samson

CHRONIC ARTERIAL OCCLUSIVE DISEASE OF THE LOWER EXTREMITIES

Clinical Manifestations

Atherosclerosis is the most common cause of lower extremity arterial occlusive disease. Lesions may be asymptomatic and manifest only as abnormal pulse examinations, or they may cause symptoms including claudication, ischemic rest pain, and gangrene.

Disease patterns may be segmental or diffuse and involve the aortoiliac, femoropopliteal, and tibial arteries alone or in combination. Atherosclerosis most commonly involves the superficial femoral artery in the adductor (Hunter's) canal. It is important to remember that patients with lower extremity atherosclerotic occlusive disease may also have silent or symptomatic atherosclerosis in their coronary, cerebral, or other arteries.

Claudication is the most benign symptom of chronic arterial occlusive disease. Exercise-related muscle pain usually occurs in the calf but may also be present in the thigh or buttocks. The location of the claudication is often, but not always, indicative of the level of arterial stenosis or occlusion. Claudication has been demonstrated repeatedly to be a benign symptom that diminishes or remains stable in most patients. Unless severe disability exists and interferes with the patient's life style, treatment is conservative.

Ischemic rest pain is a more severe manifestation of peripheral vascular disease. Typically, nocturnal pain occurs in the foot and is relieved with dependency. Dependent rubor (from peripheral vasodilatation) and elevation pallor on physical examination are findings consistent with severe arterial occlusive disease. Unlike claudication, the natural history of ischemic rest pain is more ominous. Frequent progression to ischemic ulceration and impending or frank gangrene occurs and may threaten limb viability. Therefore interventional therapy for limb salvage is often indicated during these later stages.

Diagnosis

The history and physical examination are important when assessing patients with lower extremity arterial occlusive disease. The typical symptoms (intermittent claudication, ischemic rest pain, ulceration, gangrene) have already been described. Careful pulse examination, auscultation for bruits, and examination for signs of chronic ischemia (elevation pallor, dependent rubor, ulceration, trophic changes) are important aspects of the physical examination.

Arterial noninvasive studies including Doppler segmental pressures and pulse volume recordings, or plethysmography, may offer supportive information to the history and physical examination. Doppler pressures are measured with blood pressure cuffs on the thigh, calf, and ankle and auscultation with a Doppler stethoscope distal to the cuff (usually over the dorsalis pedis or posterior tibial artery). Because of the variation in systemic blood pressure, an ankle/brachial pressure index (ABPI) is determined by dividing the ankle pressure by the brachial pressure. The normal ABPI is equal to or greater than 1.0, and an ABPI less than 0.95 is suggestive of arterial occlusive disease. Typically, patients with intermittent claudication have an ABPI in the range of 0.7, and limb-threatening ischemia generally occurs only with an ABPI less than 0.5. Diabetic patients may have arterial calcification that prevents cuff occlusions of major arteries and accurate measurement. In this situation, supplemental information obtained by volume plethysmography with analysis of wave amplitude and pattern is useful. In addition, plethysmographic tracings obtained at the forefoot and toes may provide accurate information about distal circulation and aid in the planning of vascular reconstructive operations or amputations. In selected patients, noninvasive evaluation following exercise or reactive hyperemia may provide useful information about the etiology and significance of lower extremity symptoms.

Angiography gives anatomic information about arterial lesions but is not necessary in all patients. This invasive diagnostic technique is reserved for patients who, by history, physical examination, and noninvasive diagnostic studies, are considered candidates for interventional therapy. At this point, arteriography is recommended and is usually performed via a transfemoral approach. Occasionally a translumbar or transaxillary route is used. Ultimate decisions regarding optimal therapy can be made by visualizing the infrarenal aorta and the iliac, femoral, popliteal, and tibial arteries down to and including the foot vessels in appropriate patients. Digital subtraction and magnetic resonance angiography are important adjuncts to conventional angiography, as they may demonstrate suitable arteries for reconstruction that are not seen with conventional techniques.

Treatment

Initial treatment of non-limb-threatening arterial occlusive disease is conservative. Cessation of smoking and modification of diet may prevent disease progression. Graded exercise programs improve walking distances in many patients with intermittent claudication. Although vasodilators have not been effective treatment for claudicants, experience with pentoxifylline (a hemorrheologic agent) has demonstrated improvement in occasional patients.

Patients with severely disabling claudication or limb-threatening ischemia may require interventional therapy. Appropriate therapy is selected after complete arteriography. Percutaneous transluminal angioplasty (PTA) is effective treatment for most hemodynamically significant iliac artery stenoses and short-segment occlusions and for some localized femoral or distal lesions. Results with endovascular techniques, such as laser therapy and catheter atherectomy, have been disappointing and largely abandoned. Vascular stents are currently used as an adjunct to PTA primarily in the iliac artery and subclavian vein. Further study is necessary before the role of these techniques can be clearly defined.

Surgery remains the mainstay for treatment of severe lower extremity arterial occlusive disease. In patients with predominantly aortoiliac occlusive disease primary attention must be focused on the correction of these anatomic lesions. If PTA is not feasible or is unsuccessful, arterial reconstruction is required. Although some surgeons advocate extensive aortoiliac endarterectomy, most prefer aortofemoral bypass. Unilateral iliac lesions can be effectively treated with femorofemoral bypass. Patients with bilateral disease requiring operation are usually best managed with aortobifemoral reconstruction.

Dacron (woven or knitted) grafts are preferred by most surgeons. Results of aortofemoral bypass are excellent and approach 90% patency at 5 years. Occlusion of the superficial femoral artery does not appear to influence graft patency if the deep femoral artery is not diseased (85% of patients). In addition, correction of hemodynamically significant aortoiliac disease frequently relieves symptoms in more than 80% despite uncorrected superficial femoral artery occlusion.

Extraanatomic bypass has assumed a controversial role in the management of selected patients with aortoiliac occlusive disease. As mentioned above, femorofemoral bypass is an acceptable option for patients with unilateral iliac disease. In the absence of hemodynamically significant disease of the donor iliac artery, patency rates have been excellent, and arterial "steal" should not occur. Results of axillary-femoral and axillary-bifemoral bypass have been less satisfactory and should be reserved for poor-risk patients in whom conventional aortoiliac reconstruction carries prohibitive risks. Extraanatomic bypass has also been valuable for treating patients with intraabdominal graft infections (see Aneurysms, below).

Femoropopliteal and femorotibial bypass play a major role in the treatment of patients with infrainguinal atherosclerosis. Indications for femoropopliteal reconstruction include severely disabling claudication and limb-threatening ischemia. The autogenous saphenous vein, whether reversed or left *in situ,* is the graft of choice. In the absence of suitable greater saphenous vein, alternative conduits include the lesser saphenous vein, arm veins, and expanded polytetrafluoroethylene (PTFE). The popliteal artery may provide suitable outflow for a vascular reconstruction even in the absence of continuous outflow into the tibial arteries. Bypasses to isolated popliteal segments have excellent patency rates and often result in alleviation of symptoms. When the popliteal artery is unsuitable for graft insertion, femorotibial bypass is advocated. This operation is performed only for limb salvage, and autogenous vein grafts are far superior to prosthetics. Five-year patency rates of 80% have been achieved for femoropopliteal bypass, and these rates have been approached for infrapopliteal bypass when autogenous grafts are used.

Selected patients with hemodynamically significant disease of the profunda femoris artery, in addition to superficial femoral artery occlusion, may benefit from profundaplasty. However, isolated profundaplasty has a limited role in the management of lower extremity ischemia due to the excellent results of femoropopliteal and femorotibial reconstructions. Profundaplasty has most commonly been utilized in conjunction with an inflow procedure (e.g., aortofemoral bypass).

Thrombolytic therapy is occasionally useful for management of patients with chronic arterial occlusive disease. The recently reported STILE (Surgery Versus Thrombolysis for Ischemia of the Lower Extremity) trial was designed to evaluate intraarterial thrombolytic therapy for patients who require revascularization for nonembolic arterial or graft occlusion causing lower extremity ischemia of less than 6 months' duration. Surgical revascularization was more effective and safer than catheter-directed thrombolysis. A significant reduction in the complexity of planned surgical procedures was noted after thrombolysis, and a combination of the two modalities yielded the best results.

Lumbar sympathectomy has been a controversial adjunct for treatment of patients with lower extremity arterial occlusive disease. Its results as primary treatment for ischemia or as an adjunct to bypass operations have been variable. The operation has no role in the treatment of patients with intermittent claudication and is rarely useful for treatment of infrapopliteal disease not amenable to direct arterial reconstruction. The major role of lumbar sympathectomy appears to be in the management of patients with reflex sympathetic dystrophy.

Amputation

Major amputation used as the primary treatment for patients with lower extremity arterial occlusive disease is infrequently required. It remains necessary in the presence of extensive gangrene or severe sepsis, severe organic brain syndrome with gangrene, or unreconstructable occlusive disease. Minor toe or transmetatarsal amputation can be performed alone to treat infection or gangrene if hemodynamic testing reveals adequate arterial pressure to achieve wound healing (ABPI more than 0.5). Major amputation, when required, is preferred at the below-knee level to facilitate ambulation and mobility. Above-knee amputation is required for severe peripheral vascular disease or infection only when amputation at a lower level is not feasible. Although numerous methods have been described to predict the level of amputation healing, it can often be accurately assessed on the basis of clinical criteria and noninvasive laboratory testing. Concerns have arisen that a failed vascular reconstruction may lead to a higher level of amputation than would have been necessary had no revascularization been attempted. Several studies have proved this not to be the case in most patients. Newer techniques with an immediate postoperative prosthesis and rigid plaster dressings following amputation are controversial but may facilitate stump healing and rehabilitation.

ACUTE ARTERIAL OCCLUSION

The etiology of acute arterial occlusion may be thrombotic or embolic. Differentiation between the two is frequently difficult because many patients with acute arterial occlusion have severe underlying chronic atherosclerotic occlusive disease. Angiography may be of value in the diagnosis of this condition. The management of acute thrombotic occlusion involves thrombectomy or thrombolysis (usually with urokinase) and angioplasty or bypass of the underlying arterial lesion. The management of acute embolic arterial occlusion is discussed below.

Source of Emboli

Most arterial emboli are cardiac in origin and may be related to atherosclerotic heart disease with myocardial infarction, mural thrombus, or ventricular aneurysm. Rheumatic valvular disease, atrial fibrillation, and atrial myxoma are also possible sources of cardiac emboli. Emboli can also originate from proximal atherosclerotic lesions and produce major or minor episodes of distal embolization (blue-toe syndrome). Angiographic evaluation of patients with blue-toe syndrome is mandatory to identify the source of atheroembolic lesions, as the natural history of this disease is one of recurrent embolization. Emboli can also originate from arterial aneurysms, particularly those in the aorta and popliteal arteries. Paradoxical emboli are rare; they originate in the deep venous system and enter the arterial circulation via intracardiac septal defects.

Clinical Manifestations

Clinical manifestations of acute arterial occlusion include pain, pallor, absent pulses, paresthesias, and paralysis. Progressive ischemia results from distal propagation of thrombus. Rapidly progressive ischemia may threaten limb viability within 4 to 6 hours. Most arterial emboli involve the lower extremity, with 35% at the femoral bifurcation. Other common sites include the iliac and popliteal arteries. Noninvasive testing and arteriography may help confirm the diagnosis and localize the arterial occlusion.

Treatment

Immediate heparinization helps to prevent distal propagation of thrombus. Acute arterial emboli result in a high incidence of limb loss or persistent symptoms if left untreated. Angiography may help to localize emboli (which are frequently multiple) and plan an operative approach. Balloon catheter embolectomy can be accomplished via the femoral artery for aortic ("saddle"), iliac, or femoral emboli. It is often performed under local anesthesia. Popliteal emboli may require direct exposure of the popliteal and proximal tibial arteries. Thrombolytic therapy may be considered for selected patients, but in general the urgency of the situation makes operative intervention preferable. A multicenter trial of thrombolysis or peripheral arterial surgery (TOPAS) was undertaken to compare urokinase and surgery for the initial treatment of acute lower extremity ischemia. The preliminary results indicated that thrombolytic therapy was safe and effective and reduced the requirement for complex surgery after successful lysis.

Results

Results of treatment for acute ischemia depend on the duration and location of the occlusion. Muscle necrosis with calf tenderness or rigor may preclude a successful outcome. Complications include persistent ischemia, catheter-related complications, and metabolic derangements related to lactic acidosis and myoglobinemia. Mortality is high and is usually associated with underlying cardiac disease. Long-term anticoagulation may be beneficial in reducing the risk of recurrent embolization. The results of treatment are favorable if a noncardiac source of embolization can be identified and successfully treated.

DIABETIC FOOT INFECTIONS

Diabetic foot ulcers are typically produced by a combination of neuropathy. ischemia, and infection. Diabetic neuropathy may present as a diffuse sensory disturbance or as neuropathic pain. Neuropathy renders the foot more susceptible to trauma and infection. Degenerative arthropathy (Charcot joint) may be present. Once an ulcer has developed, local infection may occur. Infection is further promoted by the relative immunocompromised state of the diabetic patient. Infections are frequently polymicrobial and require aggressive treatment with appropriate antibiotics (usually intravenous) and débridement of infected and devitalized tissue.

Diabetic patients may also develop significant peripheral vascular disease. The disease is usually multisegmental, but there is a predilection for severe involvement of the infrapopliteal arteries. Evaluation of patients with diabetic foot ulcers or infections requires careful pulse examination supplemented by noninvasive hemodynamic testing. If significant disease is present, angiography and revascularization may be required to achieve healing. Although distal bypass procedures are often required, results of vascular reconstruction in diabetic patients generally parallel those in nondiabetics.

Perhaps the most important aspect of diabetic foot care is patient education and prevention. Careful attention to hygiene and appropriate footwear can avert many limb-threatening problems.

NONATHEROSCLEROTIC VASCULAR LESIONS

Popliteal Artery Entrapment

Developmental defects that displace the popliteal artery may cause arterial compression and stenosis or segmental occlusion. This syndrome is uncommon and occurs most often in young patients. Symptoms may include claudication or severe ischemia and may be unilateral or bilateral. With the most common variety of entrapment, the popliteal artery passes medial to the medial head of the gastrocnemius muscle and is subject to compression. Less commonly, a fibrous band of the popliteus muscle, deep to the medial head of the gastrocnemius, is the compressing structure. The diagnosis may be made by noninvasive hemodynamic studies with positional maneuvers to tense the gastrocnemius. In addition, angiography may demonstrate medial deviation of the popliteal artery or stenosis, occlusion, or aneurysm formation at the appropriate level. Treatment is aimed at removal of the compressing muscular structure plus popliteal artery reconstruction if necessary. Aggressive treatment of asymptomatic contralateral lesions may avert popliteal artery thrombosis and disabling ischemia.

Cystic Adventitial Disease of the Popliteal Artery

Rarely, cyst formation in the wall of the popliteal artery produces ischemic symptoms. Treatment consists of resection and graft replacement of the involved arterial segment.

Thromboangiitis Obliterans (Buerger's Disease)

Thromboangiitis obliterans is an occlusive disease of medium-size and small arteries affecting the distal upper and lower extremities. It is pathologically a seg-

mental panangiitis and affects primarily young men. The cause is not known, but a striking relation to tobacco smoking has been observed. Recurrent episodes of superficial thrombophlebitis may also be present. Angiography typically reveals multiple segmental occlusions in the small arteries of the forearm, hand, leg, and foot with many fine collateral vessels, often in a corkscrew configuration. Treatment is symptomatic and must include avoidance of tobacco. Reconstructive surgery may be difficult, and amputation is sometimes required.

Takayasu's Arteritis

Takayasu's arteritis is an inflammatory arteritis that usually occurs in young and middle-aged women. It most frequently involves the brachiocephalic vessels, renal arteries, and abdominal aorta; and it may be associated with acute nonspecific systemic symptoms. Other symptoms include stroke, upper or lower extremity ischemia, or renovascular hypertension. Retinal vasculitis was originally described and may also be present. Active disease is treated with corticosteroids, but vascular reconstructive surgery is required in selected cases. Procedures may be complex and generally involve bypass from uninvolved arterial segments.

Giant Cell (Temporal) Arteritis

Chronic inflammation of the aorta and large arteries is associated with a clinical syndrome of pain and stiffness in the trunk and proximal extremities in elderly patients. Headaches may be associated with tenderness over the course of the temporal artery. Blindness may occur if the disease is untreated. Diagnosis is made by temporal artery biopsy. Treatment with corticosteroids is recommended.

Raynaud's Syndrome

Raynaud's syndrome is defined as episodic attacks of vasoconstriction of the arteries and arterioles of the extremities in response to cold or emotional stimuli. It manifests clinically as sequential pallor, cyanosis, and rubor of the digits. Approximately 70% of patients have some identifiable associated condition, such as immunologic or connective tissue disorders (e.g., scleroderma), drug-induced syndrome (ergot, β-blockers), or obstructive arterial disease. The diagnosis can be made clinically and may be confirmed by ice-water immersion testing, measuring the recovery time to normal digital temperature. Noninvasive vascular examination of the digits with analysis of the digital pulse waveform and hand arteriography may also be helpful for diagnosing vasospastic and obstructive conditions.

Treatment consists of cold avoidance and discontinuation of offending drugs. In severe cases, nifedipine may be useful. There is little role for cervical sympathectomy.

Thoracic Outlet Syndrome

Thoracic outlet syndrome is caused by compression of the brachial plexus, subclavian artery, and subclavian vein in the thoracic outlet. These structures may be compressed between the clavicle and first rib or by a number of anatomic variations. Neurologic compression, the most common form of thoracic outlet syndrome, is discussed further elsewhere (see Chapter 20). Vascular complications of thoracic outlet syndrome occur infrequently. Arterial complications usually result from subclavian artery compression by complete cervical ribs, which may result in poststenotic dilatation of the subclavian artery with aneurysm formation and thromboembolic complications.

Treatment is aimed at decompression of the arterial stenosis combined with arterial reconstruction when necessary. Venous complications of thoracic outlet syndrome typically present as acute axillary vein thrombosis often related to vigorous exercise or trauma. Current recommendations for treatment of "effort thrombosis" include administration of lytic agents to restore venous patency, followed by anticoagulation and possible surgical decompression of the thoracic outlet to prevent recurrence.

Hypercoagulable States

As our understanding of the coagulation cascade has increased, so has our ability to diagnose congenital clotting defects, which may be responsible for unexplained venous, arterial, or graft thrombosis. Antithrombin III binds thrombin and several other activated clotting factors and neutralizes their activity. Protein C is a vitamin K-dependent glycoprotein that inhibits activated factors V and VIII and enhances fibrinolytic activity. Protein S is a cofactor of protein C and potentiates the inactivation of factor V. Congenital deficiencies of any of these factors, as well as fibrinolytic deficiencies or dysfibrinogenemia, may be responsible for hypercoagulable states. The evaluation of patients with unexplained or recurrent thrombosis should include measurement of antithrombin III, protein C, protein S, anticardiolipin antibody, lupus anticoagulant, plasminogen and plasminogen activator inhibitors, prothrombin time, partial thromboplastin time, bleeding time, and platelet count.

CEREBROVASCULAR DISEASE

Clinical Manifestations

Carotid artery disease may present as asymptomatic carotid bruits. Transient ischemic attacks (TIAs) are neurologic deficits that resolve within 24 hours. They are usually caused by microemboli of platelets, fibrin, and atheromatous material from carotid bifurcation plaques. Amaurosis fugax represents transient monocular blindness from embolization to the ophthalmic artery, a branch of the internal carotid artery. Atheromatous material visualized in the branches of the retinal artery are called Hollenhorst plaques. TIAs may also present as hemispheric ischemia with symptoms such as hemiparesis and dysphasia. Reversible ischemic neurologic deficits (RINDs) resolve within 3 days. Longer-lasting or permanent neurologic deficits are categorized as strokes.

Diagnosis

Many techniques are available for the diagnosis of extracranial carotid artery disease. Auscultation of the cervical region for bruits is a commonly used screening technique but is not specific for significant internal carotid artery stenosis. Early noninvasive tests, such as directional Doppler examination, carotid phonangiography, and oculoplethysmography, are used to determine the presence or absence of hemodynamically significant carotid stenosis. Because symptoms are often caused by microemboli from ulcerated atherosclerotic plaques, evaluation of hemodynamics alone in symptomatic patients is inadequate. Duplex scanning has replaced all previously available noninvasive techniques for evaluation of extracranial cerebrovascular disease.

These techniques combine ultrasound imaging and Doppler spectral analysis, producing both hemodynamic information and direct visualization of carotid artery lesions. Newer techniques produce color images and accurate information regarding carotid artery stenosis. In addition, transcranial Doppler techniques are available to provide information regarding blood flow in intracranial vessels. Additional imaging techniques include digital subtraction angiography, conventional arteriography, and magnetic resonance angiography (MRA). The combination of duplex scan and MRA appears to be as accurate as a conventional angiogram and has therefore replaced the latter in many centers. Although traditional standards require visualization of the aortic arch, cervical carotid arteries, and intracranial vessels prior to surgical intervention, some reports have demonstrated the safety of carotid surgery based solely on duplex scans. This area remains controversial.

Prognosis

Before treatment can be recommended, the natural history of carotid artery disease must be clarified. Controversy regarding the natural history of carotid bruits and asymptomatic carotid stenosis led to the initiation of several multicenter prospective randomized studies. The North American Symptomatic Carotid Endarterectomy Trial (NASCET) evaluated 659 patients from 50 centers with symptomatic high-grade stenosis (70% to 99%) of the internal carotid artery. Patients were prospectively randomized to medical (antiplatelet therapy) and surgical (carotid endarterectomy) groups. After 2 years the cumulative risk of stroke in the medical group was nearly three times higher than in patients who underwent carotid endarterectomy. The authors concluded that carotid endarterectomy (CEA) is highly beneficial in patients with recent hemispheric and retinal TIAs or nondisabling strokes and with ipsilateral high-grade stenosis.

The Asymptomatic Carotid Atherosclerosis Study (ACAS) was a prospective randomized study of 1,659 patients from 39 centers with asymptomatic high-grade stenosis (60% or more). After a median follow-up of 2.7 years, the authors concluded that patients treated with CEA have a reduced risk of ipsilateral stroke if surgery can be performed with less than 3% perioperative morbidity and mortality.

Treatment

Surgical therapy is currently the treatment of choice for symptomatic patients with high-grade ipsilateral stenosis of the internal carotid artery. Prophylactic CEA for patients with asymptomatic high-grade stenosis of the internal carotid artery also appears warranted to reduce the incidence of stroke. Carotid endarterectomy involves removal of atherosclerotic lesions localized at the carotid bifurcation. Moderate degrees of intracranial occlusive disease are not a contraindication to surgery. The technical aspects of the operation are critical for achieving good results. General or local anesthesia may be used. Adequate exposure of the carotid bifurcation while avoiding injury to adjacent structures (e.g., vagus and hypoglossal nerves) is important. The need for cerebral protection by intraluminal shunting during carotid clamping is controversial. Shunts may be used routinely, selectively (stump pressure, electroencephalographic monitoring, neurologic evaluation with the patient under local anesthesia), or not at all.

When properly performed, serious morbidity or mortality following CEA should occur in fewer than 2% of patients. Additional complications of local nerve injury are usually avoidable. Symptomatic recurrence from neointimal fibrous hyperplasia (6 to 18 months after surgery) or recurrent atherosclerosis (2 to 20 years after surgery) occurs in 1% to 2% of patients. Up to 15% of patients may have varying degrees of asymptomatic recurrent stenosis detected by routine postoperative noninvasive evaluation. Routine or selective closure of the endarterectomy with a prosthetic or venous patch is advocated by many surgeons to decrease the incidence of recurrent stenosis.

Although CEA for transient ischemia and asymptomatic high-grade lesions is now widely accepted, controversy exists regarding the performance of this operation for chronic cerebral ischemia and stroke-in-evolution. Total carotid occlusion is generally considered a contraindication to CEA. Although some symptomatic patients benefit from extracranial-to-intracranial (superficial temporal to middle cerebral) bypass, the results of a multicenter study showed this procedure to be ineffective in the long-term prevention of stroke in asymptomatic patients. Selected patients with internal carotid occlusion and persistent symptoms may be candidates for external carotid endarterectomy. This artery provides important collateral pathways to the brain in the presence of occlusion or high-grade stenosis of the internal carotid artery. Numerous reports document the efficacy of external carotid endarterectomy in relieving hemispheric ischemia in the presence of ipsilateral internal carotid occlusion.

Several reports have described catheter-based angioplasty techniques for the treatment of carotid bifurcation lesions. Although carotid angioplasty, with or without stenting, has the usual appeal of any nonoperative therapy, its use should be restricted to investigational protocols until sufficient data regarding its efficacy and safety are available.

Vertebrobasilar Insufficiency and Subclavian Steal

Although symptoms referrable to the carotid territory are far more common, vertebrobasilar symptoms occasionally require evaluation and consideration for surgical reconstruction. These symptoms include motor or sensory disturbances, diplopia, vertigo, and drop attacks. Many of these patients have associated carotid artery disease. If direct vertebral reconstruction is required, endarterectomy or bypass techniques have been utilized.

Vertebrobasilar insufficiency may also occur as a manifestation of subclavian steal syndrome. With this entity, a lesion in the innominate or subclavian artery proximal to the vertebral artery causes upper extremity ischemia. The vertebral artery becomes an important collateral pathway to the arm and may "steal" blood from the posterior circulation through the circle of Willis.

Treatment of symptomatic subclavian steal is by upper extremity revascularization. A number of techniques are available, including direct transthoracic endarterectomy or bypass, or extraanatomic revascularization by axillary-axillary, subclavian-subclavian, or left carotid-subclavian bypass or transposition.

Fibromuscular Dysplasia

Fibromuscular dysplasia of the carotid artery is an uncommon nonatherosclerotic condition that occurs primarily in women. It is frequently bilateral and may produce symptoms of transient cerebral ischemia. Although asymptomatic lesions require no special attention, symptomatic disease is best treated by operative resection or dilatation of the involved carotid artery. Associated intracranial aneurysms may be present.

Carotid Body Tumors

Carotid body tumors (chemodectomas) often present as asymptomatic neck masses. These lesions are highly vascular tumors that occur at the carotid bifurcation. They are frequently bilateral and usually benign, and the diagnosis can be confirmed by angiography. Treatment is by surgical resection. Preoperative embolization of large tumors may minimize the vascularity and facilitate resection. The blood supply to the tumor often emanates from the external carotid artery, and ligation of this vessel is sometimes required.

Carotid Dissection

Dissection of the cervical carotid artery may be spontaneous or traumatic. Spontaneous dissection is often related to hypertension, fibromuscular dysplasia, or arteriopathies (e.g., Marfan syndrome). Traumatic dissection may be related to cervical hyperextension or blunt cervical trauma. Angiography demonstrates a tapered narrowing of the extracranial carotid artery.

Treatment is generally nonoperative and consists of anticoagulation with heparin. Patients with persistent symptoms may require surgical intervention.

ANEURYSMS

Abdominal Aortic Aneurysms

Abdominal aortic aneurysms have traditionally been described as atherosclerotic aneurysms because of the variable finding of atherosclerosis within the aneurysm wall. It is now recognized that the finding of atherosclerosis within an aneurysm is coincidental and does not necessarily implicate it in the formation of the aneurysm. A high incidence of aortic aneurysms among many members of the same family suggests a genetic role in the pathogenesis of aneurysms. Alterations in the metabolism of collagen and elastin have been found in the walls of aortic aneurysms and are caused by altered gene expression. The precise cause of aneurysms remains unknown, but it likely involves a combination of altered gene expression, alterations in inflammatory response, and to a limited degree atherosclerosis. Occasionally, aneurysms are mycotic (infected) or traumatic. Aortic aneurysms appear predominantly in men, and most are infrarenal. The risk of rupture of infrarenal aortic aneurysms is significant for aneurysms larger than 5 cm in anteroposterior or transverse diameter, or three times the diameter of the normal proximal aorta.

Diagnosis

Most asymptomatic abdominal aortic aneurysms can be detected by palpation on routine physical examination. Only 50% of aneurysms have calcifications, allowing detection on plain abdominal radiographs. Computed tomography (CT) and ultrasonography are reliable diagnostic tools and accurately define aneurysm size. CT may be especially useful for evaluating symptomatic aortic aneurysms and is sensitive for the detection of rupture. Although aortography is a poor test to evaluate aneurysm size (laminated thrombus may limit contrast to the lumen), it is useful to identify associated renal, visceral, or peripheral arterial occlusive disease. Magnetic resonance imaging (MRI) may also be useful for preoperative evaluation of the vascular anatomy relative to abdominal aortic aneurysms.

Treatment

Small aneurysms may be followed by serial ultrasound examinations. Studies suggest that the average growth rate of small aneurysms is 0.3 to 0.5 cm per year, but it is variable. Treatment of asymptomatic abdominal aneurysms larger than 5 cm in diameter in good-risk patients is recommended to prevent rupture. Aneurysmectomy and graft replacement (straight tube or bifurcation) is the standard operative approach. Selected patients require preoperative cardiac evaluation. Routine cardiac screening of patients with aneurysms but no risk factors for coronary artery disease has not been productive. Perioperative hemodynamic monitoring is useful for optimizing cardiac function. Large aneurysms in poor-risk patients have been managed by a retroperitoneal approach to the aorta to avoid the cardiopulmonary complications of transperitoneal dissection. Occasional patients have been managed by iliac artery ligation, angiographically controlled thrombosis of the aortic

aneurysm, and extraanatomic bypass. However, rupture of thrombosed abdominal aortic aneurysms has been reported, and this approach is of questionable value.

Ruptured abdominal aortic aneurysms may present with abdominal or back pain, syncope or hemodynamic instability, and a pulsatile abdominal mass. Emergency operative intervention is required. Prompt, uncomplicated proximal aortic control is the key to successful management of this critical condition. The rupture is usually contained by the retroperitoneum. Intraperitoneal rupture carries an exceptionally grave prognosis. As previously mentioned, CT may be useful in the occasional symptomatic patient who is hemodynamically stable.

Aneurysms, on rare occasions, rupture into adjacent structures. An aortocaval fistula results from rupture of an aneurysm into the inferior vena cava and manifests as high-output cardiac failure, a continuous abdominal bruit, and lower extremity ischemia with venous engorgement. Rupture into the left renal vein has also been reported and may present with hematuria. Operative treatment requires control of the abdominal aorta, but dissection of hypertensive venous structures is hazardous and should be avoided. Treatment is by graft replacement of the aortic aneurysm and repair of the inferior vena cava from within the lumen of the aorta.

Aneurysms can also rupture into the gastrointestinal (GI) tract, producing GI hemorrhage. The usual site of fistula formation is the duodenum. Repair of these primary aortoenteric fistulas is by aortic graft and repair of the duodenum or involved bowel. This protocol is different from the traditional management of secondary aortoenteric fistulas resulting from a previously placed aortic graft (see below).

Endovascular stent-grafts have found increasing use over the past few years for treatment of aortic aneurysms. With this technique the graft is secured to the aorta by a self-expanding or balloon-expandable metal stent that is deployed under fluoroscopic guidance. The carrier is introduced through a femoral artery cutdown, thereby avoiding the laparotomy, retroperitoneal dissection, and aortic clamping and suturing required for conventional aneurysm repair. These devices have been used to treat thoracic and abdominal aortic aneurysms, occlusive disease of the aorta and iliac arteries (transfemoral endoluminal bifurcation grafts), and occlusive disease and trauma in the upper and lower extremities. Despite the attractiveness of this technique, endovascular stent-grafts should be used only under investigational protocols until their long-term efficacy and safety have been demonstrated.

Complications

Although the risk of major morbidity or mortality from elective aneurysm resection is less than 5%, there are many potential complications. Bleeding, peripheral embolization, and lower extremity ischemia may occur. Impotence may result from neurologic or vasculogenic causes. Avoidance of the presacral neural plexus and maintenance of pelvic blood flow through the hypogastric arteries should minimize this complication. Paraplegia is a rare but devastating complication of abdominal aortic surgery, resulting from spinal cord ischemia. It occurs more commonly after surgery for a ruptured abdominal aortic aneurysm. Colonic ischemia can be minimized by preoperative evaluation of visceral arterial anatomy and preservation of hypogastric and inferior mesenteric blood flow when feasible. Postoperative rectal bleeding mandates prompt sigmoidoscopy for inspection of colonic mucosa. Mucosal ischemia can be managed conservatively, but transmural intestinal ischemia requires aggressive operative intervention.

Aortic graft infection is an uncommon but serious complication of surgery for both aneurysmal and occlusive disease. Prophylactic antibiotic use should minimize this complication. Graft sepsis requires removal of prosthetic material and extraanatomic revascularization. Secondary aortoenteric fistula may be a manifestation of aortic graft infection and requires graft removal. This complication can occur years after aortic graft insertion and should be suspected in any patient who presents with GI bleeding following aortic surgery. Immediate upper GI endoscopy to rule out other potential causes of bleeding is required, followed by prompt exploratory laparotomy. Rupture of the ligated aortic stump remains a potential cause of mortality following graft removal. Although controversial, recent reports describe successful management of secondary aortoenteric fistulas with aggressive surgical débridement and irrigation, *in situ* revascularization, and long-term antibiotic therapy.

Miscellaneous Problems

Thoracoabdominal aneurysms require an approach different from that used for infrarenal aneurysm resec-

tion. Aortic graft replacement and intraluminal attachment of visceral and renal arteries, as advocated by Crawford, have produced excellent results. Paraplegia is more common with thoracoabdominal aneurysms but may be minimized by reattaching large intercostal arteries that originate from the descending aorta, where the major blood supply to the spinal cord originates. Additional techniques, such as somatosensory evoked potentials and spinal fluid drainage to increase spinal cord perfusion pressure, may also be used.

Inflammatory abdominal aortic aneurysms may be identified on preoperative CT scan or intraoperatively by a typical dense retroperitoneal fibrosis overlying the aorta. The conduct of the operation must be modified to avoid hazardous dissection of the duodenum or other adherent structures off the aneurysm. Although partial or (rarely) complete ureteral obstruction may be present, ureterolysis is usually unnecessary because the retroperitoneal inflammation tends to subside after repair of the aneurysm.

Horseshoe kidney in association with aortic aneurysm is an uncommon but interesting problem. Because the kidney may interfere with aneurysm dissection, and blood supply to the isthmus may originate from the aneurysm, a retroperitoneal approach and revascularization or resection of the isthmus may be required.

Coincidental malignancy discovered at the time of laparotomy for aortic aneurysm may present a therapeutic dilemma. In general, a ruptured or symptomatic aneurysm requires urgent treatment. Bleeding, perforated, or obstructing GI malignancy without impending aneurysmal rupture should take precedence. If both lesions can be dealt with electively, treatment of the aneurysm is advocated because it is imminently life-threatening. Reports of ruptured abdominal aneurysms following laparotomy for treatment of unrelated intraabdominal pathology await additional corroboration.

Peripheral Aneurysms

Peripheral aneurysms likely have the same etiology as those of the aorta. The most common peripheral aneurysms occur in the popliteal artery. These lesions typically occur in men, are bilateral in more than 50% of patients, and are associated with an abdominal aortic aneurysm in about one-third of patients. Although rupture of popliteal artery aneurysms is uncommon, thrombosis or distal embolization may produce limb-threatening ischemia. Most popliteal aneurysms can be treated by ligation and bypass. Thrombosis of popliteal aneurysms may result in occlusion of the distal tibial arteries. In such cases, prompt administration of thrombolytic therapy may result in restoration of patency of outflow arteries, which can be followed by surgical correction to prevent recurrent thrombosis.

Femoral artery aneurysms may also be bilateral, and a significant association with abdominal aortic aneurysms exists. These lesions should be sought by ultrasonography or CT. Aneurysms occur rarely in the carotid, subclavian, or other arteries. Ulnar artery aneurysms have been reported following repetitive trauma (e.g., use of vibratory tools) to the hypothenar eminence of the hand. Ligation of the ulnar artery suffices in most patients, but reconstruction may be required in the absence of a complete palmar arch.

Visceral Aneurysms

Among visceral aneurysms, splenic artery aneurysm is the most common (60%) in this uncommon group. These lesions are often associated with arterial fibrodysplasia and occur predominantly in women. They are prone to rupture during pregnancy and require treatment if symptomatic, larger than 2 cm in diameter, or diagnosed during child-bearing ages. Resection or embolization of aneurysms in the proximal splenic artery can usually be accomplished with splenic preservation.

Other visceral aneurysms are rare. Hepatic aneurysms comprise 20% of this group, and their precise cause is unknown. Superior mesenteric aneurysms comprise 5.5% of the group and are usually mycotic.

Renal artery aneurysms are uncommon and may be caused by fibromuscular dysplasia. Most are asymptomatic, but these lesions may be associated with hypertension. Rupture and dissection are potential complications, and treatment of all symptomatic aneurysms and asymptomatic aneurysms larger than 2 cm is indicated.

Infected (Mycotic) Aneurysms

Infected aneurysms of the aorta should be suspected in patients with fever, pain, and a pulsatile abdominal mass. These lesions are false (pseudo) aneurysms and may occur in patients without generalized atherosclerosis. *Salmonella, Staphylococcus,* and other organisms have been described as potential pathogens. Treatment is by excision and extraanatomic bypass.

Mycotic femoral artery aneurysms may occur in intravenous drug abusers. These false aneurysms should be treated by excision with selective vascular reconstruction. Acute limb-threatening ischemia is most common with aneurysms involving the femoral bifurcation, and revascularization is considered if control of local sepsis can be achieved.

VISCERAL ISCHEMIA

Visceral ischemia may be acute or chronic. Acute mesenteric ischemia may be caused by superior mesenteric artery embolism or thrombosis, mesenteric venous thrombosis, or nonocclusive mesenteric ischemia. The latter is usually due to low cardiac output states. Accurate diagnosis requires prompt mesenteric arteriography and appropriate surgical (e.g., embolectomy) or pharmacologic (e.g., vasodilator therapy) intervention or both. Mortality remains high for this condition, usually because of delayed recognition.

Chronic mesenteric ischemia usually requires significant disease of at least two of the three visceral arteries (superior mesenteric, inferior mesenteric, celiac). Celiac artery compression by the median arcuate ligament is an uncommon syndrome of questionable clinical significance. Symptoms of chronic mesenteric ischemia include postprandial abdominal pain (mesenteric angina), anorexia, weight loss, and diarrhea.

Treatment is by aortomesenteric revascularization and often utilizes prosthetic grafts to prevent graft kinking in the retroperitoneal position. Prophylactic mesenteric revascularization during surgery on the abdominal aorta has been suggested with superior mesenteric stenosis and a large, meandering mesenteric artery, but this subject remains controversial.

RENOVASCULAR HYPERTENSION

Renal Artery Stenosis

Renal artery stenosis accounts for less than 3% of hypertension. Approximately two-thirds of renovascular hypertension is caused by atherosclerosis and one-third by fibromuscular dysplasia. Rarely, renal artery aneurysms can cause renovascular hypertension.

Diagnosis requires a high index of suspicion in young patients or patients with recent onset of severe hypertension. Controversy exists regarding optimal screening tests to identify renovascular hypertension. Hypertensive intravenous pyelogram (evaluating renal size, contrast uptake and excretion, and ureteral notching) has generally been replaced by radionuclide renal perfusion scans. The latter, however, are plagued by an unacceptable incidence of false-negative results. Selective renal vein renin sampling, with a renin output 1.5 times the output from the normal kidney, is suggestive of renovascular hypertension. Additional support for the diagnosis can be obtained by observing a reduction in blood pressure and a rise in plasma renin activity with the use of angiotensin inhibitors (e.g., captopril). Accurate information regarding renal artery anatomy and hemodynamics is currently available using duplex scanning, and many centers utilize this modality as the noninvasive screening test of choice for renal vascular disease.

Treatment options include medical therapy (e.g., captopril), PTA, surgical revascularization, and nephrectomy. The ability of medical therapy to prevent progressive loss of renal mass and consequent renal failure has been poor. PTA has yielded excellent results and is advocated for appropriate fibromuscular and atherosclerotic lesions. Atherosclerotic orifice lesions of the renal artery are usually not appropriate for dilatation because of their high recurrence rate. Improved patency by utilizing stents after dilatation of renal orificial lesions has been reported.

Surgical therapy by endarterectomy or bypass has excellent patency rates. Transaortic endarterectomy is effective in treating bilateral orificial lesions. Aortorenal bypass may be performed with autogenous vein or prosthetic material. Because of the potential for aneurysmal dilatation of saphenous vein grafts in children, autogenous hypogastric artery is preferred. In patients with extensive aortic disease not requiring simultaneous treatment, renal revascularization can be successfully accomplished with hepatorenal or splenorenal bypass if these arteries are free of disease. Branch lesions may be treated by bench surgery and autotransplantation. Nephrectomy is reserved for end-stage disease or uncorrectable renal artery lesions. Results of renal revascularization depend on the patient's age, duration of hypertension, and kidney size.

Ischemic Nephropathy

Patients with ischemic nephropathy have severe extraparenchymal renal artery occlusive disease and renal insufficiency. Renal excretory function may be improved with the surgical techniques described above, which are applicable to two groups of patients. In some patients with normal or slightly elevated serum creatinine and a poorly or nonfunctioning kidney, the contralateral normal kidney maintains overall renal function. These individuals are often identified during a renovascular hypertension workup, and renal revascularization may salvage the dysfunctional kidney. The second group is comprised of azotemic or dialysis-dependent individuals with extraparenchymal renal artery occlusive disease. Significant improvements in glomerular filtration rates and reversal of renal insufficiency have been achieved with renal artery reconstruction in properly selected patients from this group.

Angioaccess Surgery

Patients with acute or chronic renal failure require vascular access for hemodialysis. Acute access is usually via a central venous catheter, femoral vein cannulation, or a Scribner shunt (Teflon-tipped arterial and venous cannulas).

Access for chronic hemodialysis is preferred via a subcutaneous arteriovenous (AV) fistula. This procedure was originally described as a radiocephalic AV fistula by Brescia, Cimino, and colleagues. Although it remains the preferred location, fistulas may also be created at other sites in the upper extremity. If superficial veins are unsuitable for primary AV fistulas, prosthetic AV grafts may be placed and punctured directly for access. Complications of angioaccess surgery include thrombosis, infection, aneurysm formation, venous hypertension, and ischemia secondary to arterial "steal."

VASCULAR TRAUMA

Etiology

Vascular injuries may be blunt or penetrating. A number of iatrogenic conditions can occur as well, including injuries secondary to angiography, umbilical catheters, indwelling arterial cannulas, intraaortic balloon pumps, embolectomy catheters, lumbar laminectomy (iliac arteriovenous fistula), and cardiac catheterization among others.

Principles

Pathologic lesions include transection, laceration, thrombosis, or intimal flaps. In addition, a false aneurysm or arteriovenous fistula may be present. Blunt trauma frequently produces orthopedic injury and secondary vascular trauma. The diagnosis may be difficult, particularly in the absence of significant hemorrhage or pulse deficits.

Treatment

Resuscitation of the trauma patient is described in detail in Chapter 15. Specific priorities regarding vascular injury include control of bleeding, stabilization of fractures, and repair of arterial and venous injuries. Venous repair, if possible, is recommended, particularly in the popliteal area. Primary repair of arterial injuries is advocated. If it is impossible, autogenous graft material is recommended, although recent reports suggest that prosthetic grafts (e.g., expanded PTFE) may function satisfactorily, even in potentially contaminated wounds.

Compartment Syndrome

Muscles of the extremities are encased in fascial compartments. Swelling within the compartment may increase compartmental pressure and interfere with vascular and neurologic function, eventually causing muscle necrosis. Compartment syndromes may be caused by direct trauma (e.g., fractures), hemorrhage, or prolonged compression of an extremity (e.g., crush syndrome); or they may occur after revascularization of an acutely ischemic extremity (e.g., for arterial embolus or trauma). Upper extremity compartments may be similarly affected (e.g., Volkmann ischemic contracture), but the lower extremity is the usual site of compartment syndrome. Pressure in each of the four lower extremity compartments (anterior, lateral, superficial posterior, deep posterior) can be measured by direct techniques. Pressure of more than 40 mm Hg, or within 30 mm Hg of the diastolic blood pressure, may result in cessation

of flow through capillaries and arterioles. In most cases, treatment of an elevated compartment pressure is by fasciotomy of all compartments via a single incision over the fibula or in combination with a second medial incision. The sequelae of an unrelieved acute compartment syndrome are muscle and nerve necrosis with resulting functional disability.

Specific Injuries

Although a discussion of all vascular injuries is beyond the scope of this review, several specific injuries warrant further consideration. Large acute *arteriovenous fistulas* are best closed early to prevent ischemic and hemodynamic complications. Small distal arteriovenous fistulas can be observed or embolized and require only selective operative intervention. *Carotid artery injuries* should be repaired if possible, even if minor neurologic deficits are present. Vascular *injuries in the thoracic inlet* are often lethal and require a thorough knowledge of anatomy to plan the operative exposure. *Popliteal artery injuries,* if unrecognized or untreated, are associated with a high incidence of limb loss. Posterior *knee dislocation* has a significant association with arterial injury, and aggressive angiographic evaluation of these patients is recommended. *Brachial artery injuries* may occur with supracondylar fracture of the humerus and if unrecognized can result in Volkmann ischemic contracture. *Portal vein injuries* should be repaired. If it is impossible, ligation rather than acute portasystemic shunting is recommended. A second look within 24 hours is advocated, with shunting recommended only if venous engorgement threatens bowel viability. *Intraarterial drug injection* may threaten limb viability. In general, elevation, anticoagulation, dextran, and aggressive fasciotomy can minimize tissue loss. Reference to a text devoted to vascular trauma is recommended for treatment of other injuries.

QUESTIONS

Select one answer:

1. Which of the following is true about patients with intermittent claudication?
   a. Lumbar sympathectomy effectively relieves symptoms in most patients.

b. A graded exercise program improves the walking capacity of most of the patients.

c. Arteriography is required in most patients as part of the initial evaluation.

d. Vasodilators are effective treatment for most patients.

e. Amputation is required in up to one-third of patients if left untreated.

2. Acute arterial occlusion of the lower extremity:

a. Is most often the result of femoral artery thrombosis.

b. Can never occur as a consequence of deep venous thrombosis.

c. Is never amenable to treatment with thrombolytic therapy.

d. Is most often the result of a cardiac embolic event.

e. Rarely results in limb-threatening ischemia.

3. Which of the following is true regarding renovascular hypertension:

a. It is most often caused by fibromuscular dysplasia of the renal arteries.

b. Saphenous vein grafts are preferred for aortorenal bypass in children.

c. Duplex scanning is currently the preferred screening method for renal artery stenosis.

d. Percutaneous transluminal angioplasty is effective treatment for ostial stenosis of the renal artery.

e. Hepatorenal bypass is ineffective treatment for renal insufficiency caused by renovascular disease.

4. Which of the following is true regarding diabetic foot infections:

a. They are usually caused by infection with gram-positive organisms only.

b. Surgical débridement is unnecessary when pedal pulses are present.

c. Oral antibiotics are adequate treatment in most cases.

d. Neuropathy is rarely a contributing factor in their development.

e. Revascularization may be required even if adequate surgical débridement is done and appropriate antibiotics are used.

5. Which of the following statements regarding aneurysms is true:

a. Inflammatory aneurysms of the aorta rarely rupture.

b. Splenic artery aneurysms are usually atherosclerotic in origin.

c. Thrombosis of popliteal artery aneurysms may be treated with thrombolysis only.

d. Infected aneurysms of the aorta usually require complete excision and extraanatomic revascularization.

e. Aneurysms of the hepatic artery are the most common visceral aneurysms.

6. Patients with symptomatic carotid disease:

a. May be candidates for external carotid endarterectomy in the presence of internal carotid artery occlusion.

b. Usually present with vertigo and syncopal attacks.

c. Should be given a trial of antiplatelet therapy prior to considering carotid endarterectomy regardless of the degree of stenosis.

d. Are not candidates for surgery if any intracranial occlusive disease is present.

e. Always require angiography prior to the performance of carotid endarterectomy.

7. Which of the following is true:

a. Patients with fibromuscular dysplasia of the carotid artery may have associated intracranial aneurysms.

b. Cystic adventitial disease of the popliteal artery is an uncommon inflammatory arteritis best treated with corticosteroids.

c. Popliteal entrapment syndrome usually results in lateral displacement of the popliteal artery.

d. Raynaud's syndrome is best diagnosed by arteriography.

e. Takayasu's arteritis most commonly involves the distal arm and hand arteries in middle-aged men.

8. Secondary aortoduodenal fistula is:

a. Caused by rupture of an abdominal aortic aneurysm into the GI tract.

b. Is best treated by partial removal of the synthetic graft and oversewing the remaining cuff of graft at the proximal aorta.

c. Should be managed by immediate operative intervention if endoscopy fails to demonstrate any clear cause of upper GI bleeding.

d. Is most accurately diagnosed by arteriography.

e. Is accurately diagnosed by tagged red blood cell studies in more than 80% of patients.

9. Evaluation for hypercoagulable states should include measurement of:
   a. Antithrombin III.
   b. Protein C.
   c. Protein S.
   d. Anticardiolipin antibody.
   e. All of the above.
10. Aneurysms of the abdominal aorta:
   a. Are best diagnosed by arteriography.
   b. May be associated with a genetic predisposition in some patients.
   c. Are frequently associated with unrecognized coronary artery disease.
   d. When 5 cm in diameter are at a 5% risk to rupture in 5 years.
   e. Are more common in women than men.

SELECTED REFERENCES

Baron JF, Mundler O, Bertrand M, et al. Dipyridamole-thallium scintigraphy and gated radionuclide angiography to assess cardiac risk before abdominal aortic surgery. *N Engl J Med* 1994;330:663–669.

Cambria RP, Kaufman JA, L'Italien GJ, et al. Magnetic resonance angiography in the management of lower extremity arterial occlusive disease: a prospective study. *J Vasc Surg* 1997;25:380–390.

Crawford ES, Crawford JL, Safi HJ, et al. Thoracoabdominal aortic aneurysms: preoperative and intraoperative factors determining immediate and long-term results of operation in 605 patients, *J Vasc Surg* 1986;3:389–404.

Ernst CB, Stanley JC, eds. *Current therapy in vascular surgery,* 3rd ed. St. Louis: Mosby, 1995.

Executive Committee for the Asymptomatic Carotid Atherosclerosis Study. Endarterectomy for asymptomatic carotid artery stenosis. *JAMA* 1995;273:1421–1428.

Hansen KJ, Thomason RB, Craven TE, et al. Surgical management of dialysis-dependent ischemic nephropathy. *J Vasc Surg* 1995;21:197–211.

Moore WS, ed. *Vascular surgery: a comprehensive review,* 5th ed. Philadelphia: WB Saunders, 1997.

Moore WS, for the EVT Investigators. Transfemoral endovascular repair of abdominal aortic aneurysms; results of the North American EVT phase 1 trial. *J Vasc Surg* 1996;23:543–553.

North American Symptomatic Carotid Endarterectomy Trial Collaborators. Beneficial effect of carotid endarterectomy in symptomatic patients with high-grade carotid stenosis. *N Engl J Med* 1991;325:445–453.

Ouriel K, Veith FJ, Sasahara AA. Thrombolysis or peripheral arterial surgery (TOPAS): Phase I results. *J Vasc Surg* 1996;23:64–73.

Rutherford RB, ed. *Vascular surgery,* 4th ed. Philadelphia: WB Saunders, 1995.

Scher LA, Veith FJ, Samson RJ, et al. Vascular complications of thoracic outlet syndrome. *J Vasc Surg* 1986;3:565–568.

STILE Investigators. Results of a prospective randomized trial evaluating surgery versus thrombolysis for ischemia of the lower extremity: the STILE trial. *Ann Surg* 1994;220:251–268.

Strandness DE. *Duplex scanning in vascular disorders.* New York: Raven Press, 1990.

Veith FJ, Gupta SK, Wengerter KR, et al. Changing arteriosclerotic disease patterns and management strategies in lower limb threatening ischemia. *Ann Surg* 1990;212:402–414.

9

Venous and Lymphatic Disease

Russell H. Samson and Larry A. Scher

ANATOMY

The veins of the lower extremity are divided into the deep and superficial systems. The latter system consists of the long (greater) saphenous vein, the short (or lesser) saphenous vein, and their tributaries. The greater saphenous vein courses along the medial aspect of the leg from the medial malleolus to the groin and enters the deep system at the common femoral vein. Just prior to its entrance into the common femoral vein, the greater saphenous vein receives blood from up to five tributaries. A duplicate saphenous system in the thigh is not uncommon and may be available for use as an arterial conduit even after vein stripping. The short saphenous vein courses up the posterior calf and enters the popliteal vein in the popliteal fossa. The deep system of veins consists of named venous trunks that coincide with the major arteries. It should be noted that below the knee there are often two veins for every one artery. Connecting the deep and superficial systems are the perforator or communicating veins. These vessels drain into the plexus of veins within the soleus and gastrocnemius muscles and together comprise the "muscle pump." Most of the perforators are clustered around the medial malleolus, with a few just above and below the knee.

APPLIED VENOUS PHYSIOLOGY

The veins of the lower extremity are richly supplied with valves. These bicuspid leaflets prevent blood from falling back down to the foot in the erect position. The valves within the perforator veins also prevent blood from being squeezed out of the muscle pump into the superficial system when the muscle pump is activated during walking. In the normal subject, flow in the veins is toward the heart and is dependent on respiration, arterial inflow, position, and the activity of the muscle pump. Under resting conditions in the recumbent position, venous flow is phasic with respiration. In the lower extremity flow is decreased during inspiration, because although the intrathoracic pressure becomes negative the intraabdominal pressure becomes positive. With expiration, the temporary backup of blood that occurred during inspiration is released, and venous flow increases. During walking, when the muscle pump is active, blood is squeezed out of the muscle plexus of veins toward the heart, thereby increasing flow in the deep system. Flow in the superficial system usually continues in a prograde fashion. As the muscle pump relaxes within the walking cycle, blood is sucked into the muscle pump from the superficial system, refilling the deep plexus of veins. Provided the perforator veins are competent, flow is dominantly from the superficial system into the deep system and then to the heart.

Venous pressure at rest equals the weight of the column of blood from the point of estimation to the third interspace at the sternum. It should be remembered that venous valves prevent retrograde flow in the upright position but do not impede the effects of pressure. Thus in the recumbent position pressure at the ankle is approximately 10 mm Hg, whereas in the standing position it is 86 mm Hg. Furthermore, in the standing position approximately 500 ml of blood accumulates in the veins of the leg. With exercise, the muscle pump lowers venous pressure in the dependent limb, reduces venous volume in the exercised area, and, as mentioned, facilitates venous return to the heart.

With valvular destruction and chronic venous insufficiency, the hemodynamics of venous flow in the lower extremity is severely affected. Patients with primary varicose veins in which only the valves of the saphenous system are incompetent have minimal clinical manifestations, when deep and perforator valves become incompetent, the efficacy of the muscle pump is greatly reduced because during muscular activity blood is directed not only toward the heart but also out toward the superficial system. Venous pressure measurements obtained during walking no longer show the significant reduction that occurs with muscular contractions. A state of ambulatory venous hypertension results, which may be aggravated if there is any proximal venous obstruction.

This altered physiology results in diapedesis of red blood cells through the capillaries with destruction of hemoglobin and ultimate pigmentary changes in the skin. Edema and swelling may result. If it is complicated by lymphatic obstruction from fibrotic change of the edema fluid, capillary block and ultimately skin destruction may occur, resulting in chronic venous ulceration.

VARICOSE VEINS

Varicose veins may be primary or secondary. Most of the patients suffer from primary varicose veins, perhaps as a result of prolonged standing, Women are more commonly affected than men, with the varicosities usually manifesting during pregnancy. They are probably a result of hormonal changes rather than pressure effects, as the varicose veins usually begin to manifest during the first trimester, at which stage uterine growth has barely begun.

An important congenital cause of varicose veins is the Klippel-Trenaunay syndrome, which manifests as varicose veins, cutaneous arteriovenous malformations, and occasionally gigantism of the involved extremities. Venograms of such patients may also demonstrate hypoplasia of the deep venous system. It is important to recognize these infants, as venous stripping operations are generally contraindicated.

A few patients present with secondary varicose veins as a result of some other cause of arteriovenous fistulas, such as trauma. However, most of the secondary varicose veins result from valvular destruction due to previous deep venous thrombophlebitis.

Clinical Manifestations

Most patients with varicose veins remain asymptomatic, their only concern being the cosmetic effects. Some patients do complain of an aching sensation that occurs after prolonged standing and is relieved by rest. Occasionally, varicose veins hemorrhage, especially when traumatized. First-aid treatment for such hemorrhage is elevation of the extremity with local pressure. A tourniquet should not be applied proximally, as it would increase venous pressure and result in bleeding. Superficial thrombophlebitis may also occur in a varicose vein (see below).

Treatment

Asymptomatic varicose veins require no therapy. Support stockings may decrease the sense of discomfort; but if it is persistent, or if recurrent episodes of superficial thrombophlebitis or hemorrhage have occurred, surgical treatment may be warranted. Surgical management can be achieved by compression sclerotherapy or stripping procedures.

Compression Sclerotherapy

Compression sclerotherapy involves the injection of an irritant substance into the vein while the vein wall is collapsed by elevating the extremity. Compression is then maintained by wrapping the limb with a tight bandage or using a surgical-weight support stocking. The substance most commonly used for compression sclerotherapy is 3% sodium tetradecyl sulfate.

The results of compression sclerotherapy are variable. It appears to be most useful when the veins are localized below the knee. Compression of veins in the thigh is often difficult, and the recurrence rate is higher. Complications include allergic reactions, toxic effects of an overdose of the sclerosant, thromboembolic phenomenon, ulceration of the skin from extravenous placement of the sclerosing agent, brown staining, and recurrence.

Surgery

Many variations of surgical removal of varicose veins have been described. The earliest and until recently the most widely used is a stripping operation. It involves disconnecting the greater saphenous vein from the common femoral vein (or the lesser saphenous vein from the popliteal) if these superficial veins are proved incompetent by clinical or noninvasive evaluation. The greater saphenous or involved lesser saphenous vein is then removed by pulling back on a stripping device that is passed from the groin or popliteal fossa to the distalmost vein at the ankle. The remaining varicose tributaries are then surgically excised through 1- to 2-cm incisions placed in Langer's lines. This procedure usually involves an overnight hospital stay and some time off work.

Specific complications of these operations include inadvertent stripping of the femoral artery or the deep femoral venous system, ligation of the femoral vein, and pulmonary embolism. Scarring and saphenous neuropathy are also major drawbacks to this procedure. Furthermore, because the main saphenous vein itself is seldom varicose even if it is incompetent, this procedure results in ablation of what could be a usable arterial substitute in the future.

Accordingly "vein-sparing" procedures have become more popular. Such procedures can be performed under local anesthesia or with intravenous sedation if necessary. They also allow early ambulation and minimal scarring. In general, these procedures involve high ligation of the saphenous vein and surrounding tributaries and mini-incision removal of distal varices (microphlebectomy or stab avulsion phlebectomy). The latter incisions are so small they can be closed with Steri-Strips.

If the greater saphenous is itself involved with varicosities, it should be stripped in the thigh to prevent a painful phlebitis in the disconnected segment. This procedure can also be performed under intravenous sedation.

CHRONIC VENOUS INSUFFICIENCY

The clinical syndrome of chronic venous insufficiency can result from long-standing varicose veins but more often results from venous valvular dysfunction, most commonly caused by previous deep venous thrombophlebitis. Patients complain of a sense of lower extremity discomfort that is worse in the late afternoon after standing and is relieved by lying down. Examination of the legs may demonstrate varicose veins, pitting edema and swelling, brownish skin discoloration with thickening and scaling of the skin around the medial malleolus, and ultimately venous ulceration. These ulcers usually localize around the medial malleolus but may be more extensive and involve the entire leg and foot. They are commonly painless.

Diagnosis

The diagnosis of chronic venous insufficiency can be supported by noninvasive techniques, including use of the Doppler ultrasound flow detector to determine the direction of flow in the superficial and deep venous system. Retrograde flow suggests valvular dysfunction. Photoplethysmography is increasingly being used to document chronic venous insufficiency. The photoplethysmograph measures the skin capillary blood content. In normal controls, after five active dorsiflexions are performed in the sitting position, skin capillary blood content decreases as venous blood is pushed toward the heart. If valves are competent, these parameters return to normal slowly as arterial blood supply refills the extremity. The time taken for filling to occur is called the venous recovery time (VRT). The VRT is shortened (less than 20 seconds) in patients with chronic venous insufficiency and valvular dysfunction. Primary and secondary chronic venous insufficiency can be defined by combining these tests with the use of a tourniquet placed below the knee. It can be assumed that chronic venous insufficiency is caused by superficial (rather than deep) venous dysfunction if such a tourniquet, which occludes the superficial veins, returns the VRT to normal. Failure of the VRT to improve with the use of a tourniquet suggests deep venous incompetence. Color duplex scanning has been proved to be a reliable method for demonstrating venous reflux, valve function, and the location of perforators.

Management

Symptoms in patients with chronic venous insufficiency can usually be alleviated with surgical support stockings, which offer a graduated pressure of 30 to 40 mm Hg to the extremity. Patients with advanced venous ulceration require some method of delivering external compression. Standard therapy has usually consisted of an Unna's boot supplemented by an external wrap of Elastoplast or an Ace bandage. Newer techniques include use of special dressings supplemented by compression stockings (e.g., Jobst UlcerCare). Once the ulcer is healed, stocking therapy may prevent recurrence. When these ulcers do not respond to conservative forms of therapy, hospital admission with prolonged bed rest and possible split-thickness skin grafts may be required to achieve healing.

Surgical techniques for ulcer healing include subfascial ligation of perforators, direct venous valve reconstruction by valve transposition, and valve repair using the Kistner technique. The role of the latter direct surgical reconstructions remains to be defined, but advances in endoscopic and angioscopic techniques have shown promise in expediting and decreasing the morbidity associated with these procedures.

THROMBOPHLEBITIS

The formation of blood clots within the venous system of the lower extremities is called thrombophlebitis. It may occur in superficial veins or deep veins.

Superficial Venous Thrombophlebitis

Superficial venous thrombophlebitis (SVT) is usually seen in patients who have varicose veins, although it may occur spontaneously in normal veins. If SVT is recurrent and associated with episodes of SVT in other, unusual parts of the body, a diagnosis of migratory thrombophlebitis should be entertained and a workup instituted to detect some occult malignancy or hypercoagulable state. In general, SVT is a benign condition.

Clinical Manifestations

Superficial venous thrombophlebitis manifests with all the signs of local inflammation, including redness, tenderness, local heat, pain, and swelling in the involved superficial vein. On occasion, SVT is misdiagnosed as cellulitis, but persistent fever is usually absent. The risk of pulmonary embolism is low (less than 3%).

Management

Symptomatic relief is usually all that is required for such patients. It may be achieved by an antiinflammatory analgesic such as aspirin or indomethacin. Patients should be encouraged to continue ambulation, as bed rest may contribute to stasis and further aggravate the disease. Antibiotics are not required, as bacterial colonization of thrombus has not been demonstrated. The risk of pulmonary embolism increases if the phlebitis migrates up the thigh. If this occurs, the saphenous vein in the groin should be ligated and divided. Such a procedure can be done under local anesthesia. All patients with SVT should undergo some form of noninvasive testing to exclude an underlying, unrecognized deep venous thrombophlebitis. Patients who have recurrent episodes of superficial thrombophlebitis in varicose veins are candidates for venous stripping procedures.

Deep Venous Thrombophlebitis

Deep venous thrombophlebitis (DVT) may occur spontaneously or as a result of some underlying predisposing factor. Such factors include local and general trauma, postsurgical states, prolonged bed rest, occult neoplasms (specifically those of the GI tract), pregnancy, birth control pills, psychiatric disorders, and obesity. Hip surgery is a notorious predisposing factor for DVT.

Clinical Manifestations

The clinical diagnosis of DVT is unreliable, and approximately 50% of patients present without any major clinical findings, such as swelling, pain, local tenderness, and a fever spike. A palpable cord is seldom felt, and Homans' sign (pain in the calf with dorsiflexion of the foot) is present in only 25% of patients.

Because of the difficulties involved in making the diagnosis of DVT, further testing is required. However, because venograms induce phlebitis in 2% to 5% of patients and these procedures are painful, costly, and carry a small anaphylactic risk, noninvasive diagnostic techniques have been utilized. Duplex color ultrasonography has supplanted older invasive techniques, and many of the physicians who utilize these tests as the only diagnostic method forego venography. Accuracy rates for "named vein" phlebitis approaches 95% to 98%, although venography is still required in some patients.

Management

Patients with confirmed DVT should be hospitalized with bed rest and lower extremity elevation. Anticoagulant therapy with heparin is started immediately using a loading dose of 80 to 150 U/kg followed by continuous infusion at a dose of approximately 10 to 18 U/kg/hr. The anticoagulant effect of heparin is monitored using the partial thromboplastin time (PTT). Adequate heparinization is achieved when the PTT is prolonged to 1.5 to 2.0 times baseline. Once such levels are achieved, the test may be performed on a daily basis. Platelet counts are performed every 2 to 3 days because a few patients manifest an idiosyncratic reaction whereby platelet consumption occurs with formation of platelet clots and increasing resistance to heparin's anticoagulant effect. If the platelet count falls below 50,000/mm³, heparin therapy is discontinued. In general, patients with extensive DVT require large doses of heparin to achieve adequate anticoagulation.

Once heparin anticoagulation has been achieved, coumadin therapy is initiated with 5 to 10 mg PO. Subsequent doses of coumadin are adjusted based on the prothrombin time or preferably the INR. The goal of oral anticoagulation therapy is the prolongation of these values to 1.5 to 2.0 times baseline. Once this goal has been reached, heparin therapy can be discontinued and the patient discharged. It is important that compression stockings be prescribed to decrease the incidence of chronic venous insufficiency. The duration of chronic coumadin therapy is controversial, but in general most physicians agree with a 3- to 6-month course for the first episode of a spontaneous DVT. Three months of therapy should be sufficient for an episode complicating surgery or trauma. Patients who have recurrent DVT or have had a pulmonary embolism should probably be on coumadin for life.

A subset of hypercoagulable patients has been defined. If hypercoagulability is suspected because of a strong family history, unexpected occurrence, or migratory or multiple episodes of phlebitis, the following blood tests may be ordered before starting anticoagulation: antithrombin III, protein S, protein C, activated protein C resistance, and lupus anticoagulant. Clinical evaluation for an occult malignancy may also be necessary under such circumstances.

Venous thrombectomy, although popular in Europe, is rarely performed in the United States. One indication is to prevent limb loss in patients with incipient venous gangrene caused by massive iliofemoral venous thrombosis (phlegmasia alba dolens and phlegmasia cerulea dolens). This rare complication is most often associated with DVT complicating metastatic malignancies. Urokinase and other lytic therapy has also been used with the theoretic advantage of preserving venous valve function. Definitive proof of benefit is not yet available. In young patients with iliofemoral involvement, urokinase delivered directly into the clot can provide dramatic improvement in venous function and relief of ultimate leg swelling.

Patients who have a contraindication to anticoagulation should be considered for vena caval filters (see Pulmonary Embolism, below). Such contraindications include active bleeding or recent neurosurgical procedures. Relative indications for filters include massive trauma, severe hypoxemia with increased risk of pulmonary embolism, and advanced age and instability.

Prophylaxis

Various methods for the prevention of DVT in patients undergoing surgery have been described. They include full heparinization and coumadinization as well as subcutaneous heparin, low-molecular-weight heparins, dextran, compression stockings, and intermittent sequential compression devices. Aspirin and antiplatelet drugs have also been utilized. Currently, the most popular methods of treatment involve combinations of subcutaneous heparin and lower extremity compression devices. Low-molecular-weight heparin may have advantages in orthopedic surgery.

These pharmacologic and physical methods have been shown to decrease the incidence of DVT and pulmonary embolism. Low-dose heparinization is achieved by giving 5,000 units of heparin subcutaneously two or three times daily. Such low doses of heparin exert their effect by accentuating the activities of antithrombin III on the clotting cascade. The PTT and ACT remain normal. However, because some bleeding complications may still result from such prophylaxis, most surgeons reserve it for high-risk patients (i.e., orthopedic patients), especially those undergoing hip surgery, obese or elderly patients, and patients with a history of phlebitis.

Pulmonary Embolism

Pulmonary embolism (PE) remains an important cause of postoperative mortality. The clinical manifestations vary from subclinical signs to sudden death. Postoperative unexplained tachycardia is an important clue for the diagnosis of PE. Other manifestations include tachypnea, pleuritic chest pain, and hemoptysis. Arterial blood gases may reflect respiratory alkalosis in the early stages; but with extensive pulmonary emboli, respiratory acidosis may develop. An electrocardiogram may show evidence of right heart strain with S waves in standard lead I and inverted T waves and Q waves in standard lead III. The chest radiograph may be completely normal or may show hypoperfused vascular markings. Ventilation-perfusion lung scans are valuable adjuncts in the diagnosis, but a high false-positive rate makes them of limited value. The definitive diagnosis of PE may require pulmonary angiography.

Management of such patients involves general supportive care and heparin anticoagulation. The heparin dosage is similar to that for DVT, although large doses may be required. Streptokinase and urokinase lytic therapy have also been used, but evidence of improved mortality and morbidity rates has not been conclusively demonstrated. Patients who have recurrent pulmonary emboli on adequate heparin therapy or those who have a contraindication to anticoagulation therapy require some form of caval interruption. Transvenous placement of caval filters, such as the Greenfield filter, is now the preferred method for physically preventing PE. New versions of these devices can be inserted percutaneously via the groin or the neck without the need for general anesthesia or a cutdown. Preinsertion venographic confirmation of DVT or PE (or both) is mandatory. Such a venogram can also identify patients with a suprarenal clot, large vena cava, or double vena cava that would affect filter placement.

LYMPHEDEMA

Lymphedema may be of primary or secondary origin. Primary lymphedema that occurs at birth is known as congenital lymphedema. When it occurs with a familial predisposition, the condition is referred to as Milroy disease. Lymphedema that occurs first during adolescence is much more common than other varieties and is known as lymphedema praecox. The specific etiology of lymphedema praecox is not known but is related to hypo- and hyperplastic changes within the lymphatic system of the extremities. It does not carry familial tendencies.

Acquired lymphedema is the most common form of this condition and usually results from axillary or inguinal node dissection or persistent chronic venous sufficiency. Other rare causes include tuberculosis, actinomycosis, lymphogranuloma, Hodgkin's disease, and filariasis.

Pathophysiology

Lymphatic obstruction results in failure to remove capillary fluid transudation from the tissues. Because this fluid contains protein and fibroblasts, fibrous tissue builds up, thickening the skin and subcutaneous tissue and leading to further obliteration of lymphatic vessels. Thus the natural history of lymphedema is progression. Symptoms occur because of the excess weight of the extremities. The lymphedematous limb is predisposed to recurrent episodes of cellulitis, although this is less common in the praecox variety. Recurrent cellulitis further destroys lymphatics, thereby aggravating the edema. Fungal superinfection of the thickened skin is not uncommon. Rarely, lymphangiosarcoma develops in patients with long-standing untreated lymphedema.

Diagnosis

Lymphedema is usually diagnosed on clinical grounds. Swelling often begins at the ankle and moves

80%

proximally. The edema is brawny and indurated. Often the edema is unilateral, although bilateral edema is not rare. The swelling is painless, and there is no evidence of inflammation. The temperature of the involved limb remains equal to that of the uninvolved extremities. Skin ulceration is almost never seen with lymphedema praecox. Congenital lymphedema is sometimes associated with other external abnormalities, such as yellow fingernails, Turner syndrome, and Noonan syndrome.

The "gold standard" for the diagnosis of lymphedema remains lymphangiography. This technique involves injecting a vital dye into the web space between the digits of the infected extremities. The technique involves a cutdown on the foot. Accordingly, the less invasive technique of radionuclear lymphoscintigraphy using technetium-99m sulfur colloid has also been utilized.

Treatment

The clinical course of untreated lymphedema is unrelenting progression, so attention should be given not only to local treatment but also to psychological support for the adolescent patient. In general, conservative measures suffice, including use of a custom-fitted heavy-duty elastic support, modification of activity to permit intermittent periods of leg elevation, optimal foot hygiene, and prompt treatment of cellulitis, if it occurs. Patients who suffer repeated attacks of cellulitis should be placed on antibiotic prophylaxis with penicillin 250 mg q.i.d. or erythromycin 250 mg q.i.d. for 1 week of every month. Fungal infections should be controlled, as they can lead to secondary bacterial involvement. Diuretics may also be prescribed intermittently to help decrease fluid accumulation. Surgical treatment seldom is required in the adolescent. Later in life, if the limb size becomes so extreme as to impinge on daily existence, surgical therapy may be warranted. The primary surgical techniques currently include one of two approaches: (1) debulking procedures, which involve removal of most of the subcutaneous tissue with a wound cover using raised skin flaps or split-thickness skin grafts; and (b) creation of new lymphatics by pedical flaps, omental transfer, or lymphatic venous anastomosis. The latter procedures are of dubious, unproved value.

QUESTIONS

Select one answer.

1. The best screening test for detecting deep venous thrombophlebitis of the lower extremities is:
   a. Isotope venography.
   b. Venous plethysmography.
   c. Phlebograpy.
   d. Venography.
   e. Duplex scan.
2. Most patients with varicose veins complain of:
   a. Bursting sensation in the involved leg: (1) occasional bleeding from the vein; (2) pruritus.
   b. Vague aching of the leg at the end of the day.
   c. No complaints.
3. Compression sclerotherapy:
   a. Involves injection of a sclerosant into a collapsed vein.
   b. Comprises a brief period of compression (1 to 2 days) with an Ace bandage.
   c. Can usually eradicate all varicosities even with saphenofemoral incompetence.
   d. Is associated with a high risk of thrombophlebitis.
   e. Often results in obliteration of the saphenous vein.
4. Management of uncomplicated deep venous thrombophlebitis includes:
   a. Prompt initiation of subcutaneous heparin.
   b. Close monitoring of the platelet count if heparin is used.
   c. Close monitoring of the platelet count if coumadin is used.
   d. Immediate venous thrombectomy.
   e. Early insertion of a vena caval filter.
5. Lymphedema:
   a. Is usually congenital.
   b. Is often complicated by secondary skin infection.
   c. Is most often diagnosed by lymphangiography.
   d. Usually requires surgical correction.
   e. Rarely involves the upper extremity.

SELECTED REFERENCES

Bergen JJ, Yao JST. *Venous disorders.* Philadelphia: WB Saunders, 1991.
Comerota AJ. *Thrombolytic therapy.* Orlando: Grune & Stratton, 1988.

Hirsh J, Dalen JE, Deykin D, Poller I, Bussey H. Oral anticoagulants: mechanism of action, clinical effectiveness, and
optimal therapeutic range. *Chest* 1995;108(suppl):231S–
264S.

Hobbs JT. Surgery and sclerotherapy in the treatment of varicose veins. *Arch Surg* 1974;109:793.

Nichols WL, Heit JA. Activated protein C resistance and
Thrombosis. *Mayo Clin Proc* 1996;71:897–898.

Raschke R, Reilly BM, Guidry JR, Fontana JR, Srinivas S. The
weight-based heparin dosing nomogram compared with a
"standard care" nomogram: a randomized controlled trial.
Ann Intern Med 1993;102:874–881.

Strandness DE, Summer DS. *Hemodynamics for surgeons.* Orlando: Grune & Stratton; 19;396–416.

Wolfe JHN, Kinmouth JB. The prognosis of primary lymphedema of the lower limb. *Arch Surg* 1981;166:1157.

10

Diseases of the Breast

Sam Lan

Breast cancer in the United States is the second most common cancer causing death among women (after carcinoma of the lung) and is the most common cause of death between 35 and 40 years of age. Current projections are that one in eight newborn girls will develop breast cancer at some time during her life. Epidemiologic variations are striking. Japanese women have a considerably lower incidence of breast cancer than do women in North America, but an increasing incidence is being seen in the younger generations.

LUMPS IN THE BREAST

Although inspection precedes palpation during any physical examination, the most common clinical presentation of breast cancer is a lump, detected by the patient or a physician. The etiology of breast masses is frequently related to the age of the patient.

Fibroadenomas

From puberty until the late twenties the most common cause of a discrete mass is a fibroadenoma. There may be size fluctuation, with a slight increase in size and some pain during the premenstrual period. Classically, it is a well defined mass with circumscribed edges that moves easily within the breast tissue. This mobility

resulted in fibroadenomas frequently being called a "breast mouse." The natural history of these lesions is often one of fluctuation in size with eventual hyaline changes or calcification presenting as a stony-hard nodule in the cancer age groups. Occasionally, a fibroadenoma continues to grow into a cystosarcoma phyllodes, although some pathologists believe that this tumor is distinct from the common fibroadenoma. Fibroadenomas sometimes reach large dimensions in pubertal women. They have no malignant potential, are termed giant fibroadenomas, and are distinct from cystosarcoma phyllodes. An increase in size may also occur at the time of menopause, pregnancy, or lactation. It is not advisable to assume the diagnosis of fibroadenoma for a mass first discovered after age 25, despite its suggestive clinical features. Medullary carcinoma can mimic this picture absolutely, with equally well defined edges. Fibroadenomas are presumed to be hormone-related because they can be induced in animals by estrogen administration. An increased level of estrogens has not been demonstrated in the women so affected, and here the tumors are believed to be due to a susceptible cell phenomenon.

In principle, fibroadenomas should not be excised before the breasts are fully mature unless there is undue pain or unusual growth. Most surgeons wait until patients are in their twenties before removing these masses, as the delay allows time for identification of multicentric fibroadenomas, which occur in up to 15% of patients. Most fibroadenomas can be removed under local anesthesia.

Phyllodes Tumor (Cystosarcoma Phyllodes)

The malignant variant of phyllodes tumor is the most common sarcoma of the breast; however, only one in ten is malignant. These tumors resemble fibroadenomas histologically, but the stroma is considerably more cellular. The peak incidence is during the fourth decade of life. They may present as large masses where the absence of skin, muscle, or lymph node involvement can lead one to the correct clinical diagnosis. A needle-core or incisional biopsy can confirm the diagnosis. Treatment is by wide excision with clear histologic margins; large lesions may necessitate mastectomy. Axillary dissections are rarely indicated owing to the low incidence of lymph node involvement. The malignant variety is prone to local recurrence and pulmonary metastasis, emphasizing the need for complete excision.

Fibrocystic Disease

The most common cause of a breast mass in women, particularly during their fourth and fifth decades, is some form of fibrocystic disease. Because of uncertain histologic criteria by which this phenomenon can be diagnosed it has been difficult to classify or examine its natural history to determine its role as a predisposing factor to malignancy. The clinical changes of fibrosis, epitheliosis, and cyst formation are so prevalent that the term "disease" may be a misnomer.

Predominant Single Cyst

The predominant single cysts are usually well demarcated masses in women in their thirties and forties. They may vary in size, becoming larger and more tender premenstrually. Fluctuance is usually not appreciated because these lesions are tense and often situated within fatty breast tissue. Ultrasonography can identify cysts, but a simpler procedure is aspiration utilizing a 22-gauge needle.

The criteria for accepting aspiration as the sole treatment are the following.

1. Total disappearance of the mass
2. Absence of blood in the aspirate (blood in the aspirate suggests a carcinoma with necrotic, cyst-like areas)
3. Absence of recurrence of the cyst (recurrence of the cyst after 1 month indicates that the wall is still secreting and further aspiration attempts may be fruitless)

If any of these criteria are not met, the area of the cyst should be excised. Nonbloody fluid may be sent for cytology, but many believe that the yield of malignant cells is too low to justify this test.

Lumpy Breasts

Breasts with diffuse masses associated with various manifestations of induration and multiple cyst formation represent the other extreme of fibrocystic disease. Detection of changes during the examination is critical and may be accomplished by the following:

1. Monthly breast self-examinations
2. Biannual examinations by the same physician
3. Mammography
   a. Baseline mammogram at age 35 to 40
   b. Mammograms at 1- to 2-year intervals from age 40
   c. Annual mammograms from age 50

Although the malignant potential of this process is of minimal concern, the development of carcinoma in a breast with these diffuse changes may be difficult to detect.

Fat Necrosis

Fat necrosis can occur at any age. It typically presents as a mass in a large, fatty breast and may be associated with skin retraction, irregular edges, and even suggestive calcifications on mammography that mimic carcinoma. A history of trauma is present in only about half the cases and cannot be taken as a reliable diagnostic indicator.

Plasma Cell Mastitis

Plasma cell mastitis presents typically as a hard mass in the region of the areola during the perimenopausal period. Distended ducts are found with a marked round-cell infiltrate. A chronic inflammatory response is caused by extrusion of ductal contents into the surrounding interstitial tissue.

The features of a mass suggestive of cancer are as follows.

Site: upper outer quadrant. This is the position of the major mass of breast tissue.

Size: of limited importance. A history of an increase in size over several months is significant.

Shape: irregular shape.

Consistency: a hard mass.

Surface: irregular surface.

Edge: poorly defined edges with extensions into the surrounding tissue.

Relations: attachment to skin or underlying fascia.

The above notwithstanding, the dictum still holds that any clinically definable mass detected in a woman over the age of 25 demands histologic verification of its nature. On inspection of the breast, there are several features other than asymmetry that are suggestive of breast carcinoma.

FINDINGS ON INSPECTION

Paget's Disease

Paget's disease presents as a red, thickened nipple with an eczematoid reaction. The surface can be scaly or moist. It is always associated with an underlying ductal carcinoma that has extended into the nipple–areola surface. About half are associated with an underlying mass. If no detectable underlying mass is present, Paget's disease has an excellent prognosis when treated with simple mastectomy. Histologic diagnosis should be confirmed with a wedge biopsy of the nipple–areola complex. The microscopic features of the lesion include Paget's cells in the epidermis, hypertrophy of the epidermis, and round-cell infiltration. Although clinical Paget's disease of the nipple accounts for only 1% of breast cancer, its importance stems from the fact that it is an early curable cancer than can be detected clinically.

Peau d'Orange

Peau d'orange (skin of orange) is a phenomenon caused by skin edema with apparent epithelial retraction. Follicles are anchored in the deep dermis, giving the appearance of an orange-peel surface. The phenomenon may be visible in association with cellulitis or an underlying abscess, but its notoriety rests in its association with breast cancer, where dense infiltration of subdermal lymphatics causes skin edema and portends a poor prognosis.

Skin Dimpling

As an early sign of breast cancer, skin dimpling reflects the distorting effect of the desmoplastic reaction of breast cancer on Cooper's suspensory ligaments. These ligaments suspend the breast from the chest wall and extend from the pectoral fascia to the skin.

Malignant Ulceration

Malignant ulceration is a grave sign when found in association with breast cancer. Its prognosis is similar to that of metastatic disease.

ETIOLOGY OF BREAST CANCER

The etiologic factors for the development of breast cancer have been determined through epidemiologic studies.

1. *Family history:* Clinically, the high risk group includes women with first-degree relatives (mother, sister, or daughters) with breast cancer, particularly if it has appeared during the premenopausal period or if the carcinomas are bilateral. In the few women with a positive family history, there is a clear genetic component. Two genes have been fully sequenced; *BRCA1* (on chromosome 17, also associated with ovarian carcinoma) and *BRCA2* (on chromosome 13, also associated with male breast cancer.) Mutations in these two genes account for most known inherited breast cancer. To date, genetic testing of high-risk patients has been of limited usefulness in the management of affected individuals.

2. *Menstrual history:* A prolonged menstrual history, particularly early menarche with late menopause, is associated with a higher incidence of breast cancer.

3. *Age of first full-term pregnancy:* The younger the age at which the patient has had her first full-term pregnancy, the greater is the apparent protection against the development of breast cancer.

Although these factors may be important in the etiology of breast cancer, emphasis on early detection remains the most important method of affecting the mortality rate of this disease. A considerable period often precedes the development of a clinically apparent carcinoma. The average doubling time of breast cancer on serial mammographic observations is estimated to be approximately 200 days.

MINIMAL BREAST CANCER

Diagnosis

Mammography is the most effective means of detecting early breast cancer. For screening, the American Cancer Society recommends a baseline mammogram at 35 to 40 years of age and then at 1- to 2-year intervals until age 50, after which it is done yearly. The radiation risks associated with x-ray mammography are minimal. Modern techniques allow in-depth dosage of 0.1 cGy for each of the two views (cephalocaudal and lateral) conventionally used for mammography.

Ultrasonography can distinguish cysts from solid masses but has not been shown to be useful when screening for carcinoma. *Thermography* has been largely abandoned as a screening technique.

Minimal breast cancers (less than 0.5 cm, or 27 cell doublings) are detected only as groups of suspicious calcifications in about one-third of mammographically detected cancers. Small densities with irregular speculated borders, with or without calcifications, are a typical finding. Architectural distortion and secondary signs of breast cancer such as edema, thickening, and tethering of the skin are also clues.

In the original mammographic screening trial performed by New York HIP (a health maintenance organization), mortality from breast cancer was reduced by 30%. This was confirmed in an independent Swedish trial. The evidence for benefit is greatest for women over age 50.

Histologic Diagnosis

Preoperative needle localization is performed with a 22-gauge needle using the cephalocaudal and lateral mammographic views to determine the most useful approach. Methylene blue is injected through the needle is then traced with two radiographic views. A fine hooked wire is then placed through the needle for fixation to the tissues and the needle is withdrawn. The suspicious area is removed under local anesthesia, and specimen radiography is performed to confirm that the suspicious mammographic finding is contained within the specimen.

Computer-assisted stereotactically guided needle biopsies of suspicious mammographic lesions may have an important impact on the diagnosis of minimal breast cancer. Sampling errors notwithstanding, this approach can reduce the number of "benign" needle localizations performed and avoid the need for a surgical procedure for many nonpalpable carcinomas.

Carcinoma In Situ

Ductal Carcinoma In Situ

Ductal carcinoma *in situ* represents a spectrum of diseases ranging from the frankly neoplastic comedo carcinoma to lesions of atypical ductal hyperplasia. This entity has increased in frequency in recent years and now accounts for one-third of mammographically detected carcinomas. The natural history is poorly defined, and most of the small, low-grade lesions are unicentric. The mortality rate in recently reported series is low. Although mastectomy was usually performed during the premammography era (palpable lesions), current management of lesions less than 5 cm in diameter includes wide excision (with clear histologic margins) and radiation therapy (to reduce the chance of recurrence). In addition, selective management of lesions less than 2.5 cm in diameter with wide excision without irradiation has yielded good results in limited series.

Lobular Carcinoma In Situ

Lobular carcinoma *in situ* does not present as a breast mass. It is most frequently found as a coincidental finding in a biopsy specimen excised for another reason. It has a 90% incidence of multicentricity and a 50% incidence of bilaterality. Most patients with this condition never develop invasive carcinoma. When invasive carcinoma does occur, both breasts are equally at risk, and most of the lesions are ductal carcinomas. Current standard practice is nonoperative observation with lifelong surveillance. Bilateral mastectomy is a rational alternative that should be practiced with circumspection. Because lobular carcinoma *in situ* is a rare precursor of invasive carcinoma (when compared with intraductal carcinoma), few therapeutic trials are in progress.

DIAGNOSIS OF BREAST CANCER

Diagnosis of a clinically palpable mass can be accomplished at a histologic level using incisional biopsy, excisional biopsy, or needle-core biopsies. Needle aspiration cytology is not generally accepted as definitive for the diagnosis, although recent reports are promising.

Hormone Receptors

Conventional hormone receptor studies may be performed with approximately 1 cc of tissue. Monoclonal antibodies are now available for the detection of receptors in small and fixed specimens.

Several hormone receptors have been identified. Among them, estrogens and progesterone cytoplasmic receptors have clinical importance. They are measured in femtomoles per milligram of cytosol protein. The absolute criteria for positivity and negativity varies among laboratories but usually lies between 5 and 10 fmol/mg cytosol protein.

The significance of estrogen receptors (ERs) includes the following.

1. Estrogen receptor positivity is associated with a 65% probability of metastases responding to a change in the hormonal milieu. This figure is lower in brain metastases, lymphangitic lung metastases, and liver metastases. Negativity is associated with a 5% response rate.
2. The type of adjuvant therapy may also be determined by hormone receptors in the primary tumor.
3. The prognosis is improved with ER positivity, as measured by (a) the time to metastatic recurrence, (b) the response of the metastases to hormonal manipulation, and (c) the time from the appearance of the metastases until death.

Overall, 55% of breast carcinomas are ER-positive. The figure is somewhat higher in postmenopausal women than in premenopausal patients. The measurable receptors tend to be present at a higher level in older patients. Progesterone receptor positivity tends clinically to enhance the potential indicated by ER pos-

itivity. Practically, the hormone receptor status of the primary tumor is assumed to be the same in a recurrence or a metastasis. It therefore is important to measure hormone receptor levels on all primary tumors when possible. Because fresh material is necessary for conventional study, testing should be done on the specimen obtained at the time of initial biopsy. The tissue for testing can be stored in liquid nitrogen.

SURGICAL MANAGEMENT OF BREAST CANCER

Preoperative Evaluation

The preoperative evaluation of breast cancer is directed at determining within reasonable limits whether the carcinoma is regionally confined and amenable to cure through regional therapy. Clinical assessment remains an important modality in the preoperative evaluation. Those eligible for attempt at cure with regional therapy include patients with stage I and II tumors (i.e., tumors less than 5.0 cm without evidence of skin or chest wall invasion and with or without ipsilateral mobile axillary lymph nodes). No signs of lymph node or other metastasis should be present beyond the surgically encompassable field. Careful attention is paid to complaints of "joint pain," which may represent bone metastases. For tumors less than 2.0 cm with no palpable lymph nodes, the minimum preoperative evaluation should include bilateral mammography (to seek other foci of carcinoma), a chest radiograph, complete blood count, and liver function tests. An elevated alkaline phosphatase, serum glutamicoxaloacetic transaminase, or calcium level requires further investigation. Preoperative liver and bone scans are required in the presence of large tumors or palpable lymph nodes. These scans provide important baseline data for many investigative protocols and are advocated by surgeons for all operable tumors.

Surgical Approaches

Breast-preserving operations have achieved results comparable to those seen with mastectomy for tumors less than 4 cm in diameter, with or without palpable lymph nodes in the axilla. Wide excision of the primary tumor is performed. The required margins of normal tissue are controversial. Acceptable results have been achieved with full breast quadrant removal for tumors less than 2 cm and excision with histologically free margins for tumors up to 4 cm. Radiation therapy to the remaining breast is given to a minimum of 50 Gy depth dose. The intention is to sterilize any remaining cancer cells. The major effect of the radiation has been to decrease the incidence of local recurrence in the affected breast.

Axillary lymph node dissections are indicated for staging because clinical evaluation results in 20% false-negative results. For operable tumors, the 10-year survival is 75% with histologically negative nodes and 25% with histologically positive nodes. The larger the number of involved lymph nodes, the worse the survival probability and the greater the probability that distant metastases already exist. Identification of "sentinel" nodes has been advocated as a method of reducing the requirement for full axillary lymph node dissections.

With the conventional *modified radical mastectomy,* the whole breast is removed, including the axillary tail of Spence and the axillary lymph nodes. Immediate or later plastic reconstruction may be done.

Both approaches (partial and total breast removal) are predicated on the assumption that the entire carcinoma must be removed, with the remaining breast tissue removed as part of the mastectomy or treated with radiation therapy. The goal of both treatment modalities is to remove residual cancer cells and eliminate the biologic threat of multicentric carcinomas, which have been found in 20% to 50% of mastectomy specimens.

Psychological and social aspects enter into the decision-making about local or regional treatment. Risk of local recurrence is also important. Some have suggested that extensive intraductal carcinoma in the region of the primary carcinoma predisposes to unacceptably high recurrence rates in patients treated by breast conservation measures. A large tumor in a small breast may result in such a poor cosmetic result that breast conservation is not indicated.

Radiation therapy following modified radical mastectomy has been demonstrated to decrease the incidence of local recurrence. Improvement in survival has been difficult to demonstrate, however.

Radical mastectomy, involving removal of the pectoralis major and minor muscles and a large portion of skin, is performed much less frequently today, but the results remain the standard against which all lesser procedures must be compared. The result in terms of survival appears similar to that of the modified procedures.

Extended surgical procedures (e.g., extended radical mastectomy or Urban's operation) include removal of a portion of the sternum, medial cartilages, and internal mammary lymph nodes. These procedures are not regarded as standard therapy for operable cancer but may be useful for local control of disease in selected cases.

Anatomic Considerations

Lymphatics

The normal breast, even in its medial aspect, drains predominantly toward the axilla. The medial intercostal lymph nodes are few in number (about four) and are predominantly in the first, second, and third interspaces. By contrast, the axillary lymph nodes are abundant. Although surgically they are regarded as distinct from the lower cervical lymph nodes, they form a physiologic and anatomic continuum with these nodes. The deep breast tissue drains to the submammary plexus of lymphatics lying superficial to the fascia overlying the pectoralis major. Hence removal of the fascia overlying pectoralis major is required when performing a mastectomy.

Blood Supply

The blood supply to the area is dominated by the internal thoracic (internal mammary) artery. It also includes the lateral thoracic artery and the pectoral branches of the acromiothoracic artery.

Veins

The anatomy of the veins generally follows that of the arteries. In addition, there is a communication with intercostal veins, which in turn communicate with the valveless vertebral system of veins known as Batson's plexus. This route of spread is used to explain the occasional occurrence of metastases to the ribs and vertebrae without pulmonary involvement.

Pectoral Nerves

The medial and lateral pectoral nerves are so named because of their origin from the medial and lateral cords of the brachial plexus. The medial pectoral nerve enters the deep surface of the pectoralis minor after supplying a branch to this muscle. It then enters the pectoralis major and ends by supplying the lower costal fibers. If the pectoralis minor muscle is removed during a modified radical mastectomy (Patey's operation), partial denervation of the pectoralis major muscle results. Those who advocate removal of the pectoralis minor argue that it facilitates more complete lymph node dissection. The lateral pectoral nerve penetrates the clavipectoral fascia (and hence is here medial to the medial pectoral nerve) and enters the underside of the pectoralis major.

Thoracodorsal Nerve

The thoracodorsal nerve, which supplies the latissimus dorsi, arises from the posterior cord of the brachial plexus and runs down the posterior axillary wall behind the subscapular artery. Injury to this nerve results in slight weakness of abduction and internal rotation.

Long Thoracic Nerve

The long thoracic nerve of bell arises from the roots of the brachial plexus and innervates the serratus anterior. Cutting this nerve produces a winged scapula and is often accompanied by severe shoulder pain.

Intercostobrachial Nerve

The intercostobrachial nerve arises from the second intercostal and supplies the skin of the axilla. It extends for a variable distance along the inner aspect of the arm. Section of this nerve results in anesthesia to the denervated area.

Postoperative Complications

Seroma

Seroma requires repeated aspiration. It is best avoided by removing closed-suction drains after drainage falls to less than 50 ml/24 hr.

Infection

Signs of inflammation should be vigorously investigated and treated. Episodes of infection can aggravate or precipitate lymphedema of the upper extremity.

Skin Edge Necrosis

Skin edge necrosis is a technical error caused by compromised blood supply. This complications often results from making the skin edges too thick and the base of the flaps thin. Conservative management with 1% acetic acid or dilute hydrogen peroxide soaks frequently results in good reepithelialization of defects up to 5.0 cm in diameter. Massive flap necrosis requires débridement and eventual skin graft.

Limitation of Arm Movement

Although shoulder movement usually is not restricted, active exercise following mastectomy should be avoided until the fifth postoperative day because of the increased risk of seroma and hematoma formation. After that a graduated exercise program is useful.

Arm Edema

Prevention and aggressive treatment of infections and wounds of the ipsilateral upper limb are paramount for prevention of postoperative edema. Ongoing care of the limb by excellent skin care and avoidance of intravenous lines is also important. Established lymphedema is treated with elevation, massage, compression garments, or mechanical pumps. Microsurgical procedures to reestablish lymphatic drainage pathways are generally not useful.

Lymphangiosarcoma

Lymphangiosarcoma may develop in the chronically edematous arm, frequently after radiation to the breast. On average, it occurs 9 years after mastectomy. It presents characteristically as a purple subcutaneous nodule and may grow rapidly; lung metastases often appear. The prognosis is grave, with an average life expectancy of less than 6 months. Amputation can provide local palliation.

Adjuvant Therapy

Where surgery and/or radiotherapy has removed all gross local disease, therapy designed to eliminate residual microscopic disease is known as adjuvant therapy. There is no uniform adjuvant therapy for all patients

C M F

with regionally confined breast cancer. The two most frequently used adjuvant regimens are (1) a cytotoxic combination of cyclophosphamide, methotrexate, and 5-fluorouracil administered over a period of 6 months and (b) tamoxifen given for 5 years.

Studies have indicated that the beneficial effect of chemotherapy on the time to recurrence and mortality is greatest in women under age 50. By contrast, the beneficial effect of tamoxifen is greatest in women over age 50. Because the proportional risk reduction is constant, the real clinical impact is greatest in patients with poor prognostic indicators (e.g., those with positive axillary lymph nodes). There are no reliable data for patients with tumors less than 1 cm in diameter. By inference, the clinical impact is presumed to be small.

Chemotherapy is conventionally used in premenopausal women regardless of the status of the axillary lymph nodes. Both tamoxifen and ovarian ablation have also been shown to be beneficial. Optimal combinations are still undergoing evaluation.

In postmenopausal women tamoxifen is conventionally used for ER-positive patients regardless of whether they have positive lymph nodes. Chemotherapy given to the group with lymph node involvement may further improve survival.

The postmenopausal ER-negative patients are least likely to benefit from conventional therapy, although both chemotherapy and tamoxifen have a beneficial effect. If only one modality is to be used, tamoxifen is better tolerated and is the preferred therapy.

MANAGEMENT OF METASTATIC DISEASE

Metastatic breast cancer is incurable with standard current therapy, and therapy is directed at palliation. In principle, if hormonal manipulation is indicated, it should be performed prior to chemotherapy. Hormone manipulation is indicated in patients whose primary tumors or metastatic lesions have positive hormone receptors. Patients with lymphangitic lung involvement, liver metastases, or brain metastases are usually excluded. Aggressive tumors presenting with metastases soon after primary therapy are frequently treated with chemotherapy without attempting hormonal manipulation.

Generally, tamoxifen is used as the initial hormonal therapy in both pre- and postmenopausal patients. If a response occurs, a recurrence can be managed with other hormonal agents, such as megestrol or a "medical

adrenalectomy" using aminoglutethimide and hydrocortisone. Ablative procedures such as oophorectomy and adrenalectomy are rarely performed. Traditional adjuvant chemotherapy with alkylating agents, methotrexate and 5-fluorouracil has left doxorubicin, vincristine, and the taxanes for treatment of metastases. As a single agent, doxorubicin is the most effective of the chemotherapeutic agents against metastatic breast cancer. Taxol and derivatives demonstrate promising response rates when used to treat recurrent breast carcinoma.

An interesting attempt to maximize the effectiveness of current chemotherapy involves harvesting the patient's own hematopoietic stem cells from bone marrow or peripheral blood. After delivering otherwise lethal doses of chemotherapy, the patient is rescued from bone marrow toxicity by reinfusing the autologous stem cells. Randomized trials are ongoing, and the utility of this approach is not currently known. Other attempts to increase chemotherapy doses include rescue from bone marrow toxicity with growth factors for hematopoietic stem cells.

BREAST CANCER DURING PREGNANCY

Breast masses, particularly those discovered in pregnant women over age 25, should be promptly biopsied if aspiration indicates solidity. Breast cancer during pregnancy often presents as advanced disease, resulting in an unfavorable prognosis. Localized carcinoma should be treated by mastectomy. Adjuvant chemotherapy should be delayed until at least the second trimester. Occasionally termination of pregnancy may have to be considered in those with more advanced tumors, where irradiation and chemotherapy are urgently required for the welfare of the mother. There are no therapeutic reasons for avoidance or termination of pregnancy in patients following treatment for breast cancer provided they have no evidence of recurrent disease.

CANCER OF THE MALE BREAST

Male breast cancer accounts for fewer than 1% of all breast cancers. It has an apparent increased incidence in Jewish men and those who have had mumps orchitis after age 20, and it is increased in families with mutations in the *BRCA2* gene. Most of these tumors present with a mass under the nipple–areola complex that appears clinically to involve it directly. The prognosis is worse than that for women, perhaps because of the close proximity to the chest wall, the greater age of the affected population, and the higher proportion of patients with lymph node involvement at the time of presentation.

Treatment is wide mastectomy and axillary dissection. Adjuvant tamoxifen therapy may be indicated for the more advanced cases. Most of these tumors are associated with elevated ER levels. Ablative and additive hormonal manipulation have been shown to be useful for metastatic disease.

AXILLARY NODE ADENOCARCINOMA WITH NO APPARENT PRIMARY

The search for a primary lesion must include a full physical examination. The test most likely to reveal a primary is mammography (25%). Other tests should include chest radiography, liver enzyme assays, and bone scan. Positive mucin stains tend to exclude melanoma and lymphoma. Estrogen and progesterone receptors suggest a breast primary but are not conclusive. If no primary is found, standard therapy is axillary dissection and mastectomy, although this practice is being challenged in small reported series, and lesser procedures (axillary dissection and radiation therapy to the ipsilateral breast) are being advocated. The prognosis seems better than that with detectable breast cancers with an equivalent number of involved lymph nodes.

EMBRYOLOGIC CONDITIONS

Polythelia (many nipples) is a common finding in clinical practice. It can occur anywhere along the milk line (an ectodermal thickening in the 4.0-mm embryo from the mid clavicle to the inguinal ligament). Most frequently, they present inferior and medial to the nipple. This may be accompanied by *polymastia* (many breasts), which may become evident at puberty or during pregnancy. *Amastia* or *athelia* is frequently accompanied by an underlying chest wall defect.

DEVELOPMENTAL CONDITIONS

Nipple discharge at birth is a frequent result of removal from the high estrogen and progesterone maternal environment and an increase in prolactin production. It is a self-limiting disorder.

Early female breast development may be asymmetric. Precocious breast hypertrophy may be related to hormone-producing adrenal cortical and ovarian tumors. Boys can manifest a slight enlargement of breast tissue at puberty that subsides spontaneously with time.

BREAST ABSCESS

Breast abscess occurs most commonly during the first weeks of lactation. It is often caused by coagulase-positive staphylococci and may be associated with suppuration and extensive destruction of breast tissue. These abscesses require early, aggressive drainage to remove septated pockets. In principle, an incision at the lower aspect of the abscess encourages dependent drainage. *Streptococcus* produces a cellulitis that can often be controlled with antibiotics.

QUESTIONS

Select one answer.

1. A 31-year-old woman presents with a 2-cm mass in the upper outer quadrant of the right breast. It is well defined and has been present by history for 2 months. Your initial approach to this problem is to:
   a. Order a mammogram followed by a sonogram.
   b. Insert a needle to aspirate any fluid.
   c. Schedule an open biopsy.
   d. Reschedule an appointment in 6 weeks to reevaluate the problem clinically.

2. An 11-year-old girl is brought by her parents with a unilateral 1.5-cm mass underneath the areola on the right. Your approach to this problem should be:
   a. Observation only, as it is a "breast bud," which frequently develops asymmetrically.
   b. Excision, because with growth of the child the scar becomes less noticeable.
   c. Biopsy, as lymphomas occur in this age group.

3. The long thoracic nerve:
   a. Innervates the serratus anterior muscle.
   b. Courses down posterior to the axillary artery and vein because it arises from the roots of the brachial plexus.
   c. Section of the nerve results in ipsilateral scapular prominence and shoulder pain.
   d. All of the above.

4. The incidence of breast carcinoma is lower:
   a. In the contralateral breasts of patients receiving tamoxifen.
   b. In young women.
   c. In women with no family history of breast carcinoma.
   d. All of the above.
5. Mammography:
   a. Is the most effective means of detecting minimal breast carcinoma.
   b. Is more effective in detecting minimal breast carcinomas in postmenopausal women.
   c. When normal, should not result in avoiding biopsy of a palpable suspicious breast mass.
   d. May be carcinogenic in women with the gene for ataxia-telangiectasia.
   e. All of the above.
6. Breast conservation surgery in breast carcinoma:
   a. Has resulted in major improvement in mortality and morbidity figures associated with this disease.
   b. Has resulted in durable survival data comparable to those for mastectomy for certain breast carcinomas.
   c. Should be recommended to all women suffering from breast carcinoma.
   d. Has resulted in a high incidence of serious radiation-related complications.
   e. Has resulted in diminution of the need for adjuvant chemotherapy and hormonal therapy.
7. In a patient with breast carcinoma, the clinical finding portending the worst prognosis is:
   a. Eczematous changes around the nipple–areolar complex.
   b. Skin dimpling in the area of the tumor.
   c. The presence of a palpable 1-cm node in the axilla.
   d. Peau d'orange.
8. Statistically, the most powerful predictor of prognosis is:
   a. The presence of intramammary lymphatic involvement.
   b. The grade of differentiation of the tumor.
   c. The presence of marked intraductal carcinoma around the primary tumor.
   d. The size of the primary tumor.
   e. The number of axillary lymph nodes involved with metastatic tumor.

9. Ductal carcinoma *in situ* of the breast:
   a. Is almost always bilateral.
   b. Has become more frequently diagnosed as a result of mammography.
   c. Cannot present as a palpable mass.
   d. Is frequently associated with microscopic lymph node metastases.
   e. In its most benign manifestation is the comedo form.
10. A 33-year-old woman pregnant for the third time presents at 3 months with a 2-cm mass in the inner aspect of the left breast. A needle aspiration reveals no fluid. You would:
   a. Arrange for a mammogram because multicentric lesions are common during pregnancy.
   b. Consider termination of pregnancy because chemotherapy has been shown to be useful in node-negative premenopausal patients.
   c. Expeditiously obtain a histologic diagnosis of the mass.
   d. Wait until the third trimester because surgery is safer at that time.

SELECTED REFERENCES

Bland KI, Copeland EM, eds. *The breast: comprehensive management of benign and malignant diseases.* Philadelphia: WB Saunders, 1991.

Collins FS. *BRCA1:* Lots of mutations, lots of dilemmas. *N Engl J Med* 1996;334:186–188.

Early Breast Cancer Trialists' Collaborative group. Systemic treatment of early breast cancer by hormonal, cytotoxic or immune therapy. *Lancet* 1992;1:1–15.

Fisher B, Anderson S, Redmond CK, et al. Reanalysis and results after 12 years of follow-up in a randomized clinical trial comparing total mastectomy with lumpectomy with or without radiation in the treatment of breast cancer. *N Engl J Med* 1995;333:1456–1461.

Fisher B, Constantino J, Redmond C, et al. Lumpectomy compared with lumpectomy and radiation therapy for the treatment of intraductal breast cancer. *N Engl J Med* 1993;328:1581–1586.

Goldhirsch A, Wood WC, Senn H-J, et al. Meeting highlights: International Consensus Panel on the Treatment of Primary Breast Cancer. *J Natl Cancer Inst* 1995;87:1441–1445.

Hatrris JR, Lippman ME, Veronesi U, et al. Medical progress: breast cancer. *N Engl J Med* 1992;327:319–328.

Hulka BS, Stark AT. Breast cancer: cause and prevention. *Lancet* 1995;346:883–886.

Page DL, Jensen RA. Ductal carcinoma in situ of the breast: understanding the misunderstood stepchild. *JAMA* 1996;275:948–949.

11

Principles of Surgical Oncology

Ronald N. Kaleya

As the theories of cancer progression have changed over the past decades, so have principles of the surgical management of cancer and the cancer patient. In the past, the surgeon attempted to extend the scope of resection to encompass all possible local spread of the cancer. Follow-up studies for the most part did not show that the radical and superradical procedures clearly led to better survival and decreased local recurrence. Interest then changed to include other oncologic modalities. The addition of adjuvant therapy has improved the survival and disease-free survival for several cancers. Therefore multimodality therapy has become the standard of care for most cancers. Furthermore, combination therapy has reduced the scope of resection in some cases, permitting preservation of function and cosmesis. In other cases, neoadjuvant (preoperative) therapies have made unresectable tumors resectable. As a result of these trends in oncology, the general surgeon requires an intimate knowledge of the benefits and complications of these therapies to provide the best patient care.

THEORIES OF CANCER PROGRESSION

There are essentially two theories of cancer progression. The first suggests that there is an orderly spread from the primary cancer to the regional nodes and subsequently to the systemic circulation. This simplistic theory explained several findings including the decreased survival of patients who had nodal metastases compared to those without nodal metastases. This theory was the "scientific" underpinning of the radical and superradical surgical approach to cancer. However, there was rarely a survival benefit for these enormously morbid operations, thereby undermining the validity of the theory and the resultant surgical dogma. Systemic failure, despite negative nodes and locally aggressive surgery, further discredited this approach.

The theory that local therapy treats only local disease and has no effect on metastatic disease has been popularized over the last 20 years. This alternative theory suggests that cancers usually disseminate prior to diagnosis or local therapy. This theory is the underpinning of the adjuvant therapy of cancer.

Neither theory precisely explains the progression of cancer, and reality probably lies somewhere in the middle. The process of metastasis probably requires several steps and a cell that can fulfill all of these steps. Much of the metastatic cascade has not been worked out, but at a minimum the metastatic clone must be able to dissociate from the primary tumor, generate a blood supply, pass through endothelial surfaces, implant in specific tissues, and proliferate. Biologic and genetic markers for these properties have been sought, but as yet we do not have the ability to predict the metastatic potential of a specific tumor. With elucidation of this process, the surgeon and the oncologist will be better able to determine which patients are at increased risk of local and disseminated recurrences and who will most benefit from aggressive multimodality therapy.

GOALS OF SURGICAL ONCOLOGY

The goals of surgical oncology are manyfold. Surgery cures more cancer than all other treatment modalities combined. Improvement of surgical procedures for cancer involves increased cure rates or improved functional and cosmetic results without compromise of cure rates. In addition, much of surgical practice with regard to cancer has been determined by historical convention (width of margins, lymphadenectomy, extent of resection) rather than proved efficacy. Therefore procedures or surgical conventions that do not improve survival or function must be removed from surgical practice. Most prominent among them are conservation management of breast cancer, which was vocally condemned by the surgical community for two decades. Additionally, the standard 5-cm margin for rectal cancer and melanoma have been shown to be excessive and at times even detrimental to the care of the patient. Furthermore, because the surgeon remains the central figure in the diagnosis, prevention, staging, and management of almost all nonhematologic malignancies, the surgeon must be aware of the capabilities of the other cancer specialists and must be able to assess the results of both surgical and nonsurgical treatments of cancer.

SCREENING AND PREVENTION

Screening large populations for cancer has been, in general, unrewarding. As with any test, there are a large number of patients who have a false-positive test result, necessitating an expensive and unproductive workup. Unless the population is at increased risk of developing the disease, screening programs are generally not cost-effective. Even with high-risk populations, screening may not influence the outcome of treatment. Several of the large screening programs conducted in the United States and Canada have shown that screening for occult blood in the stool is not a cost-effective means of de-

tecting early colorectal cancer. In fact, half of the documented cases of colorectal cancer do not show blood in the stool. Sputum cytology screening or periodic chest x-ray examination has not been a cost-effective manner of detecting lung cancers even in the population of smokers. Mammography has definitely increased the number of early breast cancers treated, but it is not clear that overall outcome has been changed.

Patients who have a genetic or familial predisposition to cancer are more suitable for screening. Patients with cancer family syndromes should be followed closely because they are at increased risk for the development of cancer. There is no absolute definition of a cancer family syndrome, but these lineages exhibit an excess of cancers, synchronous and metachronous primaries, and earlier onset than the sporadic variety of the disease; and they appear to have an autosomal dominant inheritance with incomplete penetrance. The more common cancer family syndromes are listed in Table 11.1. A high index of suspicion in these patients can probably lead to an earlier diagnosis and likely a higher survival.

Familial breast cancers account for about 10% to 30% of cases. They occur early and are frequently bilateral. The precise contributions of life style (i.e., excess fat in the diet) and genetics are not defined. The lifetime

TABLE 11.1. *Cancer family syndromes*

Muir syndrome
  Multiple visceral cancers
  Multiple sebaceous cysts
SBLA syndrome
  Sarcoma at young age
  Breast and brain malignancies
  Leukemia, lung cancer, and laryngeal cancer
  Adrenal cortical cancers
Multiple endocrine neoplasia (MEN)
  Type I (Werner): pituitary adenomas, parathyroid adenomas, pancreatic islet cell tumors
  Type II (Sipple): medullary carcinoma of the thyroid, parathyroid adenomas, pheochromocytomas, astrocytomas
  Type III (includes all of the features of type II): café-au-lait spots and pedunculated lesions of the tongue and eyelid
Nonpolyposis colon cancer syndrome (NPCCS)
  Younger onset
  Multiple and preferentially right-sided cancers
  Better survival than sporadic cases

risk of a women with a sister and mother with pre-menopausal breast cancer approaches 50%. Survival for familial breast cancer is better, stage for stage, than for the sporadic variety (67% versus 45% at 5 years).

Similarly, familial colon cancers comprise approximately 10% to 30% of colorectal cancers. The polyposis syndromes account for only 1% of colon cancers. The polyposis syndromes are well known because of their easily identifiable mucosal marker. The nonpolyposis colon cancer syndromes are more common but less well characterized. These cancers occur in younger patients, tend to be multiple, occur preferentially in the right colon and cecum, and are associated with a better survival than the sporadic cases. The lifetime risk of a first-degree relative of a patient with colon cancer has begun in some centers, but long-term follow-up is not yet available to determine the efficacy of screening this population.

Screening of appropriate high-risk populations in Japan and China has reduced the reported mortality from esophageal and gastric cancer. Papanicolaou cervical smears have clearly reduced the mortality from cancer of the cervix in the United States and elsewhere. Evaluations of transrectal ultrasonography and prostate-specific antigen levels are presently being evaluated in the early diagnosis of prostate cancer.

BIOPSY TECHNIQUES

Frequently the surgeon is called on to evaluate a clinically suspicious mass. A presumptive diagnosis is necessary prior to biopsy so the correct biopsy technique is employed and the tissue is handled in an appropriate manner. There are basically four biopsy techniques, including fine-needle aspiration (FNAB), core-needle biopsy, incisional biopsy, and excisional biopsy. Each technique has specific applications, benefits, and limitations.

Fine-Needle Aspiration Biopsy

Cells obtained by FNAB are aspirated through a 21-gauge needle, smeared on a glass slide, immediately fixed with 95% alcohol, and stained with a variety of stains. The specimens are examined for nuclear appearance, cellular cohesiveness, and mitotic activity. Cytologic evaluation requires a pathologist trained specifi-

cally in reading this type of specimen. Small needles retrieve too few cells, and large needles tend to aspirate cores of tissue unsuitable for cytologic examination. An adequate number of cells must be aspirated to have an accurate evaluation. Because FNAB is so easily performed, it is probably overutilized. As a result of too many FNABs, patients are encouraged to undergo definitive open biopsies to confirm an equivocal cytologic biopsy.

The FNAB is useful for evaluating a thyroid nodule, breast cancer, metastases to the liver, lung, or adrenal, and a suspected metastasis to a lymph node. The results of FNAB are often misleading in the diagnosis of suspected lymphomas, sarcomas, and intraabdominal malignancies. In addition, a negative cytologic examination may be the result of sampling error rather than the absence of tumor. Many surgeons and pathologists suggest that definitive therapy for breast cancer can be carried out on the basis of cytology, but others urge caution with regard to using cytology as the definitive diagnostic test.

Core-Needle Biopsy

Core-needle biopsies obtain a small specimen that is suitable for paraffin embedding and routine histologic staining techniques. The core can be as large as a 2 × 2 × 10 mm tissue fragment. This procedure can be done under local anesthesia without the use of an operating room. The only significant risks are the development of a hematoma and false-negative results. Core-needle biopsies are of limited utility in the diagnosis of sarcomas and lymphomas.

Incisional Biopsy

Incisional biopsies are useful for evaluating large or deep lesions, especially when ablative definitive surgery is contemplated, as in the case of melanoma or the soft tissue sarcomas. In addition, incisional biopsy is used for the diagnosis of tumors that are potential candidates for neoadjuvant therapy. Stage III and IV breast cancers and laryngeal cancers are examples of the latter.

The incision should be placed directly over the primary lesion; undermining is minimized, and the incision is planned in a fashion that allows it to be included in the larger definitive resection. Drains and hematomas are avoided because they may increase the scope of a subsequent definitive surgical procedure.

Excisional Biopsy

Excisional biopsies are useful for small, superficial tumors. When possible, a rim of normal tissue is included in the specimen. Although there are no absolute upper limits of size for an excisional biopsy, in general the excisional biopsy wound should be able to be closed primarily and be small enough to be included in a large definitive surgical field.

STAGING

The purpose of staging is to predict survival, make data collection consistent among institutions permitting comparison of data, determine subsequent therapy, and evaluate the results of therapy. The most universally accepted staging system is the TMN system as adopted by the American Joint Commission on Cancer. The general rules governing the staging system are seen in Table 11.2.

After establishing the diagnosis, the patient undergoes an appropriate extent-of-disease evaluation. This evaluation is based on the natural history of the particular cancer and the likely sites of metastatic and local spread. There are several types of staging, including clinical, surgical, pathologic, and autopsy methods. Clinical staging is particularly useful for determining the primary therapy and the potential sites of metastatic evaluation. Surgical and pathologic staging methods are better predictors of survival than clinical staging. Surgical staging is important in some cases prior to the treatment of Hodgkin's disease, prostatic cancer, and lung cancer. In the latter two cases the regional nodes are sampled before proceeding with surgical therapy.

PRINCIPLES OF SURGICAL ONCOLOGY

Local Surgical Therapy

The goal of cancer surgery is resection with a rim of normal tissue. Needless to say, the margins of resection must be pathologically free of tumor. Incomplete excision is useful only in cases where there are effective alternative therapies for the residual tumor, as in ovarian cancer. Incomplete resection is reasonable for palliation of symptoms (e.g., paraneoplastic syndromes, bleeding, or obstruction).

Lymphadenectomy

The role of regional lymphadenectomy has not been clearly defined. Regional lymph nodes are frequently the first site of metastases and are removed in the course of the primary therapy for most cancers. The presence of nodal disease may determine the need for adjuvant therapy in colorectal, breast, head and neck, and uterine cancers. Elective regional lymph node dissection may provide better locoregional control of melanoma, gastric, esophageal, breast, head and neck, and colorectal cancers. Whether regional adenectomy alters the course of the disease remains speculative.

The decision to perform elective lymph node dissection (ELND) depends on many factors. The likelihood of occult lymph node metastases must be high enough to justify the expected morbidity associated with the procedure. Furthermore, the incidence of occult metastases must be substantially higher than the risk of occult systemic metastases for the procedure to have the anticipated benefit. Although ELND has not been shown conclusively to improve survival from any cancer, support by both retrospective data and prospective trials should be available to justify the procedure. There are reports that support the use of lymphadenectomy for melanoma and for gastric, esophageal, rectal, and cervical cancer. In cases where the retrospective data do not show a survival benefit for ELND, lymphadenectomy

TABLE 11.2. *TMN staging system*

Primary tumor (T)	
Tx	Primary cannot be evaluated
T0	Primary tumor occult
T1–3	Increasing size/local extent
Regional lymph nodes (N)	
Nx	RLN cannot be evaluated
N0	No RLN metastases
N1–3	Increasing RLN involvement
Distant metastases (M)	
Mx	Metastases cannot be evaluated
M0	Metastases absent
M1	Metastases present

RLN, regional lymph nodes.

can be considered if the consequences of regional recurrence are significant. Last and most importantly, ELND is recommended when the results can change subsequent therapy.

Surgical Treatment of Metastatic Disease

Surgery for metastatic disease requires that the primary lesion can be controlled, all known metastatic deposits can be resected, and there is no other effective treatment for the disease. Workup prior to resection of a metastasis should be extensive and guided by the pattern of failure for the given disease (e.g., evaluation of the liver in cases of local recurrence of colon cancer). If the metastasis is noted synchronously with the primary lesion, the procedure with the least likelihood of complete resection should be performed first to avoid unwarranted ablative surgery, as in the case of recurrent soft tissue sarcomas requiring amputation.

Pulmonary Metastases

Among patients with a history of an extrathoracic cancer and a new lung nodule, 62% have a second primary, and 25% have a solitary metastasis. If the original cancer was a squamous cancer, most of the new nodules are new primaries. About half of the patients with a history of an extrathoracic adenocarcinoma have a solitary metastasis, whereas if the cancer was melanoma or a soft tissue sarcoma almost all are of metastatic origin.

Workup should include chest radiograph, chest computed tomography (CT) scan, evaluation of other areas of common recurrence for the given primary, bronchoscopy if the lesion is central or large to exclude involvement of the mainstem bronchus, and thoracentesis for cytology if an effusion is present. FNAB is not necessary because resection must be done regardless of whether the cytology confirms the diagnosis. The patient should have adequate pulmonary reserve and an FEV_1 greater than 1 liter.

The criteria for an indicated pulmonary metastasectomy include the ability to control all disease with the resection, the absence of extrathoracic disease, and the patient being left with adequate functional lung capacity following the procedure. All of these criteria must be fulfilled before embarking on therapy. The results of therapy are determined in part by the type of tumor, the number of metastases, the interval between treatment of the primary and the recurrence (disease-free internal), and the completeness of resection. Table 11.3 lists survival by cell type.

Brain Metastases

Patients with brain metastases have a poor long-term survival. Survival by treatment is 1 to 2 months, 2 to 3 months, 4 to 6 months, and 6 to 12 months for no treatment, steroids only, steroids plus radiation, and surgery plus radiation, respectively. Indications for neurosurgical intervention include diagnostic uncertainty, a solitary metastasis, or placement of a drug delivery device. Predictors of improved long-term survival following resection of brain metastases include (1) a disease-free interval longer than 1 year following treatment of the primary, (2) better preoperative performance status, (3) relative radiosensitivity, (4) the extent of tumor resection (complete versus partial), (5) the extent of underlying cerebral dysfunction prior to surgery, and (6) slowly progressive histologic change.

Tumor Markers

Tumor markers (Table 11.4) are useful during treatment of metastatic and primary disease. They are, for the most part, tumor antigens or products or tumor metabolism released into the general circulation. The markers are helpful in the diagnosis, monitoring, staging, localization, and treatment of several cancers. In general, the tumor markers are not good screening tools because there is too high an incidence of false-positives and a low prevalence of the tumors in the general population, leading to overutilization of diagnostic resources.

Patients with known cancer can be monitored for recurrence, and tumor markers can help predict survival.

TABLE 11.3. *Survival following pulmonary metastasectomy by cell type*

Cell type	5-Year survival (%)
Osteogenic sarcoma	40–50
Soft tissue sarcoma	25–30
Urinary tract cancers	45–60
Head and neck	45
Colorectal	15
Breast	10
Melanoma	0–30

TABLE 11.4. *Useful tumor markers*

Tumor marker	Site
Carcinoembryonic antigen	Colon, breast, lung, pancreas
α-Fetoprotein	Liver, germ cell
Human chorionic gonadotropin	Trophoblast, germ cell
Calcitonin	Medullary carcinoma of the thyroid
Prostate-specific antigen/prostatic acid phosphatase	Prostate
CA-125	Ovaries
CA 19-9/TAG 72	Colon/rectum
CA 15-3	Breast

Patients with proved colon cancer and a carcinoembryonic antigen (CEA) more than 10 ng/mL have a shorter survival, stage for stage, than patients with a lower CEA level. Patients with low CEA levels and resectable stage III gastric cancer have longer survival than patients with high CEA levels.

Both CEA and CA 19-9 have been used to follow patients with colorectal cancer. Approximately 80% to 95% of patients with a rise in the CEA titer after curative resection of colorectal cancer are found to have recurrent cancer. Of the group with recurrent disease, about two-thirds of the lesions are resectable at laparotomy. One-fourth of those who undergo resection survive 5 years. It is important to recognize that most of the recurrences are in the liver, and most of the survivors had a solitary liver metastasis. Prognostic factors associated with better long-term survival following reexploration for a rising CEA level include liver versus soft tissue recurrence, recurrence of a colon versus a rectal primary, and a disease-free interval longer than 1 year.

Presently, several tumor marker-related modalities are being explored. Radioimmunoguided surgery (RIGS) and immunoscintigraphy with radiolabeled monoclonal antibodies to CEA or a specific tumor-associated glycoprotein (TAG-72) may have a role in the treatment of primary and recurrent cancer; RIGS may detect up to 20% more lesions than conventional exploration. Immunoscintigraphy appears better able to detect extrahepatic recurrences than CT scans, magnetic resonance imaging (MRI), or conventional exploration techniques. Monoclonal imaging will probably be used for melanoma, prostatic cancer, ovarian cancer, and lung cancer over the next few years. A few trials have used monoclonal antibodies to deliver either cytotoxic agents or radiotherapy to a specific tumor.

Palliative Treatment of Cancer

Bleeding is a common complication of cancer and its therapy. It may result from the tumor itself, erosion into other structures, inflammation caused by chemotherapy or radiation therapy, or pancytopenia. It is essential to identify the bleeding site preoperatively so surgery can be limited, especially in the pancytopenic patient. Bleeding parameters are corrected prior to surgery. Surgery is not contemplated until all conservative measures including cauterization and embolization have been exhausted. Surgical intervention is indicated for continued bleeding despite conservative therapy.

Obstruction in the patient with a history of an intraabdominal malignancy but no overt evidence of recurrence is adhesive in up to 90% of cases. In patients with proved recurrence, however, malignancy is responsible for most cases of obstruction. Initial decompression should be attempted in either case. Only rarely is a malignant obstruction responsible for bowel necrosis, in contradistinction to adhesive obstructions. Bypass surgery is usually needed for malignant obstructions and is associated with 25% mortality; an additional 25% of patients are never decompressed.

Perforation is uncommon but more subtle in the immunocompromised host. It is treated similarly to nonmalignant perforations, although ostomies are used more liberally, and mortality is high.

Inflammatory lesions are common following chemotherapy or radiation therapy. Because these inflammatory lesions can result in perforation of a hollow viscus or prolonged ileus, close observation is mandated. Typhlitis or neutropenic enterocolitis is common in leukemia patients treated with high-dose ara-C. Observation on antibiotics is the prudent course of therapy. Neutropenic sepsis and ileus are treated with antibiotics and observation. Diarrhea is common following several of the chemotherapy regimens and can be treated symptomatically with antidiarrheal agents, a somatostatin analog, and intravenous alimentation. These episodes are generally self-limited but can mimic ischemic or infectious colitis with an acute abdomen. Again, unless overt signs of an intraabdominal catastrophe are present, nonoperative therapy is appropriate.

CHEMOTHERAPY

Chemotherapy has become a mainstay of cancer treatment in the adjuvant, neoadjuvant, or advanced setting. There are no biochemical pathways exclusive to cancer cells; therefore chemotherapeutic agents must take advantage of quantitative and qualitative differences between cancer and normal cells to achieve a selective effect. Better uptake by the tumor cell, increased metabolic demand for a substrate because of more active cell division, inadequate salvage pathways for needed metabolites, and the inability to repair sublethal damage are some of the differences used to enhance tumoricidal versus normal cell injury. Most agents are active during cellular division; tumors have a high fraction of dividing cells and therefore are sensitive to chemotherapy. Resistance to chemotherapy may result from selection of resistant clones by the chemotherapy. Tumor cells tend to have chromosomal instability and have more mutations, which may cause drug resistance.

Cells are generally insensitive to chemotherapy during the growth phase G_0 because most agents interfere with the production of nucleic acids. As a result, as more tumor cells go into this phase as a result of decreased blood supply and limitation of nutrients (gompertzian kinetics), the entire tumor becomes more resistant to chemotherapy. Small, highly vascularized tumors tend to grow by exponential kinetics and are more sensitive to the actions of the cytotoxic agents.

Medical oncologists therefore prefer to treat patients with a small tumor burden, treat to the maximum tolerable dose (MTD), use multiple agents with nonoverlapping toxicities, and escalate the dose if the patient can tolerate it. Chemotherapeutic agents are listed in Table 11.5.

Alkylating Agents

Alkylating agents cause direct cellular death, mutations, and late carcinogenesis. They also cause interstrand cross-linking by alkylating the N^2 position of guanine, thereby preventing transcription and translation of DNA and RNA. There is a high incidence of late second malignancies. The major toxicities include pancytopenia, hemorrhagic cystitis, and gastrointestinal complaints.

The nitrosoureas cross the blood–brain barrier and are therefore used for brain tumors. DTIC has marginal activity in melanoma and the soft tissue sarcomas.

TABLE 11.5. *Common chemotherapeutic agents*

Alkylating agents
  Nitrogen mustard, cyclophosphamide, ifosamide
  Alkyl sulfonates: busulfan
  Ethylenamine: thiotepa
  Nitrosoureas: carmustine (BCNU), lomustine (CCNU)
  Triazines: dacarbazine (DTIC), streptozocin
Vinca alkaloids
  Vincristine, vinblastine, vindesine
Antibiotics
  Doxorubicin (Adriamycin)
  Daunorubicin
  Bleomycin
  Dactinomycin
  Mitomycin C
Antimetabolites
  Methotrexate
  5-Fluorouracil (5-FU)
  Cytarabine (ara-C)
  5-Fluorodeoxyuridine (FUDR)
  6-Thioguanine (6-TG)
  6-Mercaptopurine (6-MP)
Hormonal agents
  Tamoxifen
  Megestrol acetate
  Medroxyprogesterone acetate
  Leuprolide
  Aminoglutethimide
Biologic response modifiers
  Interferon (α, β, γ)
  Interleukin
  Tumor necrosis factor

Thiotepa is used for intravesical treatment of bladder tumors.

Vinca Alkaloids

The vinca alkaloids inhibit spindle formation, causing metaphase arrest. Cells caught in a prolonged metaphase die. The major toxicities include leukopenia and stomatitis. In addition, a peripheral neuropathy that is often permanent is seen frequently. The surgeon is often consulted because of an autonomic neuropathy that causes prolonged ileus. It is treated expectantly with nasogastric decompression and parenteral nutrition.

Antibiotics

The anthracycline antibiotics are intercalating agents that disrupt translation and transcription. They are not cycle-specific and are active in many solid tumors. They cause severe bone marrow suppression, alopecia, and mucositis. Cardiotoxicity following doxorubicin administration is pronounced at doses greater than 550 mg/m^2.

Antimetabolites

The antimetabolites work at different steps in the production of nucleic acids. 5-Fluorouracil inhibits thymidylate synthetase; methotrexate inhibits dihydrofolate reductase; and ara-C inhibits DNA polymerase. These agents act basically by inhibiting enzyme systems because of their similarity to physiologic substrates; they can also be incorporated as false bases into the DNA or RNA. These agents may cause mucositis and myelosuppression.

Platinum Compounds

Platinum compounds bind to DNA, causing inter- and intrastrand cross-linkages, thereby disrupting DNA and RNA synthesis. Cisplatinum causes severe nephrotoxicity, and ototoxicity, and a nonreversible peripheral neuropathy. There is minimal myelosuppression, whereas bone marrow suppression is severe with carboplatinum. These agents are used primarily for ovarian cancer, non-small-cell cancer of the lung, and the non-seminomatous germ cell tumors.

Tamoxifen

Tamoxifen is a synthetic estrogen analog with minimal estrogenic activity and a high affinity for the cytosolic estrogen receptor. It can replace estrogen from the receptor and inactivate the receptor complex. It is associated with hot flashes, nausea, vomiting, and menstrual irregularities. It is useful in receptor-positive breast cancer and is presently being studied as a chemopreventive agent in patients at high risk for the development of breast cancer.

Megestrol

Megestrol bind to the progesterone receptor and interferes with its function. It is more effective for patients with breast cancer with an increased progesterone receptor assay level. It has been reported to be useful for treatment of cancer cachexia and in some cases of endometrial cancer.

Leuprolide

Leuprolide is a gonadotropin-releasing hormone analog that acts to decrease the secretion of luteinizing hormone and follicle-stimulating hormone. It also decreases the production of androgens in the testicle and adrenal. Leuprolide is the medical equivalent of an orchiectomy for the treatment of metastatic prostate cancer. This drug has indications similar to those for diethylstilbestrol (DES) but causes fewer complications.

Aminoglutethimide

Aminoglutethimide has been called the medical adrenalectomy. At high doses it decreases the conversion of cholesterol to pregnenolone in the adrenal, and at low doses it inhibits the conversion of androstenedione to estrone (a precursor of estrogen) peripherally. It is given with hydrocortisone to suppress the production of ACTH. It is useful as second-line therapy in postmenopausal or oophorectomized women with metastatic estrogen receptor-positive breast cancer. Half of the patients who responded to hormonal manipulation respond to this agent.

Biologic Response Modifiers

Biologic response modifiers alter the host's response to cancer. They are endogenous chemotherapeutic agents used in pharmacologic dosages.

Interferon enhances the antitumor activity of killer lymphocytes and macrophages. It enhances the expression of certain tumor antigens and alters enzyme systems involved with DNA synthesis. The major toxicities are a flu-like syndrome, leukopenia, and hepatic dysfunction. Its only approved use is for hairy cell leukemia, but it is being tried in combination with 5-FU for the treatment of metastatic colorectal cancer with good results.

Interleukin is a lymphokine produced by T cells after antigen stimulation. It stimulates the production of lymphokine-activated killer (LAK) cells. Interleukin is effective in renal cell cancer and melanoma.

TABLE 11.6. *Tumors curable in their advanced stages with chemotherapy*

Choriocarcinoma
Hodgkin's disease
Lymphoblastic lymphoma
Testicular cancer
Wilms' tumor
Embryonal rhabdomyosarcoma
Ewing's sarcoma
Neuroblastoma
Ovarian cancer
Small-cell lung cancer

TABLE 11.8. *Tumors poorly responsive to chemotherapy*

Osteogenic sarcoma
Pancreatic cancer
Renal cell cancer
Thyroid cancer
Colorectal cancer
Non-small-cell lung cancer
Melanoma
Hepatocellular carcinoma

Principles of Adjuvant Chemotherapy

Tumor recurrence after curative resection suggests that there is microscopic residual disease despite an adequate scope of resection. It is against these few cells that adjuvant chemotherapy is directed. There must be effective agents against the specific cancer for adjuvant chemotherapy to be considered. In addition, the patients at risk for recurrence should be able to be identified by prognostic factors and staging. This therapy is purported to be effective only during the immediate postoperative period when the tumor burden is low and the cellular growth kinetics are exponential. Furthermore, the risk of therapy must be low. Adjuvant chemotherapy is standard for node-positive breast cancer, some node-negative breast cancer, osteogenic sarcoma, colon cancer (Astler Collier B3, C1, C2, C3), and rectal cancer with concurrent radiotherapy.

TABLE 11.7. *Tumors responsive to chemotherapy[a]*

Chronic myelogenous leukemia
Bladder cancer
Gastric cancer
Cervical cancer
Sarcomas
Head and neck cancer
Endometrial cancer
Adrenocortical cancer
Medulloblastoma
Prostate cancer
Breast cancer

[a]Used only for symptomatic disease, inoperable disease, or rapidly progressive disease.

Treatment of Advanced Cancer

Several cancers are curable by chemotherapy in their advanced stage (Table 11.6). The use of chemotherapy in advanced disease is indicated if there are marginally effective agents, the tumor is unresectable or the patient is nonoperable, the metastases are symptomatic, or the disease is progressing rapidly. This is generally called palliative chemotherapy. Cancers responsive to chemotherapy in the advanced stages include those seen in Table 11-7. Tumors poorly responsive to chemotherapy should be treated only in protocol settings (Table 11-8). Though done frequently, the routine use of ineffective chemotherapy in the advanced setting is inappropriate.

Neoadjuvant Chemotherapy

Neoadjuvant chemotherapy is actually preoperative chemotherapy. It is an attempt to make a tumor that is otherwise unresectable resectable or to preserve function by decreasing the scope of surgery. None of the studies has shown significant benefit. Areas of special interest are laryngeal cancers, soft tissue sarcomas, and rectal cancers.

RADIATION ONCOLOGY

Irradiation causes chromosomal breaks, directly or via free radicals generated from oxygen or water by the radiation. The irradiated cell appears normal until it attempts to divide. At the time of cell division the irradiated cell may die because of the aberration in the chromosomes; it may produce nonviable progeny; it may not be able to divide but may remain viable; it may divide for several generations before dying; or it may be unaffected. Cells are most sensitive to radiation during G_2 and metaphase. The effectiveness of radiation therapy may be enhanced by oxygen or radiosensitizers. The therapeutic index can be further enhanced by different fractionation methods or delivery methods, including hyperfractionation (multiple small doses), accelerated fractionation (multiple normal doses), accelerated fractionation (multiple normal doses), or interstitial therapy (brachyradiotherapy). The dose and fractionation schemes are designed to enhance tumoricidal activity and minimize local tissue destruction.

Radiotherapy (RT) is considered equivalent to surgery for early-stage laryngeal cancer and precludes the need for laryngectomy. With advanced laryngeal cancer, RT in combination with chemotherapy and salvage surgery has been shown to be as effective as wide-field laryngectomy with preservation of the larynx. It is part of most therapies designed to preserve function (Table 11-9). Like surgery, RT generally affects the local recurrence rate without having a significant impact on overall patient survival.

In patients with head and neck cancer, nodal involvement in the neck is treated with adjuvant RT. The dose varies with the extent of nodal involvement, but usually 50 to 70 Gy is given. Toxicity in the head and neck area includes mucositis, pain, xerostomia, radiation caries, and osteoradionecrosis.

Chest irradiation is frequently undertaken in the adjuvant setting following curative resection of lung cancers without proved benefit to the patient. Doses of 40 Gy to one lung or 20 Gy to both lungs can cause severe radiation pneumonitis. The manifestations of radiation pneumonitis include cough, dyspnea, fever, and chest pain. It generally responds to steroid therapy.

Radiotherapy has been shown to reduce the local recurrence rates following resection of rectal carcinoma. In combination with chemotherapy, RT is the treatment of choice for squamous carcinoma of the anus, with

---

TABLE 11.9. *Routine uses of radiation therapy*

Advanced-stage cervical cancer
Adjuvant for node-positive head and neck cancers
Decrease local recurrence of breast and rectal cancer
Equivalent to surgery for early laryngeal cancer
Potentially useful as adjuvant for gastric cancer
Neoadjuvant for rectal cancer

---

cure rates that markedly exceed those of proctocolectomy for this disease. Severe radiation colitis is seen after 50 Gy and presents with symptoms of bleeding, tenesmus, and pain. Proctosigmoiditis is common during RT given for cancer of the uterus and uterine cervix. The effects of radiation are usually self-limited; however, steroid enemas and a low-residue diet may be helpful in the acute setting.

Radiation enteritis frequently occurs after only 40 Gy to the pelvis or abdomen. It causes severe nausea, vomiting, crampy abdominal pain, and occasionally bleeding. Chronically, it may result in fistulas, obstruction, or malabsorption. The acute symptoms are treated with antispasmodics and antidiarrheal agents. The malabsorption can be severe and may require short- or long-term parenteral nutrition.

QUESTIONS   10/11

Select one answer.

1. Which of the following mass screening tests for cancer has proved effective for reducing mortality?
   a. Occult blood in the stool.
   b. Chest radiographs in smokers.
   c. Mammography is women above age 35 years.
   d. Cervical Papanicolaou smears.
2. Which of these diagnostic tests is best for evaluating a thyroid nodule?
   a. Incisional biopsy.
   b. Fine-needle aspiration.
   c. Excisional biopsy.
   d. Thyroid scan.
3. For which of the following cancers is elective lymph node dissection not indicated?
   a. Melanoma.
   b. Gastric.
   c. Esophageal.
   d. Seminoma.
4. Which of the following tests is most sensitive for detecting extrahepatic metastatic colon cancer?
   a. MRI.
   b. CT scan.
   c. Sonography.
   d. Immunoscintigraphy.
5. Which of the following mechanisms does not account for the higher sensitivity of tumor cells to chemotherapeutic agents?

    a. Increased metabolic activity.

    b. Increased mitotic activity.

    c. Poor blood supply.

    d. Inadequate salvage pathways for metabolites.

6. For which of the cancers is radiation therapy equally as effective as surgery?

    a. Testicular cancer.

    b. Breast cancer.

    c. Laryngeal cancer.

    d. Lymphoma.

Match the following agents and their appropriate mechanisms of action.

    b   7. Alkylating agents   a. Medical adrenalectomy

    d   8. Vinca alkaloids   b. Interstrand cross-linkage

    c   9. Tamoxifen   c. Binds to cytosolic estrogen receptors

    e   10. 5-Fluorouracil   d. Inhibits spindle formation

    a   11. Aminoglutethimide   e. Inhibits thymidylate synthesis

SELECTED REFERENCES

Devita VT, Hellman S, Rosenberg SA, eds. *Principles and practice of oncology.* Philadelphia: JB Lippincott, 1990.

Economou SG, ed. *Adjuncts to cancer surgery.* Philadelphia: Lea & Febiger, 1991.

McKenna RJ, Murphy GP, eds. *Fundamentals of surgical oncology.* New York: Macmillan, 1986.

Sabiston DC, ed. *Textbook of surgery: the biological basis of modern surgical practice.* Philadelphia: WB Saunders, 1991.

12

Benign Gynecologic Disorders

Vicki L. Seltzer

Occasionally the general surgeon is called on to provide care for patients with gynecologic disorders. In the author's experience, the three most common gynecologic diseases with which the general surgeon may become involved are the tubal ectopic pregnancy, salpingo-oophoritis (pelvic inflammatory disease), and ovarian neoplasia. The first two disease entities are the subject of this chapter. The topic of ovarian neoplasia is addressed in Chapter 13.

ECTOPIC PREGNANCY

The term ectopic pregnancy indicates that a pregnancy is implanted other than in its normal location in the uterus. Although ectopic pregnancies are most commonly found in the fallopian tube, they have also been reported in a variety of other locations, including the cervix, ovary, and elsewhere in the peritoneal cavity.

The incidence of ectopic pregnancy varies with the patient population served and the likelihood of patients having high-risk factors, such as previous pelvic infection, which predisposes to the development of abnormal tubal transport and tubal ectopic pregnancy. The incidence has been noted to be as low as 0.5% and as high as 5.0% in various series.

Ectopic pregnancy is a serious public health problem. It is responsible for many deaths each year in the United States, usually because of inaccurate or late diagnosis. As much as 5% to 7% of maternal mortality may be caused by complications of ectopic pregnancy. Early diagnosis of the tubal ectopic pregnancy is essential, as it makes it more likely that appropriate surgery can be performed to preserve future fertility and the patient's safety and life are not jeopardized.

Significant History

Although the presenting history may have great variability, three common components are pain, abnormal vaginal bleeding, and pregnancy-related symptomatology. If the patient is a reasonably good historian, and if she maintains a menstrual calendar, she can usually report that she missed one or more periods, that she experienced bleeding at an unexpected time during her menstrual cycle, or both. Frequently, patients have pregnancy-related symptomatology (e.g., nausea and breast engorgement). Most patients are seen with a chief complaint of pelvic or lower abdominal pain. If the ectopic pregnancy has ruptured and significant intraperitoneal bleeding has occurred, the patient may have shoulder pain as well.

Physical Findings

The findings present on physical examination are variable, depending on whether the ectopic pregnancy has ruptured. The woman who has a ruptured ectopic pregnancy with significant intraperitoneal bleeding has tachycardia and hypotension. The abdomen is distended and diffusely tender, and bowel sounds are hypoactive. The woman who has an unruptured ectopic pregnancy, on the other hand, usually has normal blood pressure and pulse, and tenderness to deep palpation is often confined to the lower abdomen. Findings on pelvic examination depend on the duration of the ectopic gestation, the location of the pregnancy in the fallopian tube or uterine cornua, and whether the pregnancy has ruptured. The cervix is somewhat tender when it is manipulated, and it frequently has a bluish hue. The uterus may be soft and somewhat larger than normal. If the ectopic pregnancy is unruptured, it can often be palpated as a mass in the fallopian tube or in the uterine cornua.

Laboratory Findings

The hematocrit is normal in the patient with an unruptured ectopic pregnancy, begins to fall in a patient with a leaking tubal gestation, and drops significantly once the ectopic pregnancy ruptures and is accompanied by significant intraperitoneal bleeding. Most patients have normal white blood cell (WBC) counts. An unusually high WBC count is more consistent with a diagnosis of pelvic inflammatory disease (PID) and would rarely be seen in a case of ectopic pregnancy. Although the latex fixation slide test for pregnancy is positive in only about half the patients who have an ectopic pregnancy, the β-subunit is positive in almost all such women. Although this information does not reveal whether the pregnancy is intrauterine or extrauterine, it does indicate whether a pregnancy is present.

Differential Diagnosis

The most common diagnoses from which an ectopic pregnancy must be differentiated include an intrauterine gestation, a corpus luteum cyst, and PID. Other pathology that less commonly mimics ectopic pregnancy includes missed abortion, incomplete abortion, appendicitis, uterine anomalies, and ovarian neoplasia.

Diagnostic Procedures

Ultrasonography is a useful procedure in cases of suspected unruptured ectopic gestation. By 6 to 8 weeks of normal pregnancy, a gestational sac should be visible in the uterus by ultrasonography. If at this time a patient who is clearly pregnant and has a positive β-subunit does not have a gestational sac in the uterus, the diagnosis of ectopic pregnancy is highly likely.

Culdocentesis can indicate whether there is free blood in the peritoneal cavity. With the patient in stirrups and a speculum in the vagina, the cervix is grasped with a tenaculum, and the cul-de-sac is painted with povidone-iodine (Betadine). An 18-gauge spinal needle attached to a 10-ml syringe is then passed through the cul-de-sac, and the syringe is held on tension. If there is blood in the cul-de-sac, 8 to 10 ml is aspirated and placed in a red-topped tube to make certain it does not clot. This finding constitutes a positive culdocentesis and indicates that the patient has had an intraperitoneal bleed. Aspiration of free peritoneal fluid that is straw-colored constitutes a negative culdocentesis.

If in a given situation the main differential diagnosis is between an intrauterine gestation and an ectopic pregnancy, and the patient does not wish to be pregnant, dilatation and curettage (D&C) can be performed. If chorionic tissue is present, an intrauterine gestation is diagnosed. The simultaneous presence of an intrauterine and an ectopic gestation is rare. Patients who have ectopic pregnancies can have a wide range of findings on curettage, including Arias-Stella reaction, decidua only, and proliferative endometrium. Dilatation and curettage should not be performed to rule out an ectopic pregnancy in a patient who wishes to keep the pregnancy should she have an intrauterine gestation.

The patient who is reliable and desirous of maintaining the pregnancy if it is a viable intrauterine gestation may be observed carefully for the progression of her β-subunit values. If they do not rise normally, or if there is other evidence that an ectopic gestation is present, surgery is performed.

Laparoscopy is helpful both as a diagnostic aid and for treatment of ectopic pregnancy. Figure 12.1 presents an algorithm for the management of a patient with a possible ectopic pregnancy that is used in one hospital's emergency department.

Treatment

In the past, ectopic pregnancy was treated by removing the fallopian tube. The gynecologic surgeon is now attempting to avoid such radical therapy. Occasionally,

Patient presents with pelvic pain or vaginal bleeding

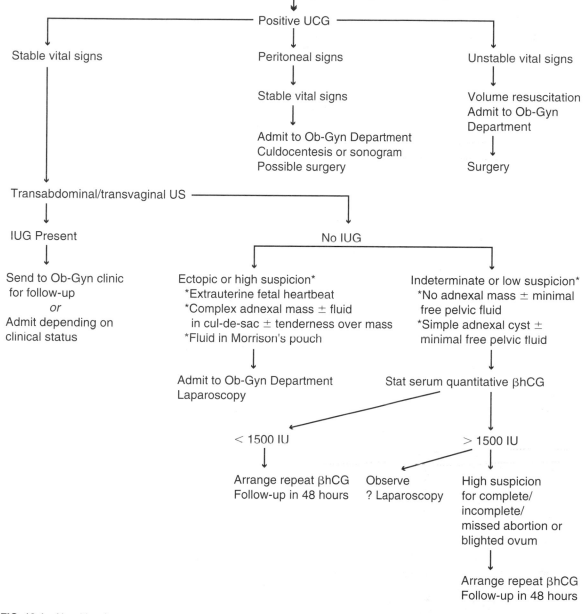

FIG. 12.1. Algorithm for emergency room management of possible ectopic pregnancy. Note that the UCG pregnancy test is *always* performed in patients of reproductive age. If there is first trimester bleeding, rule out ectopic pregnancy. *US,* ultrasonography; *IUG,* intrauterine gestation; *βhCG,* beta-subunit of human chorionic gonadotropin; *IU,* first or third standard international units.

the tubal anatomy is so abnormal as a result of the rup- tured ectopic pregnancy or former infection that the tube cannot be salvaged. For cases of unruptured ec- topic pregnancy, the patient can frequently be treated conservatively by linear salpingostomy. A linear inci- sion is made over the segment of tube that harbors the ectopic gestation. The pregnancy is then extruded and hemostasis obtained. This process can be undertaken by laparoscopy or laparotomy. At other times, segmental resection of the fallopian tube may be necessary (partial salpingectomy). In some centers, ectopic pregnancy is treated without surgery utilizing methotrexate.

Prognosis

About 5% to 7% of maternal deaths each year are caused by complications related to ectopic pregnancy. They usually involve late diagnosis with massive blood loss. With a high index of suspicion, most ectopic preg- nancies can be diagnosed before the tube has ruptured, utilizing ultrasonography and the β-subunit assay. If the diagnosis is made prior to rupture of the fallopian tube, not only does it diminish the likelihood of mortality, it improves the chance of conservative surgery being suc- cessful.

SALPINGITIS AND SALPINGO-OOPHORITIS (PELVIC INFLAMMATORY DISEASE)

Pelvic inflammatory disease is a major public health problem in the United States. Each year more than a half-million new cases are diagnosed, and the cost of treating this illness has been estimated to be more than $2 billion annually. Pelvic inflammatory disease pre- sents a spectrum of disease, the earliest manifestation of which is mild salpingitis (tubal inflammation). As the condition progresses, the ovaries frequently become involved as well (salpingo-oophoritis). The inflamma- tory process may then evolve into a tuboovarian ab- scess, which may ultimately rupture, resulting in peri- tonitis and possible death.

Significant History

The patient's chief complaint is almost always pelvic pain. The onset frequently occurs during the early pre-

menstrual phase of the menstrual cycle, and patients commonly complain of dyspareunia (painful coitus). Patients who have more severe cases of PID complain of fever, chills, and general malaise. As noted above, the process can progress, in which case the patient may experience nausea, vomiting, and ultimately the stig- mata of peritonitis.

Physical Findings

Findings on physical examination depend on when during the course of the disease process the patient is examined. Patients who have mild salpingitis may have only a low-grade fever, whereas the patient with an un- ruptured or ruptured tuboovarian abscess may have a fever as high as 105°F. Patients commonly exhibit tachycardia. Patients who have a tuboovarian abscess may begin to become hypotensive; and if the abscess ruptures, producing peritonitis, the patient ultimately manifests septic shock.

Abdominal findings approximately parallel the ex- tent of the inflammatory process. Patients with mild salpingitis have only pelvic tenderness on deep abdomi- nal palpation. As the infectious process progresses, they develop diffuse pelvic tenderness with rebound tender- ness, abdominal distension, and absent bowel sounds. Significant findings on pelvic examination include a purulent vaginal discharge and extreme pain when the cervix is moved. When an unruptured tuboovarian ab- scess is present, it is frequently palpable. However, be- cause of abdominal distension and extreme tenderness, a tuboovarian abscess may not be palpable on pelvic ex- amination. In such a case, it is unwise to exert undue force in an attempt to palpate a mass, as doing so may cause an unruptured tuboovarian abscess to leak or rup- ture. If a mass is present but not palpable by pelvic ex- amination, it can usually be identified by rectal exami- nation, as commonly a tuboovarian abscess is adherent in the cul-de-sac.

Laboratory Findings

In most cases of PID the WBC count is elevated, with an increased percentage of polymorphonuclear leuko- cytes and immature forms. The erythrocyte sedimenta- tion rate then rises, and it is not uncommon to have val- ues higher than 100 mm/hr.

Differential Diagnosis

The inflammatory processes of the fallopian tubes and ovaries must be differentiated from other inflammatory processes, including urinary tract infection, pyelonephritis, appendicitis, diverticulitis, Crohn's disease, and septic abortion. They must also be distinguished from several noninfectious entities including ectopic pregnancy, endometriosis, torsion of the adnexae, and ovarian neoplasia.

Diagnostic Procedures

Although the diagnosis can usually be made clinically, there are two diagnostic procedures that may prove useful: ultrasonography and laparoscopy. Ultrasonography cannot be used to diagnose PID. However, if it identifies other pathology (e.g., ectopic pregnancy), it has been useful for ruling out salpingo-oophoritis. If a woman has a clear-cut pelvic inflammatory process, an ultrasound scan can demonstrate that it has evolved into a tuboovarian abscess.

Several groups have suggested that salpingitis is overdiagnosed, and that many women with normal fallopian tubes have been initially misdiagnosed as having salpingitis and then repeatedly rediagnosed as having recurrent salpingitis. Because of this observation, it has been recommended by some that in all but the absolutely clear-cut cases patients should undergo laparoscopy to confirm the diagnosis of PID prior to initiation of therapy. Those who disagree with this approach do so on the ground that the laparoscopic procedure itself may exacerbate the pelvic inflammatory process and could potentially result in rupture of an unruptured tuboovarian abscess. Performing laparoscopy in all cases of possible PID to confirm the diagnosis is considered somewhat controversial, but it is being done at some centers.

Microbiology

Classic teaching had been that the fallopian tube was primarily infected with *Neisseria gonorrhoeae*, the initial damage rendering the tube more susceptible to subsequent infection by a variety of other aerobic and anaerobic organisms. In recent years, in part because of improved technology in the field of microbiology and in part as a result of changes in infectious etiology, it has been shown that likely this is not in fact always the case. Organisms that have frequently been implicated as being causative in cases of salpingo-oophoritis include *N. gonorrhoeae, Chlamydia trachomatis,* anaerobic bacteria (including *Bacteroides* and gram-positive cocci), *Escherichia coli* and other gram-negative rods, *Actinomyces israelii,* and *Mycoplasma hominis.* At present, in many parts of the United States the most commonly implicated etiologic organism is *C. trachomatis.* Because the etiologic agent or agents may be difficult to isolate, therapy is frequently based on our knowledge regarding the agents most commonly responsible for causing the disease.

Treatment

Whenever possible, treatment of PID avoids laparotomy during the acute phase unless the patient has a leaking or ruptured tuboovarian abscess. For the latter cases, surgical therapy may need to be extensive, including total abdominal hysterectomy with bilateral salpingo-oophorectomy, antibiotics, and pelvic drainage. This is done usually because the tubes and ovaries are severely infected bilaterally. In a young women of low parity who has apparent unilateral disease, the operating surgeon should perform more conservative surgery (e.g., unilateral salpingo-oophorectomy) in an attempt to preserve reproductive function. Even when severe bilateral infection is present, some surgeons attempt to preserve the uterus if it appears normal and the patient is desirous of future fertility, as the field of assisted reproductive technology has progressed rapidly.

Patients with acute PID have friable tissue, and the surgery is often difficult. Therefore for patients who do not have purulent material free in the peritoneal cavity but, rather, have an intact tuboovarian complex, it is usually considered preferable to treat with antibiotics primarily. The appropriate antibiotic therapy for PID depends on the severity of the illness. Some believe that patients with acute salpingitis must always be treated in an inpatient setting. However, when one considers the cost of inpatient therapy, it becomes obvious that it is impractical to treat all patients who have salpingitis in the hospital. Patients who have mild disease can be treated as outpatients.

The Centers for Disease Control and Prevention (CDC) recommendation for the outpatient treatment of acute salpingitis is cefoxitin (2 g IM) or ceftriaxone (250 mg IM) plus doxycycline (100 mg p.o. twice daily for 10 to 14 days). Patients can be considered as candidates for outpatient therapy for salpingitis if their temperature is below 100°F, their abdominal findings are minimal, and they do not have a tuboovarian abscess. They also must be well motivated to complete their course of therapy, as the best prognosis for future fertility is when the disease is diagnosed early and treated properly.

Patients who have a higher temperature or significant abdominal findings should be admitted to the hospital. The antibiotic treatment regimen of choice for these women has not been clearly established, as no single agent is active against the entire spectrum of potential pathogens, and for any individual the organism(s) responsible for disease are usually unknown. The CDC suggested that the following combinations may be some of the most effective in the inpatient treatment of the disease.

Regimen I: during hospitalization, cefoxitin (2 g i.v. q6h) or cefotetan (2 g i.v. q12h) plus doxycycline (100 mg p.o. or i.v. q12h). After discharge, the patient continues with doxycycline (100 mg p.o. twice daily to complete 10 to 14 days total therapy).

Regimen II: during hospitalization, clindamycin (900 mg i.v. q8h) plus gentamicin (2.0 mg/kg load followed by 1.5 mg/kg i.v. q8h in patients with normal renal function). After discharge, the patient continues with doxycycline (100 mg p.o. twice daily to complete 10 to 14 days total therapy).

Patients who have a tuboovarian abscess that is neither leaking nor ruptured should be admitted to the hospital, placed on aggressive combination antibiotic therapy, and kept NPO and at bed rest. Vital signs, urine output, and abdominal findings must be evaluated frequently. If there is any indication that the tuboovarian abscess has started to leak or has ruptured, it becomes a life-threatening surgical emergency.

Some patients do not respond to aggressive antibiotic therapy and, despite adequate trials with several aggressive antibiotic regimens, remain febrile or have a persistent tuboovarian abscess. These patients require laparotomy and may need a total abdominal hysterectomy and bilateral salpingo-oophorectomy. If the patient is young, desires future fertility, and has a unilateral tuboovarian abscess with a normal tube and ovary on the opposite side, she can be treated with a unilateral salpingo-oophorectomy. There is some risk to this procedure in that a small percentage of women so treated develop an infection in the conserved adnexa postoperatively. Even when bilateral disease is present, if the uterus is uninvolved and the patient is desirous of preserving reproductive potential, the uterus can sometimes be left *in situ,* as the field of assisted reproductive technology has made such rapid advances.

Sequelae

When salpingitis is diagnosed early and treated effectively, the prognosis for the patient is fairly good. All patients are at risk for subsequent complications related to the initial episode of PID. However, the sequelae are worst when the primary disease process is extensive. Following one episode of PID 10% to 12% of women become infertile; following two episodes approximately 25% of women are infertile; and following three episodes almost half of the women are infertile. It has been estimated that almost half of the ectopic pregnancies that occur result from the existence of previous salpingitis. Almost one-fourth of women who have had salpingitis have another episode of the infection. In addition, many women who have had salpingitis suffer from chronic pelvic pain.

QUESTIONS

Indicate whether each statement is true or false.

1. The incidence of ectopic pregnancy is the same in all areas of the United States.
2. Mortality due to complications of ectopic pregnancy almost never occurs.
3. If a patient has an ectopic pregnancy, the entire fallopian tube should always be removed.
4. By 3 weeks' gestation, the sonogram should demonstrate an ectopic pregnancy.
5. An ectopic pregnancy may be found in the abdomen or ovary.
6. *Chlamydia* is frequently the etiologic agent in salpingitis.
7. The treatment for a tuboovarian abscess is immediate laparotomy.
8. Previous salpingitis predisposes a woman to having an ectopic pregnancy.

9. Laparoscopy may be useful for confirming the diagnosis of salpingitis.

10. A woman who has bilateral tuboovarian abscesses has no potential for future fertility.

SELECTED REFERENCES

Ackerman R, Deutsch S, Krumholz B. Levels of human chorionic gonadotropin in unruptured and ruptured ectopic pregnancy. *Obstet Gynecol* 1982;60:13.

Berkley AS, Ledger WJ. Ectopic pregnancy: update on diagnosis and surgical management. *Infect Surg* 1983;2:431.

Brumstead JB. Managing ectopic pregnancy nonsurgically. *Contemp Obstet Gynecol* 1996:43–56.

DeCherney AH, Kase N. The conservative management of unruptured ectopic pregnancy. *Obstet Gynecol* 1979;54:451.

Eschenbach DA, Buchanan TM, Pollack HN. Polymicrobial etiology of acute pelvic inflammatory disease. *N Engl J Med* 1975;293:166.

Jacobson L. Differential diagnosis of acute pelvic inflammatory disease. *Am J Obstet Gynecol* 1980;138:1006.

Pelosi MA, D'Amico RJ, Goldstein PJ. Improved accuracy in the clinical diagnosis of ectopic pregnancy by the simultaneous use of pelvic ultrasonography and a radio receptor assay of human chorionic gonadotropin. *Surg Gynecol Surv* 1979;149:539.

Peterson HB, Walker CK, Kahn JG, et al. Pelvic inflammatory disease: key treatment issues and options. *JAMA* 1991;266:2605.

Seigler AM, Wang CF, Westoff C. Management of unruptured tubal pregnancy. *Obstet Gynecol Surv* 1981;36:599.

Stangel JJ, Reyniak V, Stone ML. Conservative surgical management of tubal pregnancy. *Obstet Gynecol* 1976;48:241.

Stovall TG, Ling FW, Gray LA. Single dose methotrexate for treatment of ectopic pregnancy. *Obstet Gynecol* 1991;77:754–759.

Wasserheit JN, Eschenbach DA. Pelvic inflammatory disease: etiology, epidemiology, and clinical manifestations. *Clin Gynecol Briefs* 1983;4:1.

13

Gynecologic Malignancy

Vicki L. Seltzer

OVARIAN NEOPLASIA

To have a thorough understanding of ovarian neoplasia, it is helpful to consider the disease in five categories based on histogenetic classification and embryologic etiology. The five major classes, which are considered individually, are (a) neoplasms derived from celomic epithelium, (b) neoplasms derived from germ cells, (c) neoplasms derived from specialized gonadal stroma, (d) neoplasms derived from nonspecific mesenchyme, and (e) neoplasms metastatic to the ovary.

Incidence and Age Considerations

Once a woman has started to menstruate, the presence of an ovarian mass is frequently physiologic. A woman between the ages of 20 and 30 who has an adnexal mass has less than a 10% chance that it is malignant. By the time a woman reaches the ages of 35 the incidence of malignancy starts to increase considerably; and if an ovarian mass is present in a woman 50 years of age or older there is a 50% chance that it represents a malignancy. If a girl has an ovarian mass diagnosed before she begins to menstruate, the likelihood may be 20% or more that it represents a malignancy. Because the most common etiology of an ovarian mass varies

according to the patient's age, the appropriate management also relates to this factor.

Each year in the United States there are approximately 25,000 new cases of ovarian malignancy diagnosed, and approximately 13,000 women die of the disease. Only about one in three women diagnosed as having ovarian cancer will be alive 5 years later. Although ovarian cancer is not the most common of the pelvic gynecologic malignancies (endometrial cancer is the most common), ovarian cancer will be more women each year than cervical and endometrial cancer combined and is responsible for approximately half of all deaths from malignancies of the female genital tract. On the other hand, only 20% of ovarian neoplasms are histologically malignant.

Diagnosis of Ovarian Cancer

The major reason the prognosis for women with ovarian cancer is so poor is that the disease is diagnosed in most instances when it is at an advanced stage (Table 13.1). Whereas a patient who has stage I disease has a better than 75% likelihood of surviving for 5 years, the patient with a stage III tumor has only a 10% to 25% chance of being alive 5 years later. In most series, more than two-thirds of these patients are diagnosed when the disease has advanced and is stage III or IV. It is ob-

TABLE 13.1. *Staging of ovarian cancer*

Stage I	Growth limited to the ovaries
Ia	Growth limited to one ovary; no ascites or tumor on external surface; capsule intact
Ib	Growth limited to both ovaries; no ascites or tumor on external surfaces; capsules intact
Ic	Tumor involving one or both ovaries with tumor on ovarian surface or with capsule ruptured or with ascites present containing malignant cells or with positive peritoneal washings
Stage II	Growth involving one or both ovaries with pelvic extension
IIa	Extension and/or metastases to the uterus and/or tubes
IIb	Extension to other pelvic tissues
IIc	Tumor either stage IIa or IIb, but with tumor on surface of one or both ovaries; or with capsule(s) ruptured; or with ascites present containing malignant cells or with positive peritoneal washings
Stage III	Ovarian cancer with peritoneal implants outside the pelvis and/or positive retroperitoneal or inguinal nodes or with superficial liver metastases; tumor limited to the true pelvis but with histologically proved malignant extension to small bowel or omentum
IIIa	Tumor grossly limited to the true pelvis with negative nodes but with histologically confirmed microscopic seeding of abdominal peritoneal surfaces
IIIb	Ovarian cancer with histologically confirmed implants of abdominal peritoneal surfaces, none exceeding 2 cm in diameter; nodes are negative
IIIc	Abdominal implants more than 2 cm in diameter and/or positive retroperitoneal or inguinal nodes
Stage IV	Distant metastases; if pleural effusion is present, there must be positive cytology to allot a case to stage IV; parenchymal liver metastasis equals stage IV

vious that the overall 5-year survival could be immediately improved simply by identifying a method for early diagnosis.

Patients usually do not become symptomatic until late in the course of the disease, and it has been estimated that 10,000 pelvic examinations would have to be performed in asymptomatic women to diagnose one ovarian cancer. When patients do become symptomatic, they have vague gastrointestinal complaints, usually relating to increasing abdominal girth from ascites, and early satiation following unusually small meals. It is therefore essential that for all women, particularly those over the age of 40 who have vague gastrointestinal (GI) symptomatology, a pelvic examination must be performed and a transvaginal sonogram considered; ovarian cancer must be carefully considered in the differential diagnosis of patients with vague abdominal symptoms.

It had been hoped that monoclonal antibodies would aid in the diagnosis of ovarian cancer by providing a specific screening technique for early disease. Although Bast's work with CA-125 is promising, many patients who have small amounts of disease (those who could conceivably benefit most from sophisticated sensitive and specific screening if it were available) have titers below the abnormal range. In addition, false-positive elevations may occur secondary to endometriosis, liver disease, and so on.

The 1994 NIH Consensus Statement on Ovarian Cancer: Screening, Treatment, and Follow-up concluded that the benefits of screening a woman who has one or no first-degree relatives with ovarian cancer are unproven. The PLCO screening study is currently under way to evaluate this.

At present, a high index of suspicion for patients with vague GI symptomatology is essential. In addition, each time a patient is seen by a physician for a general physical examination, she must have pelvic and rectovaginal examinations as part of the general evaluation.

Functional Cysts

Commonly when an ovarian mass is diagnosed, whether cystic or solid it is removed because it is impossible to be certain that an ovarian tumor is benign without subjecting it to pathologic evaluation. A significant exception to this statement is that functional cysts almost always resolve spontaneously within 3 months and therefore should not be treated operatively unless they rupture and produce significant intraperitoneal bleeding.

The functional cyst most commonly seen is the corpus luteum cyst, which is usually unilateral, cystic, and freely mobile. These cysts occur in women who are ovulating. There should be no nodularity in the cul-de-sac and no ascites or other findings suggestive of a possible ovarian malignancy. If a patient has an ovarian cyst and meets all the criteria, she can be observed for three menstrual cycles. If the cyst enlarges, does not resolve during three menstrual cycles, or does not meet all the aforementioned criteria, the patient usually requires surgery. Spanos evaluated 286 young ovulating women who had ovarian cysts and placed them on oral contraceptives for 6 weeks. The cyst resolved in 6 weeks in 205 of the women. The remaining 81 patients underwent an exploratory laparotomy: 76 had benign ovarian neoplasms, 5 had malignant ovarian neoplasms, and none had functional cysts. Once a functional cyst can be ruled out, the patient usually has an exploratory laparotomy or laparoscopy because neoplastic lesions do not resolve spontaneously, and without pathological evaluation it is not always possible to distinguish a benign from a malignant ovarian neoplasm. Because of the availability of sonography, certain small cystic lesions are being followed so long as the patient fully understands the risks and benefits.

Occasionally a corpus luteum cyst ruptures. Although this may result in just a small trickle of blood in the peritoneal cavity, it may also result in a massive hemoperitoneum, which cannot be distinguished clinically from a ruptured ectopic pregnancy. Either cause of massive hemoperitoneum would require immediate surgery, so it is not essential that the two conditions be distinguished or that the definitive diagnosis be made preoperatively. If the condition requires surgery to control bleeding, it can usually be treated by removing the cyst and repairing the residual normal ovarian tissue. It is almost never necessary to remove the ovary in a case of a ruptured or unruptured corpus luteum cyst.

In addition to the corpus luteum cyst, there are other types of functional ovarian masses: follicular cyst, polycystic ovaries, theca lutein cyst, and pregnancy luteoma.

Germinal Epithelial Tumors

It is thought that the histogenesis of germinal epithelial tumors is via invagination of the flattened layer of mesothelial cells of the ovarian surface, with subsequent proliferation of these cells. Germinal epithelial tumors are the most common ovarian neoplasms. Tumors in this group may be benign, malignant, or border-line tumors of low malignant potential. Benign tumors in this group include the serous cystadenoma, mucinous cystadenoma, cystadenofibroma, and the Brenner tumor.

The most common ovarian malignancies are the germinal epithelial tumors. These neoplasms account for up to 70% of all ovarian malignancies. The most common is the serous cystadenocarcinoma. Other malignancies in this group include mucinous cystadenocarcinoma, clear-cell cancer, endometrioid cancer, and undifferentiated cancer.

The appropriate operative management of these women is of paramount importance. The events at the initial operation frequently determine whether a patient can ultimately be cured. There are two aims of surgery: thorough surgical staging so decisions regarding subsequent therapy can accurately be made and thorough debulking, with an attempt to remove all gross malignancy.

When the peritoneal cavity in a patient with an adnexal mass is entered, if any ascites is present it must be sent for cytologic evaluation. If no ascites is present, peritoneal washings are obtained. Saline (50 mL) is used to irrigate the pelvis, the right and left paracolic gutters, and between the liver and the right hemidiaphragm. It is then aspirated for cytologic evaluation. As many as one-fourth of the patients who have stage I and II lesions have cytologically positive peritoneal washings. These washings may be important in determining therapy, particularly in patients who otherwise appear to have limited disease.

After peritoneal washings have been obtained, the abdomen is systemically explored. In 10% to 15% of cases otherwise thought to represent stage I disease, tumor is demonstrated to be present on the peritoneal surface between the liver and the diaphragm. The pelvic and paraaortic nodes should be carefully explored, as it is not an uncommon event that a woman who was otherwise thought to have a stage I lesion is found to have nodal metastases as her only extraovarian pathology. Nodal metastases from ovarian cancer occur most commonly via the infundibulopelvic ligaments to the paraaortic region, although, pelvic metastases and less commonly inguinal node metastases also occur.

Obviously the peritoneal washings and nodal evaluation are much more important clinical considerations in a patient who seems to have early disease, as this information may modify the decision regarding the extent of the surgical procedure performed and plans for subsequent chemotherapy. If a woman has a massive stage III ovarian cancer, the presence of positive paraaortic nodes and cytologically positive peritoneal washings would not have the same clinical significance as if these findings occurred in the woman who clinically appeared to have a small cancer confined to one ovary.

The omentum is usually removed in cases of ovarian cancer, even when it does not clinically appear to contain metastatic disease. The rationale for this decision includes the fact that the omentum occasionally harbors subclinical metastases, which are found by the pathologist on sectioning the specimen.

Classic surgery for the patient with ovarian cancer includes removal of the uterus, cervix, ovaries, fallopian tubes, and omentum; peritoneal washings; biopsy of lymph nodes; careful upper abdominal exploration; and removal of as much malignant disease as can safely be resected ("debulking surgery").

There are some instances in which it is reasonable to perform less than complete extirpative surgery in a patient who is young and appears to have a IA lesion. Conservative surgery consists of a thorough abdominal and pelvic exploration through an appropriate incision, unilateral salpingo-oophorectomy, wedge biopsy of the opposite ovary, omental biopsy, evaluation of the pelvic and paraaortic nodes with biopsy of any suspicious nodes, and peritoneal washings.

The following is a list of the requirements for performing conservative surgery. The patient should have a IA lesion with no ascites and negative peritoneal washings. The tumor must be of a favorable histologic type, that is, borderline or well-differentiated ovarian cancer or a pure dysgerminoma, granulosa cell tumor, or arrhenoblastoma. The cancer must be encapsulated and should not be ruptured at surgery. There should be no surface excrescences or adhesions and no invasion of the capsule or mesovarium. Obviously, if the wedge biopsy of the opposite ovary, the omental biopsy, or the nodes contain tumor conservative surgery is inappropriate, and the patient must be reexplored and total abdominal hysterectomy and bilateral salpingo-oophorectomy completed. To treat a patient conservatively, she should be a young woman of low parity, desirous of further childbearing. Even if the woman is in her early twenties, if she has completed her family she should undergo complete extirpative surgery.

It is preferable not to rely soley on frozen section diagnosis of an ovarian mass when a patient is young and the decision is being made regarding whether complete extirpative surgery be performed. Frozen sections of ovarian lesions are frequently difficult to interpret, and it would certainly be a serious error to remove all of a young woman's reproductive organs on the basis of frozen section, only to find on permanent section that the lesion is benign.

If in a young woman it is not clear whether an ovarian lesion is benign, it is appropriate to remove the ovary and tube on the affected side and to do a complete staging operation (peritoneal washings, node biopsies, omental biopsies, biopsy of the contralateral ovary, biopsy of the undersurface of the diaphragm, multiple biopsies of peritoneal surfaces) but not to perform a total abdominal hysterectomy with bilateral salpingo-oophorectomy. If the lesion is determined to be malignant following the final pathology evaluation, all the staging information was obtained at the primary operation. Based on the data appropriately obtained at the time of the primary surgical procedure plus the availability of the official pathology report on all this material, the decision can be made regarding whether the patient meets all the criteria for conservative surgery. If she does, she can be considered treated and continue to be observed. If she does not, she requires a second laparotomy at this time to remove her internal gynecologic organs.

A problem arises when a patient is found to have an adnexal mass at laparotomy, has the mass removed without having the appropriate staging procedures performed, and the mass is subsequently determined to be malignant. If no peritoneal washings were taken, the upper abdomen was not explored, the omentum was not biopsied, or the contralateral ovary was not biopsied, the patient deserves the benefit of a repeat operation and proper surgical staging. If the disease is, in fact, IA, she can be treated conservatively. If she has more extensive disease, as is often the case, complete surgery is done followed by appropriate chemotherapy. The younger the patient, the more she has to lose if she is undertreated.

This problem often occurs when a patient has a McBurney incision for what is thought to be appendicitis, but an ovarian neoplasm is found. If it is malignant on frozen section, the incision is extended so appropriate surgical exploration and therapy can be carried out. When this is not done, the patient invariably requires repeat laparotomy for staging and therapy over the ensuing weeks.

Because of the advent of advanced reproductive technologies, sometimes in young women who have stage Ib disease the uterus can be preserved for a subsequent pregnancy. This is an uncommon decision and is reserved for young women desirous of future fertility whose lesions have been properly surgically staged.

Patients with stage I disease in whom conservative surgery is not applicable are treated by total abdominal hysterectomy and bilateral salpingo-oophorectomy. The uterus is removed because it may be the source of occult metastases, patients with ovarian cancer are also at high risk for developing endometrial cancer, and the presence of the uterus may make it more difficult to evaluate recurrent pelvic tumor.

For stage II disease, surgery is done utilizing a retroperitoneal approach, similar to the approach utilized for radical hysterectomy, so the tumor can be removed *en bloc.*

What is the proper operative approach to the abdomen that is explored and found to be filled with ovarian tumor? The surgical effort must be determined and aggressive. It has now been shown fairly conclusively that tumor debulking makes a great difference in the patient's 5-year survival. As reported by Kolstad, a patient with a fully debulked stage III lesion has a better prognosis than the patient with a stage II lesion that has not been debulked. Griffiths and Fuller found that conscientious attempts at optimal surgical cytoreduction followed by intensive combination chemotherapy improved the 5-year survival of those with stage III disease from 5% to 40% in their series.

As would be expected, the best results are achieved when the tumor is maximally debulked. If by resecting one or more intestinal segments most of the patient's cancer can be fully debulked, it should be done. For this reason, it is important that the patient suspected of having ovarian cancer have a bowel preparation preoperatively.

There appears to be no point in performing potentially complicated surgery with multiple bowel resections if despite these efforts the patient is left with a large amount of residual tumor. Data suggest that unless the tumor is debulked to less than 2 cm in largest diameter at any site, debulking may not markedly improve the likelihood of cure.

One possible explanation for the effectiveness of aggressive tumor debulking in the therapy of ovarian cancer, despite the fact that it does not improve survival in other types of malignancies, is that there is effective chemotherapy for germinal epithelial ovarian cancer. The success of subsequent chemotherapy is usually inversely proportional to the amount of tumor left in the abdomen at the conclusion of the initial debulking sur-

gery. The aggressive surgical approach not only is beneficial, it permits subsequent chemotherapy to be much more effective. In most instances it is the combination of aggressive surgery and aggressive chemotherapy together that contributes to prolonged survival of the ovarian cancer patient. The most commonly used first-line chemotherapy for patients who have ovarian cancer combines platinum and taxol. The response rate with this combination of agents is over 80%. The duration of response is vastly improved when compared with single-alkylating-agent therapy, and the quality of life for the patients is generally good.

Second-Look Laparotomy

After patients complete chemotherapy for epithelial ovarian cancer and have no clinical or laboratory evidence of persistent disease, some patients are candidates for second-look laparotomy. It is done to determine if any tumor persists that had not been detectable by other means; patients can immediately be treated with second-line therapy if this is the case. Even when a second-look laparotomy is completely normal, approximately 30% of patients develop recurrent ovarian cancer. Not all patients should have a second-look laparotomy. It is done only if additional therapy exists that can be offered to the patient if the surgery demonstrates tumor persistence. In addition, some believe that second-look laparotomy should be reserved for patients on protocols.

Proper technique for second-look laparotomy is essential to reduce the possibility of a false-negative result. If the uterus or ovarian tissue is still present, it should be removed and peritoneal washings obtained. Residual omentum should be removed. A meticulous intraperitoneal exploration must be performed, with particularly careful focus on, and biopsies of, areas where persistent ovarian cancer is most likely to be present (undersurface of the right hemidiaphragm, surface of the bowel or mesentery, nodes, areas of adhesion, pelvic peritoneum, and areas in which tumor was previously found). Even if there is no clinical evidence of disease, multiple biopsy specimens from these areas must be obtained.

Germ Cell Tumors

The second most commonly noted ovarian malignancy is the germ cell type. This group consists of all the ovarian neoplasms derived from the primitive germ cells of the embryonic gonad.

Fortunately, the most common germ cell tumor is the benign cystic teratoma ("dermoid"). The dermoid is bilateral in approximately 15% of cases. The surgical procedure for these lesions consists of removing the dermoid cyst only and reconstructing the residual ovary. It is almost always unnecessary to remove the entire ovary. This is particularly significant because the patients are usually young and the lesion may be bilateral at the time of the primary surgery, or the woman may subsequently develop a dermoid of the opposite ovary.

Malignant germ cell tumors are less frequent occurrences than the benign variety of the group of lesions. Malignant germ cell tumors most commonly occur in young girls; and despite the fact that they are usually diagnosed when they are confined to one ovary, the prognosis may be poor. The most common malignant germ cell tumor, the dysgerminoma, has a 5-year survival rate of 70%. The less common lesions—the embryonal cancer, endodermal sinus tumor, immature teratoma, primary ovarian choriocarcinoma—are often aggressive tumors that may result in mortality for girls and young women. Tumors in this group may secrete human chorionic gonadotropin or α-fetoprotein. They may cause girls to have vaginal bleeding, precocious pseudopuberty, and positive pregnancy tests. One commonly employed chemotherapy regimen for these tumors is velban, bleomycin, and cis-platinum.

Gonadal Stromal Tumors

Gonadal stromal tumors comprise approximately 5% to 10% of ovarian tumors. They arise from the specialized ovarian gonadal stroma and are frequently hormonally active. The granulosa–theca tumors frequently secrete estrogen, and patients often present with the stigmata of excess estrogen. This tumor is most commonly found in perimenopausal and postmenopausal women, who often exhibit abnormal vaginal bleeding caused by abnormal estrogen levels and may even develop endometrial hyperplasia or cancer. Rarely, the granulosa cell tumor occurs in young girls, in whom it may present with vaginal bleeding.

Another variety of gonadal stromal tumor, the Sertoli-Leydig tumor, secretes testosterone; and the patients, who are commonly young women, present with signs of masculinization, such as hirsutism, temporal balding, hypertrophy of the clitoris, hoarseness, and

breast atrophy. The gonadal stromal tumors are usually nonaggressive malignancies and have a good prognosis.

Neoplasms Derived from Nonspecific Mesenchyme

Neoplasms derived from nonspecific mesenchyme arise in tissue that is not specific to the ovary and therefore could arise anywhere in the body. The most common ovarian tumor derived from nonspecific mesenchyme is the benign ovarian fibroma, which may be large and clinically symptomatic. Malignant lesions in this group are unusual, but when they do occur the most common is the primary ovarian lymphoma.

Neoplasms Metastatic to the Ovary

Approximately 5% of women who have a clinically significant malignancy of the ovary do not have primary ovarian tumors but metastases from other sites. A common misconception is that all tumors metastatic to the ovaries are Krukenberg tumors. This is not the case. Krukenberg tumors are usually bilateral lesions that may be quite large, are usually freely mobile, and retain the shape of the ovaries. Histologically, they contain mucin-secreting signet ring cells, in which the mucin pushes the nucleus to one side of the cell and flattens it, so the cell takes on the appearance of a signet ring. The original tumor Krukenberg described was metastatic from the stomach to the ovaries.

Clinically significant metastases to the ovaries most commonly arise from primary tumors of the GI tract, breast, and uterus. Because 5% of what preoperatively appears to be ovarian malignancies are actually metastases from other tumors, it is important to give this point due consideration preoperatively when evaluating a patient with an ovarian mass.

The clinical situation in which this information is most commonly of concern is when the metastases are from the GI tract. As has been discussed, patients who have ovarian cancer often have as their chief complaint GI symptomatology. Therefore the patient who has an ovarian mass and GI symptomatology may be assumed to have these symptoms because of the presence of an ovarian malignancy. Even at laparotomy, the clinical distribution of the disease may make it mistakenly appear that the patient has ovarian cancer, and the subsequent surgery and chemotherapy may therefore be directed toward that diagnosis. Occasionally the fact that the ovarian tumor is the result of a primary GI malignancy is not recognized until months later, when the patient presents with bowel obstruction. To avoid inappropriate therapy, it is essential that all patients who have suspected ovarian tumor but have GI symptomatology undergo an upper GI series and barium enema (one or both, depending on symptomatology) or endoscopy prior to laparotomy. In addition, any patient diagnosed histopathologically as having a mucinous ovarian cancer (which is rather uncommon and may be histologically indistinguishable from a GI cancer) should have a complete GI workup postoperatively if one had not been performed preoperatively.

Conclusion

At present, the overall prognosis for women with ovarian cancer is grim, the 5-year survival being in the range of 35%. These data can be favorably affected by maintaining a high index of suspicion so the disease can be diagnosed earlier and performing aggressive surgical debulking procedures so the chance for cure with subsequent aggressive chemotherapy is increased.

UTERINE TUMORS

Endometrial Cancer

In the United States, endometrial cancer is the most common malignancy of the female genitalia, with approximately 40,000 new cases reported annually. Fortunately, it is a disease with an excellent prognosis. In most series, at least 75% of women are diagnosed when they have stage I disease, and the overall 5-year survival is usually reported to be at least 75%.

Endometrial cancer generally affects older women. Approximately 80% of women with the tumor are postmenopausal, and only 5% are under the age of 40. Patients at high risk to develop this lesion are obese, have no children, are hypertensive, are diabetic, and have had a late menopause.

Symptoms

The hallmark symptom of endometrial cancer is abnormal bleeding. Any woman who has vaginal bleeding after menopause should be considered to have a malignancy somewhere in the genital tract unless proved oth-

erwise. In some series almost 20% of women who had postmenopausal bleeding harbored a gynecologic malignancy. The most likely type of tumor in the woman presenting with postmenopausal bleeding is an endometrial adenocarcinoma, although uterine sarcoma or cervical squamous cell carcinoma may also be the cause.

Diagnostic Procedures

If a woman is not pregnant and has abnormal bleeding, the endometrium should be sampled utilizing an outpatient office procedure such as endometrial biopsy or pipelle. In addition, if a woman has postmenopausal or abnormal perimenopausal bleeding or is at increased risk for significant pathology and the aforementioned procedures do not demonstrate the presence of a malignancy, and she continues to bleed, she should undergo hysteroscopy and fractional dilatation and curettage (D&C). Obviously, some patients have abnormal bleeding because of cervical cancer, and this possibility must also be evaluated.

Although a D&C is a minor surgical procedure, there are a few crucial points to underscore. Prior to initiating the procedure, a careful examination must be performed.

The first step in performing a fractional D&C is endocervical curettage, a procedure in which the endocervical tissue is scraped in a systematic fashion with a small curette. Then the uterus is sounded to determine the length of the uterine cavity. The cervix is then dilated, and systematic curettage of the endometrial cavity is performed. Polyp forceps are then introduced into the uterine corpus so endometrial polyps or floating tissue that had been freed by the curettage can be removed. The cervix is then stained with Lugol's solution, and biopsy specimens of nonstaining areas are obtained.

Histology

More than 90% of endometrial cancers are adenocarcinomas. Adenosquamous cancers have areas of both glandular and squamous malignancy, and they have a worse prognosis than the pure adenocarcinomas. Adenoacanthomas contain a malignant glandular component and benign squamous metaplasia. They are almost always well-differentiated lesions, and they have a good prognosis. Primary squamous cell carcinoma of the endometrium is an extremely uncommon lesion and has been reported rarely.

Staging

For most patients who have endometrial adenocarcinoma, the primary therapy is surgical. Most of the women have stage I disease (see Table 13.2 for staging), for which the recommended therapy at the author's hospital is an exploratory laparotomy with total abdominal hysterectomy, bilateral salpingo-oophorectomy, peritoneal washings, and lymph node sampling. Postoperative radiation therapy to the pelvis (5,000 rad in 5 weeks) is given to patients who have tumor metastatic to pelvic lymph nodes, poorly differentiated tumors, invasion of the endometrial cancer deep into the myometrium, or occult cervical involvement with tumor. Women who have paraaortic lymph node metastases also receive extended-field radiation if supraclavicular nodes are negative and there are no other distant metastases. The appropriate therapy for patients who have positive peritoneal cytology is controversial; however, these women are at increased risk for recurrence, and most physicians agree that they should receive ad-

ditional treatment. Women with papillary serous tumors or with disease outside the treatment field often receive combination chemotherapy as well.

The overall prognosis for women with endometrial cancer is excellent, with many series reporting the 5-year survival as 75% or better. Factors that adversely affect prognosis include the presence of deep myometrial invasion, poorly differentiated tumors, papillary tumors, lymph node metastases, positive peritoneal cytology, and disease that is at a more advanced stage.

Prognosis

Although the prognosis for women with stage I disease is excellent, the 5-year survival for women with stage II disease is approximately 50%. For those with stage III disease it is approximately 30% and for patients with stage IV disease only 10%.

Uterine Sarcoma

Uterine sarcoma is an uncommon lesion and accounts for fewer than 5% of uterine cancers. As is true for endometrial adenocarcinomas, the uterine sarcoma tends to occur in older women; unlike the patient with endometrial adenocarcinoma, the prognosis for the woman who has a uterine sarcoma is poor. Patients who have uterine sarcomas usually have vaginal bleeding as a presenting symptom. A uterus that enlarges rapidly after menopause suggests the presence of a uterine sarcoma. Patients may also complain of pain.

Histology

There are several types of uterine sarcoma. The mixed müllerian sarcoma contains elements of both carcinoma and sarcoma and contains at least one element that is not normally found in the uterus (e.g., cartilage). The carcinosarcoma contains areas of carcinoma as well as sarcomatous elements, but all the tissue present is that which is normally indigenous to the uterus. The endometrial stromal sarcoma is a pure lesion (having only sarcoma but no carcinoma present) and is a tumor that arises from connective tissue of the endometrium rather than from the myometrium. It is a relatively uncommon type of sarcoma. The leiomyosarcoma is a pure myometrial lesion that often arises in a

TABLE 13.2. *Staging of uterine cancer*

Stage I	Growth limited to the uterus
IA G123	Tumor limited to endometrium
IB G123	Invasion to less than one-half of the myometrium
IC G123	Invasion to more than one-half of the myometrium
Stage II	Disease involving the cervix
IIA G123	Endocervical glandular involvement only
IIB G123	Cervical stromal invasion
Stage III	
IIIA G123	Tumor invades uterine serosa and/or adnexae and/or positive peritoneal cytology
IIIB G123	Vaginal metastases
IIIC G123	Metastases to pelvic and/or para-aortic lymph nodes
Stage IV	
IVA G123	Tumor invasion of bladder and/or bowel mucosa
IVB	Distant metastases including intraabdominal and/or inguinal lymph node

fibroid. It tends to occur in a somewhat younger group of women than the other uterine sarcomas and is found more often as a stage I tumor, which explains why its prognosis is better than that of the other sarcomas. Other types of sarcoma, which occur rarely, include the rhabdomyosarcoma (a striated muscle sarcoma), chondrosarcoma, osteosarcoma, liposarcoma, fibrosarcoma, and angiosarcoma.

Diagnosis

The diagnosis is most commonly made when a D&C has been done for the complaint of postmenopausal or abnormal perimenopausal bleeding. It is important to note that, although this is the way in which a uterine sarcoma is most commonly diagnosed, the malignancy that would most often be found when a D&C has been performed for bleeding is an endometrial adenocarcinoma. Uterine sarcomas (particularly the mixed müllerian sarcoma) also may be diagnosed on pelvic examination because tissue from this tumor may protrude through the cervical os, giving a distinct clinical appearance. Occasionally a uterine sarcoma is diagnosed during hysterectomy done for a rapidly enlarging uterine mass in a postmenopausal woman.

Therapy

At the author's institution, uterine sarcomas are treated by primary surgery. The surgical procedure performed is an exploratory laparotomy with total abdominal hysterectomy and bilateral salpingo-oophorectomy. Peritoneal washings are obtained, and lymph nodes are sampled. The upper abdomen is evaluated for occult disease, which frequently is found. Uterine sarcomas that preoperatively appeared to be confined to the uterus are commonly found at laparotomy to have metastasized extensively. In this case, if hysterectomy can be performed without undue morbidity, it should be done because doing so may reduce the likelihood of the patient having pelvic pain, bleeding, and infection.

For patients who have sarcoma confined to the pelvis, some oncologists advocate preoperative or postoperative pelvic irradiation. It appears that the main contribution of pelvic irradiation for these women is a reduction in the incidence of pelvic recurrence, but it does not improve overall survival. Because it is common at laparotomy to find that disease that preopera-

tively appeared to be stage I has metastasized to the upper abdomen, the author recommends that if radiation is to be utilized at all it be done postoperatively.

Occasionally patients who are medically inoperable have been treated by irradiation alone. This practice significantly decreases the likelihood that the patient will be cured.

Chemotherapy has not been demonstrated to be curative for patients with uterine sarcoma. However, it has been demonstrated to have activity in patients with this disease and should be utilized for those who are found to have spread of disease at laparotomy or who have recurrent tumor that is not treatable by surgery or irradiation.

Prognosis

The overall 5-year survival for patients with uterine sarcoma is approximately 30%. Although half of the women who have stage I tumors live for 5 years, only 10% of women who have stage II to IV lesions are alive at 5 years.

CERVICAL CANCER

Because of the availability and widespread use of the Papanicolaou (Pap) smear in the United States, cervical cancer is no longer the most commonly diagnosed gynecologic malignancy. Fortunately, because of programs of regular screening by Pap smear, most cervical lesions are diagnosed in a premalignant phase. In addition, cervical cancer has been reduced from being the most common to the eighth leading cause of cancer death in American women.

The mean age for women with invasive cervical cancer is in the 45- to 55-year-old range. However, it is not uncommon to diagnose cervical cancer in a woman in her twenties, and rare patients have been found to have cervical cancer while still in their teens. Although the likelihood of finding invasive cervical cancer diminishes somewhat in the much older woman, it is not a rare event to diagnose the lesion in a woman in her eighties or nineties.

Diagnosis

Early cervical cancer may be totally asymptomatic and may be diagnosed solely because of an abnormal

Pap smear. The first symptom of cervical cancer is usually painless bleeding, commonly occurring after intercourse. Pain usually appears as a late symptom.

It is a fortunate patient whose diagnosis is made because an abnormal Pap smear in the presence of a grossly normal cervix has led her physician to perform a colposcopy and to diagnose invasive disease. More commonly the tumor is diagnosed because the clinician finds a gross cervical abnormality on pelvic examination and performs a biopsy. It is essential that all cervical abnormalities be biopsied even when the patient has a normal Pap smear. In most large series, the Pap smear has a 15% to 20% false-negative rate in diagnosing cervical neoplasia. Patients who have invasive cervical cancer may have such extensive shedding of inflammatory cells that neoplastic cells arc not present on the Pap smear. Therefore if a lesion is present on the cervix, regardless of the findings on Pap smear, it should be biopsied.

Cervical conization (removal of a cone-shaped portion of the cervix) is a surgical procedure utilized as a diagnostic technique. It is used in the patient who has an abnormal Pap smear in whom colposcopy and biopsy have not diagnosed invasive cervical cancer but have been inadequate in ruling it out. A large loop excision of the transformation zone (LLETZ) procedure may also be utilized for this purpose.

Histology

More than 90% of cervical cancers are squamous cell lesions. Approximately 5% to 7% of cervical cancers are adenocarcinomas that arise higher up, in the endocervix. Less commonly, patients have mixed adenosquamous tumors, such as the aggressive glassy-cell cancer. Rarely, tumors such as sarcomas and lymphomas are found on the cervix.

Pretreatment Evaluation

The appropriate pretreatment evaluation depends on the extent of local disease on pelvic examination (see Table 13.3 for staging cervical cancer). The patient who has a 1-cm cancer that is clinically confined to the cervix is unlikely to have distant metastases, and the required workup therefore does not need to be overly extensive. For the patient who has such a clinically early lesion, required workup prior to treatment includes a chest radiograph, intravenous pyelogram (IVP) or com-

TABLE 13.3. *Staging of cervical cancer*

Stage 0 Carcinoma *in situ*
Stage I Carcinoma confined to the cervix (extension to the corpus should be disregarded)

Ia	Preclinical carcinoma of cervix, diagnosed only by microscopy
Ia1	Minimal microscopic stromal invasion.
Ia2	Measurable microscopic disease; the upper limit of measurement must be no more than 5 mm in depth or 7 mm in lateral spread; larger lesions staged as Ib
Ib	Lesions of greater dimensions than stage Ia2 regardless of whether seen clinically

Stage II

IIa	Involvement of the vagina but not the lower one-third
IIb	Parametrial involvement, but not to the pelvic side wall

Stage III

IIIa	Involvement of the lower third of the vagina
IIIb	Extension to the pelvic wall and/or hydronephrosis or nonfunctioning kidney

Stage IV Carcinoma extends beyond the true pelvis or clinically involves the mucosa of the bladder or rectum

IVa	Spread of the growth to adjacent organs
IVb	Spread to distant organs

puted tomography (CT), complete blood count (CBC), SMA-18, and urinalysis. The patient who has locally more extensive disease, stage IIB or more, requires an extensive pretreatment workup, including chest radiography, CT, cystoscopy, sigmoidoscopy, CBC, SMA-18, and urinalysis.

Therapy

Appropriate therapy for cervical cancer is dependent on the stage of disease and the patient's age and general health. The treatment for stage IA1 and early IA2 cervical cancer is a hysterectomy (removal of the uterus and cervix). There is no indication for oophorectomy unless the patient is more than 45 years of age or has ovarian pathology.

Patients who have either more advanced IA2 disease or stage IB or IIA cervical cancer can be treated with radiation or surgery with no difference in the likelihood of cure. The benefit of surgery for the younger patient is that the use of radiation may cause vaginal stenosis and the ovaries to atrophy, with the result that the premenopausal patient becomes menopausal. Occasionally, following radical surgery the patient still requires pelvic irradiation (because at surgery the patient was found to have four or more positive pelvic nodes, tumor at the margin of surgical resection, disease in the parametrium, or other evidence of more advanced disease).

For women who are young, in good health, have advanced IA2 disease or stage IB or IIA cervical cancer, and elect to have surgery rather than radiation therapy, the appropriate procedure is an exploratory laparotomy with careful abdominal exploration and paraaortic node biopsy. If those findings are negative, a radical hysterectomy and bilateral pelvic lymphadenectomy is done. If there is tumor metastatic to the paraaortic nodes or elsewhere in the abdomen, radical hysterectomy should not be performed, as it will not result in cure of the patient. The young woman who has a radical hysterectomy and bilateral pelvic lymphadenectomy for cervical cancer does not require oophorectomy for the treatment of this disease because early cervical cancer almost never metastasizes to the ovaries.

Radical hysterectomy and bilateral pelvic lymphadenectomy involves removal of the uterus, cervix, upper vagina, parametria out to the pelvic side wall, and the pelvic lymph nodes (external iliac, internal iliac, common iliac, and obturator nodes).

In addition to the common potential complications of major pelvic surgery, 1% of patients who have had a radical hysterectomy develop a ureterovaginal fistula at approximately 10 days postoperatively as a result of devascularization of the ureter at surgery.

On the other hand, potential side effects of radical radiation therapy to the pelvis include vaginal stenosis, radiation enteritis, proctosigmoiditis, and possible rectovaginal fistula. Vesicovaginal fistula, ureterovaginal fistula, and ureteral stenosis are rare complications of radiation therapy. All patients who have had radical pelvic irradiation without prior surgery to bring the ovaries to the upper abdomen out of the radiation field have total ovarian failure and, in the previously premenopausal patient, onset of menopausal symptomatology.

Pelvic exenteration (anterior, posterior, or total exenteration) on rare occasions is utilized as primary therapy for a patient who has cervical cancer that is localized to the pelvis, does not involve the pelvic side walls, but has extended anteriorly to the bladder, posteriorly to the rectum, or along the length of the vagina toward the vulva. More commonly, pelvic exenteration can be utilized as salvage therapy for the patient who has been treated with radical irradiation for cervical cancer but subsequently develops a central pelvic recurrence. Such a patient must have no disease outside the pelvis, no extension of tumor to the pelvic side wall, and no pelvic nodes that grossly contain tumor.

If patients are appropriately selected, the 5-year survival rate for those treated with pelvic exenteration for cervical cancer that has recurred following irradiation is approximately 30%. Morbidity with this procedure is high, but mortality in most centers is below 5%.

Chemotherapy for recurrent or advanced cervical cancer frequently results in short-term responses, but no combination of chemotherapeutic agents has been shown to result in long-term survival or cure of cervical cancer. Several studies are presently in progress to evaluate the role of chemoradiotherapy in the treatment of primary advanced squamous cell cervical carcinoma.

Prognosis

The prognosis for the patient who has early cervical cancer is excellent. The 5-year survival for the woman who has stage I disease is 85% to 90%. For stage IIA it is 75% to 80% and for stage IIB approximately 60%. About 30% to 40% of patients who have stage III disease survive for 5 years, and approximately 10% of women who have stage IV disease are alive at 5 years.

Although the overall prognosis for the woman with invasive cervical cancer is quite good, the fact remains that there are likely almost 5,000 deaths from cervical cancer in the United States each year. With appropriate screening most of these tumors could be diagnosed and eradicated prior to their becoming invasive or at an earlier stage, providing the patient with a better opportunity for cure. Hence there remains an enormous amount that must be done with respect to patient and physician education regarding Pap smear screening.

VAGINAL CANCER

Primary vaginal cancer is a rare lesion, comprising fewer than 2% of gynecologic malignancies. Cancer in the vagina is more commonly a secondary lesion, either from direct extension of a cervical or vulvar cancer or from metastasis of an endometrial adenocarcinoma.

Histology

Most primary vaginal cancers are squamous cell tumors, and although there is a wide age range the typical patient is between 40 and 70 years of age. The tumor is usually in the upper half of the vagina. Primary squamous cell carcinoma of the vagina most commonly occurs in a woman who has previously had a squamous neoplasm of the cervix or vulva.

In the past, several hundred cases of clear-cell vaginal adenocarcinoma had been reported in girls and young women (ages 7 to 29; mean age 19) who were exposed to diethylstilbestrol (DES) *in utero* as a result of maternal ingestion of the drug during pregnancy. It is estimated that millions of fetuses were exposed to the drug *in utero,* but only a small number later developed vaginal adenocarcinoma. The risk for a woman who was exposed to DES as a fetus ultimately developing vaginal adenocarcinoma is 0.14 to 1.4 per 1,000. Vaginal adenocarcinoma has also been reported rarely to occur in older women, and in these cases it has been unrelated to DES exposure.

Vaginal sarcomas occur uncommonly. An unusually aggressive lesion, sarcoma botryoides, is a rhabdomyosarcoma that affects infants and young children. It presents as a polypoid tumor, occasionally protruding through the vagina and producing vaginal discharge and bleeding.

An exceedingly rare vaginal tumor is the malignant melanoma, which accounts for few than 1% of all vaginal malignancies.

Staging

The staging of vaginal cancer is similar to the staging of cervical cancer (Table 13.4).

Diagnosis

Patients who have vaginal cancer usually present with symptoms of bleeding or discharge. Rarely the woman is asymptomatic, and the disease is diagnosed because of an investigation that ensued as the result of an abnormal Pap smear. If a lesion is present in the vagina, it must always be biopsied. When no lesion is present but the Pap smear is abnormal, a colposcopic evaluation should be performed.

Two groups of women are known to be at high risk for developing vaginal cancer. If a woman has previously had a squamous cell cervical or vulvar neoplasm, she is at high risk to develop vaginal cancer. Therefore all women who have been treated for cervical or vulvar neoplasia, even if they have had a hysterectomy, must have regular Pap smears performed at least at 6-month intervals. Women who had been exposed to DES *in utero* must be screened regularly for vaginal adenocarcinoma, because they are at high risk for the development of this tumor.

Pretreatment Evaluation

Because the vagina is in close proximity to the bladder and rectum, a pretreatment evaluation for a patient with vaginal cancer must include investigation of these organs. Depending on whether the vaginal cancer is located anteriorly or posteriorly or is diffuse, the patient requires cystoscopy and/or proctosigmoidoscopy and barium enema. All patients with vaginal cancer should undergo an IVP and chest radiography as well as a CBC, SMA-18, and urinalysis. Patients who have extensive local disease can benefit from a CT scan to look for the presence of nodal or intraperitoneal metastases.

Therapy

Invasive squamous cell vaginal cancer is usually treated by radiation therapy. Occasionally a woman who has a lesion in the upper vagina is treated by exploratory laparotomy, radical hysterectomy, upper vaginectomy, and pelvic node dissection; and a woman who has a lesion in the most distal portion of the vagina may be treated by radical vulvectomy, distal vaginectomy, and node dissection. The woman who has previously received pelvic radiation (e.g., as therapy for cervical cancer) and who now has vaginal cancer may require exenteration if an attempt is to be made to perform curative surgery.

Whereas invasive squamous cancer of the vagina is usually treated with radiation, clear-cell adenocarcinoma of the vagina usually occurs in young women and is therefore treated with surgery whenever possible; when the tumor involves the upper vagina and is stage I

TABLE 13.4. *Staging of vaginal cancer*

Stage I	Cancer limited to vagina
Stage II	Cancer involving subvaginal tissue but not extending to the pelvic side wall
Stage III	Cancer extending to pelvic side wall
Stage IV	
IVa	Involvement of the bladder or rectum
IVb	Distant metastases

(i.e., cancer limited to the vagina), the patient is treated with radical hysterectomy, upper vaginectomy, and bilateral pelvic lymphadenectomy. Depending on the location of the cancer in the vagina, the patient may require a total vaginectomy and creation of a neovagina (for which a segment of colon may be utilized). When the disease has progressed beyond stage I, patients are usually treated with radiation therapy.

Prognosis

Considering the difficulties noted when treating vaginal cancer because of its proximity to the bladder and rectum, reports of 5-year survival rates between 40% and 55% are surprisingly good.

Patients who have clear-cell vaginal adenocarcinoma have a somewhat better prognosis. This may be in part because so many of the lesions are diagnosed when the patients have stage I disease.

CANCER OF THE VULVA

Vulvar cancer is the fourth most common of the pelvic gynecologic malignancies, accounting for only 5% to 10% of these tumors. It is a lesion that occurs predominantly among older women, although recently there has been an increasing incidence in younger women as well.

Histology

More than 85% of the tumors are squamous cell lesions. Melanomas are the second most common vulvar cancers, comprising approximately 5% of the tumors in most series. The remaining lesions are sarcomas, basal cell tumors, and adenocarcinomas.

Lymphatic Dissemination

The spread of vulvar cancer is usually via lymphatic dissemination. It generally proceeds in an orderly fashion, first involving superficial inguinal nodes and Cloquet's node and ultimately involving the external iliac and deep pelvic nodes. Although in most instances the involvement of nodes occurs with an orderly progression, lesions involving the clitoris or the perineum oc-

casionally have been reported to involve the deep pelvic nodes without first affecting the more superficial node groups.

Therapy

Vulvar cancer had traditionally been treated by radical vulvectomy with bilateral groin dissection. Deep pelvic lymphadenectomy or irradiation of the deep pelvic nodes is usually done if there is groin node involvement, the disease involves the clitoris or perineum, the primary lesion is large, or there is another reason to suspect that the deep pelvic nodes might be involved.

Women with early vulvar cancer (up to 2 cm in diameter and 5 mm or less in depth) have more recently been treated with wide local excision with a 3-cm margin of normal skin and adequate subcutaneous tissue and unilateral superficial groin node dissection on the side of the lesion. If node metastasis is present on histologic evaluation, a classic radical vulvectomy and bilateral inguinal lymphadenectomy may be performed.

Treatment of stage III and IV disease (Table 13.5) must be individualized depending on both the distribution of disease and the patient's general health. For early stage III disease, radical vulvectomy with bilateral groin and deep pelvic node dissections is often adequate. Although the patients are frequently elderly, when the disease involves the rectum, bladder, or most of the length of the vagina but distant disease is absent

---

TABLE 13.5. *Staging of vulvar cancer*

Stage I	Cancer 2 cm diameter or less; confined to the vulva; with no clinically suspicious groin nodes.
Stage II	Cancer more than 2 cm in diameter, confined to the vulva, with no clinically suspicious groin nodes.
Stage III	Vulvar cancer that has spread to the urethra, anus, vagina, or perineum and/or groin nodes that are clinically suspicious (enlarged and firm but mobile and not fixed).
Stage IV	Vulvar cancer involving the bladder mucosa or rectal mucosa and/or fixed to bone and/or with other distant metastases and/or with fixed or ulcerated groin nodes.

p/10

appropriate therapy may be pelvic exenteration (anterior, posterior, or total, depending on the distribution of disease) plus radical vulvectomy and groin dissection. Five-year survival with this radical surgical therapy for locally advanced vulvar cancer is excellent. If such extensive surgery is contraindicated for medical reasons, some patients possibly can be cured with radiation therapy alone or irradiation plus a less extensive surgical procedure. Studies are presently under way to evaluate chemotherapy in conjunction with irradiation for these lesions. The preliminary data are promising.

Complications of Surgery

Despite the fact that radical vulvectomy plus node dissection is a lengthy procedure that is commonly performed for elderly patients, serious surgical morbidity is uncommon, and mortality is unusual. Despite the fact that the surgery is extensive, radical vulvectomy and node dissection form an operation that is totally extraperitoneal, which reduces the potential for major serious morbidity. Most patients have wound breakdown, frequently with local infection. Patients occasionally develop lymphedema of the legs and may develop a lymphocyst. Patients often complain of spraying of urine or stress incontinence and sometimes develop a cystocele or rectocele. Operative mortality in most series is less than 2% despite the advanced age of many of the patients.

Prognosis

The corrected 5-year survival for patients with stage I and II disease treated by surgery has been reported to be as high as 90%. When lymph nodes contain metastatic tumor, survival diminishes dramatically; the likelihood of recurrence is correlated with the number of involved nodes and whether node involvement is bilateral. About 40% to 50% of women who have metastases to groin nodes are cured by the surgical procedure, but only 20% of women who have tumor in the deep pelvic nodes are disease-free at 5 years.

The prognosis for the patient with melanoma depends on the depth of the lesion, as is the case with melanomas in other areas of the body. If tumor has metastasized to lymph nodes, survival is rare.

Basal cell carcinoma, which requires only wide local excision for therapy, has an excellent prognosis.

QUESTIONS

Indicate whether each statement is true or false.

1. Ovarian cancer is the most common pelvic gynecology malignancy.
2. If an exploratory laparotomy is done and extensive ovarian cancer is found, a biopsy should be done and the abdomen closed.
3. Patients who have large amounts of residual tumor following ovarian cancer surgery should be treated with radiation.
4. Most ovarian cancer is diagnosed when patients have stage III or IV disease.
5. The most common symptom of endometrial cancer is postmenopausal bleeding.
6. In the United States since the early 1980s invasive cervical cancer has decreased in frequency, and invasive endometrial cancer has increased in frequency.
7. Appropriate therapy for a stage IB cervical cancer is total abdominal hysterectomy with bilateral salpingo-oophorectomy.
8. Patients with stage I endometrial cancer should receive preoperative radiation therapy.
9. Vulvar cancer is commonly found in older women, and therefore there is high operative mortality.
10. Ovarian cancer results in more deaths in the United States each year than endometrial and cervical cancer combined.

SELECTED REFERENCES

Aure JC, Hoeg K, Kolstad P. Clinical and histologic studies of ovarian carcinoma. *Obstet Gynecol* 1977;37:1.

Barber HRK. Relative prognostic significance of pre-operative and operative findings in pelvic exenteration. *Surg Clin North Am* 1969;49:431.

Barclay DL. Carcinoma of the vagina after hysterectomy for severe dysplasia or carcinoma in situ of the cervix. *Gynecol Oncol* 1979;8:1.

Griffiths CT, Fuller AF. Intensive surgical and chemotherapeutic management of advanced ovarian cancer. *Surg Clin North Am* 1978;58:131.

Herbst AL, Ulfelder H, Roskunzer DC. Adenocarcinoma of the vagina: association of maternal stilbestrol therapy with tumor appearance in young women. *N Engl J Med* 1971;284:878.

Jones HW. Treatment of adenocarcinoma of the endometrium. *Obstet Gynecol Surv* 1975;30:147.

Krupp PJ, Bahm JW. Lymph gland metastases in invasive squamous cell cancer of the vulva. *Am J Obstet Gynecol* 1978;130:943.

Morley GW. Infiltrative carcinoma of the vulva: results of surgical treatment. *Am J Obstet Gynecol* 1976;124:874.

NIH Consensus Statement. Ovarian Cancer: screening, treatment, and follow-up, vol 12, no 3, April 5–7, 1994.

Rutledge FN, Smith JP, Wharton JT, O'Quinn AG. Pelvic exenteration analysis of 296 patients. *Am J Obstet Gynecol* 1977;129:881.

Seltzer V, Kaplan B, Vogl S. Adriamycin and cisplatinum in the treatment of advanced uterine sarcomas. *Cancer Treat Rep* 1984;68:1389.

Seltzer VL, Sall S, Castedot M, Murian-Davidian M, Sedlis A. Glassy cell cervical carcinoma. *Gynecol Oncol* 1979;8:141.

Seltzer VL, Vogl S, Kaplan B. Adriamycin and cisdiaminedichloroplatinum in the treatment of metastatic endometrial adenocarcinoma. *Gynecol Oncol* 1984;19:308.

Spanos W. Pre-operative hormonal therapy of cystic adnexal masses. *Am J Obstet Gynecol* 1973;116:551.

Vogl SE, Seltzer VL, Camacho F, Calanog A. Dianhydrogalactitol and diaminedichloroplatinum II in combination for advanced cancer of the uterine cervix. *Cancer Treat Rep* 1982;66:1809.

Vogl SE, Seltzer V, Calanog A, Moukhtar M, Camacho F, Kaplan BH, Greenwald E. "Second-effort" surgical resection for bulky ovarian cancer. *Cancer* 1984;54:2220.

14

Pediatric Surgery

Gerard Weinberg

The aim of this chapter is to acquaint the general surgeon with some of the key points regarding major problems in general pediatric surgery. For more detailed information, the interested reader can refer to one of several excellent textbooks of pediatric surgery.

CARE OF THE PEDIATRIC PATIENT

Monitoring

All infants and children who undergo general anesthesia need the following monitors.

1. Precordial or esophageal stethoscope
2. Blood pressure cuff, manual or automated (Dynamap, Infrasonde)
3. Electrocardiogram
4. Temperature probe
5. Pulse oximeter

Additional monitoring aids may be necessary in selected cases. These include an arterial line, central venous catheter, and urinary catheter. In rare situations (open heart surgery) a pulmonary artery catheter is useful.

Temperature

Infants' relatively large body surface area in proportion to their weight in combination with little subcutaneous fat render them highly susceptible to rapid loss of heat. This problem is magnified if the child is exposed to an usually cold operating room and undergoes surgery during which body cavities are opened. These manipulations result in heat loss through radiation, evaporation, and convection. To compensate for the heat loss, infants increase their metabolic rate, but a small baby or seriously ill child may not have the energy stores to increase its caloric output to maintain normothermia. The resulting hypothermia can cause respiratory and myocardial depression.

Therefore all children who undergo surgery with anesthesia should have a temperature probe inserted and the core temperature monitored. Appropriate places to monitor are the rectum or the esophagus. Skin temperature should be monitored as well. Every effort should be made to reduce heat loss, including keeping the extremities and the head covered whenever possible. The operating room should be warmed, and the immediate area surrounding the patient can be heated with infrared heating lights, especially during induction of anesthesia and when lines and monitors are being placed. The child is placed on an appropriately controlled heating mattress; all anesthetic gases are heated, as are all intravenous fluids and blood products. Older children need to have their temperature monitored as well to alert the anesthesiologist to the onset of malignant hyperthermia.

Fluids

Infants have a resting metabolic rate approximately three times that of an adult, or about 100 kcal/kg/day. Their fluid needs therefore are correspondingly about three times that of the adult (Table 14.1).

In addition to the above, all ongoing losses such as nasogastric, ileostomy output, and severe diarrhea should be measured and replaced by the appropriate electrolyte-containing fluid. Adequacy of fluid replacement can be monitored by following urine output and specific gravity. Normal urine output in a child is approximately 0.5 to 1.0 ml/kg/hr. Newborns have immature renal tubules that are not able to concentrate the glomerular filtrate as thoroughly as those of older infants. Urine specific gravity over 1.015 therefore indicates that the kidney is concentrating urine maximally and that fluid replacement should be increased. In addition to water needs, the infant has electrolyte and glucose requirements. Sodium and potassium maintenance is 2 to 3 mEq/kg/day. Neonatal glucose levels are lower than those of the older child, hypoglycemia being defined for this age group as a serum glucose of less than 30 mg/dL. The infant is dependent on the glycolysis of existing glycogen homeostasis. Stress such as surgery, sepsis, or trauma can rapidly deplete these stores, resulting in hypoglycemia with subsequent seizures and brain damage. Therefore all infants should have blood glucose levels monitored. All intravenous solutions given to them should contain glucose. Premature or small-for-gestation-age (SGA) infants may require a continuous 10% glucose solution to maintain normoglycemia.

Calories

The surgeon caring for the infant or child is often faced with treating a patient whose gastrointestinal (GI) tract is unable to accept enough calories to maintain normal growth and development. Prolonged inadequate nutrition in the infant may have severe consequences. The immune system, already not well developed even in the normal, healthy young infant, is compromised further, and sepsis is more likely to occur with devastating results. Wound healing is impaired, which can lead to anastomotic leaks, disruption, and wound dehiscence. In addition, prolonged malnutrition may have adverse long-term effects on the brain, which is undergoing rapid development during the early months of life. Intravenous alimentation for a period exceeding 1 week should be started in any child in whom adequate enteral nutrition cannot be given. One can use either the peripheral or central route and infuse approximately 100 cal/kg/day. If the central route is to be used, a Silastic catheter is inserted percutaneously or via cutdown so the tip of the catheter lies at the junction of the superior vena cava and right atrium. When intravenous alimentation is initiated, periodic determinations of serum glucose, electrolytes, calcium, and liver function are needed. Although most children do quite well on intravenous alimentation, even for prolonged periods, some problems do occur with this technique, the most common of which is liver dysfunction. Cessation of the alimentation usually reverses the complications if they are diagnosed early.

SURGICALLY CORRECTABLE CAUSES OF RESPIRATORY DISTRESS

Choanal Atresia

Atresia of the nares is a rare anomaly occurring in approximately 1 : 60,000 live births. If not recognized promptly, choanal atresia may result in severe respiratory distress in the newborn. This condition results from a bony obstruction of the posterior nares behind the palate at the level of the sphenoid bone. Because the newborn is an obligatory nose-breather the obstruction

TABLE 14.1. *Maintenance fluid needs in infants*

Weight (kg)	Fluid needs (ml/kg/day)
1–10	100
11–20	50 (+1,000 ml)
21 +	20 (+1,500 ml)

effectively blocks the upper airway. Diagnosis is based on the inability to pass a feeding tube through the nose into the pharynx. Further information can be obtained by instillation of a water-soluble contrast agent into the nose with the patient lying supine.

Initial treatment is aimed at providing a secure airway for neonates until they can breathe spontaneously through the mouth. In most cases this can be accomplished by inserting an oral plastic airway, which is taped securely in place. In the interim, feeds are accomplished through a small feeding tube placed through the mouth. After several weeks most infants learn to breathe by mouth, and the airway can be removed and normal feeds started.

Definitive surgery for choanal atresias is usually postponed until the child is about 1 year old. Two approaches are used, each having its proponents: the transnasal and the transpalatal. The results in either case are usually highly satisfactory. Most children undergoing surgery to correct this condition lead a normal life without further problems.

Congenital Diaphragmatic Hernia

Congenital diaphragmatic hernia is one of the most common conditions causing respiratory distress in the newborn that is amenable to surgical correction. In most series the reported incidence is approximately 1 : 4,000 live births. In the usual case, a hernia of variable size at the posterolateral foramen of Bochdalek, most commonly on the left, results in protrusion of the abdominal contents into the chest, thereby compressing the ipsilateral lung and causing a shift of the mediastinum to the right. Studies have shown that both the ipsilateral and contralateral lung are affected, with a diminution in the number of alveoli. The pulmonary arterial vasculature is deficient as well, because its development parallels that of the airways. In addition, the pulmonary arteries have hypertrophic muscles in their media making them highly sensitive to hypoxia, hypercarbia, and acidosis.

Although most infants with diaphragmatic hernia present shortly after birth and quickly experience severe respiratory distress needing ventilatory assistance, others become symptomatic only during the next 24 hours. A few infants who suffer from diaphragmatic hernia are just mildly symptomatic with occasional grunting and tachypnea, and the diagnosis may not be made for several weeks after birth. Many fetuses with diaphragmatic hernia are being diagnosed by means of ultrasonography. These babies are then delivered in a major medical center where expert neonatology and pediatric surgical services can expedite treatment. *In utero* repair of the hernia is feasible and has been done in more than 20 patients at one medical center; this technique is appropriate in selected fetuses with a large hernia where the lung will become severely hypoplastic if the hernia is not repaired early.

On physical examination the infant with a congenital diaphragmatic hernia usually has a scaphoid abdomen. Auscultation reveals a heart that is displaced to the right and absent bowel sounds on the left. Peristaltic sounds are heard occasionally on the affected side. A chest radiograph reveals a left hemithorax filled with air-filled loops of bowel and a shift of the mediastinum to the right with compression of the right lung. Occasionally, cystic adenomatoid malformation mimics a diaphragmatic hernia; if any doubt exists, an upper GI series with barium can clarify the diagnosis. Once the hernia is diagnosed, a nasogastric tube in inserted and placed on suction to prevent gaseous distension of the bowel, which would further compromise the lung. If the infant is in respiratory distress, he or she should be intubated and placed on a respirator. Ventilation by mask in contraindicated.

An arterial catheter is inserted to determine the acid-base balance and the PO_2. Every effort is made to combat hypoxia and hypercarbia, as these conditions are potent stimuli for pulmonary vasoconstriction. It may necessitate placing the child on either a conventional or high-frequency respirator and starting inotropic support. If these modalities prove unsuccessful, there are several other options available, including the use of vasodilators, the most potent of which is tolazoline (Priscoline), or starting the infant on inhaled nitric oxide. Should these measures fail, the child is placed on extracorporeal membrane oxygenation (ECMO), a complex, labor-intensive technique available only in major medical centers. Briefly, the child's internal jugular vein and common carotid artery are cannulated and connected to a membrane oxygenator, bypassing the infant's inadequate lungs. The procedure reverses the acid–base and oxygen problems without subjecting the baby to severe barotrauma and allows the severe pulmonary vasoconstriction to reverse. Some centers operate on the infants while they are on ECMO. The more conservative approach is to wean the infant off ECMO and then operate. Almost all surgeons now believe that, in all cases, the baby should be stabilized for about 12 to 24 hours after birth before undertaking surgery. There is no need or place for emergency middle-of-the-night surgery in these babies.

Most surgeons use a transverse abdominal incision. The abdominal contents are removed from the chest, and any sac present is excised. The diaphragmatic defect is closed with interrupted nonabsorbable sutures. A chest tube is left in the pleural space and connected to a water-seal apparatus; suction should not be used. No attempt is made to hyperinflate the hypoplastic lung. Some surgeons insert a chest tube in the contralateral pleural space prophylactically, as many infants are subject to pneumothoraces during the postoperative period when high ventilatory settings may be necessary. The viscera are inspected for atresias or other obstructions (e.g., Ladd's bands). If found, they are repaired. The abdominal contents are then returned to the peritoneal cavity, and the abdominal wall is closed in layers. Occasionally this presents a difficult challenge, as the peritoneal cavity is often markedly underdeveloped because the bulk of the viscera were in the chest during fetal development. In such a case a temporary Silastic chimney closure may be needed (see Omphalocele and Gastroschisis below). For most cases, however, layered closure of the abdominal wall is possible.

Removal of the abdominal contents from the chest and closure of the diaphragm results in marked improvement of the respiratory condition in most children. Some have a transient improvement in their condition, the so-called "honeymoon period," and then begin to deteriorate. In most of these cases, the lung volume is adequate for survival, but a progressive right-to-left shunt due to pulmonary vasoconstriction is occurring. If therapy with vasodilators and conventional ventilators fails, infants are started on inhaled nitric oxide; should that fail, they are placed on ECMO.

Survival of infants with congenital diaphragmatic hernia who are symptomatic during the first 12 hours of life has improved somewhat with the advent of ECMO. Some centers are reporting an almost 80% survival rate, but some of these children have severely compromised lung function and may well need lung transplantation as they get older. Reduced-size transplants using lobes have been performed in a number of centers with encouraging results. Another new technology being eval-

uated and undergoing clinical trials is perfluorocarbon ventilation. These new agents produce little toxicity and have been shown to reduce lung pathology and improve gas exchange. They may have an important role to play in the treatment of congenital diaphragmatic hernia (1).

Tracheoesophageal Fistula

Anomalies that occur during development of the trachea and esophagus are common causes of respiratory problems in neonates. The types most commonly found are atresias of the esophagus, often associated with a fistula between the esophagus and the trachea. Several anatomic variants are extant (Fig. 14.1).

Signs and Symptoms

There may be a history of maternal polyhydramnios. Ultrasonography during the third trimester of pregnancy may reveal a dilated upper esophagus in the fetus, making the diagnosis highly likely. The infant usually presents in the newborn nursery as a "mucousy" baby needing frequent oral suction; a choking or cyanotic spell may occur when the baby is first fed. An attempt to place a nasogastric tube is unsuccessful because the tube meets resistance in the midthorax. Physical examination of the baby may reveal an SGA neonate. The abdomen may be scaphoid if an isolated atresia is present or distended if there is a large fistula between the esophagus and trachea. About 10% of these infants have an imperforate anus. Other conditions found in association with tracheoesophageal fistula are congenital heart disease, Down syndrome, and renal anomalies.

The diagnosis can be confirmed by radiography with a radiopaque nasogastric tube left in place as far as it will advance. The catheter typically stops at the level of the fifth interspace. The proximal esophagus may be seen as a slightly dilated air-filled pouch. If a fistula is present between the trachea and the esophagus, air is present in the stomach and bowel. Isolated atresia without fistula is seen as a gasless abdomen. Additional findings that may be noted on radiographs are vertebral anomalies, a pulmonary infiltrate, or an abnormally shaped heart shadow. If the clinical picture is still unclear, 0.5 ml of liquid barium can be instilled in the nasogastric tube, the radiograph obtained, and the barium quickly aspirated back. Under no circumstances should water-soluble contrast be used. In the most common

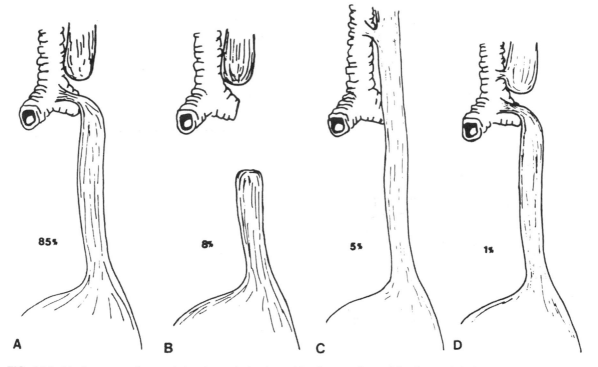

FIG. 14.1. Most common forms of esophageal atresia and tracheoesophageal fistulas and their percentage of occurrence. **A:** Proximal esophageal atresia with a fistula between the distal esophagus and the trachea, present in 85% of all cases. **B:** Isolated esophageal atresia without a fistula, present in 8% of all cases. **C:** H-type tracheoesophageal fistula without esophageal atresia, found in 5% of cases. **D:** Esophageal atresia with fistulas between the upper and lower esophageal pouches; occurs in 1% of all cases.

form of esophageal atresia, the blind upper esophageal pouch is clearly delineated. In rare situations a fistula is found between the upper esophagus and the trachea. Babies with an H-type fistula present later in life (several months old) with recurrent pneumonia.

Treatment

Once the diagnosis has been established, the child is moved to an intensive care unit with the head elevated. The pharynx and proximal pouch are kept empty of secretions by placing a Replogle tube in the upper pouch and maintaining it on continuous suction. Administration of broad-spectrum antibiotics is begun. If there are no contraindications, definitive surgery is performed.

An extrapleural approach is used through a right thoracotomy. The tracheoesophageal fistula is divided, and an end-to-end esophagoesophagostomy is performed. Many surgeons add a feeding gastrostomy during the same operation to enable early postoperative enteral feeding, bypassing the anastomosis. Definitive surgery is deferred if the child's condition does not permit such a major procedure (i.e., prematurity, pneumonia, or severe congenital heart disease). In such cases a feeding gastrostomy can be performed even under local anesthesia if necessary to prevent aspiration of highly acidic gastric contents into the trachea until the fistula can be closed. The fistula is closed at a later time through a thoracotomy. The child can then be fed and his or her condition stabilized until esophageal continuity can be established.

In some instances, especially in cases of pure esophageal atresia, the long gap between the upper and lower esophageal pouches makes primary repair difficult. Additional length on the upper pouch can be obtained by performing one or more circular myotomies on the upper pouch. As a last resort, if the distance cannot be bridged, one can perform a cervical esophagostomy (spit fistula) as a first stage repair and then a colon interposition when the child reaches the age of about 1 year.

Complications following repair of esophageal atresia are relatively common: leaks, strictures, disruptions, and recurrent fistula. They usually result from performing the anastomosis under tension. Most small leaks seal spontaneously. Strictures are usually managed by repeated dilatations. Recurring strictures may indicate that the baby has significant gastroesophageal reflux, a condition that occurs in up to 30% of these infants. Gastroesophageal reflux is often difficult to treat by medical means only and may require an antireflux operation (Nissen fundoplication). In otherwise normal full-term infants, the survival rate with tracheoesophageal fistula and esophageal atresia is 80%. The long-term prognosis for these children is excellent. The keys to good results are early recognition of the condition and intensive care during the perioperative period.

GASTROINTESTINAL TRACT OBSTRUCTION

Infantile Hypertrophic Pyloric Stenosis

Pyloric stenosis is a common condition, with an incidence of about 1 : 900 live births in the white population and 1 : 2,000 live births in the black population. Its etiology is unknown. It is not a congenital lesion and is rare during the first week of life. Male infants with pyloric stenosis outnumber female infants 4 : 1, and the firstborn boy is the most common infant stricken. Some hereditary factors have been noted; infants of mothers who have had pyloric stenosis as infants are more likely to develop the condition. The pathophysiology is unknown. When examined histologically, the pyloric muscle is hypertrophic and edematous. Some believe that the triggering mechanism is an allergic response to milk curd proteins hitting a spastic pylorus.

Signs and Symptoms

These otherwise healthy infants usually present at about 4 to 6 weeks of age with increasingly frequent vomiting of undigested formula shortly after feeds. The vomiting intensifies over the course of several days to several weeks, becoming more projectile and causing the infant to lose weight. Careful examination of the conjunctiva may show evidence of mild jaundice. Peristaltic waves may be seen crossing the upper abdomen. The careful examiner can feel an olive-shaped mass in the upper abdomen in about 85% of all cases. Finding this mass is pathognomonic of pyloric stenosis and constitutes sufficient evidence to warrant surgery. In infants where careful examination has failed to reveal the pyloric tumor, a barium swallow is done carefully with the physician looking for the characteristic elongated, markedly narrowed pyloric channel. Ultrasonography has proved accurate for delineating the dimensions of the thickness and length of the pylorus and is useful in infants in whom the olive is not felt on physical examination. Infants with prolonged vomiting have a hypokalemic, hypochloremic metabolic alkalosis; a certain percentage of infants are jaundiced with elevated indirect bilirubin. The latter is probably caused by a deficiency in hepatic glucuronyl transferase.

Treatment

After fluid and electrolyte deficits have been appropriately corrected, a pyloromyotomy is performed using the Ramstedt technique. This is a highly rewarding procedure associated with low morbidity and essentially no mortality. Fluids are slowly resumed about 12 hours after surgery and are gradually increased in strength and volume. Most infants can be discharged 4 to 5 days after surgery. Some vomiting during the postoperative period is common, but it settles down once the stomach regains normal tone. Complications, which are rare, include perforation of the mucosa, usually at the duodenal end of the pyloric tumor, and incomplete pyloromyotomy resulting in persistent postoperative vomiting. The prognosis for children with pyloric stenosis is extremely good, and they should lead normal lives.

Duodenal Obstruction

Obstruction of the duodenum occurs once in about 5,000 live births. The obstruction can be total, which is termed an atresia, or the lumen may be patent but markedly constricted, resulting in a stenosis. Most of the obstructions occur at the second portion of the duodenum, usually distal to the ampulla of Vater. A duodenal obstruction occasionally seen is annular pancreas, in which the duodenum is circumferentially surrounded by pancreatic tissue. An intrinsic atresia or stenosis is common with this condition.

Signs and Symptoms

In some cases the diagnosis is suspected antepartum if the mother is noted to have polyhydramnios. The condition can be confirmed by means of ultrasonography. The neonate usually presents during the first day of life with vomiting, most often bilious, as the usual obstruction is distal to the ampulla. There is usually little abdominal distension because the distal bowel is completely collapsed. The neonate may have normal stools even if the duodenum is atretic.

Physical examination is usually not helpful. One should check for the stigmata of Down syndrome, as about one-third of all neonates with duodenal obstruction are found to have this chromosomal abnormality. Other anomalies found occasionally are esophageal atresia and imperforate anus.

The diagnosis is simple to establish. Plain films of the abdomen reveal the classic "double bubble" sign (i.e., gas-filled distended stomach and proximal duodenum). There is no reason to use a contrast agent unless the plain films are inconclusive, as occurs in some cases of duodenal stenosis.

If surgery is delayed (for evaluation of a murmur, possible Down syndrome), a contrast x-ray study is performed to eliminate the possibility that the baby does not have a midgut volvulus, a life-threatening condition that can present as a double bubble much like duodenal atresia.

Treatment

The child is positioned with the head elevated, and the stomach is decompressed using an appropriately sized nasogastric tube. Dehydration is corrected with intravenous fluids. Supplemental fluids may be needed to compensate for ongoing nasogastric losses. Because the stomach can be effectively decompressed with a nasogastric tube, there is no reason to perform emergency surgery. If one strongly suspects a chromosomal abnormality, the infant can be maintained on this regimen until chromosomal studies are carried out and the parents are informed of the diagnosis with certainty.

Operation is performed as soon as the child's condition is stable and the appropriate facilities are ready. Two operations are commonly used: duodenoduodenostomy and duodenojejunostomy. They are both side-to-side anastomoses that bring together the proximal dilated duodenum and the small intestine beyond the obstruction. One should not dissect the duodenum excessively, because inadvertent damage to the common duct may result. If possible, one should avoid performing a gastrojejunostomy in a newborn because it carries with it the well known risk of future ulcer development. Many pediatric surgeons add a Stamm-type gastrostomy to the operation to help keep the stomach empty during the first few days until the anastomosis is patent and the child is able to tolerate oral feeds. A formula containing small curds such as Nutramigen may help speed oral feeding. Some vomiting may occur for up to 2 weeks postoperatively, but it should settle down as the stomach regains normal tone and edema resolves. If there are no other serious anomalies, the prognosis is excellent, and the infant should lead a normal life.

Intestinal Atresia

Atresias of the jejunum and ileum occur commonly. Relative to the length of the ileum, atresias are much more common there than in the jejunum. Their pathogenesis has been worked out quite well by Louw and Bernard, who showed that subjecting fetal puppies to intrauterine selective mesenteric arterial ligation results in atresia of that segment of the bowel supplied by the corresponding arterial branch. It is believed that a large percentage of intestinal atresias result from intrauterine vascular accidents to the mesenteric vasculature. Several types of atresia are found, ranging from an atretic segment that may involve just the mucosa, with an intact seromuscular coat, to a more common type where there is loss of continuity of an entire segment of bowel, often with an associated gap in the intervening mesentery. A rarer type is a proximal atresia with a markedly shortened bowel and mesentery, the so-called apple-peel atresia, with a precarious arterial blood supply arising from distal branches of the superior mesenteric artery.

Signs and Symptoms

The signs and symptoms depend to a great extent on the site of the atresia. Many of the mothers have not had polyhydramnios, which is only found in about one-fourth of cases. Bilious vomiting is common, occurring in about 85% of all cases of jejunal atresia. The more distal the atresia, the more pronounced is the abdominal distension. Infants with more proximal atresia vomit earlier than those with more distal atresia and may pass normal meconium. Physical examination usually shows a distended abdomen. Otherwise the examination may be completely normal. Other anomalies are relatively uncommon.

Plain films of the abdomen show distended gas- and fluid-filled loops of small bowel with air-fluid levels on the upright view. In the newborn, it is difficult to differentiate between small and large bowel on plain films. Therefore to be sure that the loops seen on plain films are those of small bowel, one should perform a barium enema. The enema shows a small, unused colon (microcolon), confirming the presence of small bowel obstruction.

Treatment

Once the diagnosis has been established, a nasogastric tube is passed and connected to suction; fluid and electrolyte losses are corrected. When the infant's condition has stabilized, surgery is performed expeditiously. It is important to remember than it is virtually impossible to decompress the distal small bowel adequately with a nasogastric tube. Therefore any unnecessary delay in surgical decompression may result in necrosis of the intestine.

At surgery, the entire intestinal tract is explored to make sure that no other atresias or stenoses are present. The bulbous dilated end of the atretic bowel is resected, and an end-to-end anastomosis is performed; any mesenteric defect found is closed. Before completing the anastomosis the surgeon inserts a catheter into the distal bowel and injects saline to be sure that there is no distal atresia.

Once the postoperative ileus is resolved, feeds are begun slowly. If a major section of bowel is missing, or if the ileocecal valve has been sacrificed, a short-gut syndrome may be encountered, in which case it may take several weeks to several months for the residual intestine to adapt. Parenteral nutrition or, in less extreme cases, predigested formulas such as Alimentatum may be necessary.

Malrotation

During embryonic life the intestinal tract elongates rapidly and undergoes a complex rotational process that, among other things, accounts for the small bowel mesentery being diagonally based, running from the ligament of Treitz in the left upper quadrant to the cecum in the right lower quadrant. This broad base allows the small intestine enough motility for normal peristalsis while preventing it from twisting to the point where it compromises its blood supply. Abnormalities in this rotational process are not uncommon and may lead to several entities, by far the most common of which is midgut volvulus. In this condition the entire midgut from the duodenum to the midtransverse colon is suspended from a narrow pedicle, rendering it unstable and subject to twisting. During the course of normal peristalsis the intestine rotates on its pedicle, thereby compromising its blood supply. If the condition is not recognized quickly, the bowel infarcts, leaving the baby totally dependent on parenteral nutrition unless he or she is given a bowel transplant.

Signs and Symptoms

The most common symptom is bilious vomiting in a previously well infant. Most of these infants are about 1 month old or younger, but children (or for that matter even adults) of any age can be affected. Because the obstruction occurs in the third portion of the duodenum, abdominal distension need not be present. Guaiac-positive nasogastric aspirates or stools may or may not be present. Some infants quickly go into shock if gangrenous bowel is present.

If one suspects midgut volvulus (i.e., bilious vomiting by an infant), the diagnosis must be confirmed or ruled out expeditiously because bowel viability is at stake. A plain abdominal radiograph is not usually helpful, especially at an early on stage. The most direct approach to the diagnosis of this condition is by an upper GI series. Barium flows into the proximal duodenum, and the flow is cut off in a bird's beak shape at the twist of the midgut. Even if there is no obstruction to flow (i.e., a midgut volvulus), if the duodenum does not have its characteristic C shape with a ligament of Treitz in the left upper quadrant, the baby has intestinal malrotation. The infant should be prepared for immediate surgery. An upper GI series is much more definitive than a barium enema, as it shows the cecum in a position other than the right lower quadrant, suggesting malrotation and possible volvulus.

Treatment

An upper transverse abdominal incision is used. The first thing one usually sees is small bowel with the transverse colon lying posteriorly. The entire bowel is delivered into the incision and the volvulus derotated, usually in a counterclockwise direction. Several turns may be necessary to obtain complete derotation. Only obviously necrotic bowel is resected; marginally viable bowel is left *in situ* unless it is only a small segment. In all cases where marginally viable bowel is left in place, a second-look operation is planned for 24 hours later. One next divides all peritoneal bands running across the duodenum to the right parietal peritoneum, the so-called Ladd bands. All kinks in the duodenum must be straightened. In some cases there is an intrinsic stenosis of the duodenum, and it should be dealt with in the usual manner. The pedicle of the small bowel mesentery is splayed out so the duodenum lies in a straight, vertical line to the right of the vertebral column and the ascending colon on the left. Every effort is made to make the root of the mesentery as wide as possible to prevent recurrence of the volvulus.

Because the procedure results in the cecum coming to rest in the left abdomen, an appendectomy is performed. Most surgeons do not fixate the bowel to itself or to the abdominal wall, pointing out that such procedures are not necessary, as recurrence of volvulus is rare. Others disagree and advocate that the distal small bowel be sutured to the left colon thereby ensuring that the root of the mesentery remains broad-based.

Once the postoperative ileus has resolved, the infant is begun on progressive feeds. Unless a large percentage of the small bowel has been removed, the prognosis should be excellent. Fortunately, as mentioned above, recurrence of this condition is rare.

Meconium Ileus

Meconium ileus is an entity in which the neonate's meconium becomes inspissated in the ileum, causing an obturator-type obstruction. The cause for this condition usually is pancreatic insufficiency secondary to muco-viscidosis or cystic fibrosis. Two forms of the disease are recognized: simple meconium ileus, occurring in about two-thirds of patients, and complicated meconium ileus, occurring in the remaining one-third. Infants with simple meconium ileus show signs of intestinal obstruction during the first 2 days of life: abdominal distension, bilious vomiting, and absence of meconium stools. Rubbery, dilated loops of bowel are often seen and palpated. The anus may appear stenotic, and examination may reveal a tight rectum with only a small amount of sticky meconium present. Plain abdominal radiographs show dilated loops of bowel without air–fluid levels because the inspissated meconium is too viscous to layer out. Instead, a ground-glass appearance may be noted, representing gas and meconium in the ileum.

Complicated meconium ileus represents the complications of the disease: volvulus, atresias, perforations, peritonitis, and pseudocysts. These infants are much sicker, presenting with symptoms shortly after birth. Abdominal distension is marked; and the abdominal wall is often edematous and erythematous. A mass is found occasionally. Abdominal radiographs may show free air, a large mass, calcifications, or a large, formless intestinal loop representing a gangrenous loop of small bowel.

Diagnosis

Treatments for simple and complicated meconium ileus differ greatly, so it is of utmost importance to diagnose the infant's condition as quickly as possible. If the infant's condition suggests simple meconium ileus, a barium enema is performed. The colon appears small (microcolon), as little or no meconium has passed into it during fetal life. Some pellets of inspissated mucus may be seen. Refluxing the barium through the ileocecal valve reveals inspissated meconium in the ileum, confirming the diagnosis. The enema helps differentiate meconium ileus from the other entities that present in similar fashion, such as Hirschsprung disease, ileal or jejunal atresia, meconium plug syndrome, and hypoplastic left colon syndrome.

Treatment

Simple Meconium Ileus

Helen Noblett, an Australian pediatric surgeon, introduced a method for nonoperative decompression of the small intestine by means of a hyperosmotic radiopaque enema. This technique has dramatically decreased the mortality of this condition.

The infant is started on intravenous fluids until good urine output is obtained, and parenteral antibiotics are begun. The stomach is decompressed with a nasogastric tube. The agent used, meglumine diatrizoate (Gastrografin), is extremely hypertonic, having an osmolarity of 1,900 mOsm/L. When given as an enema, the sudden increase in intraluminal osmolarity draws water into the intestine at the expense of the intravascular volume. It is therefore of critical importance to carefully monitor the infant's vital signs, hematocrit, serum electrolytes, and osmolarity during and after the enema. The influx of fluid within the small intestine loosens inspissated meconium and thereby relieves the obstruction.

The enema is usually followed by passage of liquid meconium and gas over several hours. Abdominal distension should decrease as the obstruction is relieved. If no relief is obtained, a second enema may be performed. The risk of perforation increases with repeated enemas, and so they should be done only by experienced pediatric radiologists. If, despite a technically successful enema, the obstruction is not relieved, the intestines must be decompressed surgically.

If the Gastrografin enema has been successful, infants are started on acetylcysteine (Mucomyst) via nasogastric tube, and once they are able to tolerate a diet they are placed on pancreatic enzyme supplementation and on formulas containing medium-chain triglycerides such as Portagen. A sweat test is performed on the infant to confirm the diagnosis. Because the condition is hereditary, being passed on by an autosomal recessive gene, the parents are given genetic counseling because the chances of a subsequent child having cystic fibrosis are 1 : 4.

Complicated Meconium Ileus

Children with complicated meconium ileus are often critically ill, being septic, hypovolemic and acidotic, and in shock. The intense abdominal distension may interfere with diaphragmatic movement and may cause respiratory embarrassment. Several hours of intensive care is needed to stabilize these infants, restore the circulating blood volume, and combat the acidosis. Broad-spectrum antibiotics are begun, and a nasogastric tube is inserted. If need be, these children are intubated and placed on a respirator. They are then taken to the operating room, and the abdomen is explored. Sites of obstruction, perforation, or necrosis are identified, and all obviously nonviable bowel is removed.

Atresias, sometimes multiple, may be found and should be repaired in end-to-end fashion. If an obstruction of the ileum is present, an enterotomy is performed over the most dilated loop and the contained meconium evacuated. A 4% solution of acetylcysteine is flushed into the obstructed bowel to help free the highly tenacious meconium from the mucosa. This procedure may have to be repeated until the obstruction is relieved. There are several options for the management of the opened bowel. Most surgeons favor bringing out the bowel as an enterotomy until bowel function returns to normal. Equally good results are obtained by a double-barreled ileostomy or by an end-to-side enterostomy of the Bishop-Koop or Santulli types. Once GI function has recovered, the infant is started on pancreatic enzymes given by mouth to enhance absorption. Medium-chain triglyceride-containing formulas are more easily tolerated by these infants and are the preferred choice. Gastrointestinal tract continuity should be restored only after the infant is making steady weight gain and has a well adjusted caloric intake.

These children have a lifelong tendency to manifest GI problems, including meconium ileus equivalent, intussusception, and rectal prolapse as well as cirrhosis and portal hypertension. Although the prognosis of these children is guarded in view of the systemic nature of the underlying disease and its serious consequences, aggressive medical and surgical management has made marked advances in prolonging their lives so that middle-age adults with cystic fibrosis are now alive.

INTUSSUSCEPTION

Unlike most of the other conditions discussed above, intussusception rarely affect infants during the first month of life; this age group accounts for only 0.3% of all cases. The peak incidence in several large series was at 7 to 8 months of life, with the incidence dropping off rapidly after 1 year of age. Intussusception is the invagination of a portion of intestine into itself. The portion by far most commonly affected is the ileum, which is intussuscepted into the ascending colon. On occasion the intussusception extends all the way to the rectum.

Signs and Symptoms

The classic case involves a child who is usually well, perhaps having had a viral-like condition 1 or 2 weeks prior, and is awakened from sleep with sudden severe abdominal pain causing him or her to cry and draw up the legs. The bout may last a few minutes and then stop. These attacks are almost always accompanied by vomiting, and most infants pass normal stools either during or shortly after the attack. Following the attack the infant becomes well, taking feeds until another attack begins. These attacks then occur at more frequent intervals, with the stools becoming mixed with blood, so-called current jelly stools. If the attacks are allowed to continue, the infant becomes lethargic and dehydrated, and abdominal girth begins to increase.

On examination early in the course of the condition, the child may look well and have a soft, nontender abdomen without evidence of peritonitis. A mass can be palpated in more than 85% of cases. The mass is usually in the right side of the abdomen, although on occasion it is present on the left side as well. It is usually sausage-shaped. In cases of very long intussusception a rectal mass can be palpated. There are reports of intussusception being mistaken for rectal prolapse. It is important to emphasize that early in the course of intussusception the child has a soft, nontender abdomen. An acute abdomen manifests in cases where intestinal necrosis has already occurred. Low-grade fever is not uncommon and is most often found in the young infant.

Laboratory examinations are not helpful early in the course of the condition. A plain abdominal radiograph sometimes suggests a mass in the right lower quadrant. Other suggestive findings on radiography are absence of gas in the transverse colon, absence of stool in the left colon, and signs of small bowel obstruction. The mainstay of diagnosis is the history; if the history is suggestive of the condition, one should go ahead with further diagnostic maneuvers regardless of what the radiograph shows.

The child is started on intravenous fluids, and if there are signs of small bowel obstruction a nasogastric tube is inserted to decompress the stomach. Appropriate blood samples are obtained, including one for typing and one to hold. The pediatric surgeon is notified, who then contacts the operating room so no unnecessary delay is encountered should the child need emergency surgery.

Diagnosis and Treatment

Since it was introduced in the United States by Ravitch in 1947, the barium enema has been the main diagnostic and usual therapeutic modality for children with uncomplicated intussusception (i.e., in whom there is no obvious peritonitis). More and more pediatric centers are now using other modalities for diagnosis and treatment. A more modern approach for suspected intussusception is abdominal ultrasonography, looking for the characteristic doughnut sign. A positive ultrasound scan is then followed by hydrostatic reduction using an air enema performed under fluoroscopic control. The air enema is less expensive than the traditional barium enema and is associated with fewer complications should perforation occur. This technique is still relatively new, and many radiologists may be unfamiliar with it and wish to resort to barium. If so, the guidelines set forth by Ravitch and McCune in their classic study on the subject (2) should be closely followed to avoid bowel perforation. The enema can or bag should be raised no more than 3.5 feet above the child's abdomen, and the abdomen is not manipulated in any way whatsoever. The enema is stopped if there is no advance of the column of barium after 10 minutes. One must be sure that there is reflux of barium into the distal ileum before being confident that the intussusception has been completely reduced. In most reported series the intussusception was reduced about 75% of the time by hydrostatic means alone. Once the reduction is accomplished, the child is kept in the hospital overnight, as a small percentage of cases tend to recur during the first 12 hours following reduction.

Infants for whom hydrostatic reduction is unsuccessful are taken to the operating room for operative reduction. A right transverse abdominal incision is made, and the intussusception is identified. The bowel just distal to the intussusception is compressed, driving the intussuscepted bowel proximally. The proximal bowel should not be pulled on because it invariably leads to a tear and spillage of intestinal contents. Failure of reduction often indicates the presence of gangrene, usually at the lead point, in which case a limited resection and primary anastomosis is performed with care to minimize spillage. Most surgeons recommend performing an appendectomy at the time of operative reduction.

The older the child, the more likely it is that an anatomic lead point will be found. Among the conditions causing intussusception are Meckel diverticulum, intestinal lymphoma, cystic fibrosis, polyps, and intramural bleeds as found in Henoch-Schönlein purpura. Older children (those above 4 years of age) should have a workup for these conditions even if the barium enema was successful. The mortality for intussusception should be minimal. Prompt diagnosis of the condition enables most of these children to undergo successful hydrostatic reduction, obviating the need for surgery.

HIRSCHSPRUNG DISEASE

Hirschsprung disease is a congenital megacolon caused by the absence of ganglia within the mesenteric and submucosal plexi of the distal large bowel. The zone of aganglionosis is just proximal to the dentate line and extends for a variable distance proximally. Most cases involve the rectosigmoid only. Total colonic aganglionosis, however, is by no means rare, representing about 15% of the cases. Aganglionosis extending up to the jejunum, and even more proximally, has been reported. Most of the involved infants are full term and otherwise healthy. The most common associated anomaly is Down syndrome. Some evidence suggests that a hereditary factor is involved. The incidence reported is approximately 1 : 10,000 live births, depending on the series studied. The usual rectosigmoid Hirschsprung disease is three to five times more common in male infants than female infants.

Signs and Symptoms

The most common presenting symptom is an abnormality in the passage of meconium, usually delayed passage. Ninety percent of healthy full-term infants pass their first meconium within the first 24 hours of life. More than 95% have passed meconium by day 2. Some infants with Hirschsprung disease pass a small, hard piece of meconium and then nothing else, except following rectal stimulation.

Other signs and symptoms seen are those of intestinal obstruction (i.e., vomiting, often bile-stained, and ab-

dominal distension). Rectal examination in the typical case of Hirschsprung disease may be helpful in making the diagnosis. Typically, the distal rectum is narrow and empty, and the proximal rectum or rectosigmoid is dilated and stool-filled. Upon withdrawal of the examining finger, an explosive evacuation of stool and gas takes place, often resulting in decompression of the distended abdomen.

A plain abdominal radiograph shows distended air- and fluid-filled loops of bowel. In the neonate it is impossible to distinguish between large and small bowel on plain films. Because unrelieved large bowel obstruction can be quickly followed by enterocolitis, which is associated with significant morbidity and mortality, it is of utmost importance to make the diagnosis expeditiously. The first examination usually performed is a barium enema. Again, the barium enema should be the infants's first enema. It is totally inappropriate to perform saline enemas in the neonate without having first done a carefully performed barium enema. A plain catheter is introduced into the rectum just above the internal sphincter, and barium is injected slowly by means of a syringe under the guidance of image intensification and fluoroscopy. In older infants one should see a dilated proximal colon that tapers down to a cone-shaped transitional zone representing the beginning of the aganglionosis. The distal aganglionic bowel is narrow and does not contract. One frequently sees an area of sawtoothing and spasticity in the bowel just proximal to the transitional zone. This may be seen even in the neonate. In normal infants the barium is usually evacuated within 24 hours. Barium retained beyond this period is suggestive of Hirschsprung disease.

In the neonate, where the barium enema may not be diagnostic of Hirschsprung disease, a rectal biopsy is done. (One may dispense with this procedure in the older child with a classic history, examination, and barium enema.) The biopsy may be done at the bedside using a suction apparatus. Because there is normally a narrow zone of aganglionosis just proximal to the dentate line, the biopsy is performed at least 1.5 cm above the dentate line. This type of biopsy is deep enough only to obtain submucosa. The fresh specimen is stained for cholinesterase activity. A positive biopsy demonstrates increased uptake of the stain in the hypertrophic nerve fibers present, confirming the diagnosis of Hirschsprung disease. If the pathologist is unable to make the diagnosis, a full-thickness biopsy of the rectal wall is performed under general anesthesia. In the older infant (over 2 weeks of age) Hirschsprung disease can be diagnosed using anorectal manometry. In the normal individual, distension of the proximal rectum results in relaxation of the internal sphincter. This reflex is mediated by the intramural ganglia. In Hirschsprung disease no such relaxation occurs. The test is not accurate in infants less than 12 days of age and therefore cannot be relied on to make the diagnosis.

Treatment

Most pediatric surgeons favor performing a decompressing colostomy when Hirschsprung disease is diagnosed. It can be either a transverse colostomy or a sigmoid colostomy just above the area of aganglionosis. A piece of colonic wall is sent to the pathologist at the time of colostomy to be sure that ganglia are present. At this time one may perform multiple seromuscular biopsies to determine the level of aganglionosis (the so-called leveling colostomy), thereby helping and guiding the surgeon for the next stage. Between ages 6 months and 1 year, an elective pull-through operation can be performed. The most widely used procedure today is the endorectal pull-through operation as modified by Boley et al. (3). The procedure involves resecting the aganglionic bowel segment, performing a rectal mucosectomy to just above the dentate line, bringing normally innervated intestine through the seromuscular cuff created, and performing an end-to-end anastomosis 1.5 cm above the dentate line. The procedure gives a highly satisfactory result with minimal morbidity.

This tradition approach, which requires three separate operations, has been modified by many pediatric surgeons in recent years to eliminate the need for multiple operations. A number of centers are now advocating performing a primary pull-through operation without colostomy in otherwise healthy neonates who are stable and can be decompressed with enemas prior to surgery (4). A number of surgeons have reported performing the pull-through procedure using laparoscopic techniques, obviating the need for an extensive laparotomy (5).

IMPERFORATE ANUS

Even though one would think that infants with imperforate anus would be diagnosed immediately after birth, there are numerous instances of the diagnosis being delayed for 1 to 2 days. The incidence of imperforate anus

is about 1 : 5,000 births. There are several manifestations of the condition, and the operative correction of the condition depends on the type found.

Types of Imperforate Anus

Anal Stenosis

Anal stenosis is similar in female and male infants. The rectum has descended in normal position, but the anal canal is stenotic. The diagnosis is easy, and treatment is straightforward. A simple anoplasty is performed during the neonatal period, and the results are generally good. As with all other deformities of the anus and rectum, there may be associated anomalies within the urologic, cardiac, or skeletal system. A screening workup is therefore done before these children are discharged, including radiographs of the sacrum and ultrasonography of the kidneys and heart.

Membranous Imperforate Anus

In membranous imperforate anus, the embryonic membrane covering the anus has not disappeared. On examination, the anal dimple appears normal, but the lumen of the anus is covered by a thin membrane. Often meconium is seen bulging underneath the membrane. Treatment is straightforward and involves incising the membrane. This condition is similar in female and male infants. The usual screening workup is done before discharge.

Rectal Agenesis

The next two types of imperforate anus are low (infralevator) rectal agenesis and high (supralevator) rectal agenesis. The anatomy of these two conditions is different in male and female infants, so each sex is discussed separately.

Low Imperforate Anus

Male Infants. Examination of the perineum reveals no orifice. An anal dimple may be seen, or, in some cases, heaped-up tissue at the site of the normal anus. Stimulation of the area may result in the normal anal wink reflex. The external genitalia are usually normal.

With these low lesions there is usually no communication between the rectum and the urinary system, so the examination of the urine is normal, not showing the presence of meconium (Fig. 14.2).

Female Infants. The term low imperforate anus in these children is a misnomer. The rectum does have an opening, but it is ectopic, usually anterior at the fourchette. Careful examination of the vulvar area reveals a small orifice in the posterior wall of the vulva. The opening can be catheterized with a small feeding tube and meconium expressed (Fig. 14.3).

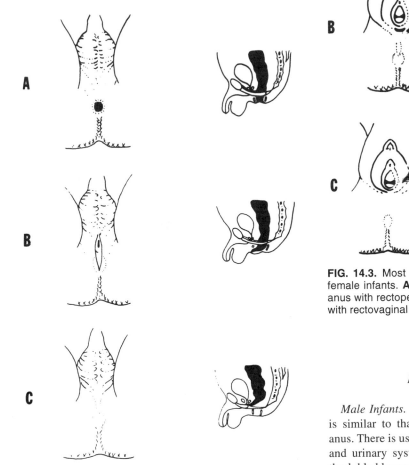

FIG. 14.2. Most common forms of imperforate anus in male infants. **A:** Normal anatomy. **B:** Low imperforate anus with rectoperineal fistula. **C:** High imperforate anus with rectourethral fistula.

FIG. 14.3. Most common forms of imperforate anus in female infants. **A:** Normal anatomy. **B:** Low imperforate anus with rectoperineal fistula. **C:** High imperforate anus with rectovaginal fistula.

High Imperforate Anus

Male Infants. The external appearance of the infant is similar to that of the infant with low imperforate anus. There is usually a fistula between the rectal pouch and urinary system, however, most often at the urethral–bladder neck junction. A careful urinalysis shows meconium in the urine. On occasion, meconium is seen at the tip of the penis, confirming the presence of a fistula.

Female Infants. The fistulous opening of the rectum is high in the vagina. Vaginoscopy can be performed using an otoscope or cystoscope and the rectal orifice found and cannulated. Rarely, one encounters a recto-cloacal fistula or the so-called one-hole perineum where only one orifice is present in the perineum. This common cloacal channel may extend for several centimeters as one tract before it branches, giving off the urethra, vagina, and rectum.

Diagnosis

The most important part of the workup for an imperforate anus in the neonate is determination of the level of the end of the rectum and whether a fistula to the urinary or genital system is present. Anomalies in which the rectum has descended below the level of the levator sling can be managed by a perineal anoplasty without colostomy. The high (supralevator) conditions are best managed by a diverting colostomy. Definitive correction is deferred until the child is older, weighing about 8 to 10 kg.

If the baby has passed meconium in the urine, the diagnosis is a high imperforate anus. No other diagnostic studies are necessary. Either a transverse or sigmoid colostomy is performed. Because a fistulous tract between the rectum and urinary system exists, it is important to irrigate the distal bowel at the time of colostomy to decrease the chance of persistent urinary sepsis.

If there is no meconium in the urine, one must differentiate between a low lesion and a high lesion. The most widely accepted method is the Rice-Wangensteen radiographic technique. This examination is done after the baby is at least 6 hours old, and the swallowed gas has had a chance to reach the rectum. A radiopaque marker is placed on the perineum where the anus should be, and the baby is turned upside down in a lateral position with the hips flexed. This position allows the gas in the rectum to rise as high as possible. A line is drawn between the posterior portion of the pubis and the lowest portion of the sacrum, the so-called pubococcygeal (PC) line. If air is seen to pass beyond this line on the radiograph, the infant has a low (infralevator) lesion, which can be treated by an anoplasty without a colostomy.

If air is not seen beyond the PC line, the infant is presumed to have a high lesion, and a colostomy is performed. This examination is not foolproof, however;

gas may not pass all the way to the end of the rectum, especially in young neonates. Thus one may perform an unnecessary colostomy in an infant for a low lesion. If air does seem to extend past the PC line, however, one can be confident that the bowel has traversed the levator sling. To be absolutely sure before proceeding with an anoplasty, some surgeons advise performing a perineal tap with a large-bore needle to gauge the thickness of the intervening tissue before finding meconium. Unless one is absolutely confident that the child has a low lesion, it is better to perform a colostomy than to risk damaging the delicate pelvic musculature, which would result in lifelong incontinence.

Treatment

Definitive surgery is postponed until the baby is thriving and weighs about 8 to 10 kg. A variety of surgical techniques exist. The important point of any procedure is to identify the levator sling of the puborectalis muscle and pass the bowel through it before bringing it down to the perineum.

The operative technique used at present by most pediatric surgeons is posterior sagittal anoplasty. A midline presacral incision is made down to the external sphincter. The voluntary muscle complex is identified and divided in the midline. The blind end of the rectum is identified, the fistula to the urinary tract is ligated and divided, and the rectum is tapered and brought down through the muscle and sutured to the perineum. Once the anal anastomosis has healed well and is of adequate caliber, the colostomy is closed. Complications of surgery for high imperforate anus are not uncommon. The most common is an everted anus with rectal mucosa protruding beyond the skin, causing a wet anus that becomes chronically irritated and finally ulcerates. The second, even more serious complication is incontinence. Many children with high imperforate anus have delayed continence of stool and flatus. Sometimes continence is achieved only when the children reach puberty. The reasons for this delay are not known. Even sophisticated testing cannot pinpoint the specific problem. Occasionally the cause for the incontinence is that the bowel has not been brought through the levator sling. In such cases a second pull-through is done, again being careful to identify the levator complex.

The low or ectopic imperforate anus in the female infant can be treated during the neonatal period by a simple cutback procedure. The anal opening close to the fourchette is brought farther posteriorly by incising the perineal skin. The rectal mucosa is then sutured to the skin with interrupted absorbable sutures. As the child gets older, the anal opening tends to separate from the vulva, giving an acceptable cosmetic result.

The overall results of surgery for children with imperforate anus are good. Most have a good result with no soiling. About 12% in a large series from The Children's Hospital of Pittsburgh were considered to have a poor result after long-term follow-up.

NECROTIZING ENTEROCOLITIS

Necrotizing enterocolitis (NEC) has become one of the most common abdominal emergencies for the newborn and is the most common abdominal surgical emergency in the premature infant. The condition occurs almost exclusively in newborns who are stressed or premature. Its causes are multifactorial and include decreased blood flow to the mesenteric vessels, increased bacterial proliferation in the gut, and the presence of incompletely digested feeds in the bowel. The small and large intestines become edematous and ischemic and can undergo liquefaction necrosis and perforate. Early in the course of the disease, the infant's signs are vague and nonspecific: lethargy, temperature instability, apneic or bradycardic spells, ileus, and then occult blood and mucus in the stools. As the disease progresses, there may be increased abdominal distension, erythema, and edema of the abdominal wall. Radiographs may show distended loops of bowel, pneumatosis intestinalis, and portal venous gas. If perforation has occurred, there is free air.

When the diagnosis is established, the infant is resuscitated, the stomach is decompressed with a nasogastric tube, and broad-spectrum systemic antibiotics covering GI tract flora are given. Serial abdominal radiographs are obtained every 6 to 8 hours to look for evidence of perforation. If perforation has occurred, laparotomy is performed; the obviously gangrenous bowel is resected, and the ends of viable bowel are exteriorized. Any marginally affected bowel is left *in situ* to prevent a short-gut syndrome later on. With aggressive medical care, NEC can be treated by medical means alone in 50% of cases. The mortality and morbidity from NEC are still high but have improved as critical care of the premature

infants has become more effective in salvaging this at-risk population.

ABDOMINAL WALL DEFECTS

Omphalocele and Gastroschisis

There are several defects of the abdominal wall at or near the umbilicus. A fair amount of confusion exits as to the exact terminology and embryology of these defects.

Omphalocele is a defect in the development of the abdominal parietes at the umbilical cord. Most investigators believe that this condition is explained by failure of the normally herniated abdominal viscera to return to the embryonic celom during the third week of development. Clinically, one finds a newborn with a large percentage of the small and large intestines present within a sac at the umbilicus. The umbilical cord emerges at the apex of the sac. The extent of the defect is variable. Large defects are not uncommon, and the liver may be found within the sac. The sac may be intact or may have ruptured during pregnancy or delivery.

Gastroschisis is a defect in the development of the abdominal parietes lateral to the umbilical cord. The cord is usually normal, and the defect is to its right. There is never a peritoneal sac. Unlike omphalocele, in gastroschisis the only extruded organs are the large and small intestines.

Associated anomalies are much more common with omphalocele than with gastroschisis. They include trisomy 21, trisomy D, cardiac defects, diaphragmatic hernias, and bladder extrophies. In addition, all neonates with omphalocele have nonrotation of the midgut. The anomalies one sees with gastroschisis are related to the defect itself. They are usually areas of atresias or stenosis of the bowel, probably resulting from compression of the bowel between the abdominal wall and the extruded viscera.

Diagnosis of these conditions is obvious. The most important points in the management of the babies are keeping them normothermic and well hydrated. The exposed viscera should be covered with warm saline pads, over which a plastic sheeting is placed to prevent evaporative water loss. A nasogastric tube is inserted to prevent the intestines from filling up with swallowed gas. Antibiotics are started, and a rapid review of systems is begun. Newborns with omphalocele are especially prone to develop hypoglycemia. Intravenous infusions with 10% dextrose are administered.

The small defects are easily corrected with layered closure of the abdominal wound. Closure of the large defects is accomplished by most surgeons using the technique pioneered by Schuster (6). Dacron-reinforced Silastic sheeting is sutured to the fascial ring circumferentially, creating a pouch for the viscera. This pouch is covered with antiseptic solutions such as providone–iodine (Betadine), and meticulous attention is paid to sterile technique. All attendants who handle the infant wear masks, gloves, and gowns. Over the next 10 to 14 days, starting at day 2, the viscera are progressively reduced out of the pouch and returned to the peritoneal cavity, which gradually expands. This is done in the intensive care unit under sterile conditions. The infant is then brought back to the operating room for removal of the pouch and closure of the abdominal wall.

Other techniques used are the creation of large skin flaps bilaterally and placing the viscera in the large ventral hernia created, closing only the skin. When the child is older, usually at age 2 years, a secondary operation is done to close the abdominal wall defect. For cases of an intact omphalocele, Gross devised a technique of painting the intact sac with 2% aqueous mercurochrome solution. A solid eschar is formed followed by slow epithelialization of the sac.

Most surgeons use the Silastic pouch technique even though there are potentially serious complications: separation of the pouch from the fascia, sepsis, and intestinal gangrene from pressure on the bowel against the Silastic pouch at the fascial ring. Infants with gastroschisis or omphalocele often have a prolonged ileus and intestinal dysmotility. It may take weeks to months until they are able to tolerate oral intake, during which time intravenous alimentation is necessary.

The prognosis for these conditions has improved dramatically with the advent of total parenteral nutrition and with the introduction of the Silastic pouch techniques. Most of the infants who die do so as a result of the cardiac defect or chromosomal abnormality.

Inguinal Hernia

Inguinal hernias during infancy result from failure of the processus vaginalis, which is normally open in the fetus, to close. The open processus allows small intestine or other abdominal viscera to protrude, incarcerate, and strangulate. The incidence of inguinal hernia during infancy is high, and hernia surgery is by far the most common general surgical procedure performed on infants. Three times as many boys as girls are affected; right inguinal hernias are more common than left.

The diagnosis of inguinal hernia in infants is straightforward. The mother or pediatrician notices a groin bulge, especially when the infant cries or strains. If the patent processus is complete and extends to the scrotum, the infant has an inguinal-scrotal hernia.

The complications of hernias are frequent and serious, and they vary inversely with the age of the infant: the younger the infant, the more likely are complications. The most frequent is incarceration of intestine leading to strangulation and necrosis. Pressure of the incarcerated intestine on the delicate spermatic vessels running through the inguinal canal can also lead to ischemic necrosis of the testicle. Therefore all inguinal hernias should be repaired surgically when discovered. No minimum age or weight is used to determine suitability for surgery. In the case of the premature infant, most surgeons operate when the infant is ready for discharge from the nursery.

Infants older than 50 weeks postconception can be operated on a same-day surgery basis. They are admitted in the morning to a separate unit; a physical examination, blood count, and urinalysis are performed; and if they are normal the infant is taken to the operating room; most can be discharged the afternoon of surgery.

Infants who were born prematurely have a tendency to develop postanesthesia apneic spells and should be observed at least 12 hours postoperatively; some surgeons advocate hospitalizing this group of patients overnight following a general anesthetic. This problem can be avoided by performing the hernia repair under spinal anesthesia, a technique that is becoming more widespread. Children with medical problems (e.g., upper respiratory tract infections or anemia) should have their surgery deferred until the condition is resolved.

As mentioned earlier, *incarceration* of the inguinal hernia is not an infrequent problem. The infant presents with a tense, somewhat tender inguinal bulge that may extend to the scrotum. Frequently the abdomen is distended, and the infant may have vomited before the parents sought medical attention. Unless there is evidence of peritonitis, one may attempt reduction of the hernia.

The older infant is sedated and kept in bed with the legs and pelvis elevated. The simple combination of sedation and the effects of gravity are often enough to reduce the incarcerated viscus. Should these measures fail, taxis on the hernia can reduce it in most cases. The infant is then admitted, and the edema is allowed to subside for about 12 to 24 hours before repair is undertaken. If attempts at reduction are unsuccessful, immediate surgery is needed. This can be an extremely difficult operation because of the edema and friability of the tissues. Extreme care is needed not to injure the vas deferens and the spermatic vessels.

Controversy exists even today as to the advisability of operating on the contralateral side. The younger the child, the greater the likelihood of finding a contralateral hernia that has gone unnoticed. As the infant gets older, a hernia, if present, would have been obvious, so a contralateral exploration on an older child tends to be less rewarding. Some surgeons explore the other side in a child up to age 5. Others perform a bilateral exploration on a child as old as 12 to 13 years.

Complications of hernia surgery include injury to the vessels or to the vas deferens. Recurrence is rare and results from incomplete removal of the sac infection or from a ligature that is too distal. In experienced hands, these complications should be minimal.

Hydroceles are common during infancy. In most cases, the fluid is slowly resorbed over the first several months after birth, so that by the time an infant is 1 year old the hydrocele is completely resorbed. An additional number of hydroceles resolve over the second year of life. Hence hydroceles need not be operated on during the first year. Some surgeons operate on them when they have persisted beyond the first year, but others wait until the child's second birthday. In all cases, the hydrocele should be explored through an inguinal incision, because the most common cause of a persistent hydrocele in the child is a small patent processus vaginalis that allows peritoneal fluid to trickle down into the scrotum while the child is up and about.

Umbilical Hernia

Umbilical hernias are common during infancy but unlike inguinal hernias are usually asymptomatic; the likelihood of intestinal obstruction or strangulation is extremely low. Most of these hernias close progressively as the child gets older. With few exceptions, umbilical hernias need not be repaired until the child reaches school age. The parents should be discouraged from taping over the protuberant hernia as it can cause skin irritation.

BILIARY ATRESIA

There are several causes of persistent hyperbilirubinemia in the infant. Among them are liver dysfunction secondary to an infection such as toxoplasmosis, rubella, or cytomegalovirus; metabolic causes; and anatomic causes (i.e., biliary atresia). Advances in the surgical management of the child with biliary atresia have lent a great deal of urgency to the importance of an early diagnosis. Unfortunately, no single or combination of examinations enables the clinician to make the diagnosis with any degree of certainty, so there is still a place for exploratory laparotomy in the child with persistently elevated direct bilirubin levels.

Signs and Symptoms

The infant with biliary atresia is usually full term, with no other congenital anomalies. The jaundice may be mild at first and masked by the physiologic jaundice most neonates have. The early stools may be normal meconium and may contain bile pigment. The infant is usually discharged and is brought to the pediatrician with jaundice after several weeks at home.

On examination, the infant appears well. The liver and spleen are usually of normal size. Rectal examination shows acholic, clay-colored stools. The urine is dark. A variety of laboratory examinations have been used to differentiate jaundice on the basis of biliary atresia from that due to other nonsurgical conditions. They include radiologic techniques such as the rose bengal nuclear medicine scan and the HIDA scan. These two tests show no excretion of the radioisotope by the liver into the bowel. Unfortunately, they are not specific for atresia, as severe neonatal hepatitis with cholestasis but a normally patent biliary tree gives the same results. Among the more promising serum tests is an enzyme test for lipoprotein-X, which is severely elevated in biliary atresia and mildly elevated in nonsurgical conditions. Unfortunately, there is a fair amount of overlap between values obtained in those with biliary atresia and those with severe hepatitis.

Several centers have reported accurate diagnosis using real-time ultrasonography. An experienced ultrasonographer should be able to identify the gallbladder and common duct and their dimensions in a normal infant. The common duct in biliary atresia is atretic, enabling the ultrasonographer to make the diagnosis. More experience must be obtained before we can rely on this test for the diagnosis. In the interim, the most accurate test is the operative cholangiogram at laparotomy.

Treatment

It is the author's belief that all infants with persistent direct hyperbilirubinemia with acholic stools require a laparotomy. If the laparotomy confirms the diagnosis, hepaticoportoenterostomy is performed. Because the results of this operation are markedly poor after the age of 12 weeks, the laparotomy must be done before the child is 2 months old. At laparotomy the gallbladder, if present, is cannulated; a cholangiogram is obtained and the biliary tree anatomy delineated. The atretic common duct is identified and dissected proximally as high as the bifurcation of the portal vein. A Roux-en-Y loop of jejunum is brought up to the transected portal tract and is there anastomosed.

The results of the operation depend in part on the histology of the bile ductules at the level of the anastomosis. Patients who have bile ductules larger than 150 μm at the time of the portoenterostomy have a good prognosis, generally obtaining good bile flow and no cirrhosis. Those patients in whom the bile ductules are less than 50 μm or in whom no epithelial-lined ductules are found have a poor prognosis, with poor bile flow, recurrent bouts of cholangitis, and ultimately progressive cirrhosis. The younger the patient, the greater are the chances that favorable histology will be found.

The prognosis following surgery for biliary atresia remains guarded. About half the children have sustained bile drainage after portoenterostomy. In most series, though, half of these patients have progressive biliary cirrhosis leading to portal hypertension and ultimately liver failure. These children should be referred to a center specializing in pediatric transplantation. Liver transplantation has proved successful, with 76% of children alive and well at 5 years with no signs of rejection.

QUESTIONS 7/10

Select one answer.

1. A newborn infant begins having bilious vomiting on day 2 of life. Which of the following investigations is most likely to give the proper diagnosis?
   a. Sonogram.
   b. HIDA Scan.
   c. Upper GI series.
   d. Barium enema.
   e. CT scan.

2. Which of the following is likely to be found in a 6-week-old with a 4-day history of nonbilious projectile vomiting.
   a. Cl = 110.
   b. pH = 7.30.
   c. HCO$_3$ = 30.
   d. K = 4.8.
   e. PO$_2$ = 70.

3. A full-term infant fails to pass meconium at 48 hours of age. Which is the most likely diagnosis?
   a. Duodenal atresia.
   b. Jejunal atresia.
   c. Hirschsprung disease.
   d. Esophageal atresia.
   e. Colonic atresia.

4. Which of the following anomalies is the most common?
   a. Proximal esophageal atresia with a tracheoesophageal fistula to the distal pouch.
   b. H-Type tracheoesophageal fistula.
   c. Isolated esophageal atresia without a fistula.
   d. Esophageal atresia with tracheoesophageal fistulas to the proximal and distal pouches.
   e. Esophaeal atresia with a tracheoesophageal fistula to the upper pouch.

5. Which of the following is not true of babies who have duodenal atresia?
   a. About 30% have Down syndrome.
   b. Most of the atresias are distal to the ampulla of Vater.
   c. There is a strong likelihood that other atresias will be found.

d. The correct operation to repair the anomaly is duodenoduodenostomy.

e. The mother may have had polyhydramnios.

6. Which of the following techniques should be used to reduce an incarcerated inguinal hernia in a 6-month-old?

a. Sedation.

b. Traction.

c. Elevation.

d. Ice packs.

e. All of the above.

7. A 2-year-old girl has an umbilical hernia. Which of the following is the recommended plan of treatment?

a. Surgery within the next few months.

b. Surgery at age 5 years.

c. Strapping the umbilical defect.

d. Surgery only if the hernia becomes incarcerated.

e. Surgery at age 12 years.

8. An 1,800-g premature infant presents with abdominal distension, lethargy, and stools positive for occult blood. Which of the following investigations needs to be done?

a. Radiography of kidneys and upper bladder.

b. CT scan.

c. Sonogram.

d. HIDA scan.

e. Barium enema.

9. A 2,000-g infant with necrotizing enterocolitis is found to have portal venous gas. Which of the following procedures is in order?

a. Continued medical therapy.

b. Abdominal paracentesis.

c. HIDA scan.

d. Immediate surgery.

e. Adding Cipro to the antibiotic regimen.

10. A 2-week-old infant is found to have a hydrocele. Which is the best course of treatment?

a. Surgery at age 6 months.

b. Surgery at age 2 years.

c. Aspiration of the hydrocele.

d. Transscrotal hydrocelectomy at age 2 years.

e. None of the above.

REFERENCES

1. Harrison MR, Adzick NS, Flake AW. Congenital diaphragmatic hernia: an unsolved problem. *Semin Pediatr Surg* 1993;2:109.

2. Ravitch MM, McCune RM Jr. Reduction of intussusception by hydrostatic pressure, an experimental study. *Bull Johns Hopkins Hosp* 1948;82:550.

3. Boley SJ. A new operative approach to total colonic aganglionosis. *Surg Gynecol Obstet* 1984;159:481.

4. Langer JC, Fitzgerald PG, Winthrop AL, et al. One-stage versus two-stage Soave pull-through for Hirschsprung's disease in the first year of life. *J Pediatr Surg* 1996;31:33.

5. Georgeson KE, Feunfer MM, Hardin WD. Primary laparoscopic pull-through for Hirschsprung's disease in infants and children. *J Pediatr Surg* 1995;30:1017.

6. Schuster SR. A new method for the staged repair of large omphaloceles. *Surg Gynecol Obstet* 1967;125:837.

SELECTED REFERENCES

Boley SJ, Lafer DJ, Kleinhaus S, et al. Endorectal pull-through procedure for Hirschsprung's disease with an anastomosis. *J Pediatr Surg* 1968;3:258.

Breaux CW Jr, Rouse TM, Cain WS, Georgeson WE. Improvement in survival of patients with congenital diaphragmatic hernia utilizing a strategy of delayed repair after medical and/or extracorporeal membrane oxygenation stabilization. *J Pediatr Surg* 1991;26:333.

Kleinhaus S, Weinberg G, Gregor MB. Necrotizing enterocolitis in infancy. *Surg Clin North Am* 1992;72:261.

Pena A. *Surgical management of anorectal malformations.* New York: Springer-Verlag, 1990.

Pringle KC. Fetal diagnosis and fetal surgery. *Clin Perinatol* 1989;16:13.

Vacanti JP, Shamberger RE, Eraklis A, Lillehei CW. The therapy of biliary atresia combining the Kasai portoenterostomy with liver transplantation: a single center experience. *J Pediatr Surg* 1990,25:149.

Welch KJ, Randolph JG, Ravitch MM, et al, eds. *Pediatric surgery,* 4th ed. Chicago: Year Book Medical Publishers, 1986.

15

Trauma

Ronald J. Simon

Trauma is not something that happens to the other person or in "that" part of town. It is something that touches each of us directly, as a victim or family of a victim, or indirectly, as the one responsible for the care of an injured person. The statistics remain staggering. According to the preliminary statistics from the Centers for Disease Control (CDC) in 1995, death relating to trauma was the fifth most common cause of death at *all* ages. Its incidence was more than twice that of acquired immunodeficiency syndrome (AIDS)-related deaths. Trauma is the number one cause of death in the 0 to 44 age group. Although statistics from the Federal Bureau of Investigation (FBI) show a 3% reduction in violent crimes, 1.8 million violent crimes were still reported. One of every five people in major metropolitan areas are subjected to a violent crime. The frequency with which accidents and violence occur in our society necessitates a complete knowledge of the management of patients who have been traumatized.

This chapter highlights the management of patients after sustaining injury. It starts with the ABCs of resuscitation and evaluation and then moves to the management of injuries in specific body regions. It must be remembered that this chapter serves as an overview. More complete descriptions of management issues can be found in books referenced at the end of the chapter.

INITIAL EVALUATION

It is good to know that a few things you learned as a resident still hold true today. Specifically I am referring to the ABCs of the initial evaluation of the trauma patient. *A*irway and *b*reathing—assessing the adequacy of the airway and the effectiveness of one's breathing—are the initial priorities after arrival of a trauma patient. Do not be lulled into a false sense of security by the presence of an endotracheal tube placed in the field. It is amazing, considering the conditions under which these tubes are placed, that so many are done correctly. There is a real percentage that are not, however, so always assess the placement of these tubes. The second benefit of assessing the airway is that it allows you to do a quick minineurologic examination. If a patient does not follow commands, the airway may need to be secured. A general rule of thumb is that patients with a Glasgow Coma Scale (GCS) of less than 10 should have airway control.

If control of the airway is necessary, endotracheal intubation is the method of choice. Nasotracheal intubation of a spontaneously breathing patient is no longer considered the treatment of choice. In-line traction of the neck is required if there is the possibility of a spinal injury. Most people now agree that intubation with in-line traction is adequate protection for the cervical spine. If intubation cannot be performed because of massive facial injuries or other factors, a surgical airway via a cricothyrotomy tube is recommended. One of the more difficult decisions we have to make is when to abandon attempts to obtain a standard airway and perform a surgical one. I allow three attempts; if they are unsuccessful, I opt for a surgical airway.

Once the airway has been controlled and breathing established, one's attention turns to the adequacy of *circulation* and establishing intravenous access. Although pulse and blood pressure are the most accessible measures, they are not the best for determining the adequacy of circulation. (A discussion on shock and resuscitation follows this section.) After most injuries intravenous access should be established regardless of whether you believe the circulation to be adequate.

The location of intravenous line placement depends on the type of injury and the patient's condition. It is recommended that two intravenous lines be inserted. Their location depends on the mechanism and location of the injury. The basic principle is that the insertion point should not be distal to an injury. After blunt injury, intravenous lines are placed above and below the diaphragm, as one is not sure if an injury exists and where it is. After a penetrating injury the lines are placed between the injury and the heart. Intravenous lines should be short and large, with 14- to 16-gauge angiocaths being optimal for peripheral lines. Triple-lumen central venous pressure (CVP) lines are inadequate as their length and small lumen size make them unsuitable for rapid-volume infusions.

Cutdowns have joined the ranks of nasotracheal intubations. If peripheral access is unobtainable, central access using a 7 French Swan introducer via a subclavian, internal jugular, or femoral approach is the method of choice.

The next phase of the initial evaluation is assessment of disability, which in essence is a minineurologic examination. It involves assessment of mental status, calculation of the GCS, and checking motor function in all four extremities.

The final phase is a quick full body examination. Make sure that the patient is fully exposed and that areas such as the axillae and groin creases have been checked for injuries. This is especially true for a patient who has sustained penetrating injury.

After this initial phase, which should take only a few minutes, radiographs are obtained. After penetrating injury the need for radiographs depends on the nature and

location of the injury. The evaluation of a patient after blunt injury is less focused, as it is designed to evaluate for occult multisystem injury. The initial survey consists of three films: chest, pelvis, and cervical spine. I always insist on a chest radiograph first because the most immediately life-threatening injuries would be in the chest (i.e., pneumothorax or hemothorax). Three views are required to evaluate the cervical spine: anteroposterior (AP), lateral, and odontoid. If the patient is nontender without distracting injuries, these three are all that are required. If there is cervical spine midline tenderness and the three views are negative, flexion and extension views are indicated to rule out ligamentous injury. If there is no time or the films are unsatisfactory, it is safer to leave the cervical spine collar in place until one is sure. Remember the series is not complete unless the top of T1 is visualized.

SHOCK AND RESUSCITATION

Blood pressure and pulse are poor indicators of the shock state. It is not that a hypotensive patient is not in shock, he is. It is that the normotensive patient can fool you. Shock is defined as a state in which oxygen delivery is inadequate to meet demand. When less than 25% of blood is lost, the blood pressure is maintained by systemic vasoconstriction, and blood is shunted away from nonvital organs such as the gut. A prolonged reduction in gut blood flow has been implicated in the development of multiple system organ failure (MSOF). Thus despite a normal blood pressure, there can be isolated organ ischemia that if not treated may result in an adverse outcome.

If blood pressure and pulse are poor indicators for shock, what is better? The most available indicator is base excess, which has been shown in numerous studies to be a good indicator for the presence of shock. What appears to be most helpful is not the numeric value itself but the trend of the numbers and the speed with which these numbers normalize. The presence of a base deficit by itself suggests the recent presence of anaerobic metabolism. If the base deficit increases with time despite resuscitation, it suggests that anaerobic metabolism is still occurring and there is either on-going bleeding or the efforts at resuscitation have been inadequate to restore perfusion. A good rule of thumb is that the base deficit should be resolved or at least reduced by half within 24 hours.

The lactate level is another measure of value for predicting the level of shock and the adequacy of resuscitation. It usually takes some time to see the test results, though, which may limit its usefulness. As with base deficit, the direction and rate at which the values move provide important information about the status of the patient and the resuscitation.

There has been recent interest in fluid management during initial resuscitation in the emergency department (ED). The major controversy is about how much fluid to give a hypotensive patient after a penetrating truncal injury. Several studies have shown in both animals and humans that giving volume when bleeding is uncontrolled results in increased blood loss and higher morbidity and mortality. Many believe that patients with penetrating truncal injury should not spend time in the ED being resuscitated. The place for this patient is in the operating room with rapid control of bleeding. Similarly, in a patient who sustained a significant blunt injury, a rapid and diligent search for, and control of, bleeding is essential for optimal patient outcome.

The next issue is *what* to give. This problem is much simpler. If a patient is hypotensive, the fluid of choice is blood. Otherwise, crystalloid (0.9% normal saline or lactated Ringer's solution) can be used as the initial resuscitation fluid.

MANAGEMENT OF SPECIFIC INJURIES

Head Injury

Head injuries are the major cause of death in trauma patients. The diagnosis is usually straightforward. Any patient admitted after a traumatic event with altered mental status undergoes head computed tomography (CT). Do not make the mistake made by hundreds of inexperienced physicians: assuming that altered mental status is secondary to drugs or alcohol only to find out several hours later when a pupil blows that this intoxicated patient also has a large subdural hematoma that has caused herniation. My teaching is that a patient is never drunk until he has a negative head CT scan. Whether to obtain a head CT scan on every patient with a transient loss of consciousness (LOC) but who has a GCS of 15 on arrival in the ED is controversial. Some argue that if the head scan is negative and there are no other injuries the patient can be discharged. Others prefer to admit the patient overnight for observation with-

out a CT scan. Any change in mental status indicates the need for CT. Of course the middle ground also exists, where all people with a brief LOC undergo head CT scanning and are admitted for observation. Neither of these protocols is right. The one you follow must depend on the reliability of the patient population and whether admitted patients are observed or simply "housed" in the hospital.

The indications for surgical repair vary with the neurosurgeon. There is no disagreement that a subdural or epidural hematoma that is causing a mass effect with midline shift should be decompressed, but a 1-cm subdural hematoma in a neurologically intact patient is now simply observed by many. Whether to débride a gunshot wound of the head is unclear. Most neurosurgeons believe that the débriding process removes more viable tissue than it saves and so do not débride these wounds.

Medical management of intracranial hypertension has recently changed. The American Association of Neurological Surgery has come out with new guidelines for management of the head-injured patient. Hyperventilation is no longer done unless the patient is herniating or has refractory intracranial hypertension. If hyperventilation is to be used, the PCO_2 is kept between 30 and 35 mm Hg. This change has come about because of changing attitudes toward the benefits of increased blood flow versus the potentially adverse affects of reduced blood flow during hyperventilation-induced vasoconstriction.

Few words raise my blood pressure more than hearing a neurosurgeon say "keep them dry." That thinking again is based on the misconception that low pressure is good even at the sacrifice of flow. Head-injured patients must be kept **euvolemic** to optimize blood flow to ischemic areas of the brain. Euvolemia, though, does not mean hypoosmotic. Serum osmolality should be kept around 300 to 310 mmol/dL, which can be achieved with mannitol or furosemide (Lasix). Neither should be given to a hypovolemic patient, as it may cause hypotension, which along with hypoxemia are the nemesis of head-injured patients.

Neck Injuries

When discussing penetrating neck injuries the zone of injury must be located. As demonstrated in Figure 15.1 the zones are defined as the following: zone 1,

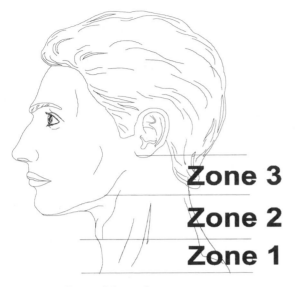

FIG. 15.1. Zones of the neck.

manubrium to cricoid cartilage; zone 2, cricoid cartilage to the angle of the mandible; zone 3, angle of the mandible to the base of the skull. The presence of hard signs of injury indicates the need for surgery in all areas of the neck. Hard signs include hemodynamic instability, active bleeding, enlarging hematoma, hoarseness, difficulty breathing, and subcutaneous air.

Zone 1 injuries are the most life-threatening. Obviously if any hard signs of a vascular or aerodigestive tract injury are present, emergent surgery is indicated. If there is evidence of a vascular lesion and the patient is hemodynamically stable, an angiogram of the great vessels may be indicated to define which vessel is injured. This may be important for determining the location of the incision. Whereas proximal control of most vessels in the neck can be achieved via a median sternotomy, injuries to the left subclavian artery are best approached via a left thoracotomy.

If hard signs are not present, zone 1 injuries should be studied. Angiography is usually considered mandatory, as vascular injuries may remain occult. Probably the most important organ to evaluate is the esophagus. Penetrating injuries to the esophagus may remain hidden until a raging mediastinitis develops. If the diagnosis is missed for 12 hours, mortality is 5% to 25% and increases with time. Whether one performs esophagoscopy (rigid or flexible) or esophagraphy depends on the expertise available at the time.

If hard signs are present in zone 2, neck exploration is mandatory. Angiography is not indicated, as proximal control is straightforward. Still controversial is what to do with injuries in this area without hard signs. Options include (a) operate on all and accept a 30% to 90% negative exploration rate; (b) perform angiography and endoscopic evaluation of the aerodigestive tract; and (c) observe the patient.

The major concern for zone 3 injuries is the presence of a vascular injury. If a hard sign is present, injuries in the proximal vessels can be approached surgically. On occasion the mandible must be dislocated for exposure. For more distal injuries angiographic control and embolization may be the only therapeutic option.

Thoracic Injuries

Rib fractures remain a common entity for the traumatologist. Management of a patient with multiple rib fractures remains a challenge, especially in the elderly. The standard of care for these patients is the use of an epidural catheter, which provides the best long-lasting pain relief. Rib block, although effective for one or two isolated fractures, is not helpful when there are multiple fractures. The pain relief obtained from it is short-lived and for prolonged control would involve two to three blocks per day. This is beyond the time capabilities of most surgeons and would be tolerated by only the most masochistic patient.

Ribs broken in two places create a flail segment. The problem with this flail segment is that it moves in a paradoxical fashion relative to the rest of the rib cage. That is, during inspiration it moves inward and during expiration it moves outward. This abnormal movement increases the work of breathing. If the flail segment is large, the work of breathing may be so increased as to require that the patient be intubated. Adequate pain relief is probably the best way to avoid unnecessary intubation. It was once believed that the paradoxical motion resulted in hypoxemia, but has been shown not to be true. If hypoxemia is present it appears to be related to the pulmonary contusion underlying the flail segment.

First and second rib fractures no longer mandate angiography to rule out a great vessel injury. It is true that these fractures call for a high level of suspicion, but the incidence of associated vessel injury is not great enough, without other signs, to warrant angiography.

The remaining myth in the management of patients with rib fractures and pulmonary contusions is how to manage the fluid status. In the past it was thought that patients with a pulmonary contusion should be kept dry. This is not true. It is correct that hypervolemia should be avoided in the presence of pulmonary contusion. Maintaining a euvolemic state allows adequate organ perfusion while limiting third space fluid accumulation in the injured segment.

Cardiac Contusion

It is now thought by most that an aggressive search to rule out cardiac contusion is unnecessary and often wastes precious intensive care unit (ICU) beds. The major concern with cardiac contusion is the development of arrhythmias, which has led to admitting patients in whom the diagnosis is entertained to an ICU for monitoring. This practice has been demonstrated to be overkill. At a recent meeting of the Eastern Association for the Surgery of Trauma, guidelines for such an evaluation were suggested. Based on an extensive literature the following conclusions were reached: patients in whom the diagnosis is suspected should have an electrocardiogram (ECG) on admission. If the ECG is normal no further diagnostic maneuvers are needed, as the diagnosis is ruled out. If the ECG is abnormal, the patient should be admitted for 24 to 48 hours for observation. If a patient is unstable echocardiography appears to be the best test to detect wall motion abnormalities. Creatine phosphokinase (CPK) values are not helpful for predicting complications. Another guideline concerned management of the patient with a documented contusion: If surgery is necessary, it can be performed so long as filling pressures are monitored; whether a central venous pressure (CVP) or a pulmonary artery (PA) catheter is preferred has not been defined.

Cardiac Rupture

Cardiac rupture is rarely diagnosed in the ED, as most of these patients die in the field. Ventricular ruptures are uniformly fatal, though rupture of the atria has been successfully repaired. The key to salvage is early recognition. If an unstable patient arrives, and a source in the abdomen, pelvis, and chest has been ruled out, this diagnosis must be considered. Evaluation for Becks' triad (elevated CVP, muffled heart sounds, and hypotension) should be done, but the diagnostic tests of choice are an emergent ultrasound, pericardial window or left thoracotomy, depending on the patient's

stability. As more surgeons become comfortable performing abdominal ultrasonography for trauma, this modality can be used to evaluate for tamponade. Transthoracic or transesophageal echocardiography can also be used if rapidly available. If the patient is extremely unstable an anterolateral thoracotomy may be used as a last ditch effort to salvage the patient.

Aortic Rupture

Although blunt rupture of the aorta and other great vessels in the thorax are not uncommon, it is uncommon to see them in the ED. About 80% to 90% of patients with a great vessel injury die before reaching the hospital. The most important factor in making this diagnosis is a high index of suspicion based on the mechanism of injury and some key clinical findings. Table 15.1 lists some of these high risk factors. Once one's awareness has been raised, the most commonly used screening test is the chest radiograph. Common findings of great vessel injuries are listed in Table 15.2. It must be remembered that a negative chest radiograph does not rule out the diagnosis. As many as one-third of patients with rupture may have an initially normal chest radiograph.

The role of CT scanning in the diagnosis of great vessel injury is controversial. Many believe that it is most useful as a screening tool. CT evaluation includes examining the mediastinum for evidence of a hematoma. If there is no hematoma and there is a low suspicion for injury, the patient can be observed with the knowledge that aortic rupture may still be present. If there is a mediastinal hematoma, further evaluation is necessary as there is a high incidence of false positives caused by bleeding from lung or chest wall injuries. In most centers the gold standard for this diagnosis is aortography. It must be kept

TABLE 15.1. *Clinical features suggesting possible traumatic rupture of the aorta*

High-speed deceleration injury
Multiple rib fractures
Fractured first or second rib
Fractured sternum
Hoarseness or voice change without laryngeal injury
Hypertension, especially in the upper extremities
Superior vena cava syndrome
Systolic murmur, especially interscapular
Pulse deficits

TABLE 15.2. *Some chest radiographic findings associated with traumatic rupture of the aorta*

Superior mediastinal widening
Loss of definition of the aortic knob
Obliteration of the outline of descending aorta
Deviation of esophagus to the right at T4 more than
    1.0–2.0 cm
Obliteration of the aortopulmonary window
Tracheal deviation to the right
Apical cap
Depression of left main stem bronchus more than 40 degrees
Widened paravertebral stripe
Fracture of first or second ribs
Fractured sternum, especially in younger individuals
Thickened and/or deviated paratracheal stripe

in mind that even this modality can give both false-positive and false-negative results. Some centers prefer transesophageal echocardiography to angiography. Its use is highly dependent on the availability of an interested echocardiologist. Although we prefer aortography, we have used transesophageal echocardiography in the operating room (OR) in patients who had to be taken rapidly to the OR for bleeding control and required prolonged OR procedures. In this scenario, echocardiography can be performed in a semiemergent setting. If it is negative, definitive operative procedures can be performed. If it is positive, some thoracic surgeons still require an aortogram, whereas other are willing to operate based on the echocardiographic results. Without this procedure temporizing procedures may need to be done so a timely angiogram can be obtained.

The most common site for injury of the aorta is at the aortic isthmus, which is the area between the left subclavian artery and the ligamentum arteriosum. The second most common site is in the ascending aorta. Once the location has been determined, if and how to repair the problem becomes important. There are two ideas on how to repair the aorta: bypass and clamp-and-sew. The major concern with the latter procedure is the development of paraplegia during cross-clamping. What is apparent from the literature is that the incidence of paraplegia is related to expertise and not how the procedure is done. If the repair can be performed with 30 minutes or less clamp time, the incidence of paraplegia rivals that using bypass. Therefore the recommendation is that unless there is expertise in the rapid repair of such injuries, some type of bypass should be utilized.

Of interest is the notion and supporting evidence that not all of these injuries must be repaired. There is increasing experience that delayed or non-repair of injuries *in high risk patients* has a better outcome than attempting repair. Some authors have gone so far as to say that in stable patients over the age of 55 years nonoperative management is the treatment of choice. This is not yet the consensus opinion.

If there is going to be a delay in treatment, medical management is important. The cornerstone of such management is the reduction of shear forces on the aorta, which is achieved by tight control of blood pressure using β-blockers. Systolic blood pressure should be maintained below 120 mm Hg. Preventing gagging due to nasogastric tube manipulation or suctioning with its resultant transient rise in blood pressure is also important.

The management of associated injuries is the last topic of controversy. In an unstable patient with a widened mediastinum and a grossly positive ultrasound scan or diagnostic peritoneal lavage, the decision to go to the OR for control of intraabdominal hemorrhage is easy. What is less clear is what to do with the patient who has associated injuries that are not immediately life-threatening. There seems to be an increasing voice first to repair the aorta rapidly and then to take care of these less severe injuries.

Penetrating Injuries to the Chest

According to careful reviews in the literature, thoracotomy in the ED is a procedure that provides little benefit to the patient and incurs high risk to providers and high cost to the system. Careful analyses have shown the subgroups of patients who may benefit from this procedure. Overall survival varies from 0 to 20%. The highest survival rates are in patients who arrive *in extremis* after a penetrating cardiac injury. No matter what the mechanism, patients with no signs of life in the field have no chance of survival, and thoracotomy should not be performed in the ED. The group of patients who appear best served by this procedure are those with penetrating injury to the chest or extremities who have signs of life either during transport or after ED arrival. These patients fare significantly better than those with penetrating injury to the abdomen because rapid control of bleeding is possible in the chest or the extremities. Although one may restore vital signs in patients with severe intraabdominal injuries, these patients just rebleed once blood pressure has been restored and die before or soon after definitive control of the bleeding is established.

Indications for operating room thoracotomy in the patient **not** *in extremis* are (a) chest tube output more than 1500 mL after insertion; (b) chest tube output of 200 to 300 mL/hr for 3 hours; (c) chest radiograph with significant retained hemothorax after chest tube insertion; and (d) large air leak with hypoxemia. Whether to perform a left or right thoracotomy or a median sternotomy is determined by the location of the injury and the expected organ injured.

Figure 15.2 demonstrates another area of concern in patients who are stable after sustaining penetrating thoracic injuries. The outlined box represents an area where the risk of cardiac injury is the highest. Reports of unsuspected injuries as high as 23% have been reported in patients sustaining penetration in this area (especially after stab wounds). Although the pericardial window has been the mainstay in the diagnosis of these injuries, many centers are resorting to transthoracic echocardiography in these patients as a means of noninvasive, rapid evaluation. When there is the additional concern of a mediastinal injury, some centers evaluate both the heart and the mediastinum using thoracoscopy.

Transmediastinal gunshot wounds often present a dilemma. These patients usually present in one of two ways: (a) *in extremis* after sustaining an injury to the heart, pulmonary hilum, or great vessel; or (b) in stable condition with minimal evidence of life-threatening injury. Concern involves four basic structures: heart, great vessels, tracheobronchial tree, and esophagus. Gunshot wounds to the heart and great vessels are rarely occult, unlike stab wounds to these organs. Angiography to rule out an unsuspected injury is usually not necessary. Concern over occult injuries to the heart after high-risk trajectories can be evaluated by either echocardiography or pericardial window. Bronchoscopy is usually not necessary unless there is evidence of a significant air leak. On the other hand, the esophagus must be evaluated in all patients with this type of injury. Esophageal injuries are notoriously subtle on initial presentation and often fatal when they present in a delayed fashion. Mandatory evaluation of these injuries is especially easy when the test involved (esophography or esophagoscopy) carries almost no risk. Mortality rates for esophageal injuries if repaired within 12 hours vary from 5% to 25% depending on associated injuries. If repair is delayed 12 to 24 hours, the mortality doubles, and it triples if repair is delayed more than 24 hours.

The approach to operative repair depends on the location of the injury. If the wound is in the proximal or midesophagus, operative repair should be via a right posterolateral thoracotomy. Injuries to the distal third of the esophagus are best approached via a left posterolateral thoracotomy. It is best to repair the esophagus in

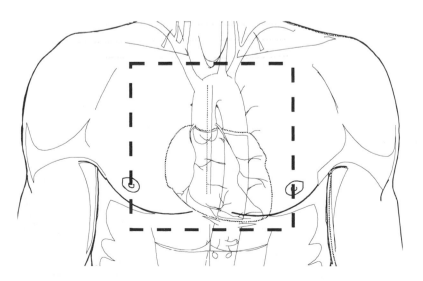

FIG. 15.2. Cardiac zone of risk.

two layers and to buttress the repair. In the upper esophagus this can be achieved with either a wrap of pleura or intercostal muscle. In the lower esophagus a gastric fundal wrap may be used.

Blunt Abdominal Injuries

Thorough evaluation of the abdomen after blunt injury remains a critical part of the evaluation of the trauma victim. Missed intraabdominal injury remains the most common cause of *preventable* trauma deaths. The methods used to determine the presence of an injury depends on patient stability and available resources. Although diagnostic peritoneal lavage (DPL) is still the "gold standard," most centers perform many more CT scans than DPLs. New to the armamentarium of the American traumatologist is ultrasonography. Though the gold standard in Europe for years, it has only recently caught on in the United States as a quick and easy way to detect the presence of free fluid.

The general criteria for evaluating the abdomen are listed in Table 15-3. These criteria simply suggest that evaluation is necessary; they do not define the type of evaluation needed. That is determined by the clinical condition of the patient. DPL could be used for all of the outlined criteria. Table 15.4 lists the strengths and weakness of DPL. The only absolute contraindication for DPL is when there is an obvious need for laparotomy. Relative contraindications include third-trimester pregnancy and multiple previous abdominal operations. The criteria for evaluating the results of DPL are listed in Table 15.5.

Table 15.6 reviews the good and bad aspects of CT scanning. Because it is noninvasive it is the preferred method by which to evaluate the stable trauma patient. It is also the *last* method for evaluating the unstable patient because it is almost impossible to resuscitate a patient during a CT scan and one's ability to monitor such a patient is greatly limited. With the high incidence of

neurologically impaired blunt trauma patients (due to ethyl alcohol, drugs, brain injury) it is no surprise that the overwhelming number of CT scans done are normal. Scanning this large group of patients who are at low risk for injury but cannot be adequately assessed clinically requires significant resources in physician and technician time with little gain. Ultrasonography (US) has gained acceptance for this reason. Its ability to screen for the presence of free fluid appears to reduce the need for CT.

Table 15.7 lists the strengths and weaknesses of US. In most centers US plays two roles. The first is in stable patients with equivocal examinations or who are neurologically impaired. In those cases if the US shows no free fluid, a CT scan is not performed. Any change in

TABLE 15.4. *Strengths and weaknesses of DPL*

Strengths
  Rapid
  Easy to teach
  Highly sensitive to the presence of injury
  May detect bowel injury
  Inexpensive
Weaknesses
  Invasive
  Iatrogenic complications
  Misses retroperitoneal organ injuries
  High rate of unnecessary laparotomy
  Nonspecific
  Difficult to do in obese or uncooperative patients

TABLE 15.3. *Criteria for evaluating the abdomen*

Unexplained hypotension
Equivocal or unreliable examination
Inability to observe patient (need for surgery for associated injury)
Multiple lower rib fractures
Pelvic fracture

TABLE 15.5. *Criteria for interpretation of lavage results after blunt abdominal trauma*

Positive findings
  Aspiration of 5 ml blood
  Lavage fluid comes out Foley catheter or chest tube
  RBC > 100,000/mm³
  WBC > 500/mm³
  Amylase > 175 U/mL
  Presence of bile, bacteria, and/or particulate matter
Indeterminate findings
  Aspiration of < 5 ml of blood
  RBC 50,000–100,000/mm³
  WBC 100–500 mm³
  Amylase 75–175 U/mL
Negative findings
  No blood aspirated
  RBC < 50,000/mm³
  WBC < 100/mm³
  Amylase < 75 U/mL

TABLE 15.6. *Strengths and weaknesses of CT scan*

Strengths
  Noninvasive
  Good for retroperitoneal injuries
  Organ-specific
  Provides grading of solid organ injury
Weaknesses
  Never scan unstable patient
  Misses bowel injuries
  Expensive
  Time-consuming
  Need cooperative patient
  Weight limitations

condition warrants a repeat US scan. If fluid is seen, CT is performed to detect the presence of organ injury. In the unstable patient the presence of fluid on US is adequate indication that there is intraabdominal hemorrhage, and the patient is taken to the OR. This protocol obviates the need for DPL.

Management of Blunt Solid-Viscus Injury

Although conservative management of blunt *splenic* injury was initiated in children, it rapidly became the standard for management in the adult. The major criteria for nonoperative management in adults are that the patient be hemodynamically stable and that there be no concern for hollow-viscus injury. If the injury extends into the hilum on CT (grade 4) or there is a blush of contrast in the injured area, conservative management cannot be effective and an operative approach should be pursued. Although some surgeons operate if the CT

TABLE 15.7. *Strengths and weaknesses of ultrasonography*

Strengths
  Noninvasive
  Rapid
  Inexpensive
  Repeatable
  Sensitive for the presence of fluid
  Can evaluate heart
Weaknesses
  User-dependent
  Misses bowel injuries
  Need cooperative patient
  Weight limitations
  Nonspecific

shows evidence of bleeding, others first attempt angiographic embolization of the source of bleeding. The latter approach requires an aggressive interventional radiology department. Proponents of early surgery for splenic injury have demonstrated a high splenic salvage rate when operation is done early rather than when conservative management has failed.

Nonoperative management of *hepatic* injuries uses basically the same criteria as for the spleen. Injuries near the porta hepatis carry a higher failure rate than more peripheral injuries. Active bleeding demonstrated by hemodynamic instability or a blush on CT should be treated with laparotomy or angiographic embolization. Severe liver injuries remain a surgical challenge. I believe in the adage that "if it isn't bleeding, don't touch it." Stirring up bleeding in the depths of the liver can have disastrous consequences. Less severe injuries can often be controlled with direct pressure and patience. On occasion, liver sutures and an omental pack may be effective. With severe injuries vascular control using the Pringle maneuver (clamping the porta hepatis) may be necessary, followed by the finger fracture technique to reach the site of bleeding. Lateral injuries can be treated with resectional débridement. It is important to drain most injuries of moderate and greater degree because bile leaks are common after these injuries and may not be evident immediately.

Blunt and penetrating injuries to the *pancreas* are handled in a similar fashion. The key concept is conservative operative management. There is no role for nonoperative management. The location and extent of the injury usually determine the treatment. Proximal and distal injuries that do not involve the duct can usually be managed by drainage alone. If there is involvement of the distal duct, distal resection is the treatment of choice. Splenic salvage is recommended only in the stable patient with isolated injury. Proximal injuries that involve the pancreatic duct are more complex to manage. Distal pancreatectomy is inappropriate for injuries to the right of the superior mesenteric vessels, as it would produce a state of pancreatic insufficiency. How the proximal pancreas is handled is determined by the status of the duodenum. If the duodenum is badly injured, pancreaticoduodenectomy is indicated, which is rarely performed. Many would argue that a full pancreaticoduodenectomy should not be performed at the initial operation. Bleeding and any intestinal spillage should be controlled at the first operation and the patient stabilized and resuscitated. The definitive operation can then be performed during the initial 24 to 48 hours after injury. If the duodenum is not injured, the proximal duct is ligated and a distal pancreatic enteric anastomosis is performed. As for liver injuries, it is important to drain all pancreatic injuries. There is support in the literature for the use of somatostatin after pancreatic injury to reduce the incidence of fistula formation.

Penetrating Abdominal Trauma

Management of penetrating abdominal injuries depends on numerous factors, including the mechanism of injury, the location of the injury, and the clinical status of the patient. Gunshot wounds (GSWs) are different from stab wounds (SWs). The mortality due to GSWs (5% to 15%) is significantly higher than that due to SWs (1% to 2%). The incidence of intraabdominal injury is also higher with GSWs (92% to 98% vs. 15% to 25%). All GSWs that penetrate the abdomen require surgery because of the high incidence of injury. Such is not the case for SWs, as the abdomen is regionalized to determine optimum management.

Stab wounds to the **anterior abdomen** create no intraabdominal injury in 20% to 40% of cases. If all patients with injury to this area were explored, an unacceptably high negative laparotomy rate would occur. If one limits exploration to those with hypotension, evisceration, or peritonitis, the negative laparotomy rate is reduced to 15%. How best to evaluate those who do not meet those criteria is controversial. DPL is not helpful for SWs to the anterior abdomen because DPL may be negative in the presence of injuries to the bowel and diaphragm or positive in patients with small liver and spleen injuries that have stopped bleeding. Laparoscopy can be performed but requires general anesthesia, and running the small bowel can be time-consuming. We believe in careful observation. In a series by Ivatury et al., hemodynamically stable patients with benign abdomens were followed by serial examinations. They found that 75% did not need laparotomy, and the negative laparotomy rate was 3%. There did not appear to be any morbidity or mortality associated with observation.

There is more debate over the management of stab wounds to the flank and back. These injuries are special because of the risks associated with retroperitoneal colon injuries. There are proponents for doing triple-contrast CTs, DPL, and laparoscopy. I believe that CT and laparoscopy can be useful in specific patient groups. For stab wounds to the flank that are between the anterior and midaxillary line, laparoscopy may be useful for evaluating peritoneal penetration and colon injuries. Any hematoma or air seen near the colon mandates exploration. This method is especially useful for left upper quadrant and thoracoabdominal SWs where the risk for occult diaphragm injury is present.

For stab wounds to the back the preferred method of evaluation is the CT scan. There is a belief that the optimal way to perform this scan is with oral, rectal, and intravenous contrast. This preference is often met with resistance from radiologists, and the scans are performed with intravenous and oral contrast alone. If it is performed in this manner it is critical that enough contrast is given and time is allowed to obtain adequate filling of the colon. Any air or hematoma seen around the colon dictates the need for laparotomy.

Penetrating injury to the area of the thoracoabdomen has its own scheme of management. Studies have shown a 20% to 30% incidence of occult diaphragm injury after penetrating injury to this region. The morbidity and mortality of diaphragmatic hernia from a missed injury has led some to advocate mandatory laparotomy for all patients with injury to this area. If followed, a 75% negative laparotomy rate would result, making this kind of approach less than optimal. Others advocate the use of DPL in this setting. The choice again is less than perfect as positive lavage can occur from small injuries to the liver and spleen, and there have been many reports of a false-negative DPL in the presence of a diaphragmatic injury. I believe that the optimal method for evaluating penetrating injury to the thoracoabdominal area is laparoscopy. It is minimally invasive and highly sensitive for detecting diaphragmatic injuries. Injuries to the right thoracoabdominal area are probably not an issue, as the liver seals the diaphragmatic hole, and the risk of herniation is low.

Management of Colon Injuries

Repair of a penetrating injury to the colon, like most other injuries discussed so far, is determined by patient stability and the extent of the bowel injury and contamination. Injuries to the right and transverse colon should be primarily repaired under most circumstances. Primary repair or resection plus anastomosis are acceptable procedures. If a left colon or sigmoid injury is present, a primary repair can be performed if the patient is stable, there is minimal contamination, and there are no major associated injuries (pancreatic injury is probably the worst). Although primary repair is the preferred method for reconstruction, if one is unsure colostomy is the safest choice.

DAMAGE CONTROL: OPERATIVE STRATEGY IN THE UNSTABLE PATIENT

It is important to know when injuries should *not* be definitively repaired but should be observed and the final treatment delayed. This is the concept of "damage control." The basic philosophy follows three points: (a) the OR is a bad place for resuscitation; (b) resuscitation takes precedence over definitive repair; and (c) cold, acidotic, coagulopathic patients do not do well in the OR. When a hypotensive, acidotic patient is in the OR, the operative strategy would be to control hemorrhage and intestinal contamination and then move the patient to the ICU for resuscitation. Bowel repairs should be limited to simple repairs or stapling of injured segments to stop spillage. Intestinal continuity should not be restored at this time. The abdomen should be closed rapidly once these repairs are achieved. Closure is accomplished with towel clamps, an intravenous bag, or a prosthetic patch (e.g., Gortex or Vicryl).

The underlying theory is that these patients remain in a state of shock with progressive acidosis and organ injury. If this cycle continues, even if the patient eventually makes it off the table, there is a significantly increased risk of developing multiple organ failure. Using the principles of damage control, resuscitation is accomplished in the ICU under a more controlled setting and at a more rapid pace. Once the patient has been resuscitated, definitive repairs can be performed in the OR under optimal circumstances. This method of treatment has been shown to salvage severely injured patients with a significant reduction in morbidity and mortality.

PELVIC FRACTURES

No chapter on trauma management would be complete without a discussion on the management of pelvic fractures. This injury often complicates our ability to manage a multiply injured patient. The usual issue is whether an unstable patient with a pelvic fracture is bleeding from vessel injury in the pelvis or an associated intraabdominal injury, which occurs in about 5% to 10% of patients with these fractures.

The key management principle is rapid evaluation of the abdomen. The gold standard for this evaluation is DPL. When DPL is performed in the presence of a pelvic fracture, a supraumbilical tap using the open technique should be used to avoid entering the pelvic hematoma, which would result in a false-positive tap. Another alternative is ultrasonography. If the ultrasound scan shows evidence of free fluid, it can be presumed that the instability is from an intraabdominal source and the patient taken to the OR for exploration. If the DPL or ultrasound scan is negative, it can be presumed that the bleeding is from the pelvis.

The optimal method for control depends on the type of pelvic fracture. The four major classifications are open book, lateral compression, vertical shear, and a combination of these types. With an open book fracture pattern there is an increase in pelvic volume. The bleeding vessels with this type of injury are usually veins from the sacral plexus. The best way to control this bleeding is by placing an external fixator on the pelvic rim to reduce the pelvic volume. This reduction in volume often increases the pressure on the pelvic veins enough to stop the bleeding. If placing such a fixator on the pelvis does not control the bleeding, it is presumed that the bleeding is from an arterial source and an angiogram is obtained with the hope of visualizing and embolizing the source of bleeding.

If one of the other fracture patterns is present, the pelvic volume is not increased and external fixation is not a viable alternative. With these fractures, bleeding from small arteries such as the pudendal or obturator artery is more common. Unstable patients with these injuries should have their abdomens rapidly evaluated by DPL or ultrasonography and, if negative, be taken emergently for angiography for evaluation and potential treatment.

CONCLUSIONS

This chapter reviews basic management principles for the trauma patient. The most important reminders are a high level of suspicion and attention to detail. Current data suggest that arresting hemorrhage and re-

suscitation should take priority over definitive therapies.

QUESTIONS 9/10

1. A 25-year-old man arrives after sustaining a GSW
to the right lower quadrant. He is explored and
found to have a 3-cm laceration to the right colon.
He is hemodynamically stable, and there is minimal local contamination. The correct procedure
would be to:
   a. Perform an ascending loop colostomy.
   b. Resect the injury and bring up an end-colostomy
   and mucous fistula.
   c. Exteriorize the repair and drop it back in after 5
   to 7 days if intact.
   d. Perform a primary repair.
   e. Perform a resection and anastomosis.

2. A complete cervical spine evaluation after a motor
vehicle accident should include:
   a. Careful clinical examination.
   b. Lateral radiograph including the top of T1.
   c. Anteroposterior view.
   d. Odontoid view.
   e. All of the above.

3. The first priority during evaluation of a multiply injured patient who is hypotensive is to:
   a. Establish intravenous access.
   b. Obtain blood for crossmatch.
   c. Perform a minineurologic examination.
   d. Assess the airway.
   e. Search for occult bleeding.

4. A 36-year-old woman arrives with stable vital signs
after sustaining a stab wound to the neck just lateral
to and above the cricoid cartilage. There is a slowly
expanding hematoma lateral to the wound. The
next step in management would be:
   a. Observation.
   b. Angiography to better define bleeding source.
   c. Neck exploration
   d. Esophography and observation.
   e. CT scan.

5. A 34-year-old man arrives at the ED hypotensive
after being involved in a motorcycle accident. He
has an angulated right femur, facial trauma, and a
tender abdomen. Initial films revealed an unre-

markable chest radiograph, normal lateral cervical
spine, and an open-book pelvic fracture. Despite 2
liters of crystalloid he remains hypotensive. The
next step in management is:
   a. Exploratory laparotomy.
   b. CT scan of the abdomen.
   c. DPL.
   d. Angiography.
   e. None of the above.

6. The preferred fluid for a patient who arrives at the
ED hypotensive after sustaining a GSW to the chest
is:
   a. Normal saline 0.9%.
   b. Ringer's lactate solution.
   c. 5% Albumin.
   d. Whole blood.
   e. 5% Hetastarch.

7. The most important determinant for the need for
aortography in a patient at risk for blunt aortic injury is:
   a. Clinical suspicion.
   b. First rib fracture.
   c. Morphology of aortic knob.
   d. Sternal fracture.
   e. Myocardial contusion.

8. The best indicator for the presence of hemorrhagic
shock is:
   a. Blood loss at the scene.
   b. Blood pressure.
   c. Pulse.
   d. Central venous pressure.
   e. Base deficit.

9. A 68-year-old man is involved in a high speed motor vehicle accident. He is unconscious and hypotensive with systolic pressure of 80 mm Hg on
arrival at the ED with a distended abdomen. Initial
radiographs reveal a minimally displaced pelvic
fracture and normal cervical spine; the chest radiograph shows a widened mediastinum, loss of aortic contour, and deviated nasogastric tube. Despite
blood transfusion he remains hypotensive. DPL reveals 10 mL gross blood. The next step in management is:
   a. Head CT scan.
   b. Pelvic angiogram.
   c. Aortogram.
   d. Emergency thoracotomy.
   e. Exploratory laparotomy.

10. A 48-year-old man is stabbed in the right upper quadrant. He arrives in the ED hypotensive and with abdominal tenderness. He is taken emergently to the OR for laparotomy. At exploration he is found to have a 3-cm laceration to the dome of the liver that is not bleeding but appears deep. No other injuries are found. The next step in managing this injury would be:

    a. Pringle maneuver.
    b. Pringle maneuver and finger fracture exploration of the injury.
    c. Exploration of the injury.
    d. Drain injury and close the abdomen.
    e. Close the abdomen.

SELECTED REFERENCES

Ivatury RR, ed. Cavitary endoscopy in trauma. *Trauma Q* 1993;10(4).

Ivatury RR, ed. Critical care in the trauma patient. *Trauma Q* 1996;12(3).

Ivatury RR, Cayten CG, eds. *The textbook of penetrating trauma.* Baltimore: Williams & Wilkins, 1996.

Maull KI, ed. *Advances in trauma and critical care.* St. Louis: Mosby, 1994.

Statistics on violence in America. National Center for Health Statistics and FBI Web pages: http://www.cdc.gov/nchswww/nchshome.htm and http://www.fbi.gov/publish.htm.

Wilson RF, Walt AJ, eds. *The management of trauma: pitfalls and practice.* Baltimore: Williams & Wilkins, 1996.

16

Transplantation

Dean Kim, Stuart Greenstein, Richard S. Schechner, and Vivian A. Tellis

Progress in human transplantation continues at a brisk pace. Transplantation of the kidney, heart, and liver have become so safe and effective as to be the standard of treatment for many conditions. Transplantation of pancreas and lung has increased rapidly, and increasing numbers of small bowel transplants have been reported. In 1995 alone, 20,182 organs were transplanted. Problems remain, however. The availability of organs for transplantation lags far behind the need. The number of potential donors in the population has been estimated at 50 per million, even after exclusion of those with contraindications. The actual number of cadaveric or donors in the United States in 1994 was 5,100, a fraction of the possible number. In November, 1995 there were 43,370 people on waiting lists. This figure represents only a fraction of the problem because many of those awaiting hearts, lungs, and livers die before an organ becomes available. It follows that the failure to retrieve transplantable organs from all potential donors results in the preventable death of those who might have received them. Attempts to deal with the inadequacy of donors have been varied. For *cadaver donors* indications have been extended to include older donors and those with concurrent diseases; the use of *live donors* has been extended to virtually all relatives, as well as *emotionally related* donors (unrelated volunteer donors with a strong bond, such as spouses or long term

family friends). Finally, *xenografts* have been brought into the realm of the possible.

A single chapter on a subject as vast as transplantation can have only a limited purpose. We provide an overview of the immunologic basis for the immune response and the related topics of rejection and immunosuppression. The indications, contraindications, and results of transplantation of various organs, the complications of surgery and of immunosuppression, and the role of various regulatory agencies are also addressed.

INDICATIONS FOR TRANSPLANTATION

The potential recipient should have the prospect of a significant improvement in quality of life with a transplant and improved life expectancy. There should be no clearly defined contraindication, such as infection or malignancy, which could spread in an explosive manner under the influence of immunosuppression. In treatable situations, such as an abscess that could be drained or a hepatoma that could be extirpated by removing the entire liver, the patient might still be considered a candidate. However, disseminated sepsis, extreme debility, or psychosocial problems (e.g., noncompliance or self-destructive behavior) could result in exclusion of a potential candidate.

Another factor to be considered is whether there is a safe alternative to transplantation. This could include corrective cardiac surgery, partial liver resection, or administration of exogenous insulin for uncomplicated diabetes. If another method of treatment can be successfully applied, the risks of immunosuppression attendant on transplantation may not be justified. Various aspects of transplantation are discussed here with kidney transplantation as the model because kidneys are the most commonly transplanted organ. The similarities and differences relative to transplantation of heart, liver, lung, and pancreas are addressed.

INDICATIONS FOR RENAL TRANSPLANTATION

Although patients with end stage renal disease (ESRD) can be maintained on dialysis, life expectancy (particularly among diabetics) has been shown to be improved after transplantation. The most common indication for renal transplantation is ESRD due to glomerulonephritis; among African-Americans, hypertension is a common cause. Diabetic nephropathy accounts for up to one-third of kidney recipients. Other common indications for renal transplantation are listed in Table 16.1. Although all of the 125,000 patients with ESRD are potential candidates, most are ruled out because of severe coexisting multiorgan disease. The presence of circulating antibodies (e.g., from active lupus nephritis or Goodpasture syndrome) could damage a new kidney and may cause a patient to be temporarily excluded until the antibody has disappeared.

Most renal transplant recipients are on maintenance dialysis at the time of transplantation. Transplantation can be carried out before dialysis becomes necessary ("preemptive" transplantation), particularly if a suitable living donor is available. The median age of both donors and recipients is rising, and age is no longer a major de-

TABLE 16.1. *Common indications for renal transplantation*

Chronic glomerulonephritis
Chronic pyelonephritis
Diabetes mellitus types I and II
Hypertensive nephrosclerosis
Polycystic kidney disease
Obstructive uropathy

termining factor. Transplants are being performed on infants as well as septuagenarians. Transplantation in children must be aggressively pursued, as physical and emotional growth become stunted on dialysis.

PREPARATION FOR TRANSPLANTATION

For the average adult who has been well until the onset of renal failure, little preparation is required in addition to investigations common before any major operation: chest radiograph, electrocardiogram (ECG), and the usual laboratory tests. Of particular importance are *serologic tests,* the results of which may cause a patient to be excluded [hepatitis B, human immunodeficiency virus (HIV)]or that may have an impact on management [cytomegalovirus (CMV)]. Hepatitis C is an increasing problem because it is widely encountered in donors and recipients. In many centers the patients with hepatitis C antibodies undergo a liver biopsy, which guides the decision whether to accept the patient as a candidate. Other investigations are prompted by circumstances. *Stress tests* are advisable for older recipients, diabetics, and those with abnormal ECGs. Those with a history suggestive of **gastrointestinal or genitourinary** problems may need investigation of the appropriate organ system and treatment of any discovered pathology (e.g., peptic ulcer disease) before transplantation. *Skin testing* for tuberculosis and a search for ova and parasites in stools is important in patients who have lived abroad or come from large urban populations. The patient's own kidneys are usually left alone; nephrectomy is reserved for indications such as severe ureteropelvic reflux, massive calculus disease, or infection, which if left untreated may pose a problem after transplantation.

Immunologic Testing and Preparation

The term "tissue typing" is loosely applied to a series of tests that may have a bearing on the choice of donor and on the patient's chances of receiving and retaining an organ.

Red Blood Cell Agglutinin Testing

Organ distribution follows rules similar to those for blood transfusion: type O kidneys may be transplanted into all recipients, but type O recipients can receive only type O kidneys, whereas AB-type recipients can receive kidneys of all blood types. In practice, kidneys are generally allocated to the type-specific recipient. With the scarcity of organs, it is particularly inappropriate to transplant type O kidneys into recipients who can receive organs of other types.

Histocompatibility Testing

The cells of every organism carry proteins known as major histocompatibility (MHC) antigens, which are different for each individual. The greater the differences between individuals, the greater the chance the recipient will reject the tissues or organs from the donor. Other mechanisms also participate in the destructive process. Grafts between perfectly matched pairs can be rejected, whereas those between disparate pairs may survive. With clinical transplantation, the effort is to minimize the differences between donors and recipients to prevent rejection.

In humans, MHC antigens are encoded by a set of genes located on chromosome 6 and designated human leukocyte antigens (HLAs). The antigens are distributed at several loci (A, B, C for class I; DR, DP, DQ for class II). The greatest importance appears to be attached to matching at the A, B, and DR loci. There are more than 120 antigenic specificities known. Not all antigens can be clearly identified, as cross reactions do occur. Each person inherits a "set" of antigens (one A, B, and DR) known as a "haplotype" from each parent. For most individuals, it is possible to identify all six antigens at the A, B, and DR loci. These haplotypes, identified by HLA serotyping, are used to determine the degree of similarity between prospective donors and recipients. This simplifies the process of identification of possible donors within a family, as only four possible permutations exist for the two "halves" of each parent. When a patient has several siblings, there is a 25% chance that one of them is identical at all loci (six-antigen match), a 25% chance of a total mismatch, and a 50% chance of being haplo-identical (half-matched). Obviously, matches between parents and offspring can only be haploidentical (except in small populations in which inbreeding has resulted in a limited gene pool).

Matching has important connotations. Before the availability of cyclosporine (CsA), the results of transplantation between relatives were proportional to the degree of matching. Six-antigen matches continue to have the best long term results and require the least amount of immunosuppression. Graft survival is excellent for six- and five-antigen matched cadaver kidneys; with lesser degrees of matching the data are conflicting. Currently, if a medically suitable six-antigen matched recipient is identified for a kidney anywhere in the United States, it is mandatory for the kidney to be offered to the recipient. For all other kidneys, a computer-assisted allocation is made, based on HLA matching, time waiting, and degree of sensitization.

It must be stressed that typing of HLA antigens does not give any indication of compatibility. It is important to determine whether a potential recipient has soluble antibodies against a potential recipient.

Cytotoxic Crossmatch

In a direct test of compatibility, the serum of a potential recipient is incubated with the lymphocytes of potential donors. Care must be taken to exclude autoantibodies [some patients have immunoglobulin M (IgM) antibodies that react universally and have no bearing on transplantation] and to confirm that the reaction occurs at room temperature. Lysis of the donor cells (a "positive crossmatch") signifies the presence of a circulating antibody that is destructive to the donor. Therefore the crossmatch is essential before any renal transplant, living or cadaver. Transplantation despite a true positive crossmatch usually leads to the aggressive, immediate loss of the graft (hyperacute rejection). With liver transplantation, a positive crossmatch does not seem to be of importance, possibly because destructive antibodies are phagocytosed within the Kupffer cells of the liver itself. Due to time constraints, crossmatching generally has not been utilized for heart transplantation, although it does not seem to have major significance. However, because catastrophic hyperacute cardiac rejections have been reported in sensitized recipients and with retransplantation of the heart, crossmatching is selectively practiced.

Antibody Testing

Antibody status is assessed using a panel of lymphocyte donors, representing the most commonly occurring HLA antigens. The sera of potential recipients are tested against this panel to determine the percentage of panel donors cells that are lysed by the recipient serum. This percent panel-reactive antibody (% PRA) provides a measure of the reactivity of the patient; a patient with a high PRA (sensitized patient) has difficulty obtaining a compatible kidney and may be at high risk for graft loss. Causes of such sensitization include previous transplants, blood transfusions, and pregnancy. The test is carried out when a patient is first placed on the waiting list and at intervals thereafter.

Blood Transfusion

At one time patients who had received blood transfusions were noted to have improved graft survival. Improved results in the CsA era have removed the advantage of transfusion; the deliberate use of blood transfusion as an immunosuppressive technique has all but disappeared. This is also true of "donor-specific transfusion" in which a live donor's blood was given to the recipient over several weeks before transplantation.

Other Investigations

Additional tests are carried out as necessary. A mixed lymphocyte culture (MLC) involves simultaneous incubation of donor and recipient lymphocytes to determine the degree of reactivity. In the current immunosuppressive era, it has little practical value. Patients suspected of having circulating antibodies may be tested for anti-vascular endothelial antibodies.

Choice of Donor

A kidney may be obtained from a cadaveric donor or from a living donor (related or unrelated). Several factors must be taken into account to make a reasonable and prudent choice. First, kidneys can function equally well whether from living or cadaveric donors, so long as the donor is free of renal disease, hypertension, and systemic disease. However, the survival of kidneys transplanted from living related donors (LRD) is superior to that from other sources. This difference is best appreciated in terms of "half-life": the mean time that elapses for 50% of a cohort of transplanted kidneys to cease functioning. For cadaver kidneys the half-life is 9 years, for one-haplotype LRD kidneys 12 to 14 years, and for identical living LRD kidneys 24 years. It has become

unexpectedly clear that kidneys from **living unrelated donors (LURD)** have results comparable to those with haplo-identical live donors (1 year survival 90% to 95%, half-life 12 to 15 years) and superior to those with cadaver donors. Spouses comprise most LURDs. For the recipient, the long-term benefits of live donor kidneys include less immunosuppression and a reduced risk of rejection and loss of the kidney. Additional advantages of LRD/LURD are minimal waiting time and immediate diuresis (and consequently avoidance of dialysis and a shorter hospital stay). The disadvantage is that a healthy person (donor) must undergo a major operation without tangible benefit. The operative mortality risk for the donor is 3 : 10,000. There is also a small (less than 1%) risk of complications, such as infection or bleeding. A live donor has a normal life-span, as can be noted from the fact that life insurance companies do not increase the premium payments of kidney donors.

Live Donors

The willing donor who is crossmatch compatible must undergo extensive preoperative evaluation, including a history and physical examination, chest radiography, ECG, and routine blood tests. The donor should be in excellent health and a grade I anesthetic risk. There must be no systemic disease that threatens the donor or the kidney. Tests of renal function, such as renal scan, urinalysis, urine cultures, and intravenous urography must also be carried out. The crossmatch is repeated, and if it still shows compatibility the final step before the transplant is an angiogram to determine the anatomy of both kidneys and the number of arteries on each side. Spiral computed tomography (CT) is being used in many centers in place of transfemoral arteriography; it is reported to provide similar anatomic information without invasion and with reduced expenditure of time and money.

The *operative technique* for live donor nephrectomy is an operation unlike any other in surgery. A healthy person undergoes the risk of a major operation for no direct benefit. Maximum care in handling tissues must be exercised, both for the sake of the donor and so the kidney functions immediately upon reimplantation in the recipient.

After induction of anesthesia, the patient is placed in the lateral position over a kidney rest with a central venous line and Foley catheter in place to monitor fluid balance. A flank incision is made and carried through the bed of the twelfth rib. The peritoneum is retracted medially and Gerota's fascia opened. The ureter is dissected as far distally as possible. The renal artery and vein are dissected to their connections to the great vessels. For the left kidney, the adrenal and gonadal veins are divided between ligatures. If the right kidney is being removed, the mobilization must go right up to the vena cava. During dissection, urine output is carefully monitored, and fluids and diuretics are administered as necessary to ensure a brisk diuresis.

When donor and recipient teams are ready, the ureter is divided. In some centers, heparin is given before vascular clamps are placed across the renal artery and vein (on the right, the venous clamp is placed on the vena cava). The vessels are divided with the maximum possible length compatible with safety. The kidney is removed from the field, flushed with cold electrolyte solution, and taken to the recipient operating room. The stumps of donor vessels are secured. If heparin was given, it is reversed with protamine. Hemostasis is carefully ensured, and the wound is closed.

In some centers the classic approach is being replaced by laparoscopically assisted nephrectomy. A small incision is made that stops short of the peritoneum. The patient is placed in the lateral position and four or five ports are used to carry out the dissection. When all is ready, the artery and vein are stapled and divided, and the kidney is removed from the previously made incision, which is now carried into the peritoneal cavity. In its early stages, this approach may take longer but is reported to have less morbidity, with patients being discharged within 2 to 3 days, and returning to activity almost immediately.

Cadaver Donors

Organ Recovery and Distribution Network

Because most of the costs of renal transplantation are borne by public funds through Medicare coverage, the U.S. government has asserted its interest in and authority over the acquisition and distribution of organs. The Health Care Financing Administration (HCFA) awarded the contract to the United Network for Organ Sharing (UNOS), which has responsibility for all organ recovery and distribution. The 50 states are divided into 11 geographic regions. Representatives of each region, including donor and recipient advocates, surgeons, med-ical specialists, ethicists, and representatives of health organizations form the national policy-making board.

Within each region are one or more organ procurement agencies (OPAs), which are responsible for organ recovery in their geographic areas; distribution of organs occurs first on a regional and then on a national basis, according to definitive criteria, which differ with the organs concerned. The complexities of donor identification, declaration of death and maintenance, and organ distribution have given rise to a group of professionals, the transplant coordinators, with expertise in the field. In most cases the personnel in an institution who recognize that a patient may be a potential donor need only to call their regional OPA, and much of the subsequent responsibility (as detailed below) is then assumed by them, thus freeing busy physicians and nurses to pursue their own tasks.

Organ Donor Identification

Organ donation should be considered whenever death is imminent in an individual free of transmissible disease, such as sepsis and malignancy. It should be possible to sustain perfusion of the vital organs until the final determination is made. In practical terms, the cause of death is usually a sudden intracranial event, such as trauma or a cerebrovascular accident. There is no absolute age requirement; organs from 80-year-old donors have been successfully transplanted. Although one organ may be known to be diseased, others may be salvageable (e.g., the kidneys from an alcoholic with cirrhosis). Any organ that is to be used must have normal function and be unaffected by disease or trauma. A kidney donor must generally be free of renal disease, hypertension, or systemic diseases known to affect kidneys. Different criteria apply for donation of other organs (Table 16.2). For example, in addition to absence of disease affecting the organs, heart, liver, and lung transplants must be matched in size to the prospective recipient. Finally, consent of the next of kin is required in the United States before organs are removed. In some European countries, organ removal is permitted so long as the family does not raise an objection.

Declaration of Death

In the United States cadaver donors are determined to be dead by cerebral criteria ("brain death"), but circulation and ventilation are artificially maintained until or-

TABLE 16.2. *Criteria for exclusion of organ donors[a]*

Criterion	Kidney	Heart	Liver	Pancreas
Age (years)	>70	>50	>70	>50
Malignancy	+	+	+	+
Sepsis	+	+	+	+
Intravenous drug abuse	+	+	+	+
+Hepatitis B or C, HIV	+	+	+	+
Prolonged hypotension	+	+	+	+
DIC	+	+	+	+
Donor size incompatible	−	+	+	−
Abnormal ECG	−	+	−	−
Abnormal BUN, creatinine	±	−	−	−
Abnormal LFT	−	±	+	−

HIV, human immunodeficiency virus; DIC, disseminated intravascular coagulopathy; ECG, electrocardiogram; BUN, blood urea nitrogen; LFT, liver function tests.

[a]The crisis in organ availability prompts continued reevaluation of criteria. For example, kidneys from older donors or those with known hypertension or diabetes may not be ruled out. A biopsy is often done; and based on the degree of glomerular senescence or arteriolar disease, a decision may be made to use the kidney for an older recipient. Some have advocated using two suboptimal kidneys in a single recipient to provide adequate renal mass.

gan removal. The advantage of pronouncement by cerebral criteria is that the operative procedure is carried out under controlled circumstances, and retrieved organs are therefore in better condition. Without such criteria, donors are taken to the operating room, artificial support is discontinued, and organs are harvested after cessation of heartbeat. Under these circumstances, the chance of retrieving viable organs is reduced dramatically.

Cerebral criteria for death are as follows: (a) The cause of brain damage must be known. (b) There must be no brain-generated response to any neural stimulus (Table 16.3). These findings must occur under circumstances of normothermia and in the absence of drugs that may depress brain function, such as alcohol and barbiturates. When these clinical criteria are met, they can be confirmed by the finding of an isoelectric electroencephalogram (EEG) or a radionuclide scan or cerebral arteriogram that demonstrates an absence of cerebral blood flow. There is a clear distinction made between death and coma. However hopeless the prognosis for recovery of cerebral function, the diagnosis of death cannot be made unless all criteria are rigidly observed.

Maintenance of the Potential Donor

Once a potential donor has been identified, considerable time may elapse before death can be diagnosed with certainty and consent obtained. During this time, care and maintenance of the donor is critical. Most donors by this time are dehydrated, so massive fluid infusion is required. There may have been blood loss, which must be replaced, and the administration of colloid, together with diuretics, may be indicated. The choice of intravenous fluid is dictated by the circumstances; initially, isotonic solutions such as normal saline or lactated Ringer's solution may be required. If diabetes insipidus has set in, sodium is avoided, and dilute glucose solutions are used; if the volume of dilute urine is too great to be effectively replaced, the administration of pitressin may be necessary. The need to maintain good diuresis to preserve kidney function must be balanced against the possibility of fluid overload, which may compromise the heart or liver. The use of vasopressors also requires discretion. In all patients, meticulous asepsis must be observed in the care of catheters, endotracheal tubes, and so on. Blood chemistries should be obtained to monitor the function of liver, kidneys, and pancreas; cultures of blood and of other sites should be obtained to determine the presence

TABLE 16.3. *Criteria for absence of brain function*

No pupillary response to light
No corneal reflex
No eye movement with doll's eyes or caloric testing
No motor response to supraorbital pain
No cough reflex
Apnea

of infection. Finally, serologic tests for hepatitis B and C, CMV, and HIV should be obtained. When all the preliminaries have been completed, the donor is sometimes pretreated with cytotoxic drugs, such as cyclophosphamide and methylprednisolone in the hope of favorably influencing the kidneys after transplantation by destroying "passenger leukocytes."

Retrieval of Organs

As with any other surgical operation, cadaver donor nephrectomy must be conducted with maximum care, minimum blood loss, and preservation of all vital structures. This is even more important (and more difficult) when multiple organs are retrieved, which is increasingly the norm.

An incision is made from the sternal notch to the pubis. The chest and abdomen are opened simultaneously. A thoracic team isolates the great vessels and passes vessel tapes around them in preparation for removal. Simultaneously, an abdominal team dissects and isolates the blood supply to the liver: The isolation of hepatic artery or arteries and portal vein must be done without compromise to other viscera, such as the pancreas and kidneys. The distal aorta is encircled, and supraceliac dissection is done for placement of a clamp. When all preliminary dissection has been completed, the patient is heparinized, the distal aorta is cannulated, the aorta is cross-clamped above the celiac axis, and preservation solution is flushed into the distal aorta, cooling all abdominal organs. Outflow is provided by venting the vena cava above the diaphragm. The thoracic team simultaneously cools and removes the heart. The abdominal organs are removed sequentially, with the blood vessels to each being carefully preserved. Once the needed organs are removed and packaged, the spleen and a large number of lymph nodes are also removed to provide a source of lymphocytes for HLA typing and crossmatching.

When the kidneys alone are to be retrieved, the abdomen is opened through a full midline incision, which may be converted to a cruciate incision. The right colon is mobilized and, together with the small intestine, retracted above and to the donor's left. The aorta and vena cava are visualized and traced up to the renal arteries and veins. The superior mesenteric artery is identified, ligated, and divided. Dissection is continued cephalad on the aorta to allow room for a clamp or a tie proximal

to the renal arteries. Both kidneys are mobilized, so they are attached only by the renal vessels to the aorta and vena cava. Care is taken to preserve the ureters throughout their length and to leave a sheath of adventitial tissue attached to them. The ureters are divided close to the bladder. The donor is given 20,000 units of heparin, and the distal aorta is cannulated. The aorta and vena cava are ligated and divided distally and then mobilized cephalad by dividing pairs of lumbar vessels between clips until both kidneys are now completely free and attached only by the proximal aorta and vena cava. At this point a clamp is placed across the proximal aorta, and cold preservation solution is flushed through the aortic cannula. The vena cava, which is also clamped proximally, is opened distally to provide outflow. In this fashion, both kidneys may rapidly be flushed free of blood and cooled. Once cooling is accomplished, the aorta and vena cava are transected proximally; the kidneys are removed, immersed in cold solution, and then separated and packaged in sterile insulated containers immersed in ice for transportation.

Preservation

Preservation of solid organs is based on the premise that deep hypothermia reduces metabolic requirements. The initial step is for all solid organs to be flushed *in situ* using iced preservation solution (via cannulation of the distal aorta in the donor, as already discussed). Reduction of the core temperature to 0°C causes cellular metabolism to slow by a factor of 12 to 13 and the requirements for ATP and oxygen to be reduced markedly. However, the anaerobic state leads to acidosis and paralysis of the Na-K pump, which increases interstitial edema and causes cell swelling and ultimately cell death.

The ideal preservation solution minimizes cell swelling, prevents intracellular acidosis, and restricts interstitial expansion during the perfusion period. It also prevents injury from oxygen-derived free radicals and provides a substrate for the generation of high energy phosphate compounds during the reperfusion period. The solution that comes the closest to achieving these goals is the University of Wisconsin (UW) lactobionate solution. It contains impermeable osmotic agents (potassium lactobionate and raffinose) that minimize cell swelling and exert an effective oncotic pressure to reduce interstitial swelling, a hydrogen ion buffer (phosphate), and precursors for ATP production (adenosine). It also contains glutathione and allopurinol to counteract oxygen free radical injury. Preservation time using UW solution has been extended up to 72 hours for the kidney and pancreas and up to 30 hours for the liver. Therefore UW solution has largely supplanted Collins solution for solid organ preservation.

The University of Wisconsin preservation solution has the following ingredients:

Component	Action
Potassium lactobionate	Osmotic agent
Raffinose	Osmotic agent
Phosphate	Buffer
Adenosine	Precursor to ATP production
Glutathione	Free radical scavenger
Allopurinol	Free radical scavenger

As an alternative to cold storage, kidneys may also be preserved by pulsatile perfusion. After being flushed and cooled, the kidneys are connected via a cannula in the aorta or renal artery to the pulsatile perfusion apparatus. A plasma solution or modified UW solution is perfused through the cannula; it emerges through the renal vein and is collected in a chamber in which flow can be measured. After filtration and aeration, it is recirculated. Temperature is maintained at 4°C. In addition to providing a longer preservation time, this method permits measurement of pressure and flow and can thus provide a means of assessing viability. Preservation for more than 72 hours is regularly achieved. These extended preservation times allow a kidney to be sent anywhere in the world. It should be cautioned, however, that in prospective randomized clinical trials comparing perfusion and static storage in matched-donor pairs little significant difference has been shown between the two methods. Therefore from an immunologic, economic, and functional point of view, for routine preservation static storage is the norm.

SURGICAL TECHNIQUES FOR RENAL TRANSPLANTATION

The standard approach for transplantation of the kidney is through an extraperitoneal incision in the iliac fossa. The peritoneum is retracted medially, and the iliac vessels are exposed. The renal vein is usually anastomosed end to side into the external iliac vein. The renal artery may be similarly anastomosed to the external iliac artery or anastomosed end-to-end to the divided hypogastric artery. The vascular clamps are then released. When good flow to the kidney is confirmed, the ureter is attached to the bladder using an antireflux implantation. Modification of the technique may be required because of the presence of vascular disease, urologic abnormalities, or gross disparity in size, such as an adult kidney in an infant. In the latter case, the vascular anastomoses are done to the aorta and the vena cava through a standard midline incision. Care must be taken that hemostasis is absolute. If possible, division of large lymphatics is avoided; if unavoidable, these lymphatics must be ligated to prevent the occurrence of a lymphocele. Frequent, liberal irrigation of the wound is carried out with antiseptic solution. If surgical drains are used, they should be of the closed suction variety.

Of equal importance to surgical technique is management of the recipient before and during the operation. Most patients should be dialyzed within the 24 to 48 hours preceding the operation to ensure optimum body chemistry. Perioperative prophylactic antibiotics are given. Some immunosuppressives are more effective if started preoperatively. Caution should be exercised in the use of anesthetic agents that are predominantly excreted by the kidney, with special reference to muscle relaxants: A patient with acute tubular necrosis may otherwise have respiratory paralysis for an extended period. Attention must also be given to adequate fluid management. Despite renal failure, recipients may be fluid-depleted as a result of preoperative dialysis, intraoperative blood and insensible loss, and perhaps a large urine volume from the newly transplanted kidney. Inadequate administration of fluid may result in renal shutdown. We routinely monitor the central venous pressure as a guide to fluid and diuretic therapy. It is customary to administer diuretics after the vascular clamps are released in the recipient. Mannitol and furosemide are usually given singly or in combination. Finally, those who have not received any immunosuppressive agents prior to the procedure should receive them during the operation.

TRANSPLANTATION IMMUNOLOGY

The long-term success of transplantation depends on the prevention of graft rejection while at the same time preserving the ability of the recipient to respond to other foreign antigens. For the most part, the immune process is mediated through the actions of lymphocytes. Totipotent cells of the bone marrow differentiate into precursors of the various cellular elements of the blood. Lymphocytes undergo maturation in the thymus (T cells) or in various areas, such as bone marrow, spleen, and Peyer's patches (B cells). B cells are large and short-lived, whereas T lymphocytes are small and long-lived.

The multiple roles of T cells may be classified according to function: cytotoxic cells (T_C) whose principal function is to effect destruction; helper cells (T_H), which aid in the differentiation of other lymphocytes; and suppressor cells (T_S) which curb cytotoxic functions and thus permit tolerance. The T_S cells act as a balance to the T_C cells. T lymphocytes are better classified by specific cell surface antigens, known as cluster of differentiation (CD) receptors. Many CD antigens exist, but CD4 and CD8 are probably the best known. They generally, but not absolutely, correspond to the functional description of the T cells. Generally, T_H cells are CD4+ and react with class II molecules (e.g., HLA DR), whereas T_C cells are usually CD8+ and react with class I molecules, HLA A and B. All T cells also carry the cell antigen recognition complex, CD3+.

The T cells diffuse through body tissues, entering the bloodstream from the thymus. They enter the lymph nodes through venules and afferent lymphatic channels. Lymphocytes leave the nodes via efferent lymphatics, which merge with other channels, to enter the bloodstream via the thoracic duct. Because lymph flowing into the nodes also contains antigens and dendritic cells, the stage is set for the first encounter in the immune response. Foreign antigen can directly stimulate small numbers of T_H, T_C, and B cells to perform their respective functions, but rejection appears to depend mostly on the effects of lymphokines (Fig 16.1.).

Normally quiescent, T cells require two separate signals to become activated. A foreign antigen is ingested by an antigen presenting cell (APC), usually a macrophage or dendritic cell, which processes it in a way that permits recognition by the clone of T_H cells that possess the CD3 complex specific for that antigen. With the double signals from the APC and the antigen, interleukin (IL)-1 is secreted, stimulating the clone of T_H cells to proliferate and release IL-2. This is a critical point in the process. IL-2 is essential for the further differentiation and proliferation of antigen-stimulated T_C cells. It also acts as a stimulus for the further prolifera-

tion of T_H cells, escalating the process and becoming self-perpetuating. IL-2 stimulates interferon (IFN), which mobilizes macrophages and causes many cells to increase their expression of MHC antigens on the surface, thereby increasing their vulnerability. Finally, IL-2 is necessary for the stimulation of resting B cells to proliferate and differentiate into plasma cells, which produce antibodies. Inhibition of IL-2 may therefore play a significant role in the abrogation of the immune response. In addition to the processes described, some T_H cells remain as memory cells for future response to the same antigen; T_S cells are also stimulated to proliferate and act as a balance to the cytotoxic cells.

The CD4+ T lymphocytes have been subdivided into two groups: T_H1 and T_H2. It is hypothesized that the T_H1 cells produce IFNγ, which stimulates the endothelial cells and the APCs, and that they secrete IL-2, which stimulates the activation of T cells. The second group of CD4+ cells is the T_H2 cells. These cells produce IL-4 and IL-10, both of which inhibit differentiation of the T_H1 cell line. The importance of this division of the CD4+ cells is that the propagation of the T_H1 cell line may be responsible for acute cellular rejection, whereas maturation of the T_H2 cell line may induce tolerance, or at least nonresponsiveness (anergy), to the allograft. Much work is being done to further elucidate this process.

Cell adhesion molecules are now recognized as integral in the acute rejection process. The activation of T cells and endothelial cells causes up-regulation and expression of various cell adhesion molecules. These cell adhesion molecules are part of the integrin family and are important not only in the migration of T cells but also in promoting activation of the lymphocytes. One such molecule is CD28. The interaction between this T cell antigen with the B7 molecule on APCs is thought to be important for the activation of T cells. A soluble homolog of the CD28 molecule, CTLA4, is currently being actively investigated in an attempt to induce nonresponsiveness to the allograft. Some of the other common cell adhesion molecules are listed in Table 16.4.

If unchecked, the immune process continues until the antigen is destroyed by two mechanisms: cellular rejection, through the agency of lymphokines (e.g., tumor necrosis factor); and humoral rejection, caused by soluble antibodies released through the activation of B cells. Numerous lymphokines (including interleukins) have been identified. The acquisition of this knowledge

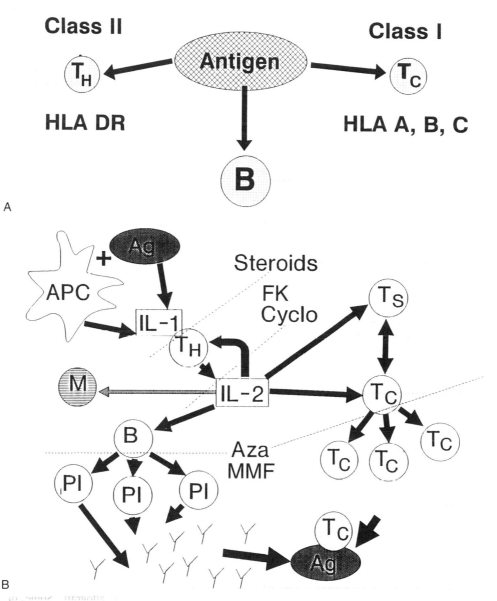

FIG. 16.1. A: Immune response: antigen-activated cells. Class I molecules of the antigen (usually HLA A,B,C) stimulate CD8+cytotoxic cells (Tc); class II (HLA DR) stimulate CD4+helper cells (T$_H$). B cells are also stimulated directly. **B:** Immune response: lymphokine activated cells. Action of immunosuppressive agents. Antigen (Ag) and antigen-presenting cells (APC) send separate signals, which cause interleukin (IL)-1 to be secreted by the helper (T$_H$) cell. T$_H$ secretes IL-2, which (i) stimulates further proliferation of T$_H$; (ii) stimulates B cells to differentiate into plasma cells (Pl), which secret antibody; (iii) stimulate cytotoxic (T$_C$) cells to proliferate; (iv) cause T$_S$ cells to proliferate while maintaining a balance with T$_C$ cells; and (v) causes some T$_H$ cells to become memory cells (M) to react to future stimuli. *Dotted lines* show action of drugs: Corticosteroids act by blocking production of IL-1, cyclosporine (*Cyclo*) and tacrolimus (FK) by blocking IL-2, and Azathioprine (*AzA*) and mycophenolate mofetil (MMF) by inhibiting cell proliferation.

TABLE 16.4. *Common cell adhesion molecules*

T cells	Antigen-presenting cells
LFA-1 (CD 11a/18)	ICAM-1 (CD 54), ICAM-2
CD 28	B7–1 (CD 80), B7–2 (CD 86)
CTLA4	B7–2 (CD 86), B7–1 (CD 80)
VLA-4 (CD 49d/29)	VCAM-1 (CD 106)

has provided numerous opportunities for intervention, which can be considered under two categories: *prevention* of rejection and *treatment* of rejection.

PREVENTING REJECTION

Except between identical twins, transplantation without immunosuppression is uniformly unsuccessful. The earlier approaches—massive steroid doses, total body irradiation, and thoracic duct drainage—have largely given way to more selective immunosuppression, in smaller doses.

Until 1984, two drugs (prednisone and azathioprine) formed the cornerstone of immunosuppressive therapy; since then cyclosporine has become the mainstay. In addition, polyclonal and monoclonal antibodies, although mainly used to treat rejection, are also used as part of induction protocols. Cyclosporine is the drug of choice; it is usually given with low-dose steroids, often in combination with azathioprine (Table 16.5).

1. *Corticosteroids.* These agents block the activation of IL-1 and thus indirectly IL-2. They also have an anti-inflammatory effect, which may help minimize the rejection injury (IL-1 was previously called endogenous pyrogen). Most centers now use a low-dosage schedule (e.g., total daily dose of 25 mg/day achieved within the first month), which has resulted in a significant decline in complications while kidney and patient survival has improved. The dose is tapered until a low maintenance level is achieved. In children and selected adults, total withdrawal of steroids may be possible.

2. *Cyclosporine.* Cyclosporine (CsA), a fat-soluble extract of fungal origin, has revolutionized transplantation since the first reports of its clinical use in 1978. It blocks secretion of IL-2, the essential stimulus to the further proliferation and differentiation of T cells. Cyclosporine has been found to work only on resting T cells, not activated ones. CsA binds to its intracellular binding protein, cyclophilin. Cyclophilin is an example of a class of intracellular receptors found in T cells known as immunophilins. Two such proteins have been described: cyclophilin and FK binding protein (see below). This CsA–cyclophilin complex, in turn, inhibits calcineurin. Calcineurin is an enzyme involved in the activation of genes responsible for the immune response by a mechanism that has not yet been elucidated. By inhibiting calcineurin, CsA blocks secretion of IL-2. It must be administered intravenously or orally in an oil-based solution or in capsules.

It was initially hoped that CsA alone would be effective, but rejection usually ensues unless a second agent is given. In the United States CsA is used with small doses of corticosteroids. Unfortunately, CsA is nephrotoxic, and its use in renal transplantation can cause clinical dilemmas. With cadaver kidneys, early graft dysfunction often occurs; and to avoid toxicity it is common not to use CsA until good renal function has been established. During this period of uncertainty, the use of antilymphocyte globulin (ALG or ATG) or

TABLE 16.5. *Immunosuppressive agents*

Agent	Action	Toxicity
Corticosteroids	Blocks IL-1	Physical appearance, hyperglycemia, avascular necrosis of bone
Cyclosporine A	Blocks IL-2	Hepatotoxicity, nephrotoxicity, hirsutism, gingival hyperplasia, hypertension
Azathioprine	Blocks cell proliferation	Bone marrow suppression, hepatotoxicity
Antilymphocyte globulin (ALG)	Lymphocytolytic	Thrombocytopenia, leukopenia, fever, serum sickness
OKT3	Blocks T cell effector function	High fever, chills, GI symptoms, pulmonary edema
Tacrolimus (FK506)	Blocks IL-2	Tremors, headache, nephrotoxicity, glucose intolerance, hyperkalemia
Mycophenolate mofetil	Blocks cell proliferation	Nausea, vomiting, diarrhea

muromonab cd3 (OKT3) offers a high degree of protection against rejection until the kidney has recovered sufficient function for CsA to be started. Later in the course, an elevated serum creatinine level may pose a problem: It may be due to CsA toxicity, which would require reduction of CsA dosage; or it may be secondary to acute rejection, which would mandate augmented immunosuppression. When the clinical circumstances are unclear, measurement of blood levels of CsA may be helpful; needle biopsy of the kidney can also be useful by establishing the presence or absence of rejection.

3. *Tacrolimus (FK 506)*. Tacrolimus is a macrolide antibiotic derived from a fungal source. Although structurally dissimilar to CsA, its mechanism of action is similar. Essentially, both work by blocking IL-2 expression and production. Like CsA, FK 506 works by binding to its cytoplasmic receptor, FK binding protein (FKBP). In a mechanism similar to that described for CsA–cyclophilin, FK–FKBP inhibits the T cell's calcineurin, which in turn renders the T cell unable to produce IL-2. Tacrolimus is approximately 500 times more potent than CsA.

Originally used to rescue patients suffering from steroid- or OKT3-resistant rejection, FK 506 has become one of the basic immunosuppressive agents used for liver allograft recipients. In the renal allograft recipient, FK 506 has mainly been used to treat patients as rescue therapy (i.e., to rescue patients with steroid- or OKT3-resistant acute rejection). Several prospective, randomized clinical trials have demonstrated that the efficacies of CsA and FK506 as initial therapy after renal allograft transplantation are similar. These studies have shown that (a) the nephrotoxicities of the two agents were similar; (b) there was decreased hypertension, cholesterol, gingival hyperplasia, and change in physical appearance; but (c) there was increased neurotoxicity (e.g., headaches, paresthesias) and pancreatic beta-cell toxicities (insulin requiring diabetes mellitus) with FK506.

Tacrolimus may be given as an initial intravenous dose but usually is switched within 24 hours to an oral formulation. Tacrolimus and CsA are not given together, as their mechanisms of action are similar, and when used in combination they may have an increased nephrotoxic effect. Like CsA, FK506 is metabolized in the liver. The therapeutic window for this agent is narrow so it is important to monitor the blood levels in patients on FK506.

Cyclosporine and FK are both metabolized through the cytochrome P-450 enzyme system of the liver, as are many commonly used therapeutic agents. Thus the use of erythromycin or ketoconazole may result in augmentation of the effect of CsA and FK and possibly toxicity, whereas rifampin and diphenylhydantoin may cause a reduction of the CsA and FK level and precipitate rejection. One must always be alert to the possibility of drug interactions in patients on either of these agents.

4. *Azathioprine*. Azathioprine (AZA), one of the earliest agents, continues to play a role in transplantation. A derivative of 6-mercaptopurine, it is an antimetabolite that acts more peripherally in the immune process by blocking DNA synthesis and by inhibiting cell division. The action is nonspecific and affects all dividing cells. Bone marrow suppression is a common complication, and the white blood cell (WBC) count must be monitored carefully.

The clinical difficulties often encountered with the use of CsA have led many centers to adopt a "triple therapy" protocol, wherein all three agents (prednisone, AZA, CsA) are used in relatively small doses, thereby minimizing the toxic effects, and the immunosuppressive effects are additive. Because each works at a different point in the process, it is an appealing approach. It also offers some protection if one of the agents must be discontinued.

5. *Mycophenolate mofetil*. A modified ester of mycophenolic acid (a fermentation product of several *Penicillium* species), mycophenolate mofetil (MMF) is effective when taken orally. Essentially, MMF blocks *de novo* purine synthesis. Unlike most cells, lymphocytes (T and B) rely on this pathway more than the salvage pathway for purine synthesis, and so MMF prevents T and B cell proliferation. MMF also appears to decrease smooth muscle proliferation within blood vessels. Its mechanism of action is similar to that of azathioprine in that both agents are antiproliferative medications. Its efficacy against acute and chronic rejection is being studied actively in clinical trials, and its immunosuppressive effects and smooth muscle effects make this agent attractive for combating chronic rejection. Currently, MMF is being used at many centers as part of the primary immunosuppressive regimen. It has also been used in patients with chronic rejection and for acute rejection that is refractory to standard therapy. Azathioprine and MMF are not used together because they are both antiproliferative agents.

There are several known adverse effects of MMF, the most prominent being gastrointestinal effects (diarrhea, nausea, vomiting) and dose-responsive leukopenia and thrombocytopenia.

6. *Antilymphocyte globulin.* Antilymphocyte globulin (ALG) or antithymocyte globulin (ATG) is an antiserum to human lymphocytes, created in animals (rabbits, horses, goats). The globulin fraction is extracted from the serum of the animal and contains a potent polyclonal antilymphocyte antibody that acts by destroying or masking T cell antigens; it may also promote the development of suppressor cells. It is relatively nonselective and has effects on other cellular elements of the blood. Administered in dilute intravenous solution into a central vein, it has three principal uses: induction therapy, initial prophylaxis during a period of graft dysfunction, and treatment for established acute rejection.

7. *Muromonab cd3 (OKT3).* Among the first of a new generation of products, OKT3 is a hybridoma product. It is engineered by fusion of a strain of immortal mouse myeloma cells with cells from a mouse immunized against human lymphocytes. Cells selected for their specific activity against the CD3 antigen recognition complex are then propagated. The resultant monoclonal antibody is specific, consistent, and predictable. It is not subject to biologic variability like the polyclonal ALG and does not affect the other cellular elements of blood. One of the disadvantages is the fact that antibodies develop against the mouse antibody (antiidiotype antibodies), which renders the product ineffective after some time. Other adverse effects are the initial physiologic reactions to the first few doses of OKT3, including fever, diarrhea, and sometimes bronchospasm, pulmonary edema, and meningeal irritation. Thus patients must be adequately prepared by diuresis or dialysis to remove excess fluid and by premedication to mitigate the severity of the initial response. OKT3 is most useful for treatment of acute rejection; but like ALG, it is occasionally used for initial prophylaxis or induction.

New Agents

Sirolimus (rapamycin). Rapamycin is another macrolide antibiotic derived from a fungal source found in Rappanui (Easter Islands). This agent is structurally similar to FK 506, but its mechanism of action is different. Unlike FK 506, rapamycin does not block IL-2 expression and production; rather, it blocks cytokine-mediated signal transduction (e.g., IL-2 and IL-2 receptors), thereby preventing cell proliferation. Because the mechanism of action is different from that of CsA, and because rapamycin and CsA appear to block cell proliferation at different steps, there is much work focusing on using these two agents in combination. It is thought that CsA and rapamycin may work synergistically, and that the dose requirements of the two agents can be reduced without compromising adequate immunosuppression. Unlike CsA and FK 506, nephrotoxicity has not been demonstrated. Currently, rapamycin is undergoing clinical trials with a great deal of success.

Deoxyspergualine and *leflunomide.* Many new immunosuppressive agents are being created and tested. Two such agents include deoxyspergualine and leflunomide. Briefly, deoxyspergualine is an agent whose mode of immunosuppression targets monocytes/macrophages rather than T lymphocytes. It is thought that this drug might be synergistic with agents already approved for organ transplantation. Leflunomide inhibits proliferation of activated T and B cells by an unknown mechanism, although different from CsA and FK 506. Clinical trials have been initiated.

Other Approaches

In addition to chemical agents, experimental efforts are being directed toward biologic methods to induce tolerance. Administration of donor bone marrow simultaneously with the organ and selective irradiation of the recipient prior to transplantation are two such ap-

TABLE 16.6. *Criteria for categorizing rejection*

Type	Mechanism	Pathology
Hyperacute	Circulating antibodies	Endothelial swelling, platelet thrombi, glomerular and arteriolar thrombosis, fibrinoid necrosis
Acute	Cell-mediated	Edema, lymphocytic infiltration, hemorrhage
Chronic	? Antibody-mediated	Endothelial thickening, fibrosis, vascular occlusion

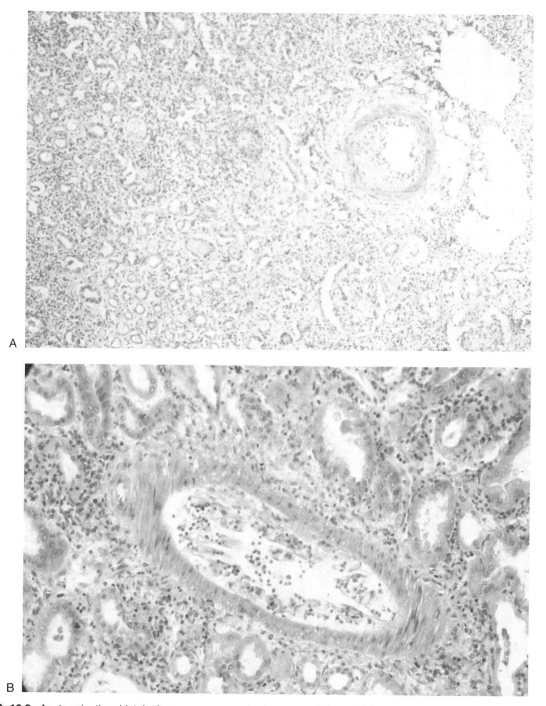

FIG. 16.2. Acute rejection: histologic appearance, under low power (**A**) and high power (**B**) light microscopy, of a core-needle biopsy specimen of kidney. Note edema and diffuse infiltration with mononuclear lymphocytes; vasculitis is manifested by infiltration and endothelial swelling and proliferation. Glomeruli show swelling, but the architecture is preserved. (H&E)

proaches. New, highly specific monoclonal antibodies are being designed to disable the mechanisms specific to the graft while leaving all other mechanisms intact. Because recognition of a foreign antigen requires two signals, blocking one of them is a potential avenue to creating tolerance. CTLA4Ig is a synthetic agent that competes for the CD-28 binding site on the lymphocyte. Because it has great avidity for the ligand, it has been successfully used experimentally to create tolerance. Clinical trials in humans are under way.

REJECTION

Classification

Total abolition of the immune response is impractical and undesirable, so rejection occurs despite prophylactic drug regimens. It is frequently simplified into "humoral" and "cellular" types, but there is considerable overlap.

Pure humoral (*hyperacute*) rejection occurs when a kidney is transplanted into a patient who has circulating antibodies to donor antigens. These antibodies attack the vascular endothelium of the graft, resulting in endothelial damage, platelet aggregation, and rapid vascular occlusion of the graft (Table 16.6).

More common is the *acute rejection* "crisis." This process requires recognition of a foreign antigen by host lymphocytes, the creation of effector cells, and finally the destruction or attempted destruction of the graft. Although more common during the first few months after transplantation, acute rejection can occur at any time. Histologic examination of acute rejection reveals massive infiltration of the interstitium, tubules (tubulitis), glomeruli (glomerulitis), and vascular endothelium (arteritis) with lymphocytes and monocytes, together with edema and some protein deposition within Bowman's space (Fig. 16.2). It should be noted that severe, transmural arteritis involving the whole arterial wall (endothelium, medial smooth muscles, media) involves not only lymphocytes and mononuclear cells, but also polymorphonuclear leukocytes. To standardize how pathologists and transplant physicians around the world define rejection and attempt to elucidate the most effective immunosuppressive regimen for patients suffering acute rejection, the Banff classification was developed. Renal biopsies are graded in ascending order depending on the severity of the acute rejection (Table 16.7).

Finally, *chronic rejection* is a process that takes place over weeks, months, or years. It consists of gradual restriction of the blood supply, starting with subendothelial thickening and fibrosis, and resulting in eventual

TABLE 16.7. *Banff classification for renal allograft biopsies*

Category	Definition	Pathology
Normal	No abnormalities	No glomerular abnormalities; no cellular infiltration; no tubulitis; no vascular abnormalities
Hyperacute rejection	Immediate rejection (within hours)	Abnormalities in glomerular and peritubular capillaries at 1 hour after transplant; subsequent endothelial damage and capillary thrombosis
Borderline changes	Suggestive of rejection (nondiagnostic)	No intimal arteritis present, but mild or moderate focal mononuclear cell infiltration seen; mild tubulitis and/or mild glomerulitis present
Acute rejection		
Grade I	Mild rejection	Moderate, focal, or diffuse interstitial infiltration and moderate tubulitis and/or moderate glomerulitis
Grade IIA	Moderate rejection	Severe interstitial infiltration and moderate or severe tubulitis (but no arteritis), and/or severe glomerulitis regardless of degree of interstitial infiltration
Grade IIB	Moderate rejection	Mild or moderate intimal arteritis irrespective of the degree of interstitial infiltration
Grade IIIA	Severe rejection	Severe inimal arteritis regardless of other changes (but lacking transmural arteritis); possibly recent infarction, interstitial hemorrhage, and capillary thrombosis
Grade IIIB	Severe rejection	Same as grade IIIA but with transmural arteritis with fibrinoid change and necrosis of medial smooth muscle cells

Source: ISN Commission on Acute Renal Failure Meeting, Banff, Alberta, Canada, 1991 (revised 3/92).

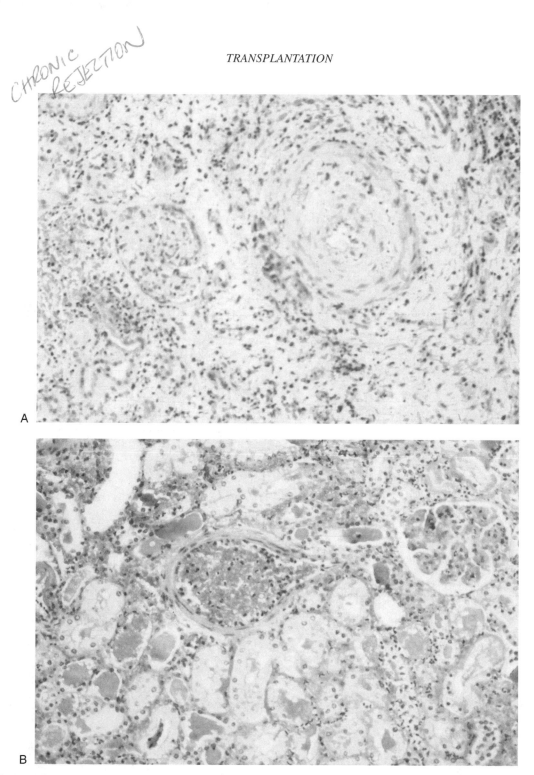

A

B

FIG. 16.3. Chronic rejection: histologic appearance of core-needle biopsy specimen of kidney under low power (**A**) and high power (**B**) light microscopy. Note in (**A**) the extensive fibrosis, almost total obliteration of the vascular lumen by proliferative endarteritis, areas of tubular atrophy, and patchy lymphocytic infiltrate. (H&E)

loss of the kidney (Fig. 16.3). It is probably caused by the action of humoral antibodies.

Diagnosis and Treatment

Hyperacute rejection, usually apparent in the operating room, presents as a rapid vascular occlusion that occurs despite an apparently patent anastomosis. The manifestations may be delayed by some hours, in which case it presents as rapid loss of function of the graft. Investigations such as radionuclide scanning, duplex sonography, and arteriography demonstrate the loss of blood supply. There is no treatment, and the syndrome requires immediate removal of the graft; it is usually, but not always, prevented by a reliable crossmatch.

Chronic rejection also has no treatment and is a diagnosis of exclusion. Care must be exercised that some treatable lesion is not missed. When a patient who has apparently had good function for a period of time demonstrates gradual deterioration of renal function, the cause must be investigated. In the absence of any other explanation, such as renal artery stenosis or ureteral stenosis, the diagnosis of chronic rejection may be assumed and can be confirmed by biopsy. Because there is no treatment, immunosuppression is continued until such time that the patient once again requires dialysis or can receive a new transplant.

An acute rejection crisis is usually an easily recognizable syndrome, consisting of the combination of an acute inflammatory response and acute renal failure. The patient may have fever, tenderness over the graft site, and leukocytosis, as well as oliguria, hypertension, proteinuria, and an elevated serum creatinine level. The clinical syndrome may be mild, such as a minimal rise in creatinine or a minor elevation in temperature with no other clinical symptomatology; and the diagnosis is sometimes difficult to establish. It is important that other causes of some of these findings are not missed. A urinary leak may cause localized pain and tenderness, fever, leukocytosis, and oliguria. Viral infection (e.g., with CMV) can similarly present with fever and creatinine elevation. Increased steroid dosage, in a mistaken attempt to treat rejection, would obviously be disastrous under these circumstances. In ambiguous clinical situations rejection may be confirmed by (a) radionuclide scans, which may demonstrate deterioration of function compared to a previous similar study; (b) duplex sonography, with which the degree of vascular re-

sistance within the kidney can be assessed; and (c) biopsy, which may reveal a classic picture of acute cellular rejection. (Abnormal fluid collections or extravasations would also be detected by these means.)

Acute rejection can usually be reversed with treatment. The most common method of treatment consists of administering high doses of steroids for a short time, orally or intravenously. If azathioprine has been used as a basic immunosuppressive agent, the dose may have to be reduced because it is partly excreted through the kidney. If steroid therapy fails, it may be prudent to biopsy the kidney, if it has not already been done, before initiating further treatment. At present, most centers use 10 to 14 daily doses of OKT3 to treat steroid resistant rejection. During this time cyclosporine is withheld, and azathioprine is given in small doses, the latter to retard the development of antiidiotypic (antimouse antibody) antibodies. Antilymphocyte globulin is also an effective method of treatment for rejection; and prior to the availability of OKT3 it was the drug of choice for steroid-resistant rejection. Because its administration requires insertion of a central venous catheter and prolonged hospitalization, its use has diminished. Additional treatment methods now include the use of tacrolimus, which may be used for treatment as well as prophylaxis of rejection. It is given orally and is not associated with the side effects associated with antibody products, so it is an attractive alternative. Mycophenolate mofetil has also been used in some centers to treat rejection.

COMPLICATIONS OF TRANSPLANTATION

Complications of transplantation may be considered in three broad categories: complications due to the immunosuppressed state, those engendered by the surgical operation, and those due to the medications used.

Complications of the Immunosuppressed State

General impairment of host defenses occurs at extremes of age, in the presence of certain malignancies, after chemotherapy for malignancy, in patients with immune deficiency syndromes, and in patients immunosuppressed after transplantation. One consequence of immunosuppression is increased susceptibility to infection from all sources, including bacterial, viral, fungal, rickettsial, protozoan, and parasitic. Vigilance is therefore required during the management of these patients.

Aggressive evaluation is carried out for minor temperature elevations, and vague syndromes such as malaise and joint pains cannot be ignored.

Most infections, if diagnosed early, can be treated effectively with the appropriate agent. If infection is life-threatening (e.g., meningitis or severe viral pneumonia), immunosuppression is terminated to allow host defenses to recover. This may result in loss of the kidney, which is preferable to the death of the patient. For less severe infections, high doses of immunosuppressive drugs are usually reduced; if doses are already low, they are usually continued unless it is apparent that the therapeutic agent is not effectively reversing the infectious process. Whenever possible the specific agent for the bacteria, viruses, or parasites involved is administered. Infections after transplantation generally fall into predictable, sometimes preventable, patterns.

First Transplant Month

During the early postoperative period infections are those that may occur in any surgical patient (e.g., pneumonia, urinary tract infection, line sepsis). Special care must be exercised to prevent their occurrence and to treat any event rapidly and aggressively. Infection during this period may also result from donor causes inadvertently transmitted with the transplanted organ. Obviously, careful screening of donors is critical.

Reactivation of latent herpes simplex virus (HSV) can also begin during the early postoperative period. Viruses of this category can be controlled, though not eradicated, with the use of acyclovir.

One to Six Months

Opportunistic infections are most likely to manifest during the first 1 to 6 months. Cytomegalovirus (CMV) is a common viral infection, the clinical presentation of which ranges from a mild nonspecific febrile illness to lethal multiorgan failure. Milder forms may require no intervention or a modest reduction of immunosuppressive agents. Serious forms require aggressive management, including blood gas determination to detect hypoxia (before chest radiographs become abnormal) and pathologic diagnosis (by aspirate, bronchoscopy, or open lung biopsy) to confirm the disease.

Treatment then consists of cessation of immunosuppression except for stress doses of steroids and the ad-

ministration of hyperimmune serum and antiviral agents such as ganciclovir or foscarnet. Other viral infections (e.g., HSV, herpes zoster, and Epstein-Barr virus) are also likely to occur during this period. Acyclovir is useful for managing some of these problems. *Pneumocystis pneumoniae* seems to be more prevalent during the current CsA era, but prophylaxis with trimethoprim–sulfamethoxazole can effectively prevent it in most patients. As with CMV pneumonia, aggressive diagnostic measures are necessary when the diagnosis is suspected. Once established, treatment consists of intravenous trimethoprim–sulfisoxazole or pentamidine; respiratory support may also be necessary. *Other infections* include those caused by *Legionella, Listeria, Mycoplasma,* and various fungi.

After Six Months

Patients with stable graft function on low dose immunosuppression are usually free of problems except for simple urinary tract infections. Patients who have received high-dose therapy or repeated rejection treatment continue to be at risk for opportunistic infection. Of note are the late consequences of hepatitis: After as long as ten years of apparently normal life there is a high incidence of cirrhosis, which progresses to end-stage disease. The issue of whether patients who are carriers of hepatitis B should receive transplants must therefore be seriously examined.

There is also an increased risk of malignancy in all immunosuppressed patients. This is particularly true of skin malignancies, such as squamous cell and basal cell carcinomas and malignancies of the lymphoid system. The former are most notable in regions of excessive sunshine, such as southern California and Australia. Patients should be carefully monitored for new skin lesions, which must be aggressively removed as they appear. In regard to posttransplant lymphoproliferative disorder (PTLD), the general incidence of lymphoma ranges from 1% in kidney recipients to 4.5% in heart–lung recipients. Lymphomas constitute 22% of all cancers in transplant recipients, compared with 5% in the general population. PTLD occurs predominantly in extranodal sites, with a particularly high incidence of involvement of the central nervous system, which is rare in the general population. Rather than being associated with a particular drug, PTLD appears to be a consequence of heavy immunosuppression. Thus patients with prolonged or repeated courses of ALG or OKT3, especially if these agents are combined with others, are at greater risk. Oncogenic viruses such as Epstein-Barr (EBV) may play a role, especially in children. In addition to reducing immunosuppressive treatment, the use of antiviral agents, such as acyclovir, may help reduce the incidence. Once PTLD has occurred, 30% of the cases regress with treatment, such as withdrawal of immunosuppression, chemotherapy, excision, or treatment with agents such as interferons.

Complications of the Surgical Operation

After surgery hematomas, seromas, infections, and disruptions can occur as with any *wound.* The patient is predisposed to these complications by virtue of poor nutrition, edema, hypoproteinemia, platelet dysfunction, and anemia; and many of these conditions are exaggerated by the effects of steroids. Extra care is therefore taken in the conduct of the operation to control all sources of bleeding, handle tissue gently, and thoroughly irrigate the wound with antibacterial agents.

Faulty technique at the arterial or venous suture lines may compromise *blood supply* to the kidney, as no collateral vessels exist. When a kidney had been undergoing active diuresis in the operating room, but concern had existed regarding the vascular anastomoses (because of factors in host vessels, the recipient vessels, or technique), any sudden fall in urine output immediately postoperatively should arouse suspicion. Although vascular problems can be confirmed by duplex scanning or arteriography, by the time the diagnosis is confirmed it may be too late to reverse the process. If the index of suspicion is high, such a patient should be taken directly from the recovery room to the operating room in the hope of correcting the problem. Arterial complications may also occur long after transplantation. When a patient has had good function for a period of weeks, months, or years and presents with new hypertension or hypertension newly difficult to control, renal artery stenosis must be suspected. It may occur with normal serum creatinine and despite a normal radionuclide scan. Preliminary duplex sonography or scintigraphy before and after the administration of captopril may assist in the diagnosis, but arteriography is the only definitive test. If a lesion is found, it must be treated by balloon angioplasty or by operation. Venous thrombosis is occasionally seen as a late phenomenon; it manifests as proteinuria and sometimes ipsilateral edema. Its presence is confirmed by duplex scanning or venography. Treatment consists of heparinization, with or without attempts at thrombectomy.

Urinary complications account for most of the noninfectious problems (3% to 5%). During the early postoperative period obstruction may occur owing to a blood clot or malposition of the ureter during implantation. Urinary fistulas may develop at the site of implantation in the bladder or because of ischemic necrosis of the ureter, now entirely dependent for its blood supply on the renal artery. Such problems obviously require urgent surgical intervention. Obstruction may be treated by percutaneous insertion of a stent or by surgical reimplantation. Urinary fistulas usually require operation, which may range from simple reinforcement of a bladder implant site to reconstruction of a sloughed ureter. Nephrectomy is sometimes the safest alternative. Ureteral obstruction, due to extrinsic compression by lymphocele or to scarring, may also occur months after transplantation. Treatment, as during the acute period, may be by percutaneous or open surgical means; it is important to investigate late rises in serum creatinine, rather than making an assumption that what is occurring is untreatable chronic rejection.

The development of *lymphocele* is a particular possibility after transplantation. The lymph may arise from lower extremity lymphatics disrupted during the operation or from the kidney. It may present as a mass, as extrinsic compression on the ureter causing an elevation in creatinine, pain, or sometimes fever. Once the fluid is confirmed to be lymph, drainage is necessary, which may be done internally into the peritoneal cavity (by open operation or laparoscopically). Less desirable is insertion of an external drain, which must be left in for an extended period, and therefore is a potential source of infection.

The diagnosis of most surgical problems at the transplant site, including those mentioned above, is usually made with relative ease. Sonography, B-mode and duplex, provides clear visualization of the normal structures and of abnormal findings such as obstruction, collections, and occlusion. Radionuclide scanning offers additional help. Occasionally, the use of CT or magnetic resonance imaging (MRI) is required.

Specific Drug-Related Complications

Corticosteroids were responsible for most of the complications of transplantation in previous years, including changes in appearance (obesity, growth retardation, cushingoid habitus), aseptic necrosis of bone, cataracts, peptic ulcer disease, glucose intolerance, and hypertension. Many of these complications are dose-related, and with low-dose steroid regimens the incidence is rapidly decreasing, although steroid-induced diabetes still occurs.

Azathioprine, if administered in excessive doses, causes nonspecific depression of the bone marrow, resulting in leukopenia, thrombocytopenia, and anemia. Because azathioprine is partially excreted by the kidney, a dose that is well tolerated by a patient with normal renal function may become excessive during rejection. It is sometimes necessary, therefore, to reduce the dose of azathioprine when rejection occurs. A late complication of azathioprine is hepatotoxicity, which appears chemically as obstructive jaundice; a liver biopsy reveals bile deposits in the canaliculi. Both of these complications are usually reversed with cessation of the drug. Some patients also experience transient alopecia.

Cyclosporine principally causes renal and hepatic dysfunction, both of which usually respond to a decrease of the dose. Minor complications are hirsutism, tremors, gingival hyperplasia, hypertension, hyperkalemia, neuropathy, and hypercholesterolemia. The unpredictability of absorption, common with the old formulation, is less of an issue with the new microemulsion formulation (Neoral). It must be used cautiously with many commonly used therapeutic agents because of drug interactions.

Tacrolimus has adverse effects similar to those of CsA. The hyperkalemia and nephrotoxicity are similar to that caused by CsA and are usually dose-dependent. Neurologic side effects are common, including headaches, tremors, and insomnia. Glucose intolerance also occurs, sometimes requiring insulin. On the other hand, hirsutism, gingival hyperplasia, and hypercholesterolemia are not commonly seen.

Muromonab cd3 (OKT3), as with all biologic agents, can induce anaphylaxis. Problems include the severe cytokine release syndrome with initial use, including fever, diarrhea, and pulmonary edema. Development of antibodies to the mouse antibody also limits the prolonged or repeated use of the product. Because it is a powerful agent there is heightened susceptibility to infection, particularly of viral origin, during and shortly after its use. There is also a risk of lymphoproliferative disorder.

Antilymphocyte globulin occasionally causes anaphylaxis and serum sickness. Fever is common, as is a drop in platelets, owing to the nonspecific effect of the serum. Viral infections can supervene with its use. Serious complications are unusual with this product, but treatment often must be terminated prematurely because of its side effects.

RESULTS

Renal Transplantation

Patients can be sustained on dialysis after failure of a renal transplant, so patient survival and graft survival are not identical. One-year patient survival after renal transplantation, inclusive of all patients, is reported to be 96%. Graft survival depends on numerous factors, which varies among transplant centers. In general, 1-year graft survival for LRD kidneys is 91% and for cadaver kidneys 81% (from 1984 to 1994) (Table 16.8). Patient mortality after the first year is relatively small and is related to general issues, such as age and cardiovascular disease. Graft survival varies with the source of the kidney. Six-antigen-matched LRD kidneys can be expected to function for decades; for cadaver kidneys, the 5-year graft survival is approximately 58%, although some have continued to function nearly 30 years after transplantation.

The greatest advantage is in quality of life. For virtually all recipients the state of chronic illness is replaced by a feeling of normalcy. Women are again fertile and can bear normal children. Children, if given transplants early, can grow normally and develop alongside their peers, without the physical and emotional restriction they endure on dialysis. Most recipients can return to a

TABLE 16.8. *One-year survival*

Organ	Survival (%)	
	Graft	Patient
Kidney (LRD)	91	97
Kidney (cadaver)	81	93
Liver	70	80
Heart	82	83
Heart–lung	62	63
Lung	71	73
Pancreas	74	90.5

Source: UNOS Facts and Statistics (10/87–12/94), based on UNOS OPTN/Scientific Registry data (1/14/97).
LRD, living related donor.

normal life, with few restrictions, despite their need for immunosuppression.

Transplantation of Other Organs

Although more than 200,000 renal transplants have been performed, comprising the bulk of clinical experience, transplantation of other organs has been steadily increasing. It is now common for multiple organs (heart, liver, pancreas, other organs) to be obtained from most donors for transplantation.

Heart, Heart–Lung, Lung

One of the most striking accomplishments of the past two decades has been the improvement in the results of cardiac transplantation, with the 1-year graft and patient survival rates in 1995 approximately 84% and 84%, respectively. The typical heart transplant patient in the United States is male (78%), over 50 years old (54%), and Caucasian (83%); the primary indication for transplant is coronary artery disease (43.5%) or cardiomyopathy (42%). It should be noted, however, that approximately 11% of all heart transplants were performed in pediatric patients (less than 18 years old).

A patient who can be fully rehabilitated by transplantation, whose life expectancy without it is less than 6 months, and for whom no other treatment option is available is a candidate for cardiac transplantation. The relative contraindications include severe diabetes mellitus, smoking, obesity, malignancy, age, and psychiatric problems. Pulmonary disease was previously considered a contraindication but may now serve as an indication for possible heart–lung transplantation. Patients accepted for transplantation, listed with UNOS by weight and blood group, are assigned to one of two status groups: status 1 (hospitalized in the ICU) and status 2 (all other patients). Status 1 patients are given priority. Approximately 20% of patients wait-listed for cardiac transplantation in 1996 died before a suitable donor was found.

Cadaver donor hearts are transported in cold storage to the transplant center where the recipient, on cardiopulmonary bypass, has been prepared by excision of the diseased heart. The new heart is transplanted orthotopically. Emphasis is placed on minimizing the ischemia time between donor cardiectomy and restoration of flow in the recipient. The usual time is 4 to 6 hours; longer periods of ischemia can adversely affect cardiac performance. Immunosuppression is similar to that for other organs (CsA, prednisone, and azathioprine). Post-transplant patients are monitored for rejection by percutaneous transvenous endomyocardial biopsies. Infection (40%) is still the most common cause of death after transplant, followed by cardiac complications (25%) and acute rejection (25%). Patients unresponsive to acute rejection therapy and those who experience accelerated coronary artery disease or chronic rejection must undergo retransplantation, their only alternative being death.

The most common indications for heart–lung transplantation are primary pulmonary hypertension (31%) and congenital lung disease (40%). Patients with end-stage lung disease today are being considered for double lung transplantation rather than heart–lung transplantation. Relative contraindications for heart–lung transplantation include previous extensive thoracic surgery and impaired liver function. The 1-year survival rate is 62% with 30% early postoperative mortality, usually associated with inadequate hemostasis and prolonged cardiopulmonary bypass time. Infection is the most common cause of late death following heart–lung transplants. Tracheal anastomotic problems are avoided by withholding the use of steroids for the first 2 weeks after transplant. The diagnosis of rejection is difficult because endomyocardial biopsy is not a good monitor for pulmonary tissue. Chest radiography, although imprecise, is the established method for diagnosing rejection. Long-term graft failure from bronchiolitis obliterans and accelerated coronary artery disease occurs in 50% of patients. Consequently, the need for retransplantation is high.

Beginning in 1983 a new era in lung transplantation was initiated by the Toronto lung transplant group. Through careful patient selection, the use of CsA, and an omental wrap for the bronchial anastomosis, they reported improved results in 15 single lung transplant patients. Most patients achieved maximal aerobic capacity within 6 months after transplant. In addition, with the development of the *en bloc* double-lung transplant method, patients with end-stage cystic fibrosis and emphysema have undergone transplantation successfully. The encouraging results have given new impetus to lung transplantation, with 1-year graft and patient survivals of 71% and 73%, respectively.

Liver

Although technically demanding, liver transplantation (LTX) has evolved into a safe, predictable surgical operation. Still controversial are issues of patient selection, surgical strategies, immunosuppression, and retransplantation. The inadequate supply of organs and the problems encountered financing LTX add to the difficulties.

Adult candidates for LTX are patients with end-stage liver disease that is not expected to recur after transplantation. Included in this group are patients with primary biliary or alcoholic cirrhosis, Budd-Chiari syndrome, and primary sclerosing cholangitis. More controversial are patients with postnecrotic cirrhosis secondary to hepatitis B or C virus, because the viral infection may recur. It should be noted, however, that the most common liver disease among adults for which LTX is performed is hepatitis C, followed by alcoholic liver disease. These conditions alone, or in combination, accounted for more than 40% of adult LTX in 1994. Patients with liver cancer, especially hepatocellular carcinoma, may undergo transplantation successfully if the tumor is strictly confined to the liver. Gallbladder carcinoma or cholangiocarcinoma are relative, not absolute, contraindications for LTX.

Acute fulminant hepatic failure has emerged as a strong indication for LTX. The predominant causes of this form of liver failure are hepatitis C, hepatitis B, and unspecified fulminant hepatitis. Indications for emergency transplantation are relentless progression of hepatic failure, severe coagulopathy, cardiovascular instability, sepsis, and grade 3 to 4 encephalopathy. The results are equivalent to those for patients given transplants for chronic liver diseases, especially in the 10- to 40-year age group.

In the pediatric patient biliary atresia is the most common indication for transplantation (54%), with inborn metabolic errors being next (13%). Because of particular difficulty finding pediatric donors, techniques have been developed that allow an adult liver to be utilized in a child. They include the "split liver technique" from cadaver livers and transplantation of segments of livers from living related donors. Extensive thrombosis of the portal, mesenteric, or splenic veins or multiple prior upper abdominal surgical procedures do not preclude LTX. Patients with bleeding esophageal varices may be better served by a liver transplant than a shunt procedure. The pool of potential recipients is increasing, and LTX is increasingly becoming the treatment of choice, rather than a last-ditch attempt, for many conditions.

Cadaver livers can be preserved for up to 24 hours, using the University of Wisconsin (UW) solution, allowing time for selection and preparation of the most appropriate candidate. The recipient's liver is removed, often the most challenging aspect of the operation; during the anhepatic phase, a venovenous bypass is often utilized, shunting the splanchnic and distal systemic venous blood into a major tributary of the superior vena cava. The donor liver has been removed *en bloc* with the vena cava, portal vein, and arterial supply, including a cuff of aorta. Grafts of donor iliac vessels are utilized to provide additional length when necessary or to convert multiple arteries into a single trunk while the liver is still "on the back-table" in cold preservation solution. The proximal and distal cut ends of the vena cava are then end-to-end anastomosed to the corresponding ends of the recipient vessels, and air is evacuated. The portal vein is then anastomosed, and finally the arterial supply is restored. Release of vascular clamps may be accompanied by acidosis and circulatory instability due to sudden changes in volume. The biliary tract is reconstructed using a choledochocholedochostomy or a Roux-en-Y choledochojejunostomy.

The main causes of death during the early posttransplant period are primary nonfunction and coagulopathy. During the ensuing weeks acute rejection and hepatic artery thrombosis become the most frequent causes of graft loss. Complications of LTX can result in a 15% to 30% graft loss and include nonfunction, technical problems, bleeding, infection, and acute rejection. In many of these cases, retransplantation is required. Bacterial infection secondary to staphylococci and gram-negative organisms are frequent. Viral infections are also common, especially with CMV and herpes simplex virus. Fortunately, an increasing number of antiviral agents (e.g., acyclovir, ganciclovir, and foscarnet) are available.

Acute rejection occurs with more than 50% of liver allografts, usually within the first 2 weeks. Accurate diagnosis is obtained by needle biopsy of the liver. The most common histologic findings are portal tract inflammation and edema and mononuclear cell involvement of portal vein branches and small bile ducts.

The 1-year graft survival rate has improved from about 50% prior to CsA to the present level of 70%. The best results are in patients aged 5 to 60 years. In many centers the results of emergency liver transplants equal those of elective liver transplants. The 5-year survival rates now range from 40% to 70%, except for patients with liver cancer, who have only a 10% to 15% survival rate at 5 years. The future for liver transplantation depends on better methods for the diagnosis and treatment of rejection and refinement of surgical techniques, which allows more frequent use of a single liver for two or three patients. The latter allows some alleviation of the greatest problem currently facing liver transplantation: the serious shortage of organs.

Pancreas

The first clinical pancreas transplant was performed in 1966 by Kelly and Lillehei. After lagging behind other organ transplants, pancreas transplantation has begun to increase, with more than 7,500 being done worldwide up to late 1995 (12/66 to 11/95). The goals of pancreas transplantation are to provide physiologic replacement of insulin and prevent the secondary complications of diabetes mellitus. These goals may be achieved by pancreas or islet cell transplantation.

In general, the risks of immunosuppression outweigh the benefits for most juvenile-onset diabetics, who can regulate their glucose with exogenous insulin. Three categories of patients, however, may be suited for pancreas transplantation. The most common indication is the uremic-diabetic patient. Because these individuals require immunosuppression for a necessary kidney transplant, a simultaneous pancreas transplant is a logical response to both problems with little added risk. The second and third groups are nonuremic: Some have already received a kidney transplant, whereas others may have early renal failure or other catastrophic complications of diabetes. All potential candidates for pancreas transplantation generally undergo cardiac evaluation in addition to the usual preparation required for a kidney transplant, as patient survival is markedly improved if significant cardiac disease, common in these patients, is diagnosed and treated before transplantation.

The pancreas is usually obtained from a cadaver donor. These organs are obtained from living related donors at a few centers, but some donors have developed glucose intolerance despite the fact that only the distal segment of pancreas is resected. The pancreas transplant is placed intraperitoneally in the iliac fossa. The recipient operation varies in the amount of pan-

creas transplanted, the site of revascularization, and management of the duct. The results are essentially the same, whether the whole pancreas or the distal segment is transplanted. The pancreas is usually revascularized by anastomoses of its blood supply to the external iliac artery and vein, but some surgeons prefer portal venous drainage. Exocrine pancreatic function can be managed by duct ligation, duct injection (with neoprene or proline), or anastomosis (to the recipient's gastrointestinal or urinary tract). Bladder drainage has the advantage of allowing direct monitoring of pancreatic function by measuring urinary amylase. A decrease in urinary amylase precedes hyperglycemia by 24 hours, providing earlier diagnosis of pancreas rejection.

In addition to immunosuppression, exogenous insulin is given to maintain serum glucose levels at less than 150 mg/dL during the early postoperative period because chronic hyperglycemia has been shown to be detrimental to the islets. Anticoagulants are given to reduce the risk (12%) of thrombosis of the splenic vessels of the transplant. Serum glucose levels, C peptide, urinary amylase, and pH are monitored. Radionuclide flow scans are performed early to distinguish between thrombosis and pancreatitis. Significant postoperative complications include pancreatitis, wound infection, ascites, and fever of unknown origin. Immunosuppression appears to prevent recurrence of the autoimmune type I diabetes mellitus in the transplanted pancreas.

A functioning pancreas transplant can lead to a normal metabolic state, with normal oral and intravenous glucose tolerance tests with the hemoglobin A1C and C-peptide levels returning to normal. Information is limited regarding the effects of a pancreas transplant on the secondary complications of diabetes. Regression of the histologic lesions of diabetic nephropathy has been demonstrated after pancreas transplantation. Alleviation of neuropathy or retinopathy, however, has not been shown. This may be because until recently only end-stage diabetics received pancreas transplants; as patients with diabetes receive pancreas transplants at an earlier stage these complications may also diminish.

The results have improved markedly over the past few years, primarily due to better immunosuppression with CsA and better preservation of the pancreas with UW solution. The international registry reports 1-year patient and graft survival to have improved to nearly 90% and 70%, respectively (from 40% and 5%, respectively, in 1966). HLA matching appears to play a role in pancreas graft survival; DR matching has been noted to have a beneficial effect. Bladder drainage appears to be associated with a higher graft survival rate than intestinal drainage or duct injection. Simultaneous kidney–pancreas transplant recipients have a higher graft survival rate than patients receiving a pancreas alone or after a kidney transplant (78% vs. 55% vs. 56%, respectively), although the patient survival rate is better for pancreas-only patients; the latter may be due to better patient selection.

An alternative to pancreas transplantation is islet cell transplantation. The first successful animal islet cell transplant was performed in 1972 by Bollinger and Lacy. It appears to be a safe, simple procedure that permits *in vitro* manipulation of the graft prior to transplantation. Despite the remarkable success of experimental studies, clinical islet cell transplantation is fraught with problems, including the difficulty of preparing sufficient quantities of human islet tissue (multiple donors are required for a single recipient) and the marked immunogenicity of these allografts. The attempts to control these problems focus on improved techniques for islet preparation. Fetal islets and xenogeneic sources for islet cells are also being evaluated. Strategies to reduce the immunogenicity of the islet include encapsulation of the islets in an artificial membrane and pretreatment of the islets *in vitro* to reduce immunogenicity. To date, long-term success of islet transplants has not been achieved, but research is continuing.

Small Bowel

Small bowel is the latest organ to be transplanted. It is indicated for patients dependent on total parenteral nutrition (TPN) because of congenital or acquired loss of absorptive capacity of the small intestine. It can obviate the significant morbidity of vascular access problems and cholestasis associated with TPN. Small bowel transplantation (SBTx) was first attempted in 1901 by Carrel; and Lillehei revived interest in the procedure in 1959. A dual problem with rejection occurs with SBTx: classic graft rejection by host T lymphocytes and graft-versus-host disease (GVHD) by donor lymphocytes. Moreover, the physiologic function of the graft can be severely impaired by the transplantation process, thereby negating the purpose of the transplant.

Cyclosporine absorption, as well as all other drug absorption, is initially impaired with an SBTx. For this reason, the CsA was given intravenously during the early postoperative period. Despite this route of administration, CsA was less effective than tacrolimus as an immunosuppressive agent. Currently, clinical transplant centers are using tacrolimus as the primary immunosuppressive agent after SBTx. Immunosuppression with azathioprine and prednisone has been ineffective in dealing with GVHD. Irradiation of the organ has reduced GVHD but often leads to radiation enteritis. Donor pretreatment with polyclonal antibodies has been used experimentally to reduce the incidence of GVHD.

Intestinal function following transplantation is monitored by tests of absorptive function and of mucosal integrity of the small bowel. Initial motility of the transplanted bowel is grossly abnormal because of graft denervation, which can be demonstrated by myoelectric activity studies. This is an important issue because salt and water absorption are under tight control by the autonomic nervous system. Diarrhea may result unless a sufficient length of bowel is transplanted. Venous drainage of the transplant into the inferior vena cava is also associated with problems due to the portosystemic shunt created, leading to increased ammonia and amino acid absorption, which is similar to hepatic encephalopathy models. Although there are many complications associated with SBTx, centers have had relative success with this solid organ transplant. The longest surviving human SBTx to date has been in place almost 7 years.

Bone Marrow

Most allogeneic bone marrow transplants have been performed using HLA-identical sibling donors. Attempts now have been made using partially mismatched donors. Bone marrow transplants are indicated for the following conditions: (a) hematologic malignancies such as acute lymphatic leukemia, acute and chronic myelogenous leukemias, and non-Hodgkin's lymphoma; (b) nonmalignant disorders such as severe aplastic anemia; and (c) hereditary disorders such as Fanconi's anemia, thalassemia, and severe combined immunodeficiency syndrome. The preparation of the recipient involves complete destruction of all functional lymphoid tissue by irradiation and chemotherapy. For this reason, there is little initial fear of acute rejection. The major early complication is GVHD. The major relative contraindications are age, sex, mismatch of the transplant, CMV infection, and neutropenic sepsis. Early immunosuppression is directed toward preventing GVHD. The future for bone marrow transplants includes the use of unrelated matched and mismatched related bone marrow donors. Better immunosuppression and anti-T cell monoclonal antibodies may improve the results. In addition, growth factors are being evaluated to improve the engraftment rate in mismatched situations or after T cell depletion.

XENOTRANSPLANTATION

Although great strides have been made in the immunobiology of transplantation, clinical transplants have been limited by the number of human organs available for the ever-growing number of potential recipients. Many alternatives are being explored, including mechanical devices such as the implantable left ventricular assist device (LVAD) for those with cardiac failure, the extracorporeal liver for those with acute liver failure, and the various osmotic pumps to deliver insulin to those with insulin dependent diabetes mellitus. Each has its limitations.

Among the options are organs from animals of different species. These organs, called *xenografts,* have the advantage that they act similarly to the recipient's own organ and do not need to be replaced unless rejection occurs. There are many barriers before xenotransplantation becomes a viable option. One of the major barriers is hyperacute rejection, which occurs between "discordant" organs (e.g., pig to baboon). This is thought to occur because of the binding of xenoreactive antibodies of the recipient to the blood vessels in the donor organ leading to activation of the complement system and the intrinsic susceptibility of the graft to injury by the heterologous complement. Another major barrier is acute cellular rejection, or "delayed xenograft rejection." In "concordant" species (e.g., baboon to human), hyperacute rejection does not occur, but the graft is then subjected to severe acute cellular rejection. The mechanism of this reaction is not well delineated at this time. Ethical and moral issues arise as well. Concordant species (nonhuman primates) are sentient, have prolonged and limited gestation periods, and some are endangered. These factors override the fact that humans do not have a natural antibody against them.

Use of the pig overcomes these objections, as the pig breeds rapidly and the species is already in widespread use for food. However, the natural antibody must be overcome. Currently, swine herds are being bred that are genetically altered to avoid initiation of the complement cascade and thus avert hyperacute rejection. Xenotransplants will continue to be experimental until these issues have been convincingly resolved.

A final issue is specific to xenotransplantation: *zoonosis,* which is the transmission of disease from animals to humans. Although a relatively rare phenomenon now, it may be of concern if xenotransplantation is widely practiced. Specific concerns include the possible transmission into the human population of diseases not currently known and to which humans have no resistance. A related concern is if such infection does occur, it may have the potential of a pandemic. These issues have been addressed in depth by national panels, and current policy is to proceed with caution, on an experimental basis, until knowledge is gained.

CONCLUSIONS

Transplantation has evolved to a degree that was unthinkable several years ago. Virtually all vascularized organs can be replaced successfully. Immunosuppression has become safer and more selective, resulting in most organ transplant recipients resuming an active role in society. Yet the recovery of organs falls far behind reasonable expectations. Waiting patients die while thousands of organs go unrecovered. Society and the medical profession have an obligation to correct this cause of preventable death.

GLOSSARY

Antibody   Soluble protein that reacts to a specific antigen; produced by B cells

Antigen-presenting cells (APC)   Cells that present antigen to initiate T cell activation; can be various cells, such as monocytes, dendritic cells

Autologous   Graft that originates from the same individual who receives it

Azathioprine (Imuran)   Immunosuppressive agent that acts by inhibiting cell division; often used with prednisone and CsA in "triple therapy"

B lymphocytes   Small white blood cells essential to

immune defenses; derived from marrow; produce antibodies

CD (cluster of differentiation) Variety of cell surface molecules each with a different function (e.g., CD3 T cell antigen receptor; CD4 helper T cells, recognize MHC class I; CD8 cytotoxic T cells, recognize class II

Cellular immunity Immunity mediated by direct action of cells (in contrast to humoral immunity)

Chimera Cell populations from one organism surviving in another

Class I and II molecules See **MHC**

Clone Groups of cells that are genetically identical

Cyclosporine (CsA) Immunosuppressive agent derived from fungal extract; prevents rejection by inhibiting production of IL-2; Two oral formulations exist: the older Sandimmune and the newer Neoral

Cytotoxic cells T lymphocytes that can kill certain target cells; usually carry CD8 surface marker

Dendritic cell White blood cell found in lymphoid organs; presents trapped antigen to T cells

Haplotype Set of genetic determinants on a single chromosome

Helper cells T lymphocytes activated early in the immune process; help generate cytotoxic T cells and stimulate B cells to form antibodies; usually carry CD4 surface marker

Heterologous Antigenic differences between species

Histocompatibility Ability to accept grafts between species

Human leukocyte antigen (HLA) Major histocompatibility genetic region in humans: self markers

Homologous Of the same species

Humoral immunity Immunity through soluble factors (e.g., antibody)

Interferons Mediators of cell function with implications for immune response, infection, and cancer chemotherapy; IFNαproduced by leukocytes; IFNβ by fibroblasts; IFN$\gamma$by T cells

Interleukins (IL) Agents involved in cell signals: IL-1, many effects, including activation of T cells to express IL-2 receptors; IL-2 , released by activated T cells, necessary for T cells to proliferate; many other ILs

Lymphokines Soluble T cell products that regulate the activation, growth, and differentiation of many cell types

Major histocompatibility complex (MHC) Genetic region in all mammals, products of compatibility responsible for rejection of grafts between individuals

MHC class I molecules Expressed on all cell types, consists of heavy αchain, associated with light βchain

MHC class II molecules Expressed on B cells, macrophages, and activated T cells; have $\alpha$and βchains, which may form a common binding site

Monoclonal antibody Homogeneous antibodies, derived from a single clone, with a specific action

Mycophenolate mofetil (MMF) Antiproliferative agent targeting lymphocytes. Actions similar to azathioprine; also known as CellCept

Natural killer (NK) Lymphocytes that recognize and destroy certain cells (e.g., virally infected, tumor)

Polyclonal antibody (ALG, ATG) Antibody usually generated against lymphocytes using horse, rabbit, or goat; action not restricted to lymphocytes

Tacrolimus (FK 506) Immunosuppressive agent; prevents rejection by inhibition of IL-2; structurally different from CsA but functionally similar; also known as Prograf

T lymphocytes Lymphocytes processed in the thymus; direct participants in immune response

Tolerance Specific immunologic unresponsiveness

Xenograft Graft between species (e.g., baboon to human, mouse to rat)

Zoonosis Disease of animals transmissible to humans

QUESTIONS

1. Seven days after cadaver renal transplantation, a patient develops a fever to 101°F, pain and tenderness over the incisional area, and oliguria. Serum creatinine has risen from 1.5 mg/dL to 1.9 mg/dL. Likely possibilities include:
   a. Acute rejection.
   b. Wound infection.
   c. Urinary leak.
   d. Wound dehiscence.
   e. All of the above.
2. The patient in question 1 should:
   a. Be rushed to the operating room.
   b. Receive high doses of steroids immediately.
   c. Be investigated using ultrasonography, nuclear scan, or both.
   d. Receive broad-spectrum antibiotic coverage.
   e. None of the above.

Possible answers for questions 3 through 6:

    a. Interleukin-2.
    b. Interferon-2.
    c. T-helper cells.
    d. T cytotoxic cells.
    e. B cells.

D　 3. These cells are usually CD8+ and recognize class I molecules.

E　 4. Stimulated by antigen or other cells, these cells ultimately produce antibody that causes graft destruction.

A　 5. Secretion that stimulates various antigen-activated cells to proliferate.

C　 6. Normally resting, these cells are stimulated by antigens and macrophages to initiate the immune response.

     7. For a through e, below, choose the best option from i through v. (choice may be repeated).

    a. Blocks interleukin-1   iii
    b. Blocks interleukin-2   i, iv
    c. Inhibits cell division   ii, v
    d. Can depress bone marrow.   ii, v
    e. Nephrotoxicity is a problem   i, iv
    i. Cyclosporine.
    ii. Azathioprine.
    iii. Corticosteroids.
    iv. Tacrolimus.
    v. Mycophenolate mofetil.

     8. True or false:

F   a. Because of high mortality, cardiac transplantation should be restricted to the terminally ill.

T   b. Patient survival 1 year after kidney transplantation exceeds 90%.

T   c. Cytomegalovirus infection is a common problem after all organ transplants.

F   d. Liver transplantation should never be considered for acute hepatic necrosis.

     9. In regard to transplant rejection:

F   a. Acute rejection is irreversible and leads to loss of the kidney.

T   b. There is no treatment for chronic rejection.

T   c. Hyperacute rejection is precipitated by circulating humoral antibodies.

    d. a, b, and c are correct.

    (e) b and c are correct.

10. The following statements are true *except:*

T   a. Deep hypothermia sharply reduces cell metabolism.

T   b. Oxygen-derived free radicals may be responsible for reperfusion injury.

T   c. Cell swelling can be minimized by the addition of impermeable osmotic agents to the preservation/perfusion solution.

    (d) Hypothermia prevents anaerobic metabolism.

T   e. With the use of UW solution, preservation of abdominal organs more than 24 hours can be regularly achieved.

SELECTED REFERENCES

Cecka JM, Terasaki PI, eds. *Clinical transplants 1995.* Los Angeles: UCLA Tissue Typing Laboratory, 1996.

Langnas AN, Shaw BS Jr, Antonson DL, et al. Preliminary experience with intestinal transplantation in infants and children. *Pediatrics* 1996;97:443–448.

Morris PJ, ed. *Kidney transplantation: principles and practice.* 4th ed. Philadelphia: WB Saunders, 1994.

Todo S, Tzakis A, Reyes J, et al. Small intestinal transplantation in humans with or without the colon. *Transplantation* 1994;57:840–848.

United Network for Organ Sharing Scientific Registry. Richmond: UNOS, 1996.

17

Pituitary and Adrenal Gland Surgery

Michael Coomaraswamy

The role of the pituitary gland as the orchestrator of virtually all metabolic processes of the body makes knowledge of the anatomy and function of the hypothalamo-hypophyseal system essential for accurate diagnosis and appropriate treatment of the myriad disorders associated with hypo-or hyperproduction of the eight pituitary hormones. The following is intended to serve as a brief overview of the anatomy and physiology of the pituitary and of the more common associated disorders.

PITUITARY

Embryology and Anatomy

The pituitary is embryologically derived from two separate ectodermal anlagen. At approximately 24 days of gestation an upgrowth of oral ectoderm termed Rathke's pouch begins an anterior migration to form the anterior pituitary lobe or adenohypophysis. The posterior pituitary lobe, or neurohypophysis, forms as a simultaneous downgrowth of neuroectoderm from the diencephalon.

The pituitary gland rests within the sella turcica, a depression in the sphenoid bone. The sella is lined by dura mater, which forms an incomplete diaphragm through which the pituitary stalk passes. Immediately lateral to the sella are the cavernous venous sinuses, within which are the carotid arteries and several of the cranial nerves. The optic chiasm decussates just anterior to the pituitary stalk.

In contrast to the anterior pituitary, which under normal circumstances becomes physically separate from its site of origin, the posterior pituitary remains connected to the midbrain via the pituitary stalk. The two polypeptide hormones of the posterior pituitary, antidiuretic hormone (ADH) and oxytocin, are produced in the supraoptic and paraventricular nuclei of the hypothalamus, respectively, and are transported directly to the neurohypophysis for release into the systemic circulation.

The hormone ADH is vital in the maintenance of normal serum osmolality and intravascular volume. In the kidney ADH receptors on the peritubular aspect of the distal convoluted tubules mediate the pore size in the luminal membrane, leading to increased water resorption from the ultrafiltrate and the formation of concentrated urine. Control of ADH release is mediated via hypothalamic osmoreceptors and to a lesser extent by volume receptors in the right atrium.

Oxytocin promotes uterine contraction during labor. It also aids in milk ejection during the postpartum period.

The anterior pituitary produces six hormones. Three are polypeptides: human growth hormone (hGH) or somatotropin, prolactin, and ACTH. The remainder—thryoid-stimulating hormone (TSH), follicle-stimulating hormone (FSH), and luteinizing hormone (LH)—are glycoproteins consisting of a common α-subunit and a unique β-subunit.

Control of the production and release of these hormones is mediated by releasing and, in some instances, inhibiting hormones produced in the hypothalamus and delivered to the adenohypophysis through the hypophyseal portal circulation.

Pituitary Disorders

Most pathologic conditions of the pituitary cause symptoms by a mass effect on the gland itself or on adjacent structures or by alterations in the levels of pituitary hormone production.

Nonfunctioning Masses

Empty sella syndrome, caused by herniation of the arachnoid through the incomplete dural diaphragm, occurs most commonly in obese, multiparous women. Symptoms are caused by a combination of mass effect and functional compromise of the gland.

Craniopharyngiomas are benign secretory vestiges of Rathke's pouch that cause symptoms by suprasellar extension (leading to the classic finding of a bitemporal hemianopsia visual field defect) and by invasion of the gland (causing panhypopituitarism). Treatment of these lesions usually involves a combination of radiation therapy and surgery.

Pituitary Adenomas

Pituitary adenomas, histologically benign lesions, are being identified with increasing frequency as imaging techniques, particularly computed tomographic (CT) scanning, improve. Many adenomas are asymptomatic, and some autopsy series show a 10% to 25% incidence of these tumors. *Chromophobe adenomas* are nonfunctioning and produce a characteristic sequential parahypopituitarism beginning with the suppression of hGH followed by FSH, LH, TSH, and ultimately ACTH. Functioning adenomas produce the characteristic syndromes outlined below.

Growth Hormone-Secreting Tumors

Excessive hGH production by acidophilic microadenomas causes gigantism if it occurs prior to long bone epiphyseal closure and acromegaly in adults. Because hGH is diabetogenic, fully 25% of these patients have an insulin-resistant diabetes. Other associated abnormalities include a proximal myopathy and a dilated cardiomyopathy. There is a high incidence of myocardial infarction as a cause of death in these patients. Treatment options include surgical hypophysectomy, usually done via a transsphenoidal approach, proton beam irradiation, and the dopamine antagonist bromocriptine, which is effective in 70% to 80% of patients.

Prolactin-Secreting Tumors

Prolactin-secreting tumors are the most commonly detected pituitary tumors. In women the triad of galactorrhea, irregular menses, and anovulatory cycles in combination with a serum prolactin level higher than 260 ng/dL is diagnostic. Oligospermia with or without gynecomastia is seen in men. Bromocriptine is effective medical treatment in up to 90% of cases.

Cushing's Disease

Cushing's disease is hypercortisolism caused by an ACTH-secreting basophilic adenoma; if iatrogenic etiologies are excluded, it is the most common cause of hypercortisolism. Short-term treatment of this condition includes metyrapone or aminoglutethimide. Definitive treatment requires surgery, proton beam irradiation, or both. TSH-, LH-, and FSH-secreting tumors of the anterior pituitary are rare.

Anterior Pituitary Failure

Pituitary apoplexy, caused by acute hemorrhage into the gland, is usually associated with adenomas, especially if recent radiation therapy has been given. Patients present with headaches, visual loss, ophthalmoplegia, and meningismus.

Postpartum pituitary hemorrhage, or Sheehan syndrome, is associated with hypotension during labor. It manifests as lactation failure or persistent amenorrhea.

Life-threatening pituitary hemorrhage is treated with stress-dose intravenous steroids and thyroxine.

Neurohypophyseal Dysfunction

Central diabetes insipidus is caused by inadequate secretion of ADH, resulting in voluminous polyuria and hypernatremia if renal losses are not replaced. Common etiologies are surgical or other forms of head trauma, and most cases are transient. Intranasal insufflation of DDAVP is the treatment of choice for prolonged deficiency states.

ADRENALS

The adrenal glands are functionally and anatomically composed of two parts: the inner medulla, which is embryologically derived from neural crest ectoderm, and the outer cortex, which is of mesodermal origin. In adults the adrenals exist as paired retroperitoneal organs overlying each kidney. Normal glands are roughly 5 g in mass. The arterial blood supply is directly from the aorta via the adrenal artery and from branches of the phrenic and renal arteries. The right adrenal vein drains directly into the inferior vena cava, whereas the left adrenal vein drains to the left renal vein. The adrenal cortex is histologically divided into three zones.

The *zona fasciculata* and *zona reticularis* produce the glucocorticoid cortisol in response to ACTH stimulation. Under normal circumstances there is tight feedback control of plasma levels of cortisol via the hypothalamic–pituitary–adrenal axis. Approximately 30 mg of cortisol is produced daily under normal circumstances. There is a diurnal variation in plasma cortisol levels with a peak during the early morning and a nadir in the evening. Glucocorticoid actions include profound effects on carbohydrate metabolism (mediated through decreased peripheral utilization and increased glucogenesis) and primarily inhibitory actions on immune function, inflammatory response, and wound healing. In addition to glucocorticoid production the zona reticularis is the site of sex hormone synthesis.

The *zona glomerulosa* produces the mineralocorticoid hormones, the most important of which is aldosterone. Approximately 150 g of aldosterone is produced daily. Aldosterone secretion is controlled by the renin–angiotensin system.

Renin is released from the juxtaglomerular apparatus of the kidney in response to conditions of decreased perfusion. It mediates the conversion of angiotensinogen to angiotensin I, which is further hydrolyzed in the lung to form angiotensin II, a powerful vasoconstrictor and promoter of aldosterone synthesis. Aldosterone causes net resorption of sodium from the proximal collecting tubule, kaliuresis, and secretion of hydrogen ion.

Adrenal Disorders

Hypoaldosteronism is usually associated with a hyporeninemic state resulting from renal disease that has damaged the juxtaglomerular apparatus. Classic features include hyperkalemic, hypochloremic, and metabolic acidosis. Mineralocorticoid replacement therapy must be undertaken with extreme caution, as it may precipitate congestive heart failure in these patients, who tend to be elderly and have atherosclerotic heart disease.

Hyperaldosteronism

Hyperaldosteronism is a rare cause of hypertension and is responsible for only 1% to 2% of cases in this population. It is associated with a hypernatremic, hypokalemic, metabolic alkalosis; consequently patients often complain of muscle weakness, cramps, and polyuria/polydipsia. There is a 3 : 1 female/male predominance, and most cases are diagnosed during the second to fifth decades of life.

In approximately 80% of cases primary hyperaldosteronism results from a benign adrenal cortical adenoma. Bilateral adrenal cortical hyperplasia is responsible for most of the remaining 20%. Adrenal cortical carcinoma is a rare cause of hyperaldosteronism.

Nonsuppressibility of urinary aldosterone secretion during a period of prolonged salt loading has emerged as the most effective screening test for this condition. An aldosterone secretion of more than 14 mg in a 24-hour urine collection when the urine sodium is at least 250 mEq/24 hr indicates nonsuppressibility of aldosterone secretion. Persistent hypokalemia during the diagnostic workup is strong evidence for an aldosterone-producing adenoma.

Preoperative localization of adenomas is vital, as these tumors are often small and not easily palpable. In addition, operative morbidity is substantially reduced if a limited posterior, rather than a transabdominal, approach can be used. A CT scan can reliably localize adenomas larger than 1.5 cm but is less helpful for smaller lesions. If CT scanning is nondiagnostic, bilateral adrenal venous sampling for aldosterone, although invasive, has been shown to have a sensitivity approaching 100%.

The treatment of primary hyperaldosteronism caused by bilateral adrenal hyperplasia is medical, with spironolactone or amiloride. Surgical treatment with bilateral total adrenalectomy yields inferior results and should be reserved for failures of medical therapy. Surgical treatment of aldosterone-producing adenomas is highly effective. Total adrenalectomy should be performed on the side of the tumor.

Cushing Syndrome

The classic features of hypercortisolism include truncal obesity, moon facies, purple abdominal striae, atrophic, easily bruised skin, and muscle weakness. Patients are often hypertensive and diabetic, and they may have severe osteoporosis with pathologic bone fractures. Myocardial infarction is a common cause of death in untreated patients.

If iatrogenic causes are excluded, hypercortisolism is caused by an ACTH-producing pituitary microadenoma in approximately 70% of cases. This form of the syndrome is termed Cushing's disease. Roughly 15% of cases result from primary adrenal pathology, including adenomas, hyperplasia, and adrenal carcinoma. In the remaining 15% tumors causing ectopic production of ACTH or corticotropin-releasing factor (CRF) are the cause of the hypercortisolism. Precise determination of the etiology of the hypercortisolism is vital to the proper management of these patients.

Diagnosis

Florid Cushing syndrome in general presents little diagnostic challenge. However, some patients have been shown to have cyclic or episodic forms of the syndrome and may have only one or a few findings suggestive of hypercortisolism. In these patients a 24-hour urine collection for measurement of urinary free cortisol has proved to be a sensitive, specific screening test. Serum cortical determinations done at 8 a.m. and 8 p.m. are

also diagnostic of the syndrome if the values are elevated and show loss of the previously described circadian rhythm. Patients with pituitary hypercortisolism generally have a positive high-dose dexamethasone suppression test. Administration of 8 mg of the high-potency steroid dexamethasone in four divided doses or as a single intravenous dose in the hospitalized patient inhibits ACTH release from a pituitary microadenoma and results in decreased plasma cortisol. Metyrapone is another agent used for diagnosis. This compound blocks the 11-hydroxylation step in cortisol synthesis. Administration of a single 3-g oral dose results in a marked increase in plasma levels of 11-deoxycortisol in patients with pituitary Cushing syndrome.

Patients with adrenal hypercortisolism have low plasma ACTH levels and do not respond to high-dose dexamethasone with decreased cortisol synthesis. Metyrapone administration does not result in increased plasma levels of the 11-deoxy metabolite because the adrenals are already maximally stimulated and are unable to augment their function when cortisol synthesis is blocked.

Ectopic ACTH-producing tumors are associated with a negative (nonsuppressible) high-dose dexamethasone suppression test, and the patients may show a decrease in 11-deoxycortisol production when given metyrapone. As expected, these patients all have extremely high serum levels of ACTH.

The diagnostic algorithm is illustrated in Fig. 17.1.

Treatment

Pituitary Cushing syndrome is treated with transsphenoidal hypophysectomy alone or in combination with heavy-particle irradiation. It is important to note that imaging studies of the pituitary, even utilizing the latest-generation CT scanners, may fail to localize the adenoma. This point should not be used in an argument against hypophysectomy. Surgical cure after hypophysectomy is achieved in roughly 80% of cases. As with other surgical treatment of this syndrome, postoperative steroids must be administered to avoid an addisonian crisis (see below); however, the function of the pituitary–adrenal axis generally recovers after subtotal hypophysectomy, and long-term maintenance steroids are seldom needed.

Adrenal hyperplasia is treated with bilateral adrenalectomy. Nelson syndrome develops in 8% to 15% of

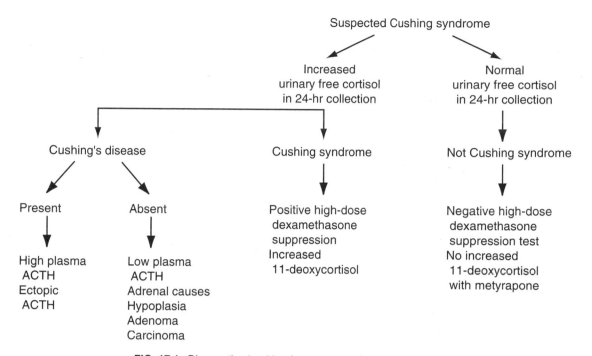

FIG. 17.1. Diagnostic algorithm for suspected Cushing syndrome

adults and in up to 35% of children after bilateral adrenalectomy. It manifests as hyperpigmentation (resulting from extreme elevations in plasma ACTH) and visual field defects if pituitary enlargement occurs. Adrenal cortical adenomas are treated with unilateral adrenalectomy. Adrenal cortical carcinomas are highly malignant tumors that are radio- and chemotherapy resistant. These tumors metastasize widely via blood and lymphatics. Surgical cure is achieved in fewer than 10% of patients. Palliation of symptoms in patients with unresectable tumors can be achieved with aminoglutethimide or metyrapone.

Treatment of Cushing syndrome caused by ectopic ACTH-producing tumors remains a vexing clinical problem. Most of these ACTH-producing tumors are highly malignant. Oat cell carcinoma of the lung and pancreatic and thymic neoplasms are most often responsible. Therapy should be directed to finding and removing the source of ectopic ACTH production. Palliation can be achieved medically with aminoglutethimide or metyrapone or surgically with bilateral total adrenalectomy in appropriate cases.

Adrenogenital Syndrome

The two most common inborn metabolic defects responsible for adrenogenital syndrome are partial and complete blockage of the C_{21} and C_{11} hydroxylation steps of cortisol synthesis. When a C_{21} hydroxylation defect is present, decreased plasma cortisol levels trigger increased ACTH release. Increased plasma levels of the androgenic 17-ketosteroids cause pseudohermaphroditism in the female infant and macrogenitosomia praecox in the male infant. Exogenous steroid administration causes normalization of plasma ACTH and a decrease in the 17-ketosteroid levels to more normal levels.

Adrenogenital syndrome in the adult is most often virilizing. It is caused by an adrenal cortical adenoma or carcinoma.

Addison Disease

Chronic adrenal insufficiency, or Addison disease, generally manifests as weight loss, hypotension, hyperpigmentation, and muscle weakness with hyponatremia and hyperkalemia. Acute adrenal insufficiency, or addisonian crisis, is a medical emergency that must be rapidly treated with high-dose intravenous steroids. Patients in addisonian crisis present with fever, hypotension, hyponatremia, lethargy, and vomiting. Surgery or trauma in the setting of a suppressed adrenal axis is the most common precipitory event. Other causes of adrenal insufficiency include the Waterhouse–Friderichsen syndrome (adrenal hemorrhage associated with meningococcal sepsis), tuberculous infection of the glands, and autoimmune and metastatic disease.

Disorders of the Adrenal Medulla

Pheochromocytoma

The adrenal medulla is derived from neural crest ectoderm, which also forms the sympathetic ganglia, paraganglia, and organs of Zuckerkandl. Remnants of this enterochromaffin tissue can be found from the base of the skull to the testes, mirroring the distribution of extraadrenal pheochromocytomas. All chromaffin tissue is capable of enzymatically converting phenylalamine to norepinephrine; however, only adrenal medullary and organ of Zuckerkandl pheochromocytomas have a functional methyltransferase enzyme capable of producing epinephrine. Norepinephrine is a relatively pure α-agonist. Epinephrine has both α- and β-agonist effects, which cause increased pulse rate, cardiac output, and systolic blood pressure, promote lipolysis, and produce elevated serum glucose levels.

Most pheochromocytomas occur in adults, with an equal sex distribution and a peak incidence during the fifth decade. Roughly 10% of these tumors are diagnosed in children; 10% are extraadrenal, 10% are bilateral, 10% are malignant, and 10% are familial, being associated with the multiple endocrine neoplasia type II syndrome. In pediatric patients or adults with a family history of pheochromocytomas, a serum calcitonin assay should be performed to rule out a coexisting medullary thyroid carcinoma.

Although pheochromocytoma is thought to be the cause of hypertension in only 0.1% to 0.2% of this population, coexistence of the symptomatic triad of excessive sweating, palpitations, and headaches should prompt a thorough diagnostic workup for this condition. Untreated pheochromocytomas can be lethal, and fatal hypertensive crises may be precipitated by pregnancy.

Diagnosis and Localization

The most reliable screening test for the presence of pheochromocytoma remains a 24-hour urine collection for assays of the catecholamine metabolites normetanephrine, metanephrine, and vanillylmandelic acid (VMA). Reliable assays for plasma catecholamines are difficult to obtain. Blood should be obtained from a resting, supine patient through a preexisting intravenous line. Nonsuppressibility of plasma catecholamines after administration of clonidine is characteristic and can help differentiate pheochromocytoma from essential hypertension.

Computed tomographic scanning is highly accurate in localizing adrenal pheochromocytomas. Intravenous contrast should not be used unless α-blockade has been established, lest a hypertensive crisis occur. Extraadrenal and metastatic pheochromocytomas can be localized by scintigraphy with ^{131}I-methyliodide benzylguanethidine (^{131}I-MIBG), which has also shown some utility in the treatment of malignant pheochromocytoma when given in therapeutic doses. Patients with pheochromocytoma of the bladder may have classic attacks of hypertension, sweating, and palpitations when urinating.

Treatment

The treatment of choice for all types of pheochromocytoma is surgical excision. Successful outcome requires meticulous operative technique, careful preoperative preparation, and skillful anesthetic management.

Preoperative management is directed to establishing α-blockade. The α-antagonist phenoxybenzamine is given in increasing doses over a 7- to 14-day period. Reversal of these patients' characteristic hypovolemia should proceed simultaneously to minimize the orthostatic hypotension that occurs with this medication. β-Blockers such as propranolol should be used only after α-blockade has been established as needed to control blood pressure and heart rate. Premature administration of β-blockers precipitates a hypertensive crisis from unopposed α-receptor-mediated vasoconstriction. A transabdominal approach should be used for removal of these tumors. This approach allows thorough bilateral retroperitoneal exploration to identify and remove bilateral or multiple tumors. Ideally, control of the venous drainage of these tumors is attained first, and manipulation of the mass is kept to a minimum to avoid an acute increase in plasma catecholamines.

Physiologic control of the patient undergoing resection of a pheochromocytoma is an anesthetic challenge. Atropine and halothane are avoided, as they are extremely arrhythmogenic in these patients. Control of the often widely fluctuating blood pressure is achieved with nitroprusside and phentolamine drips. Immediately after removal of the tumor, these patients' blood pressure characteristically requires support with volume infusion and pressors. Failure to see a hypotensive response after resection of a pheochromocytoma should prompt a thorough search for an additional tumor.

The malignancy of a pheochromocytoma can be difficult to establish in the absence of metastatic disease or obvious local invasion by the tumor. Histologic features of the tumor are not reliable, and metastases, as manifested by recurrent hypertension, may not occur for several years after removal of the primary tumor.

Irradiation and chemotherapy are of little utility for treating recurrent pheochromocytomas. Reexcision is attempted if feasible.

Management of Incidentally Found Adrenal Masses

With the increasing use of CT and MRI scanning, the incidental discovery of apparently asymptomatic adrenal masses has increased in frequency. The discovery of any solid adrenal mass should prompt a biochemical assessment, including a 24-hour urine collection to assay metanephrines and urinary free cortisol. Biologically active masses should be removed regardless of their size. Inactive masses smaller than 3 cm can be followed with serial CT scanning at 2, 6, and 18 months, with removal if any change in size is noted. An aggressive approach to nonfunctioning masses larger than 3 cm is surgical removal, as the risk of carcinoma increases with the size of the mass.

The CT-guided aspiration of cystic masses has been advocated. Clear cyst fluid is essentially diagnostic of a benign lesion; bloody cyst fluid should be sent for cytologic evaluation with removal of cystic lesions larger than 6 cm.

QUESTIONS

Select one answer.

1. The following statements regarding the embryology/anatomy of the pituitary are correct *except:*
   a. The posterior pituitary remains in direct continuity with the midbrain via the pituitary stalk.
   b. Inhibiting and releasing factors for anterior pituitary hormones are delivered via the hypophyseal portal circulation.
   c. Rathke's pouch is an upgrowth of oral ectoderm that forms the posterior pituitary lobe.
   d. The principal arterial blood supply to the pituitary is the superior hypophyseal artery.
   e. Dura mater lines the sella turcica and forms an incomplete diaphragm through which the pituitary stalk passes.

2. The following are hormonal products of the anterior pituitary (adenohypophysis) except:
   a. hGH.
   b. ADH.
   c. ACTH.
   d. LH.
   e. FSH.

3. Control of ADH secretion is primarily via osmoreceptors in the right atrium.
   a. True.
   b. False.

4. The six hormones of the anterior pituitary are glycoproteins consisting of a common α-subunit and a unique β-subunit that confers specificity.
   a. True.
   b. False.

5. Which statement is correct?
   a. Craniopharyngimas are highly malignant vestiges of oral ectoderm that are often treated with a combination of surgery and radiation therapy.
   b. Chromophobe adenomas cause a characteristic sequential parahypopituitarism starting with loss of lactogenic hormone, FSH, LH, TSH, and finally ACTH.
   c. Prolactin-secreting pituitary adenomas are less common than other functioning pituitary adenomas and generally respond to therapy with bromocriptine.
   d. hGH-secreting pituitary adenomas in adults generally cause few biochemical or physical derangements other than acromegaly.

e. Transsphenoidal hypophysectomy is contraindicated in cases of Cushing disease unless a pituitary mass can be clearly demonstrated on a CT scan.

6. All of the following statements are true *except:*
   a. Pituitary apoplexy following radiation therapy manifests as headache, meningismus, ophthalmoplegia, and visual loss.
   b. Postpartum lactation failure following prolonged maternal hypotension during labor is consistent with a diagnosis of Sheehan syndrome.
   c. Central diabetes insipidus following blunt head trauma is generally a transient phenomenon.
   d. "Empty sella syndrome" is usually described in cachectic elderly male patients.

7. The following statements concerning adrenal physiology and anatomy are correct *except:*
   a. Approximately 150 mg of aldosterone is released from the juxtaglomerular apparatus daily.
   b. Angiotensin II is formed in the pulmonary vasculature and is a promoter of aldosterone release.
   c. Cortisol is produced in both the zona fasciculata and the zona reticularis of the adrenal cortex.
   d. Aldosterone causes net sodium resorption from the renal tubes as well as potassium and hydrogen ion excretion.
   e. The arterial blood supply of the adrenal is from the aorta, phrenic, and renal artery branches.

8. The venous drainage of the left adrenal gland is directly to the inferior vena cava.
   a. True.
   b. False.

9. The following statements regarding the diagnosis of adrenal disorders are true *except:*
   a. Hyperaldosteronism is associated with a hypernatremic, hypokalemic metabolic alkylosis.
   b. Nonsuppressibility of urinary aldosterone secretion during a period of prolonged oral salt loading is diagnostic of an aldosterone-secreting adrenocortical carcinoma.
   c. Oat cell carcinoma of the lung is the most common cause of ectopic ACTH production.
   d. In approximately 70% of cases hypercortisolism is caused by a pituitary microadenoma.
   e. Administration of metyrapone results in a marked increase in deoxycortisol levels in patients with pituitary Cushing syndrome.

10. The following statements regarding the diagnosis and treatment of pheochromocytomas are correct *except:*
    a. Extraadrenal pheochromocytomas comprise roughly 10% of these tumors and can be located from the base of the skull to the testes.
    b. Epinephrine is produced only by adrenal medullary and organ of Zuckerkandl pheochromocytomas.
    c. The diagnosis of medullary thyroid carcinoma should prompt a thorough biochemical workup for the presence of an occult pheochromocytoma.
    d. Preoperative localization of these tumors should allow exploration and resection to proceed via a unilateral posterior approach.
    e. Histologically it is not possible to differentiate benign from malignant pheochromocytomas.

11. Preoperative preparation of a patient undergoing resection of a pheochromocytoma can be rapidly achieved with repeated small intravenous doses of propranolol and volume infusion.
    a. True.
    b. False.

SELECTED REFERENCES

Bravo EL, Gifford RW. Pheochromocytoma: diagnosis, localization and management. *N Engl J Med* 1984;1928.

Byyny RL. Preventing adrenal insufficiency during surgery. *Postgrad Med* 1980;67(s):219.

Carpenter PC. Cushings syndrome: update of diagnosis and management. *Mayo Clin Proc* 1988;61:49.

Civetta JM, Taylor RW, Kirby RR. *Critical care.* Philadelphia: JB Lippincott, 1988.

Copeland PM. The incidentally discovered adrenal mass. *Am Surg* 1984;199:116.

Grant CS, Carpenter PC, Van Heerden JA, Hamberger B. Primary aldosteronism, clinical management. *Arch Surg* 1984;119:585.

Jex RC, Van Heerden JA, Carpenter PC, Grant CS. Ectopic ACTH syndrome, diagnostic and therapeutic aspects. *Am Surg* 1985;149:276.

Miller, TA. *Physiologic basis of modern surgical care.* St. Louis: CV Mosby, 1988.

Scott HW, Abumral NN, Orth DN. Tumors of the adrenal cortex and Cushings syndrome. *Am Surg* 1985;201:586.

18

Thyroid and Parathyroid Surgery

Sanford Dubner, Keith S. Heller, Michael Coomaraswamy

ANATOMY AND EMBRYOLOGY

The thyroid is embryologically derived from the primitive alimentary tract, arising from the ventral wall of the pharynx in the region that becomes the foramen cecum at the base of the tongue. The main portion of the thyroid descends into the neck along a tract, a portion of which becomes the pyramidal lobe. Remnants of this tract can develop into thyroglossal cysts. The parafollicular (C) cells migrate to the thyroid from the neural crest.

The thyroid is bounded posteriorly by the trachea and larynx, the carotid sheaths, and sternocleidomastoid muscles laterally and by the strap muscles (sternohyoid, sternothyroid) anteriorly. The deep cervical fascia divides into an anterior and a posterior layer, creating a false capsule around the thyroid. Posteriorly this capsule is more dense and adherent to the trachea (ligament of Berry).

The arterial blood supply includes the superior thyroid arteries, arising as the first branch of the external carotid arteries bilaterally, and the inferior thyroid arteries, which arise from the thyrocervical trunks. Venous drainage is into the superior and middle thyroid veins (which drain into the internal jugular vein) and the inferior thyroid veins (which drain into the innominate vein). Draining lymph nodes include the pretra-

cheal (delphian), paralaryngeal, jugular, paratracheal, and paraesophageal lymph nodes.

The recurrent laryngeal nerve, a branch of the vagus nerve, passes around the aortic arch at the ductus arteriosus on the left and around the subclavian artery on the right. The nerves lie in the tracheoesophageal groove and enter the larynx through the cricothyroid membrane, innervating all of the muscles of the larynx except the cricothyroid muscle. In a small percentage of patients, the right recurrent laryngeal nerve does not loop around the subclavian artery but directly enters the larynx, crossing the neck transversely or obliquely downward (nonrecurrent laryngeal nerve). Injury to the recurrent laryngeal nerve results in hoarseness due to vocal cord paralysis and occasionally in airway obstruction if both cords are paralyzed.

The superior laryngeal nerve, also a branch of the vagus nerve, has two divisions in the neck: an internal branch that supplies sensation to the mucosa of the larynx and hypopharynx and an external branch that innervates the cricothyroid muscle. This nerve lies near the upper pole of the thyroid and the superior thyroid vessels. Injury to this nerve results in vocal fatigue and changes in the strength and pitch of the voice.

The parathyroid glands are usually four in number, weighing approximately 35 mg each. The paired superior glands are embryologically derived from the fourth branchial pouch. They descend in the neck for a short distance along with the thyroid and generally lie close to the superior portion of the lateral thyroid lobes. The inferior parathyroid glands arise from the third branchial pouch along with the thymus. They descend for a variable distance during embryologic development and may ultimately come to lie anywhere from the upper neck to the mediastinum. They are most commonly located on the lateral or posterior surface of the inferior pole of the thyroid. The second most common location is the upper portion of the thymus. As a general rule the superior parathyroids lie lateral to the recurrent laryngeal nerve and the inferior parathyroids medial to it. Anomalous locations do occur, and parathyroid glands may be found in the carotid sheath, behind the esophagus, in the thyroid, and in the anterior or posterior mediastinum. Occasional patients have more than four parathyroids. All four parathyroid glands generally derive their blood supply from the inferior thyroid artery, although it is not uncommon for the superior glands to be supplied by the superior thyroid artery.

The lateral aberrant thyroid is a rare entity, as the lateral components of the thyroid are normally incorporated into the medial thyroid derived from the foramen cecum. Therefore any lateral thyroid tissue almost always represents well-differentiated thyroid carcinoma that has metastasized to and replaced a lymph node with tumor.

Lingual thyroid is a rare entity that results from failure of the normal descent of the thyroid anlage from the base of the tongue. It may present as an asymptomatic posterior lingual mass, or it may enlarge and become symptomatic, causing dysphagia or dyspnea. It is more common in females and frequently is associated with absent thyroid tissue in the normal anatomic position, thus serving as the most common form of functioning ectopic thyroid tissue.

PHYSIOLOGY

The thyroid produces thyroid hormone and calcitonin. Although calcitonin lowers serum calcium levels, its role in human physiology is unclear. Thyroid hormone formation depends on absorption of iodine by the gastrointestinal tract. It is then distributed in the plasma as an iodide and is extracted by the thyroid or kidney, with approximately two-thirds excreted in the urine. In the thyroid it is converted from iodide to elemental iodine and linked with tyrosine to form monoiodotyrosine

or diiodotyrosine. These molecules are then linked to form triiodothyronine (T_3) and thyroxine (T_4), which are hormonally active and are stored in thyroid follicles where they are incorporated into thyroglobulin. The transfer of iodine from plasma into the thyroid is under the control of thyroid-stimulating hormone (TSH), which also affects thyroid hormone synthesis and secretion at each step. The secretion of TSH is controlled by thyrotropin-releasing hormone (TRH), which is released by the hypothalamus. Hydrolysis of thyroglobulin releases T_4 and T_3, which are bound to thyroid-binding globulin (TBG) and albumin in the serum. Most thyroid hormone in the circulation is T_4, but T_3 is four times as active as T_4; T_4 can be converted to T_3 peripherally. Both hormones are conjugated in the liver and excreted in the bile. T_3 has a half-life of 2 to 3 days, whereas the half-life of T_4 is 7 to 10 days.

PATHOPHYSIOLOGY

Hyperthyroidism represents an elevated circulating level of free T_3, T_4, or both. Its clinical symptoms include tachycardia, fever, weight loss, palpitations, heat intolerance, and emotional instability. The three most common causes of thyrotoxicosis are autonomous functioning adenoma, toxic multinodular goiter, and diffuse toxic goiter (Graves' disease).

Graves' disease is the most common cause of thyrotoxicosis. It is six times as common in women as in men and usually occurs in the 20- to 40-year age group. The syndrome is characterized by thyrotoxicosis, goiter, and exophthalmos. The hyperthyroidism of Graves' disease results from autoantibodies that bind to the TSH receptors on the cell membrane, stimulating thyroid function. The relation of the characteristic exophthalmos to this autoimmune process has not been determined.

Patients with a solitary, autonomous, functioning adenoma usually have a slow-growing mass that appears as a single hot nodule suppressing the remainder of the gland on thyroid scan. The thyroids in patients with toxic multinodular goiter contain several palpable nodules.

Thyroiditis, an inflammatory condition, may be acute or chronic. Acute suppurative thyroiditis is an uncommon condition that presents with an acute onset of neck pain, a tender, fluctuant gland, fever, and chills. Surgical drainage may be required. DeQuervain's thyroiditis is a subacute inflammation that often follows a viral upper respiratory infection. It usually presents as thyroid swelling and pain with fever, fatigue, and weight loss. Because of the disruption of the thyroid follicles with release of previously formed thyroid hormone, the patients are initially hyperthyroid. As the disease resolves they may become hypothyroid before the euthyroid condition is restored. Symptomatic treatment of pain with salicylates or steroids may be required.

Hashimoto's, or chronic lymphocytic, thyroiditis is the most common form of thyroiditis. It is characterized by diffuse induration of both lobes of the gland, although asymmetry and nodularity can occur. The disease is frequently asymptomatic but can be painful. Most patients eventually become hypothyroid, but initially thyrotoxicosis is seen. The diagnosis is based on the demonstration of lymphocytes and Hurthle cells on biopsy and by the frequent demonstration of elevated serum levels of antimicrosomal and antithyroglobulin antibodies. Treatment is symptomatic. Surgery is almost never indicated. Hyper- or hypothyroidism, of course, must be treated when it develops.

Patients with thyrotoxicosis due to excess production of thyroid hormone have elevated uptake of iodine by the thyroid. They can be treated effectively with antithyroid drugs, radioactive iodine, or surgery. The most commonly used antithyroid agents are propylthiouracil (PTU) and methimazole (Tapazole), both of which interfere with the binding of iodide to tyrosine and inhibit the coupling of iodotyrosines. Symptomatic relief usually occurs within 2 weeks of the initiation of therapy. Patients with Graves' disease treated in this fashion occasionally go into permanent remission and require no further treatment. Because these drugs cross the placenta and are excreted in breast milk, their use during pregnancy and lactation must be carefully regulated.

β-Adrenergic blockers can be used as an alternative to the thioureas. These drugs control all of the peripheral manifestations of hyperthyroidism, although serum levels of T_3 and T_4 remain elevated. They are particularly useful when preparing hyperthyroid patients for surgery. Because of the long serum half-life of T_4, it is necessary to administer βblockers for several weeks postoperatively to prevent recurrence of hyperthyroidism and thyroid storm.

Traditionally, hyperthyroid patients being prepared for thyroid surgery received oral iodine preparations. Careful regulation of antithyroid medications or βblockers usually makes the use of additional iodine unnecessary.

Patients who are noncompliant with their medication or whose thyrotoxicosis recurs after cessation of their antithyroid medication can be treated with radioactive iodine (RAI) or surgery. RAI is particularly useful for treating diffuse toxic goiter. It is administered orally at a dose based on the severity of the disease and the size of the gland with the intent of delivering approximately 8,500 rad to the thyroid. It takes several months for the effects to fully manifest. Most patients eventually become hypothyroid. Approximately 20% of patients require more than one dose to achieve a euthyroid or hypothyroid state. RAI may not be given to pregnant or lactating women because it crosses the placenta and is secreted in milk.

Radioactive iodine is the preferred treatment for Graves' disease. The risk, pain, and expense of surgery are avoided. There has been no demonstration of an increased risk of thyroid cancer or birth defects in patients treated with RAI. Nevertheless, surgery is indicated when definitive treatment during pregnancy is required and in patients unwilling to accept treatment with RAI. It is also indicated when a rapid response is desired. Surgical excision is preferable in instances of hyperfunctioning adenoma and when there is a coexisting malignant lesion.

SURGERY

Thyroid surgery is usually performed under general endotracheal anesthesia with the neck hyperextended by placing a rolled sheet underneath the shoulders. A transverse incision is made in a natural skin crease near the level of the cricoid cartilage. Subplatysmal skin flaps are elevated from the upper margin of the thyroid cartilage to the sternal notch. The gland is exposed by retracting the strap muscles. Division of these muscles is sometimes required to remove large glands. Blunt dissection around the periphery of the thyroid lobe in the loose areolar plane allows identification and division of the middle thyroid vein. The superior thyroid vessels are then ligated on the surface of the upper pole of the thyroid gland to avoid injury to the external branch of the superior laryngeal nerve. The thyroid lobe can then usually be rotated anteriorly and medially, permitting visualization of the posterior portion of the gland and the paratracheal tissues. The recurrent laryngeal nerve may now be visualized in the tracheoesophageal groove and its course traced superiorly to its entry into the larynx. It should be remembered that in few patients this nerve is not recurrent on the right side.

During dissection in the tracheoesophageal groove the surgeon should be alert to the location of the parathyroid glands. By identifying the blood supply to each parathyroid and preserving it as the parathyroid is mobilized away from the thyroid, injury to the parathyroids is avoided. The inferior thyroid vessels may now be ligated and divided distal to the origin of the blood vessels to the parathyroids. The isthmus is divided at the junction with the opposite lobe, and the lobe is sharply dissected off the trachea medially, dividing Berry's ligament between clamps.

The extent of surgery depends on the pathologic process. In hyperthyroid states the solitary toxic nodule is usually treated by thyroid lobectomy or nodulectomy. When it is necessary to operate for Graves' disease or toxic nodular goiter, a small remnant (5 to 10 g) of thyroid can be left to avoid persistent hypothyroidism. Hypothyroidism is common after surgery for hyperthyroidism.

Another important indication for thyroidectomy is to relieve compression of adjacent structures, including the trachea, esophagus, and regional veins, by an enlarged thyroid gland. This situation can be assessed clinically by a history of dyspnea, dysphagia, or facial swelling, and it can be documented by CT scan, MRI, esophagraphy, and chest radiography. Pulmonary function tests may be needed to assess the clinical significance of any tracheal narrowing seen. In these situations the extent of surgery is aimed at easing the symptoms. In the patient with significant substernal extension of the thyroid it is usually possible to perform thyroidectomy through a transcervical approach if there is a portion of thyroid extending above the clavicles and sternal notch, as the thyroid frequently mobilizes into the neck when it is hyperextended. Nevertheless, it is occasionally necessary to perform a sternotomy to remove a substernal goiter that cannot be mobilized into the neck.

The most common indication for thyroidectomy is the treatment or evaluation of a nodule for malignancy. This subject is discussed in Chapter 19.

PARATHYROID

Parathyroid hormone (PTH) is synthesized in the chief cells of the parathyroid glands. It is an 84-amino-acid polypeptide that is rapidly degraded into a biologically active N-terminal fragment and an inert C-terminal fragment. Although radioimmunoassays have been developed for both the N-terminal and midregion segments of this hormone, the latest generation assays that measure the intact hormone have the most utility. Normal values for the intact hormone range from 35 to 65 ng/dL in most laboratories.

The physiological action of PTH is mediated through stimulation of adenylate cyclase in target tissues, including kidney, bone, and intestine. PTH stimulates renal tubular resorption of calcium and increases tubular secretion of phosphate and bicarbonate; it also promotes 1-hydroxylation of vitamin D to form the more active 1,25-dihyroxyvitamin D. Under normal circumstances the level of ionized serum calcium exerts tight feedback control on the release of PTH from the parathyroid gland. Symptoms of moderate hypercalcemia (10.5 to 14.5 mg/dL) include polydipsia, weight loss, renal colic, muscular and bone pain, epigastric abdominal pain, and such neuropsychiatric disorders as depression, weakness, and insomnia. Severe hypercalcemia (Ca higher than 14.5 mg/dL) can be life-threatening and should be vigorously treated with forced saline diuresis. Dichloromethylene diphosphonate (clodronate), which effectively inhibits bone resorption, appears to have fewer side effects than mithramycin and can be given to control the calcium level while the etiology of the hypercalcemia is being investigated. Hypercalcemia in hospitalized patients is statistically most likely to be due to a malignancy, whereas elevations in serum calcium detected in an outpatient population are more likely to be due to hyperparathyroidism.

Primary hyperparathyroidism is defined as an elevated serum PTH level in the presence of hypercalcemia. A solitary parathyroid adenoma is the cause of primary hyperparathyroidism in about 85% of cases; in 12% four-gland hyperplasia is found and in about 1% parathyroid carcinoma. A small percentage of patients have multiple adenomas. Although most cases are sporadic with no known etiology, primary hyperparathyroidism is associated with multiple endocrine neoplasia (MEN) syndromes type I and II, which is in keeping with the neural crest origin of the parathyroid glands.

Secondary hyperparathyroidism is best viewed as a normal endocrine response to altered serum chemistry. It is most frequently encountered in association with chronic renal failure in which phosphate retention leads to persistently low serum calcium, which stimulates PTH production and eventually four-gland hypertrophy.

Tertiary hyperthyroidism occurs in patients with long-standing secondary hyperparathyroidism in which feedback control of PTH secretion is lost when serum calcium levels are elevated to a normal range. Complications of secondary hyperparathyroidism include debilitating bone pain, pruritus, pathologic fractures, and ectopic tissue calcifications.

Most patients with secondary hyperparathyroidism are managed medically with phosphate binders and calcium supplementation, with the aim of lowering the serum calcium phosphate product to less than 70mg/dL. About 5%–10% of patients require total or subtotal parathyroidectomy for failure of medical treatment.

Most patients diagnosed with hyperparathyroidism are noted only to have elevated serum calcium but with few or no associated symptoms. Such radiologic findings as Brown tumors, subperiosteal resorption of the phalanges, and bone cysts are rarely seen but, when present, are diagnostic of this condition. Presenting symptoms may include renal stones, peptic ulcer disease, hypertension, pancreatitis, depression, and lethargy. An elevated intact PTH level in the presence of persistent hypercalcemia and increased urinary calcium excretion are diagnostic of primary hyperparathyroidism. Preoperative localization techniques include ultrasonography, CT scanning, MRI, and scintigraphy with thallium/technetium or sestamibi. There is no consensus as to whether routine preoperative localization studies are cost-effective. Arteriography and selective venous catheterization with PTH sampling can be useful as a prelude to reexploration after an initial failed operation or when an ectopic mediastinal gland is suspected on the basis of less invasive imaging studies.

The surgical approach to the parathyroid glands is similar to that for thyroid surgery. After the thyroid gland has been exposed by mobilizing the strap muscles and dividing the middle thyroid veins, the thyroid lobe is mobilized anteriorly and medially. The parathyroid glands can often be identified in the vicinity of the recurrent laryngeal nerve as it crosses the inferior thyroid artery. The inferior gland is often found in this location, with the superior gland usually 1 to 2 cm above it, in the tracheoesophageal groove or along the posterior surface of the thyroid. All four parathyroid glands should be identified and all enlarged glands removed. When four-gland hyperplasia is found, a vascularized fragment of one gland is left in situ or several small (1 mm) portions

of a histologically confirmed gland are autotransplanted into the sternomastoid muscle or the brachioradialis muscle in the forearm. In the event that an abnormal parathyroid gland is not readily identified, the thymus is mobilized into the neck to look for an aberrant inferior parathyroid. An aberrant superior gland may be located in the retroesophageal area or the posterior mediastinum. Finally, the thyroid lobe is removed on the side of the missing gland and sectioned to rule out an intrathyroidal parathyroid gland. Median sternotomy is not performed at the time of initial surgical exploration nor are normal-appearing parathyroid glands removed. Rather, the operation is terminated, and repeat localization studies are performed.

QUESTIONS

Select one answer.

1. Imaging studies commonly used to identify parathyroid adenomas preoperatively include all of the following *except:*
   a. Technetium/thallium subtraction scan.
   b. CT scan.
   c. Sonogram.
   d. Selenium scan.
   e. MRI.
2. Surgery may be considered the treatment of choice for which of the following causes of hyperthyroidism?
   a. Solitary functioning adenoma.
   b. Graves' disease.
   c. Hashimoto's thyroiditis.
   d. Subacute thyroiditis.
3. Which of the following structures is not routinely identified during thyroid surgery?
   a. Parathyroid glands.
   b. Superior laryngeal nerve.
   c. Middle thyroid vein.
   d. Recurrent laryngeal nerve.
   e. Inferior thyroid artery.
4. The diagnosis of primary hyperparathyroidism requires knowledge of which of the following laboratory tests (more than one may be correct)?
   a. Creatinine.
   b. Phosphate.
   c. Calcium.
   d. Urinary cAMP.
   e. PTH.

5. The most common symptom of hyperparathyroidism is:
   a. Bone pain.
   b. Kidney stones.
   c. Pancreatitis.
   d. No symptoms.
   e. Ulcer disease.

SELECTED REFERENCES

Bradley EL, Liechty RD. Modified subtotal thyroidectomy for Graves' disease: a two-institution study. *Surgery* 1983;94:955–958.

Cheung PSY, Borgstrom A, Thompson NW. Strategy in reoperative surgery for hyperparathyroidism. *Arch Surg* 1989;124:676–680.

Cooper DS, Ridgway EC. Clinical management of patients with hyperthyroidism. *Med Clin North Am* 1985;69:953–971.

Fitzpatrick LA. Hypercalcemia in the multiple endocrine neoplasia syndrome. *Endocrinol Metab Clin North Am* 1989;18:741–752.

Hay ID. Thyroiditis: a clinical update. *Mayo Clin Proc* 1985;60:836–843.

Karbowitz SR, Edelman LB, Nath JH, Dwek JH, Rammohan. Spectrum of advanced upper airway obstruction due to goiters. *Chest* 1985;81:18–21.

Marcus R. Laboratory diagnosis of primary hyperparathyroidism. *Endocrinol Metab Clin North Am* 1989;18:647–658.

Scholz DA, Purnell DC. Asymptomatic primary hyperparathyroidism: 10-year prospective study. *Mayo Clin Proc* 1981;56:473–478.

Spaulding SW, Lippes H. Hyperthyroidism: causes, clinical features, and diagnosis. *Med Clin North Am* 1985;69:937–951.

19

Head and Neck Tumors

Carl E. Silver, Brigid K. Glackin, Francis J. Velez, and Helen H. Kim

An outline of the histologic tumor types that occur in the head and neck is presented in Table 19.1. This discussion centers on the three most commonly occurring epithelial tumors: squamous cell carcinoma, adenocarcinoma of the thyroid, and adenocarcinoma of salivary origin. These three types of epithelial tumor are unique in their head and neck manifestations. The behavior of lymphomas, other sarcomas, and melanoma in the head and neck is generally similar to their behavior in other parts of the body.

SQUAMOUS CELL CARCINOMA

Almost all head and neck squamous cell carcinomas (SCCs) arise in the mucosa of the upper aerodigestive tract and metastasize almost exclusively by means of lymphatics to the cervical lymph nodes, which are categorized into six regions (levels I to VI). Distant metastases tend to occur only with advanced stages of disease, particularly to the lungs. In rare instances squamous cell carcinoma may arise primarily in parotid or submandibular salivary glands or within a branchiogenic cyst. As a practical matter, SCC within a cervical mass should be considered metastatic and, depending on the location of the mass, to have arisen from a primary site in the upper aerodigestive tract, skin of the head and neck, the lungs, or the esophagus.

This discussion concerns evaluation and management of tumors that have arisen from primary sites above the clavicle: nose and paranasal sinuses, oral cavity, oropharynx, larynx, hypopharynx, cervical esophagus, and skin of the head and neck. Although lesions arising from individual primary sites may differ from one another in their natural history, treatment, and prognosis, these differences are mainly a matter of degree. Tumors in some locations tend to grow and spread more rapidly and to be more difficult to cure than in other locations. The basic principles of evaluation and management, as well as etiologic and epidemiologic factors, are similar for the entire group of mucosal squamous cell head and neck cancers. Skin cancers are similar in their pattern of spread and principles of management.

Epidemiology

In 1994 an estimated 29,600 new cases of SCC of the oral cavity and pharynx and 11,000 new cases of laryngeal SCC were reported in the United States. Incidence rates for male and female patients according to race are listed in Table 19.2. The disease tends to predominate in men by a ratio of 3:1 and occurs with greatest frequency in the white male population. In recent years the incidence of the disease in women has increased. In the white population, the incidence of the disease increases

TABLE 19.1. *Head and neck tumors*

Connective tissue tumors
  Lymphoma
  Sarcoma
Epithelial tumors
  Squamous cell carcinoma
  Adenocarcinoma
    Salivary gland
    Thyroid
  Melanoma
  Neuroepithelial tumors

with age, whereas in nonwhites, a peak incidence is reached during the fifth decade of life and is relatively constant thereafter. Prognosis of squamous cell head and neck cancer tends to be more favorable in female than in male patients for equivalent lesions and is somewhat more favorable for the white than the nonwhite population.

Etiologic Factors

The association of head and neck SCC with combined alcohol and tobacco consumption is well known. Eighty-five percent of these patients indulge in daily usage of lighted tobacco, and daily consumption of more than minimal quantities of alcohol is reported for 60% of patients. Other carcinogens associated with various head and neck (squamous cell) cancers are wood dust, radiochemical materials, nickel, nitrosamines, betel nuts, and nonlighted tobacco. Various infectious agents may be involved in some cancers. Epstein-Barr virus and human papilloma virus (HPV), specifically, HPV16,18, have been associated with SCC. Syphilis, when it was prevalent, was often associated with SCC of the involved organ, such as the larynx. Chronic infection may play a role in the development of paranasal sinus carcinoma. Other etiologic factors are nutritional

TABLE 19.2. *Incidence rates for squamous cell carcinoma*

Population	Incidence
White male	17.2/105
White female	5.6/105
Black male	13.2/105
Black female	5.2/105

deficiencies, racial and genetic factors, edentulousness, chronic trauma, and poor oral hygiene.

Premalignant Lesions

There is a spectrum of mucosal aberrations in the upper aerodigestive tract that may be precursors of infiltrating SCC. Not all such lesions are premalignant, however, and in most cases of malignancy there is no evidence that the tumor arose as a progression of a "premalignant" mucosal aberration. The term leukoplakia is generally associated with lesions thought to be premalignant. Leukoplakia, however, is merely a descriptive term and does not constitute a pathologic diagnosis. Various types of inflammatory and neoplastic lesions can present clinically as "leukoplakia." Biopsy is necessary to determine the precise diagnosis.

Many truly premalignant or early malignant lesions present as erythroplasia (red lesions), most often on the floor of the mouth and gingiva. Some patients, often habitual alcohol and tobacco abusers, have diffuse abnormalities of the oral and pharyngeal mucosa, with numerous white and red lesions representing various states of mucosal aberration.

The histology of the premalignant lesions consists of varying degrees of hyperplasia and keratosis of the epithelium. It is the keratosis that is often responsible for the white color of the lesions. Keratosis may occur with or without hyperplasia, and the reverse is true as well. Hyperplasia may occur with or without cellular atypia. Hyperplasia without atypia, whether associated with keratosis, is not considered a premalignant lesion. The important factor in the development of malignant potential is the presence of atypical changes within the cellular nuclei. In instances of marked atypical hyperplasia, there may be individual frankly malignant cells within the epithelium, but malignant changes do not extend through the full thickness of the epithelium.

When malignant cells are found throughout the entire thickness of the epithelium but do not penetrate the basement membrane, the condition is known as intraepithelial carcinoma, or carcinoma *in situ*. When a minimal degree of penetration of basement membrane by tumor is found, the lesion is termed carcinoma *in situ* with microinvasion.

There is considerable controversy concerning to what degree atypical hyperplasia and even carcinoma *in situ* may be reversible or the inevitability of progression to infiltrating SCC. It is thought by most authorities that at least some if not all of these lesions do progress to frank malignancy. Many of the less advanced lesions with atypia can be reversed by removing the cause (smoking, dental irritation). More advanced lesions can be simply treated by local excision or with surgical laser. There is some indirect evidence that carcinoma *in situ* is reversible; but treatment with local excision, cryosurgery, laser, or even radiotherapy is recommended by most authorities. The significance of microinvasion associated with carcinoma *in situ* is also questionable. Its presence, however, may encourage a more aggressive form of treatment.

Evaluation of Primary Tumor

Whether a patient presents initially with a painless neck mass, prompting a search for a primary tumor, or the presentation is for complaints relating to a lesion of the upper aerodigestive tract, the initial diagnostic measure is thorough examination of possible primary sites: inspection and bimanual palpation of the oral cavity and oropharynx; visualization of the larynx, pharynx, and nasal cavities; and complete examination of the skin and scalp. Indirect laryngoscopy to visualize the larynx and hypopharynx, nasal speculum examination (anterior rhinoscopy) after shrinking the nasal mucosa with a vasoconstrictor, and posterior rhinoscopy with a mirror to visualize the nasopharynx are the traditional examination procedures employed for the past century, and they require considerable skill for application. A variety of endoscopic instruments, the most popular of which is the short, thin flexible fiberoptic nasopharyngolaryngoscope, have greatly enhanced the ability to conduct a thorough examination in the office with topical anesthesia.

Conventional "rigid" endoscopy (direct laryngoscopy, esophagoscopy, tracheobronchoscopy) is often necessary for complete evaluation and biopsy of the index tumor in the larynx, hypopharynx, and cervical esophagus, as the incidence of synchronous lesions in the upper aerodigestive tract is in the order of 10% to 20%. Newly developed miniaturized endoscopic instruments have greatly simplified the evaluation and biopsy of lesions in the nasal cavity and nasopharynx.

New "imaging" techniques have revolutionized the ability to evaluate primary tumors of the entire upper aerodigestive tract and cervical lymph node and distant metastatic disease. Computed tomography (CT) and magnetic resonance imaging (MRI) are useful for evaluating of lesions in the base of the skull, paranasal sinuses, parapharyngeal space, pharynx, and larynx, and for evaluating cervical lymphadenopathy. Ultrasonography, scintigraphy, and angiography may be useful for evaluating various mass lesions in the neck and thyroid gland.

Evaluation of Neck Mass

Primary SCCs of the upper aerodigestive tract characteristically metastasize to cervical lymph nodes. The conventional method for evaluating the neck is palpation. The size, location, number, consistency, and degree of fixation of any palpable neck mass should be noted. CT scanning of the neck has extended our ability to evaluate metastatic cervical lymphadenopathy, particularly in obese or short-necked individuals. Present staging classifications rely on palpation for clinical diagnosis of cervical metastatic disease, although this may change in the future as our ability to identify "occult" regional metastasis has been increased by imaging studies.

In patients with metastatic SCC in cervical lymph nodes, it has long been recognized that open biopsy of these neck masses is of little value for diagnosis and is detrimental to treatment. If a primary tumor is identified and proven by biopsy, any clinically suspicious cervical mass has traditionally been considered metastatic disease for purposes of staging and treatment planning. The advent of fine needle aspiration biopsy (FNAB) with cytologic evaluation of the material has provided a simple, rapid, safe method of determining the nature of a cervical mass without incurring the disadvantages of open biopsy. The accuracy of FNAB is approximately 90% in experienced hands. The procedure is most reliable for distinguishing malignant and benign lesions and for determining tissue types in lesions of the neck. Ultrasound- and MRI-guided FNABs have assumed an increasing role in the diagnosis and staging of SCC of the head and neck region, particularly in the clinically negative (N0) neck.

In cases where the patient presents initially with a neck mass but without evidence of a primary tumor, evaluation by imaging studies and FNAB provides excellent orientation as to the nature of the tumor. Thus a neck mass may be recognized as metastatic SCC, suspicious for lymphoma, benign, due to metastatic thyroid carcinoma, or due to other metastatic malignancy. A plan for further evaluation, as outlined in Figure 19.1, can be based on such information.

Metastatic SCC is occasionally found in cervical lymph nodes, without evidence of primary tumor, despite intensive search. Often the location of the cervical node with proved SCC can provide a clue as to the origin of the primary tumor. For example, cervical nodes presenting predominantly in the supraclavicular region generally originate below the clavicles. For SCC the lung would be the most frequent primary site of supraclavicular metastases. Primary tumors originating in the mouth, pharynx, and larynx generally metastasize to lymph nodes in the upper and midportions of the neck. The nasopharynx is probably the most frequent site of origin of occult primary tumors, and small lesions in the tonsil, base of the tongue, piriform sinus, and other sites may also remain obscure for prolonged periods.

Patients with metastatic cervical SCC of occult origin should undergo a complete endoscopic and CT examination. If the examination remains negative, they may be treated in one of two ways. One alternative is to perform a radical neck dissection and continue to observe the patient for the development of a primary tumor. Another alternative is to treat the patient with radiotherapy to both sides of the neck and the entire pharynx from the base of the skull to the cervical esophagus. Neck dissection is performed if there is residual neck mass without evidence of a primary tumor. With either method of treatment, a 25% to 30% overall cure rate may be obtained. Prognosis is better in patients in whom the primary tumor is never found.

Staging

Staging of head and neck SCCs is based on the TNM system. The tumor is grouped into four stages according to the size of the tumor (T), nodal status (N), and distant metastasis (M). Staging criteria are derived by evaluating numerous variables related to the primary tumor and metastatic disease. The variations of TNM encountered are grouped into stages I to IV according to similar survival experience for each stage. The American Joint Committee (AJC) staging criteria for oral cavity tumors are outlined in Tables 19.3, 19.4, and 19.5. Staging criteria for tumors at other primary sites are generally similar. For oral cavity tumors the greatest diameter of the primary tumor (T) has been found to have the highest correlation with survival. Cervical lymph nodes (N) are classified by size, number, and whether homolateral, bilateral, or contralateral (Table 19.4). The presence or absence of distant metastasis is designated

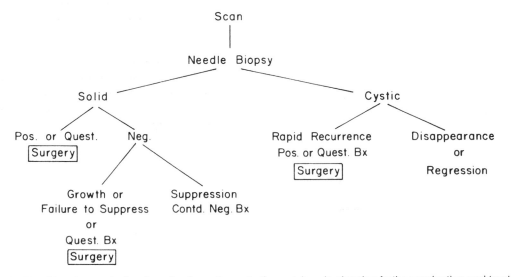

FIG. 19.1. Algorithm demonstrating the role of needle aspiration cytology in planning further evaluation and treatment of a cervical mass. (From Schneider et al., 1984, with permission)

TABLE 19.3. *Primary tumor (T) staging categories for oral cavity tumors*

Category	Description
T1	> 2 cm diameter
T2	2–4 cm diameter
T3	> 4 cm diameter
T4	Massive tumor with deep invasion of antrum, pterygoid, base of tongue, or skin

Table 19.5. *Stage groupings for oral cavity tumors*

Stage	TNM criteria
I	T1N0M0
II	T2N0M0
III	T3N0M0
	T1–3N1M0
IV	T4N0–1M0
	T1–3N2–3M0
	T1–3N0–3M1

by M0 (no evidence of distant metastasis) or M1 (clinical or radiographic evidence of distant metastasis). The various T, N, and M combinations that form stages I through IV are summarized in Table 19.5. In general, survival experience is relatively similar by stage for lesions at various primary sites. Thus 5-year survival rates for most stage I tumors range from 70% to 90%, stage II 60% to 80%, stage III 30% to 50%, and stage IV 25% or less.

Staging is important not only for determining prognosis for individual cases but also for evaluating the results of various types of treatment. It is essential that tumors of comparable stage be evaluated in any study comparing the results of one form of treatment with another.

Treatment

Treatment modalities employed for head and neck SCC are chemotherapy, radiotherapy, and surgery. Although the role of chemotherapy in treatment of head and neck cancer remains controversial, improvements in available agents and regimens show promise for treatment of both curable and incurable advanced tumors. Cisplatin in combination with one or more other agents, particularly 5-fluorouracil (5-FU), bleomycin,

TABLE 19.4. *Cervical lymph node (N) staging categories for oral cavity tumors*

Category	Description
N0	No clinically positive nodes
N1	Single homolateral node < 3 cm
N2a	Single homolateral node 3–6 cm
N2b	Multiple homolateral nodes < 6 cm
N2c	Bilateral or contralateral nodes < 6 cm
N3	Nodes > 6 cm

vincristine, and methotrexate, are the most effective and commonly employed drugs. For potentially curable tumors, chemotherapy has generally been employed in various clinical trials preoperatively (induction, neoadjuvant, or protochemotherapy), postoperatively (adjuvant), or concurrent with radiation therapy (chemoradiation). Overall survival reported in nonrandomized trials of induction chemotherapy has been statistically better with cisplatin in combination with 5-FU than with other cisplatin combinations. Prospective randomized clinical trials have not yet demonstrated improved survival, despite the relatively high (20% to 35%) achievement of complete response to chemotherapy.

The effectiveness of various postoperative regimens of chemotherapy is currently under study in prospective randomized trials. The rationale for combining cisplatin with radiation therapy for resectable and unresectable locally advanced carcinoma is based on the fact that their toxicities do not overlap and their therapeutic effects may be synergistic. Early results of clinical trials indicate improvement in the overall response rate for chemoradiation but with no difference in survival.

One application of chemotherapy has been based on the demonstration that complete response to chemotherapy serves as an accurate predictor of response to subsequent radiation therapy. It has been employed in patients with advanced laryngeal carcinoma to select patients for treatment with radiation alone, rather than total laryngectomy, which would otherwise have been required.

Radiotherapy and surgery are forms of local treatment that alone or in combination may be employed as definitive treatment (treatment for cure) of head and neck cancer. Although there is considerable controversy concerning the relative value of these modalities for treatment of various tumors, certain principles emerge that have found general acceptance and form the basis of treatment in most centers.

Early (stage I and II) head and neck cancers are usually treated by single modality (radiotherapy or surgery) therapy. When radiotherapy is employed as definitive treatment, doses of 60 Gy or higher are required for curative treatment of gross disease. In such cases, following radiation surgery is employed only to treat proved recurrent or persistent disease ("salvage" surgery). If surgery is the initial treatment, limited resection with preservation of functionally and cosmetically important tissue is usually possible for early stage cancer. Adjuvant radiotherapy is usually not employed in these cases unless there are microscopically involved margins of resection or microscopic evidence of cervical metastatic disease. Thus for early stages of SCC a choice is usually made between radiotherapy or surgery as the initial treatment modality. Considerations involved in such a choice are the age and condition of the patient, the reliability of the patient, expected functional and cosmetic results, the tumor site, and the preferences of the physician and the patient.

For advanced-stage (stages III and IV) head and neck tumors, most authorities agree that the results of planned combined radiotherapy and surgery produce results superior to treatment with either modality alone. Radiotherapy may be employed preoperatively or postoperatively. When employed preoperatively, it is generally given in doses of less than 60 Gy to minimize wound complications and radionecrosis after surgery. Most surgeons and many radiotherapists now prefer to employ high-dose radiotherapy after resection of the tumor. The reason for this preference is that surgical wounds in nonirradiated tissues usually heal rapidly with minimal postoperative complications. After healing, full-dose radiotherapy can be administered at a point at which the patient has minimal "tumor burden."

There has been little concrete statistical evidence to support many of our concepts about treatment of head and neck cancer. A few retrospective studies performed during the 1960s and early 1970s indicated some enhancement of the cure rate for advanced-stage tumors with preoperative radiotherapy. One well controlled prospective study by Strong et al. (1978) showed no difference in survival produced by preoperative radiotherapy compared with treatment by surgery alone. Several studies have shown statistically significant improvements in cure rates resulting from postoperative irradiation or strong trends indicating the same.

The standard surgical treatment of head and neck cancer is "block" resection of tumor including grossly and microscopically clear margins, with continuity between the primary tumor and regional lymph nodes when feasible. Advances in reconstructive surgery, particularly myocutaneous flaps, free revascularized transfers of soft tissue and bone, and prosthetic implants, have increased the ability of the surgeon to resect disease adequately and obtain satisfactory functional and cosmetic rehabilitation for the patient. A discussion of specific surgical techniques is beyond the scope of this general review.

During treatment of head and neck cancer consideration must be paid to the question of treatment of the neck. When evidence of metastatic cervical disease is present, a neck dissection is said to be "therapeutic." Neck dissection performed when there is no evidence of regional metastasis is termed a "staging" or "elective," neck dissection. Patients with clinically evident cervical metastasis have a greatly reduced survival rate compared with patients with equivalent primary lesions without cervical metastasis. Most authorities agree that a combined treatment modality (surgical resection followed by postoperative radiotherapy) provides the best locoregional control of disease in patients with clinically evident cervical metastasis. Extranodal spread (ENS) of lymph node disease is an indicator of poor prognosis, and the survival rate is reduced by more than 50% in such cases. ENS of lymph node disease may serve as an indication for additional adjuvant therapy.

Many primary tumors of the head and neck are associated with clinically occult microscopic metastasis in cervical lymph nodes. In recognition of this fact and in an effort to remove the tumor completely before the cervical metastasis evolves into a more advanced stage, many authorities recommend "elective" treatment of the neck in cases where the probability of occult metastatic disease is relatively large. This includes most lesions staged T3N0 and (at least) the larger T2N0 tumors of the oral cavity and pharynx. Treatment may be surgical, by selective or modified radical neck dissection. It has also been established that 50 Gy of external radiation can effectively sterilize microscopic cervical metastatic disease and may be employed in suitable cases as an alternative to surgery for elective treatment of the neck. In some instances, particularly for small oral cavity tumors treated surgically, the presence of occult cervical metastatic disease can be evaluated with a staging partial, or upper (supraomohyoid), neck dissection. The nodes most likely to be involved with metastatic cancer are removed and examined microscopically. If involvement is found, partial neck dissection may be extended to a complete radical neck dissection, or the neck may be treated postoperatively with radiotherapy.

When surgery is used for treatment of clinically evident cervical metastasis, the procedure employed is radical or modified radical neck dissection. With conventional radical neck dissection, the sternomastoid muscle, internal jugular vein, and accessory nerve are sacrificed. Modified radical neck dissection, which spares one or all of the above mentioned structures, is employed for lesser degrees of cervical involvement and particularly for elective treatment of the neck. Preservation of the accessory nerve during elective neck dissection is the most universally accepted and most frequently performed modification, as severing the accessory nerve carries the greatest morbidity associated with neck dissection.

New Frontiers

Gene therapy involves introducing DNA into host cells to induce expression of that particular gene. The most recent data concerning the use of gene therapy to treat head and neck cancer show some promise. Further research in molecular genetics has led to new insights into the diagnosis and treatment of human malignancies. The alterations of tumor-suppressor genes, such as retinoblastoma, *p53,* and others may have an important role in tumorigenesis. Mutations of *p53* have been found in most human malignancies, including head and neck cancer. The *p53* mutation in head and neck tumors is an early event and has been localized to specific chromosomal sites (codons). Although mutation and loss of heterozygosity at *p53* are important in the genesis of head and neck cancer, other mechanisms such as binding of viral and cellular proteins to P53 are also likely to play a role (Pavelic and Gluckman, 1997). Alterations in *p53* may also play a role in "field cancerization" and second primary tumors.

THYROID CARCINOMA

Pathology

For thyroid carcinoma, unlike SCC, the prognosis is predominantly related to the histologic type and de-

pends little on the stage (clinical characteristics of mary tumor and metastasis) at which the tumor presents. The relative frequencies of various histologic types of thyroid carcinoma are summarized in Table 19.6.

Papillary Carcinoma

Papillary carcinoma is the most common histologic variety of thyroid malignancy, comprising 80% of such lesions. Only 2% of thyroid malignancies are pure papillary, the remainder being mixed papillary-follicular. Nevertheless, the behavior of such mixed lesions coincides entirely with that of pure papillary carcinomas. In patients under the age of 40, even lesions that appear to be entirely follicular in morphology have the same natural history as pure papillary tumors. Many authorities consider these lesions to be a "follicular variant" of papillary carcinoma.

Papillary carcinoma occurs at a younger age than other thyroid tumors, most of them occurring before age 40. The disease preponderates in the female population by a 3:1 ratio. Clinically palpable lymph node metastasis is present in approximately 30% of cases, with occult metastasis occurring in up to 70% of carefully studied specimens in some series. The metastases are usually multicentric. Despite the frequency of occurrence, lymph node metastasis has no effect on survival: Many patients with occult metastatic lymph node involvement are never treated for their metastatic disease.

About 35% of papillary carcinomas measure less than 1.5 cm in diameter and are considered "occult" lesions, as many are not clinically palpable. About 50% of papillary carcinomas are larger than 1.5 cm but are

TABLE 19.6. *Classification of thyroid cancers*

Thyroid cancer	Incidence (%)
Papillary	62
Occult (<1.5 cm)	35
Intrathyroid	50
Extrathyroid	15
Follicular	18
Angioinvasion minimal	50
Angioinvasion moderate or marked	50
Anaplastic	14
Medullary	6

Source: Modified from Woolner et al. (1968).

contained entirely within the capsule of the thyroid gland (intrathyroidal). Another 15% of lesions extend through the thyroid capsule to invade contiguous structures (extrathyroidal spread).

The 5-year survival with papillary thyroid carcinoma ranges from 73% to 93% in most reported series, with additional mortality of 10% to 20% over a 10- to 20-year period. For occult and intrathyroidal lesions less than 5 cm diameter, survival curves are the same as for the normal population. Significant mortality from the disease generally occurs only from intrathyroidal lesions larger than 5 cm in diameter or from locally invasive tumors. Occult thyroid carcinomas are associated with virtually 100% survival. Unlike most malignant tumors, thyroid carcinomas tend to have a more favorable prognosis in young patients; the disease has a more aggressive course in patients over age 40. An exception to this rule occurs in prepubertal children, in whom 50% of thyroid nodules are malignant and whose malignancies follow a more aggressive course.

Follicular Carcinoma

Follicular carcinoma is the second most common thyroid malignancy, comprising 10% of all malignant lesions. True follicular carcinomas occur in an older age group (over age 40) than do most papillary carcinomas. The female/male ratio is 3:1, as with papillary carcinoma.

Follicular carcinomas are characterized mainly by their degree of angioinvasion. Approximately 50% of tumors demonstrate minimal angioinvasion, and the other 50% show moderate to marked angioinvasion. Unlike the situation with papillary carcinoma, lymph node metastasis is not a prominent factor in the natural history of follicular carcinoma, occurring in only 2% to 20% of cases. Distant metastases, skeletal or pulmonary, are seen in 50% to 65% of patients.

The 5-year survival of patients with nonmetastatic follicular carcinoma is approximately 70%, but it is only 22% in patients in whom distant metastasis is present at the time of initial diagnosis. The 10- to 20-year survival of those with follicular carcinoma is approximately 40%. About 50% to 60% of patients ultimately die of their tumor.

Unlike papillary carcinoma, the size of the primary tumor is not a critical factor in determining prognosis.

Prognosis is adversely affected by the presence of angioinvasion of moderate to marked degree, as well as by distant metastasis at the time of diagnosis.

Medullary Carcinoma

Medullary thyroid carcinoma (MTC) is an interesting and unusual tumor that comprises 1% to 7% of thyroid malignancies. About 80% of cases occur sporadically and are unilateral, and 20% are seen in association with multiple endocrine neoplasia type IIA (MEN-IIA) and MEN-IIB syndromes, as well as familial disease. MTC associated with MEN-IIA and MEN-IIB is usually bilateral, occurs at an earlier age, and carries a much poorer prognosis. Elevated levels of serum calcitonin are usually associated with medullary carcinoma and form a reliable "marker" for detection of occult lesions in familial cases or of recurrent disease in previously treated patients. The discovery of point mutations on the *RET* proto-oncogene responsible for MEN-II and familial MTC in 1993 has facilitated early detection and treatment.

The MTC arises from the so-called C cell, embryologically derived from the ultimobranchial body. The incidence in male and female patients is equal over a wide age range. Lymph node metastasis occurs in approximately 50% of patients. Distant metastasis tends to occur late in the course of the disease. Calcification of the primary tumor is often a prominent feature.

The 5-year survival of MTC patients has been reported to be 88% and the 10-year survival 78%. Prognosis is more favorable in younger patients. The presence of cervical lymph node metastasis has an adverse effect on survival.

Anaplastic Carcinoma

Anaplastic carcinoma comprises 1% to 5% of all thyroid carcinomas. Small-cell, giant cell, and spindle cell lesions and mixed varieties of anaplastic carcinoma exist. Anaplastic tumors occur in older patients, with the peak incidence during the seventh and eighth decades of life. No significant gender preference has been found. A multimodality treatment scheme offers the best result in terms of tumor response. It includes preoperative radiotherapy and multiagent chemotherapy followed by surgery and more adjuvant therapy. The 5-

year survival is less than 10%. Most patients die within 6 months of diagnosis.

Evaluation of Thyroid Nodules

Only a small percentage of thyroid nodules are malignant. Although some malignancies are clinically obvious, most are clinically indistinguishable from benign nontoxic nodular goiter. As most thyroid cancers have an excellent prognosis once identified and treated, the most significant problem in management of thyroid cancer consists of identifying the nodules that are malignant among the numerous benign goiters encountered in the adult population. A balance must be reached between recommending surgery in an excessively large number of cases, and so subjecting many patients with benign lesions to surgery that is of little benefit to them, and an overly conservative attitude that may result in failure to recognize and treat curable thyroid cancer. The modalities available for evaluating thyroid nodules are clinical evaluation, radioisotope scanning, ultrasonography, and needle aspiration biopsy.

Clinical Evaluation

The clinical criteria for diagnosis of thyroid cancer are outlined in Table 19.7. Such absolute criteria as the hardness and fixation of an obviously malignant lesion, vocal cord paralysis on the side of the thyroid mass, and histologically diagnosed metastatic disease are indications for surgical treatment without regard to the results of other tests and procedures. The relative criteria listed

TABLE 19.7. *Clinical criteria for diagnosis of thyroid cancer*

Absolute criteria
  Hardness and fixation
  Vocal cord paralysis
  Metastatic disease
Relative criteria
  Enlargement of "suppressed" nodule
  History of irradiation
  Obstruction of airway or esophagus
  Single nodule
  Pregnancy
  "Cold" nodules
  Solid nodules

are situations in which surgical exploration should be strongly considered but weighed with other factors such as the degree of risk presented by the patient's general condition and needle aspiration biopsy findings. Pre- and postoperative thyroglobulin levels obtained while the patient is on thyroid-stimulating hormone (TSH) suppression can be a useful tool for surveillance of well-differentiated thyroid carcinomas (i.e., papillary and follicular).

Radioisotope Scanning

Thyroid nodules that concentrate iodine poorly are more often malignant than similar lesions with normal or greater than normal function. The incidence of malignancy in hyperactive nodules is only about 2.5% and in normally active nodules 6.1%; in hypoactive (cold) nodules, the incidence of malignancy ranges from 17% to 25% in many series. The major weakness of radioisotope scanning is that whereas the sensitivity is high (few false negatives) the specificity of this test is unacceptably low because of the large number of false positives. The latter attribute minimizes the effectiveness of radioisotope scanning in precluding surgery for benign lesions. As such, the utility of obtaining a radioisotope scan preoperatively can be helpful in the setting of the "hot" nodule with an FNAB consistent with a "follicular lesion," which in most cases indicates a follicular adenoma rather than a follicular carcinoma. Technetium scanning, frequently employed because of its lower cost, is somewhat less sensitive than radioiodine scanning, and many authors advocate rescanning patients with negative (hot) technetium scans with radioactive iodine.

The chief value of isotope scanning is identification of hyperfunctioning nodules because of the extremely low incidence of carcinoma in these cases. It is important to remember, however, that there are occasional exceptions to this rule. Thus isotope scanning gives the clinician only a rough indication as to whether a thyroid nodule is benign or malignant.

Ultrasonography

With the advent of fine-needle aspiration (FNA) cytology the use of ultrasonography has diminished. A solid lesion has a greater propensity toward malignancy than does a cystic lesion, but as with "hot" nodules there are exceptions. Ultrasonography is useful for evaluating lesions that are difficult to palpate and to follow subtle changes in size during TSH suppression therapy. FNA of such lesions may be performed under ultrasound guidance.

Fine Needle Aspiration Cytology

Cytologic evaluation of specimens obtained by FNA has emerged as the primary diagnostic modality for evaluating thyroid lesions. Large-needle "core" biopsies have been largely abandoned owing to reported complications such as hemorrhage, vocal cord paralysis, and tumor implantation. Numerous large FNA series, however, have failed to demonstrate significant complications.

The results of FNA cytology are generally reported in three categories: positive (malignancy), negative, or atypical (suspicious or indeterminate). Most authors agree that "positive" cytology specimens are highly accurate, with few false-positive reports. False-negative examinations occur more often than false positives but are nevertheless infrequent, ranging from 0.5% to 7.0% in various reported series. A substantial number of biopsies are reported as questionable or indeterminate.

These specimens usually show cellular atypia or evidence of a microfollicular tumor. In the latter instance, it is generally recognized that the diagnosis of follicular carcinoma is more often based on morphologic than cytologic criteria. Thus follicular lesions detected by FNAB are considered adequately suspicious for follicular carcinoma to warrant surgical removal. In most reported series, the incidence of carcinoma within the "atypical" group of specimens has ranged from 14% to 23%.

Many authors now recommend routine aspiration of all thyroid nodules, with surgery generally recommended for specimens reported as positive or "questionable." Nodules with negative biopsies, in the absence of absolute or relative clinical criteria for thyroid surgery, are generally treated with thyroid hormone for TSH suppression and then observed, with needle aspiration biopsies repeated periodically. Surgery is usually recommended for "hot" nodules only when the biopsies are positive or strongly suspicious.

Cystic nodules are usually aspirated, with surgery recommended for large cysts that recur rapidly and for lesions with positive or questionable cytology. Needle aspiration cytology is a useful test for diagnosing malignancy in thyroid nodules, but it must be employed in conjunction with other criteria for arriving at a decision as to whether to operate (Fig. 19.2). Our use of this pro-

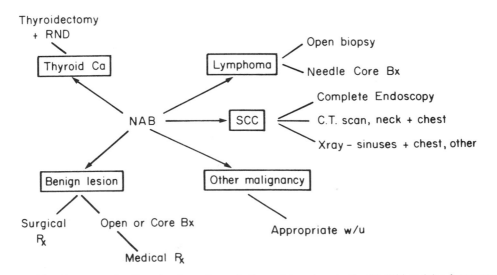

FIG. 19.2. Algorithm demonstrating the role of needle aspiration cytology in selecting thyroid nodules for surgery. (From Silver, 1986, with permission)

cedure has resulted in an increase in "yield" of malignancies on thyroid nodules operated on, from 16% prior to routine use of needle aspiration biopsy to 35% once the procedure was employed routinely.

Nonsurgical Treatment of Thyroid Carcinoma

Chemotherapy

To date, no chemotherapeutic agents have been found to be effective against thyroid cancer. Doxorubicin (Adriamycin) has been used in combination with radiotherapy, particularly for anaplastic carcinoma, but it is difficult to demonstrate a significant effect on either local control or survival.

TSH Suppression

Administration of thyroxine to suppress TSH and consequent TSH-sensitive thyroid cancer is an important adjuvant to surgery. Although not particularly effective in producing regression of clinically evident tumor, it does prevent occult disease of the contralateral thyroid lobe and metastatic disease from becoming clinical disease.

Patients who undergo total thyroidectomy require hormone replacement. Proper levels of thyroid replacement can be monitored clinically by following the patient's weight and cardiac rate, as well as periodic assays for thyroid-stimulating hormone (TSH), triiodothyronine (T_3), and thyroxine (T_4).

Radiation Therapy

Radiation therapy should not be employed to treat resectable disease in the neck when the patient is a suitable surgical candidate. External irradiation is best employed to manage residual disease in the operative field (particularly on the airway), unresectable tumor, and metastatic lesions. The mainstay of treatment for anaplastic carcinoma is external beam irradiation (after confirmation with open biopsy) plus adjuvant chemotherapy.

Ablation with radioiodine is best used to treat the functioning metastatic lesion of follicular carcinoma. A smaller percentage of papillary carcinomas may concentrate radioiodine. Many authorities obtain postoperative radioiodine scans after total thyroidectomy in all cases of well-differentiated thyroid carcinoma and ablate any residual thyroid tissue found in the neck (usually 5% to 10% of normal). Total body scanning can then be employed at regular intervals following temporary cessation of thyroid hormone administration to detect possible functioning metastases. Although some data have been presented to indicate that long-term cure rates are better in patients who have undergone radioiodine ablation of residual thyroid tissue and other adjuvant therapy following total thyroidectomy, the treatment of well-differentiated thyroid carcinoma is controversial. The value of postoperative ablation is questionable in view of the excellent cure rates for papillary carcinoma.

Surgical Treatment of Thyroid Carcinoma

Surgery is the mainstay of therapy for thyroid carcinoma. In this respect, treatment of the primary tumor and that of lymph node metastasis must be considered separately. There is considerable controversy concerning the various alternatives with regard to both of these areas.

Primary Tumor

The main controversy concerning the treatment of the primary tumor involves whether total or hemithyroidectomy should be employed for well-differentiated carcinoma. The basis of this controversy is outlined in Table 19.8. It is well known that with papillary thyroid carcinoma multicentricity of the primary tumor is frequent, as evidenced by the high incidence of occult carcinoma found in the opposite lobe in total thyroidectomy specimens. Nevertheless, many authors have reported excellent results after treating papillary carcinoma with hemithyroidectomy when total lobectomy has been performed properly and the surgery is followed by long-term administration of thyroid hormone for TSH suppression. In such instances, the occurrence of clinical carcinoma in the opposite lobe is infrequent. Advocates of total thyroidectomy point to the high incidence of microscopic involvement of the contralateral lobe, the ease of resection of the contralateral lobe at the time of initial surgery, and the inconclusiveness of all but the longest-term follow-up studies for evaluating treatment of thyroid carcinoma as reasons for recommending total thyroidectomy.

TABLE 19.8. *Incidence of multicentricity (in total thyroidectomy specimens) versus incidence of recurrence (with hemithyroidectomy) in various series*

Study	Incidence (%)	
	Multicentricity (occult carcinoma opposite lobe)	Recurrence (clinical carcinoma opposite lobe)
MacDonald & Kotin (1953)	91.0	—
Crile (1964)	—	0
Russel et al. (1975)	87.5	—
Tollefsen et al. (1972)	30.0	3.7
Rose et al. (1963)	61.7	24.4

Classification of thyroid carcinomas into low- and high-risk groups is perhaps the most commonly accepted means of determining whether hemi- or total thyroidectomy is indicated for treatment. Although the criteria for low and high risk may differ from one institution to another, age (less than 50 years), size (less than 5 cm), and lack of extrathyroidal spread generally define the low-risk group. Follicular carcinoma is generally treated similarly to papillary cancer unless there is evidence of marked angioinvasion or distant metastasis, in which case aggressive treatment is warranted.

Total thyroidectomy is considered mandatory for medullary carcinoma because of the high incidence of bilateral disease and the more aggressive course of the disease. Anaplastic carcinoma rarely is amenable to extensive surgery and is best treated with local resection, if feasible, followed by irradiation with or without chemotherapy.

The surgical approach to a thyroid nodule consists of total lobectomy on the side of the lesion with frozen section diagnosis. Further resection may be performed on the basis of frozen section diagnosis. The recurrent laryngeal nerve should be identified during every operation on the thyroid unless the procedure is confined to excision of a small nodule in the isthmus, for which an isthmusectomy may be an adequate procedure (followed by total thyroidectomy if carcinoma is found).

Lymph Node Metastasis

Two groups of lymph nodes must be considered when treating thyroid cancer: the nodes in the paratracheal and upper mediastinal areas and those in the lateral neck (carotid sheath and posterior triangle). About 90% of the lymphatic drainage of the thyroid gland is to the paratracheal and upper mediastinal nodes, with only the upper poles draining to the lateral neck. Thus metastatic disease occurs most frequently in the former group of nodes, levels II, III, IV, and VI. Clinically palpable metastatic disease in the lateral neck occurs in only a small percentage of well-differentiated thyroid cancers. Consequently, at the time of thyroidectomy the paratracheal and upper mediastinal nodes that are accessible within the field of surgery should be removed while preserving parathyroid tissue on the contralateral side. Most authors do not recommend elective resection of nodes in the lateral neck for treatment of well-differentiated thyroid cancer.

When lymph node metastasis in the lateral neck is clinically evident at the time of initial surgery or subsequently, therapeutic neck dissection is indicated. For well-differentiated thyroid cancer, modified radical neck dissection with preservation of the sternomastoid muscle, accessory nerve, and possibly the internal jugular vein is usually the preferred procedure. In cases with massive cervical metastatic lesions or in elderly or poor-risk patients it may be more efficacious to perform a standard neck dissection. It is usually not necessary to dissect the submaxillary and submandibular triangles of the neck to treat of thyroid cancer, as most metastases occur in the lower carotid sheath and posterior triangle regions.

"Berry picking" operations, where individual lymph nodes are separately resected without performing block dissection, has been occasionally advocated. In certain instances, particularly in poor-risk patients, this surgery may be appropriate, but such procedures are not recommended in most situations because of the high probability of further recurrence in the cervical area.

For treatment of medullary carcinoma, elective conventional neck dissection is advocated by many authors because of the high incidence of lymph node involvement and the known association of lymph node metastasis with poor prognosis of this disease. Other authors prefer initial treatment by total thyroidectomy without neck dissection. They then use postoperative calcitonin levels and high resolution CT scans of the neck to detect residual or persistent disease for subsequent neck dissection in patients with medullary carcinoma without clinically apparent cervical metastasis. In most cases of anaplastic carcinoma, radical neck dissection is neither effective nor feasible.

SALIVARY GLAND TUMORS

Salivary gland tumors are far less common than squamous cell and thyroid neoplasms, comprising 3% to 6% of all head and neck tumors. Table 19.9 summarizes the essential data concerning the incidence and relative occurrence of malignancy in the major and minor salivary glands. Parotid tumors are by far the most common but have the lowest incidence of malignancy. Nevertheless, because of the greater overall number of such tumors parotid malignancies outnumber all other salivary gland concerns. Minor salivary (mucous) glands occur ubiquitously throughout the mucosa of the upper aerodigestive tract, with the greatest concentration in the hard and soft palate. Minor salivary glands are subject to the same spectrum of tumor involvement as other salivary gland epithelium, although the distribution of the histologic types differs. At least half of minor salivary gland tumors are malignant. Tumors of the submandibular gland are uncommon but have a high incidence of malignancy. Sublingual gland tumors are rare, with fewer than 50 cases reported in the literature, although 80% of the reported cases were malignant.

The entire subject of salivary gland tumors is complex owing to the wide variety of histologic tumor types and the diversity of sites involved. It is characteristic that the most frequently occurring benign tumor, pleomorphic adenoma, in some cases follows a formidable clinical course, whereas most malignancies tend to be relatively low grade.

Benign Tumors

Nonneoplastic Lesions

Various nonneoplastic conditions may produce tumor masses in the parotid or other salivary glands that are clinically indistinguishable from neoplasms. In many cases, particularly in the parotid gland, such lesions must be approached in an identical manner to the approach to neoplastic lesions and so must be considered in the differential diagnosis. Such lesions include cysts and obstructive inflammatory disease. Localized lymphoepithelial lesions, which form part of the spectrum of Mikulicz's disease, or Sjögren's syndrome, may present as a mass in the salivary parenchyma. Adult immunodeficiency syndrome (AIDS) is often associated with a mass in the parotid gland. Benign lymphoepithelial cysts are almost pathognomonic for AIDS, and identification by preoperative imaging and needle aspiration of a cystic lesion filled with amylase-rich clear fluid containing lymphocytes should indicate the need to test for human immunodeficiency virus (HIV). As these lesions respond well to low-dose irradiation, surgery is rarely necessary. On the other hand solid parotid lesions associated with AIDS require tissue diagnosis. Although benign lymphoepithelial lesions and inflammatory lymphadenopathy are most often found, intraparotid lymphoma, Kaposi's sarcoma, and other malignancies may occur.

Nonepithelial Tumors

Lesions of connective tissue origin account for a small percentage of salivary gland masses in adults. In infants and children vascular tumors are the most common cause of mass or neoplastic lesions of the salivary glands. Capillary hemangiomas account for approximately 50% of parotid tumors in infants. Other salivary glands are involved far less frequently. Most of the patients are female. Cavernous hemangiomas tend to occur in older children. Hemangiomatous lesions regress spontaneously in many cases. Surgical removal is required for persistent or enlarging lesions. Lymphan-

TABLE 19.9. *Salivary gland tumors: relative incidence of total occurrence and malignancy*

Site of tumor	Incidence (% of tumors)	Malignant (%), mean and range
Parotid	76–85	35 (17–47)
Minor	10–20	50 (31–88)
Submaxillary	10	50 (31–61)
Sublingual	Rare	80

giomatous lesions (cystic hygroma and cavernous lymphangioma) also occur in infants, involving the parotid or submandibular glands in association with other cervical structures. Spontaneous regression often occurs, but surgery may be required to relieve obstruction and for cosmetic purposes.

Connective tissue lesions can arise from all the individual vascular, fibrous, muscular, and perineural structures situated in and around the parotid gland. Among these lesions, lipoma is the most common.

Pleomorphic Adenoma (Benign Mixed Tumor)

Pleomorphic adenoma accounts for approximately 65% of all parotid neoplasms. Most occur within the lateral lobe, most often in the tail, of the parotid. They account for a much lower percentage of minor salivary gland neoplasms, occurring most often in the hard and soft palate in elderly patients. Histologically, the lesions contain both glandular and connective tissue elements. The latter may be myxomatous, cartilagenous, fibrous, or osseous.

Pleomorphic adenomas, unless they have undergone malignant change (carcinoma ex pleomorphic adenoma or malignant mixed tumor), are benign, encapsulated lesions. They do not invade the facial nerve or other structures. Nevertheless, pleomorphic adenomas may be multilobulated, with pseudopods that can be amputated and left behind, serving as a nidus for recurrence if the tumor is incompletely removed. If resected totally with the capsule intact, pleomorphic adenomas are 100% curable. Recurrences result only from incomplete removal, not from any inherent malignant tendency. Once the lesion has recurred, the possibility of cure diminishes significantly because of the multifocal nature of such recurrences and the difficulty of complete extirpation, particularly in the parotid gland where attempted preservation of the facial nerve may preclude wide extirpation.

Adenolymphoma (Warthin's Tumor, Papillary Cystadenoma Lymphomatosum)

Adenolymphoma is a benign lesion that occurs only in the parotid gland, usually in older patients. It is the second most common parotid tumor, representing 6% to 10% of all such lesions, and it is frequently bilateral (70% of all bilateral tumors) or multiple within the same gland. Occasional familial cases have been reported. Malignant transformation of adenolymphoma is almost nonexistent. Histologically, the lesions consist of epithelial elements, usually papillary in nature, separated from a lymphoid stroma by a thin basement membrane. The lesions are usually thick, containing turbid or mucoid fluid.

Adenolymphomas are usually superficially situated and may attain rather large size. There is often slight fluctuation in size due to changes in the fluid content. There is little tendency for local recurrence after excision, but the lesions do not enucleate easily. They require partial parotidectomy for complete excision.

Oncocytoma

Oncocytomas comprise less than 1% of all salivary gland tumors. They occur most commonly in the parotid gland, with rare involvement of the submandibular gland and even rarer appearances in minor salivary glands. Oncocytomas tend to occur in older age groups. The tumors are encapsulated and usually noncystic, and there is a tendency for bilaterality. These lesions grow slowly and almost never recur after complete removal.

The rare oncocytomas of minor salivary gland origin are often cystic, rather than solid. A small number of malignant oncocytomas have been reported in the literature. These lesions are microscopically indistinguishable from benign oncocytomas but tend to occur in minor salivary glands, where they are solid rather than cystic. Batsakis (1981) considered solid oncocytomas of the nose, paranasal sinuses, and larynx to be malignant. Malignant oncocytomas tend to behave like other low-grade salivary gland malignancies, with favorable short-term survival and overall high long-term recurrence rates.

Monomorphic Adenomas

Monomorphic adenomas comprise a rare group of tumors of interest to pathologists in that they may represent a link, as precursor, to the far more commonly occurring pleomorphic adenoma and to adenoid cystic carcinoma. The lesions are benign, occur in parotid and minor salivary glands, and in many cases, bear a resemblance to dermal appendage tumors.

The tumor occurs in several forms. The basal cell adenoma is found predominantly in minor salivary glands, often in the lip. The membranous type of monomorphic adenoma is distinguished by its production of a membranous intracellular material, producing a cylindromatous appearance. This lesion most often involves the parotid gland. "Hybrid" forms, intermediate in appearance to pleomorphic adenoma or adenoid cystic carcinoma, also occur. The major importance of this lesion lies in the diagnostic problem of confusing benign monomorphic adenomas with malignant adenoid cystic carcinomas.

Malignant Salivary Gland Tumors

Nonepithelial Tumors

Connective tissue lesions most often involve salivary tissue secondarily, usually by continuity. This situation arises most frequently in the parotid gland. Smooth and striated muscle, fibrous tissue, and nerves account for the occasional malignancy in this area. Lymphoma is the most common nonepithelial malignancy to involve salivary gland tissue, most often the parotid. Such lesions usually arise in the intraglandular lymphoid tissue. Periparotid lymph nodes may be involved in lymphoma from other cervical lymph nodes. Occasionally, lymphomas arise in association with a previously existing lymphoepithelial lesion.

Mucoepidermoid Carcinoma

Mucoepidermoid carcinoma is the most common salivary gland malignancy and the most common malignant parotid tumor, comprising approximately 50% of parotid malignancies. It occurs less commonly than adenoid cystic carcinoma in the submandibular gland and less frequently than adenoid cystic and adenocarcinoma in minor salivary glands. The histologic characteristic of these lesions is the mixture of epidermoid and mucus-secreting cells. The lower-grade lesions tend to consist predominantly of mucoid elements, and high-grade lesions histologically resemble squamous cell carcinoma with considerable anaplasia. The tumor is more common in men than in women and occurs most often during the fourth and fifth decades of life. Approximately two-thirds of mucoepidermoid carcinomas are of the low-grade variety and have an excellent prognosis. Both local recurrences and cervical lymph node metastasis occurs infrequently. The 15-year survival is

approximately 85%. High-grade mucoepidermoid carcinomas tend to recur locally and to metastasize. The 5-year survival is approximately 30% for these lesions.

Adenoid Cystic Carcinoma

Adenoid cystic carcinoma accounts for only 7% of parotid malignancies but is the most frequently occurring neoplasm of the submandibular and minor salivary glands, comprising 35% to 40% of such malignancies. Adenoid cystic carcinoma tends to grow slowly but has a marked tendency to invade perineural lymphatics, thereby spreading along nerve sheaths and producing a high frequency of pain and facial nerve paralysis. Lymph node metastasis occurs in about 30% of patients, and 50% ultimately develop distant metastasis. Although adenoid cystic carcinoma has a relatively favorable short-term prognosis (approximately 75% five-year survival), the long-term prognosis is grave (30% at 10 years and 13% at 20 years). The prognosis is somewhat better for adenoid cystic carcinoma of the parotid or minor salivary glands than for that of the submandibular gland, paranasal sinuses, or larynx.

Malignant Mixed Tumor

Batsakis (1981) classified two types of malignant mixed tumor. The far more common variety is carcinoma ex pleomorphic adenoma, which consists of malignant transformation of a previously benign pleomorphic adenoma. The true malignant mixed tumor is much less common and represents a form of carcinosarcoma in which both epithelial and connective tissue elements are malignant.

The usual clinical course is that of sudden enlargement of a previously long-standing parotid tumor, sometimes with pain or facial nerve paralysis (or both). This type of lesion tends to occur in the older age group. The parotid gland is most frequently involved. Submandibular and minor salivary gland involvement is far less frequent.

Malignant mixed tumor has a worse prognosis than other "low-grade" salivary gland carcinomas (mucoepidermoid, adenocystic, acinic cell). Lymph node metastasis occurs in 15% of patients, and approximately 30% develop distant metastasis. The 5-year survival ranges from 40% to 50%, with a decrease to 20% at 15 years.

Acinic (Acinous) Cell Carcinoma

Acinic cell carcinomas are low-grade malignancies that occur mainly in the parotid gland, accounting for 2% to 4% of all parotid tumors and 10% of parotid malignancies. Tumor cells resemble normal salivary parenchyma, and there is a poor correlation between the histologic appearance of the lesion and its clinical behavior. Some authors use the term acinic cell tumor to describe these lesions on the theory that not all are malignant. Acinic cell carcinoma typically occurs during the fifth decade of life, although it also has a propensity to occur in children.

The typical behavior of these lesions is slow growth with late recurrence and metastasis. About 10% of tumors metastasize to cervical nodes, and distant metastasis occurs occasionally. The lesions may be locally invasive, and death may be caused by both local extension and metastasis. The 5-year cure rate ranges from 75% to 90%, declining to 55% to 60% at 15 years. The prognosis may be more reliably predicted by the clinical extent of the tumor at initial presentation than by histologic grading. Approximately 3% of parotid acinic cell carcinomas are bilateral.

Adenocarcinoma

Malignant salivary gland tumors that do not fall in the above defined specific categories (e.g., mucoepidermoid, adenoid cystic, acinic cell) are classified as adenocarcinoma. These lesions comprise 10% to 15% of parotid malignancies and generally resemble mucus-producing adenocarcinomas of other portions of the gastrointestinal tract. Parotid tumors, however, tend to be cystic and papillary.

Adenocarcinomas are divided by most authors into two or three grades of malignancy. Low-grade adenocarcinoma has a relatively good prognosis with 70% to 80% five-year survival and 50% to 55% survival at 15 years. The highest-grade adenocarcinomas have poor prognosis (10% five-year survival).

Squamous Cell Carcinoma

Primary SCCs of salivary glands are rare. Such lesions must be distinguished from mucoepidermoid carcinoma and metastatic carcinoma. With regard to the latter, it is noteworthy that lymphatic drainage from the skin of the upper two-thirds of the face is through the intraparotid lymphatics. In many instances careful questioning of a patient found to have SCC in the parotid gland reveals a history of a facial lesion excised during the past year or two. If a specimen had been submitted for pathology, it usually proves to have been SCC. True primary SCCs of the submandibular and minor salivary glands are essentially impossible to distinguish from metastatic cervical disease or primary SCC at various mucosal sites.

The prognosis of primary SCC of the parotid gland is generally poor. Ultimate survival is related to the stage of disease at the time of initial diagnosis.

Diagnosis

Clinical Factors

Malignancy is suspected in a salivary gland mass on the basis of its location, the type of salivary gland (major or minor), and the clinical characteristics of firmness and fixation. The incidence of malignancy is much higher among submandibular gland and minor salivary gland tumors than among those in the parotid gland. The rare tumor in the sublingual gland is almost always malignant. Paralysis of facial, lingual, or hypoglossal nerves in association with mass lesions in the parotid or submandibular gland is almost certain a sign of malignancy. Adenoid cystic carcinoma is highly suspected if there is nerve involvement. Lymph node metastasis may be evident, making the diagnosis obvious. An occasional patient presents with facial nerve paralysis due to a deeply infiltrating parotid tumor that is not readily palpable. Occasionally such patients are diagnosed as having Bell's palsy by inexperienced clinicians. Modern radiographic techniques, particularly MRI, plus clinical suspicion should minimize this possibility. Deep lobe parotid or parapharyngeal tumors may be discovered by intraoral evaluation, revealing medial displacement of lateral pharyngeal structures.

Radiology

Conventional sialography is not ordinarily used for the diagnosis of mass lesions, but it is helpful for defining the cause of inflammatory disease. CT and MRI are much more accurate procedures for delineating mass lesions and localizing deep or superficial lobes. The infiltrative nature of a malignant lesion may be demonstrated. Tumors of the deep lobe of the parotid may be distinguished from neurogenic tumors of the parapharyngeal space by demonstration of a characteristic fat or areolar plane in the latter. Involvement of the temporal bone and skull base may be evaluated by modern imaging techniques.

Biopsy

Open incisional biopsy is not indicted for suspected benign or low-grade malignant tumors of the parotid and submandibular glands. Accessible minor salivary gland tumors and extensive malignant lesions of the major salivary glands that require radical removal should undergo incisional biopsy with the biopsy site placed so the tumor is included well within the confines of the resected specimen.

Fine-needle aspiration biopsy may be safely employed to evaluate tumors in the parotid and submandibular glands. The procedure is particularly helpful for distinguishing lymphoid and inflammatory lesions from neoplastic masses. The procedure is not sufficiently sensitive for reliable distinction between benign and malignant epithelial tumors and so should not be used to determine the indication for surgery for neoplastic lesions in otherwise healthy patients. The sensitivity of FNAB of salivary gland lesions has been reported to be approximately 40%, whereas its specificity is approximately 90%. Needle aspiration biopsy is of value for distinguishing salivary gland tumors that present as a cervical mass, due to lymphadenopathy, metastasis, or otherwise.

Surgical Extirpation

Surgical extirpation is an important diagnostic procedure for benign and low-grade malignant tumors of the parotid and submandibular glands. It consists of conservative but complete surgical resection of the lesion by the techniques described below. Conley (1975) termed this approach "the grand biopsy." It has the advantage of not violating the tumor capsule and of providing in one step both diagnosis and complete cure for most lesions. Frozen section diagnosis should always be obtained before sacrificing an important structure if malignancy has not been confirmed by previous biopsy.

While surgical excision remains the appropriate and ultimate diagnostic procedure for benign major salivary gland tumors, it is always helpful to confirm the diagnosis of malignancy by one of the preoperative biopsy techniques in cases with obvious clinical signs of malignancy.

Treatment

Benign salivary gland tumors are 100% curable if completely removed with an intact capsule. This usually cannot be accomplished by simply enucleating the lesion but requires conservative local resection of the lesion with a margin of tissue left around the intact capsule, if feasible.

Low-grade malignant tumors are treated with wide local excision but without elective sacrifice of vital uninvolved structures, such as the facial nerve. The tendency of adenoid cystic carcinoma for perineural invasion may lead the surgeon to sacrifice a major nerve if tumor is sufficiently proximate. Considerable judgment must be exercised in each case. Elective neck dissection is not considered by most authors to be indicated for treatment of low-grade salivary gland malignancies.

High-grade tumors consist of the high grade forms of mucoepidermoid and adenocarcinoma, malignant mixed tumor with anaplastic and sarcomatous features, and primary squamous cell carcinoma. These tumors should be treated by radical extirpation, including important adjacent neurologic structures, plus elective radical neck dissection.

Spiro (1986) developed a staging system for salivary gland neoplasms that correlates with survival at least as significantly as the histologic type (Table 19.10). The 10-year survivals for stages I, II, and III are 90%, 65%, and 22%, respectively.

Radiotherapy is not employed for primary definitive treatment of salivary gland tumors unless they are unresectable. Postoperative radiotherapy may be employed as adjuvant treatment in lymph node-bearing areas after treatment of both low- and high-grade malignancy. To date, there is no specific chemotherapy available to treat salivary gland tumors.

Parotid Tumors

Most benign tumors are located in the lateral (or superficial) lobe of the parotid and should be excised by lateral parotid lobectomy, with dissection and preservation of the facial nerve. The technique described by Woods (1983) represents the standard approach employed by most surgeons. Although there are many methods for identifying the facial nerve, the most reli-

TABLE 19.10. *Staging of salivary gland tumors*

Classification	Criteria
TNM system	
T1	Tumor < 2 cm with significant local extension
T2	Tumor > 2 and <4 cm with significant local extension
T3	Tumor > 6 cm with significant local extension
T4a	Tumor > 6 cm
T4b	Any tumor with significant local extension
N0	No regional nodal involvement
N1	Palpable regional nodes
M0	No distant metastasis
M1	Distant metastasis
Stage	
I	T1N0M0
II	T3N0M0
III	T1or2N1M0
	T4aorbN0M0
IV	T3–4N1M0
	Any T,any N,M1

Source: Adapted from Spiro (1986).

able procedure is to locate the main trunk, which has a consistent relation to the adjacent bony structures (mastoid tip, bony ear canal, and styloid process) and trace it distally, separating the parotid tissue from the nerve branches as they are exposed.

For tumors in the deep lobe of the parotid, it is necessary to remove a large portion of the lateral lobe first and then mobilize the facial nerve to permit removal of the deeply situated tumor. Large retromandibular masses may require anterior dislocation of the mandible to facilitate delivery. In some cases, tumors lie partially or totally underneath a fascial tunnel created by the stylomandibular ligament. These tumors present mainly in the parapharyngeal space as extramucosal masses displacing the tonsil medially. Division of the stylomandibular ligament facilitates delivery of the lesion. (Such tumors may be distinguished from neurogenic tumors within the parapharyngeal space by preoperative imaging, as mentioned above.) Massive tumors of the deep lobe and other large lesions of the parapharyngeal space may require midline mandibulotomy for adequate exposure.

Small, benign tumors of the parotid gland confined to the tail of the gland may require only partial lateral lobectomy. Most other lesions in the lateral lobe require total lobectomy.

Low-grade malignant tumors of the parotid should be treated by subtotal parotidectomy, sparing the uninvolved facial nerve if possible. If only a branch or a portion of the facial nerve is involved, it may be selectively resected with preservation of the remaining portions of the nerve. In all cases where facial nerve is sacrificed, an attempt should be made at immediate reconstruction by free nerve grafting using microsurgical technique. The greater auricular nerve, or occasionally the sural nerve, may be used for this purpose.

High-grade malignancies, massive malignant tumors of the parotid presenting with facial nerve paralysis, and recurrent parotid malignancies should be treated by radical excision, sacrificing the facial nerve. Overlying areas of involved skin and previous surgical scars should be included in the resection. If mandible, temporal bone, or other adjacent structures are invaded, the operation should include appropriate resection. Myocutaneous flaps and skin grafts can be used for reconstruction. Nerve grafting is usually successful if the facial nerve was functional preoperatively but it is usually unsuccessful if the nerve had been paralyzed prior to surgery. Occasionally the intramastoid portion of the facial nerve can be used for the proximal graft site. In cases where cure is thought possible, elective radial neck dissection may be added to the procedure. Therapeutic neck dissection should be done in patients with clinically evident cervical metastasis.

Submandibular Gland Tumors

Benign tumors and low-grade malignancies without nerve involvement are treated by complete removal of the submandibular gland. If there is involvement of the lingual or hypoglossal nerves, or invasion into the deep structures of the floor of the mouth, a "composite" type resection involving mandibulectomy in continuity with wide resection of the contents of the submandibular triangle and mucosa of the floor of the mouth should be performed. It is more important to remove the primary tumor completely by adequate resection than to perform elective neck dissection for submandibular gland tumors.

Sublingual and Minor Salivary Gland Tumors

Tumors of the sublingual gland are treated in the same manner as other tumors of the floor of the mouth.

For malignant lesions, marginal or segmental mandibulectomy with wide excision of overlying mucosa and removal of the contents of the submandibular triangle is required for adequate resection.

Benign tumors of the hard palate present a therapeutic dilemma due to the difficulty of distinguishing benign from low grade malignant lesions on biopsy specimens. Small and moderate-size benign lesions of the hard palate may be resected intraorally, without resecting bone, if careful preoperative workup has indicated that the bone is intact. For large benign lesions and low-grade malignant lesions of the palate, partial maxillectomy involving resection of overlying palatal bone should be performed. More radical types of maxillectomy performed through an external (Webber-Furguson) approach may be required for large malignant tumors.

Other minor salivary gland tumors are treated according to the organ involved and the nature of the pathology following the principles enumerated above. Partial or total laryngectomy, segmental resection of the trachea, and various procedures in the pharynx may be required to treat minor salivary gland malignancies.

QUESTIONS

Select one answer.

1. A 29-year-old man presents to your office with a diagnosis of medullary carcinoma of the thyroid. Physical examination shows a hard mass of the right thyroid. Optimal treatment is:
    a. Subtotal thyroidectomy.
    b. Total thyroidectomy.
    c. ^{131}I irradiation.
    d. Biopsy and external beam irradiation.
2. Complications of radiotherapy include:
    a. Xerostomia.
    b. Osteoradionecrosis.
    c. Failure of cable nerve grafts.
    d. All of the above.
3. Radical neck dissection includes all of the following *except:*
    a. Sternocleidomastoid muscle.
    b. Submaxillary gland.
    c. Accessory nerve.
    d. Levator scapulae muscle.
4. The greatest morbidity of radical neck dissection is from:
    a. Lack of drainage of internal jugular vein.
    b. Deficit of sternocleidomastoid muscle.
    c. Accessory nerve deficit.
    d. Edema secondary to lymph node dissection.
5. What percentage of parotid masses are malignant?
    a. 10%.
    b. 20%.
    c. 50%.
    d. 65%.
6. A 34-year-old man has a 3.5-cm tumor on the right side of the tongue. Three nodes ranging in size from 2 to 3 cm are palpable in the ipsilateral neck. What is the stage of the carcinoma?
    a. I.
    b. II.
    c. III.
    d. IV.
7. Occult thyroid carcinoma is defined as:
    a. A carcinoma smaller than 1.5 cm.
    b. Disease isolated to one lobe without nodal metastasis.
    c. Microscopic disease, not palpable.
    d. None of the above.
8. A 62-year-old woman has a 3-cm mass in the left thyroid lobe; pathology reports indicate follicular carcinoma. Ideal treatment is:
    a. Lobectomy with ^{131}I irradiation.
    b. Total thyroidectomy.
    c. Biopsy and external beam irradiation.
    d. Enucleation.
9. A 68-year-old woman presents with bilateral parotid tumors. The most likely diagnosis is:
    a. Pleomorphic adenoma.
    b. Adenoid cystic carcinoma.
    c. Benign mixed tumor.
    d. Warthin tumor.
10. The following are true statements:
    a. Warthin duct drains the submaxillary gland.
    b. Stenson duct drains the parotid gland.
    c. Elihu duct drains the sublingual gland.
    d. Benign lymphoepithelial cysts are frequently associated with HIV.

SELECTED REFERENCES

General

Batsakis JG. *Tumors of the head and neck,* 2nd ed. Baltimore: Williams & Wilkins, 1981.

Chretien PB, Johns ME, Shedd DP, et al. *Head and neck cancer.* Philadelphia, B.C. Decker, 1985.

Mancuso A, Hanafee WN. *Computed tomography of the head and neck.* Baltimore: Williams and Wilkins, 1982.

Silver CE. *Atlas of head and neck surgery.* New York: Churchill Livingstone, 1986.

Silver CE. Head and neck procedures. In: Gliedman ML, ed. *Atlas of surgical techniques.* New York: McGraw-Hill, 1990;2–25.

Silver CE, Koss LJ, Brauer RJ, et al. Needle aspiration cytology of tumors at various body sites. *Curr Prob Surg* 1985; 22:1.

Suen J, Myers EN. *Cancer of the head and neck,* 3rd ed. New York: Churchill Livingstone, 1996.

Squamous Cell Carcinoma

Al-Sarraf M. Head and neck cancer: chemotherapy concepts. *Semin Oncol* 1988;15:70–85.

American Joint Committee on Cancer (AJCC). *Manual for staging of cancer,* 4th ed. Philadelphia: JB Lippincott, 1992.

Atula TS, Varpula MJ, Kurki TJ, Klemi PJ, Grenman R. Assessment of cervical lymph node status in head and neck cancer patients: palpation, computed tomography and low field magnetic resonance imaging compared with ultrasound-guided fine-needle aspiration cytology. *Eur J Radiol* 1997;25:152–161.

Bocca E, Pignataro O, Sasaki CT. Functional neck dissection: a description of operative technique. *Arch Otolaryngol* 1980;106:524.

Bosl GJ. Adjuvant chemotherapy in the management of stage III and IV tumors of the head and neck. *Cancer* 1983;33: 139.

Breau RL, Clayman GL. Gene therapy for head and neck cancer. *Curr Opin Oncol* 1996;8:227–231.

Decker J, Goldstein JC. Risk factors in head and neck cancer. *N Engl J Med* 1982;306:1151.

Ensley JF, Jacobs JR, Weaver A, et al. The correlation between response to cisplatinum combination chemotherapy and subsequent radiotherapy in previously untreated patients with advanced squamous cell cancers of the head and neck. *Cancer* 1984;54:811–814.

Fletcher GH, Jesse RH. The place of irradiation in the management of the primary lesion in head and neck cancers. *Cancer* 1977;39[suppl 1]:826.

Jacobs J, Al-Sarraf M, Crissman J, Valerote F, eds. *Scientific and clinical perspectives of head and neck cancer management strategies for cure.* New York: Elsevier, 1987.

Jesse RH. Management of the suspicious cervical lymph node. *Postgrad Med* 1970;48:99

Jesse RH, Perez CA, Fletcher GH. Cervical lymph node metastases: unknown primary cancer. *Cancer* 1973;31:854.

Johnson JT, Barnes L, Myers EN, et al. The extracapsular spread of tumors in cervical node metastasis. *Arch Otolaryngol* 1981;107:725–729.

Lindberg R. Distribution of cervical lymph node metastases from squamous cell carcinoma of the upper respiratory and digestive tracts. *Cancer* 1972;29:1447–1449.

Loverme PJ, Rush BF, Legaspi A, et al. Combined therapy in advanced squamous cell carcinoma of the head and neck. *Am J Surg* 1982;48:197.

Mantravadi R. Radiation therapy for subclinical carcinoma in cervical lymph nodes. *Arch Otolaryngol* 1982;108:108.

Masberg A, Morrsey JB, Garfinkel L. A study of the appearance of early asymptomatic oral squamous cell carcinoma. *Cancer* 1973;32:1436.

Murthy P, Laing MR, Palmer TJ. Fine needle aspiration cytology of head and neck lesions: an early experience. *J R Coll Surg Edinb* 1997;42:341–346.

Nahum AM, Bone RC, Davidson TM. The case for elective prophylactic neck dissection. *Laryngoscope* 1977;87:588–599.

Pavelic ZP, Gluckman JL. The role of *p53* tumor suppressor gene in human head and neck tumorigenesis. *Acta Otolaryngol Suppl (Stockh)*, 1997;527:21–24.

Rice DH, Spiro RH. *Current concepts in head and neck cancer.* Atlanta: American Cancer Society, 1989.

Righi PD, Kopecky KK, Caldemeyer KS, et al. Comparison of ultrasound–fine needle aspiration and computed tomography in patients undergoing elective neck dissection. *Head Neck* 1997;19:604–610.

Schneider KL, Schreiber K, Silver CE. The initial evaluation of neck masses by needle aspiration biopsy. *Surg Gynecol Obstet* 1984;159:450.

Silver CE. Management of the primary site: larynx and hypopharynx. In: Pillsbury H, Goldsmith M, eds. *Operative challenges in otolaryngology/head and neck surgery.* Chicago: Year Book Medical Publishers, 1990;322–345.

Silver CE, ed. *Laryngeal cancer.* New York: Thieme Medical Publishers, 1991.

Silver CE, Croft CB. Elective dissection of the neck. *Surg Gynecol Obstet* 1979;149:65.

Silver CE, Glackin BK, Brauer RJ, Lesser ML. Surgical treatment of oral cavity carcinoma. *Head Neck Surg* 1986;9:13.

Silver CE, Moisa II. Elective treatment of the neck in cancer of the oral tongue. *Semin Surg Oncol* 1991;7:14–49.

Silver CE, Moisa II. The role of surgery in treatment of cancer of the larynx. *CA Cancer J Clin* 1990;40:134–147.

Slaughter DP, Southwick HW, Smejkal W. "Field cancerization" in oral stratified squamous epithelium: clinical implications of multicentric origin. *Cancer* 1953;6:963.

Spiro RH, Strong EW. Epidermoid carcinoma of the oral cavity and oropharynx, elective vs. therapeutic radical neck dissection as treatment. *Arch Surg* 1973;107:382–384.

Stern WB, Silver CE, Zeifer BA, Persky MS, Heller KS. Computed tomography of the clinically negative neck. *Head Neck* 1990;12:109–113.

Strong MS, Vaughan CW, Kayne HL, et al. A randomized trial of preoperative radiotherapy in cancer of the oropharynx and hypopharynx. *Am J Surg* 1978;136:494.

Thawley SE, Panje WR. *Comprehensive management of head and neck tumors. Part IV. Tumors of the oral cavity.* Philadelphia: WB Saunders, 1987;460–613.

Vandenbrouch C, Sancho-Garnier H, Chassagne D, et al. Elective versus therapeutic radical neck dissection in epidermoid carcinoma of the oral cavity: results of a randomized clinical trial. *Cancer* 1980;46:383.

Vikram B, Strong EW, Shah T, Spiro RH. Elective post-operative radiation therapy in stages III and IV epidermoid carcinoma of the head and neck. *Am J Surg* 1980;140:580.

Thyroid

Ashcraft MW, Van Herle AJ. Management of thyroid nodules. *Head Neck Surg* 1981;3:297.

Beargie JM, Brown CL, Doniach I, et al. Primary malignant tumors of the thyroid: the relationship between histological classification and clinical behavior. *Br J Surg* 1976;63:173.

Block MA. Surgery of thyroid nodules and malignancy. *Curr Probl Surg* 1983;20:136–204.

Block MA, Miller JM, Horn RC. Medullary thyroid carcinoma of the thyroid: surgical implications. *Arch Surg* 1968;96:521.

Block MA, Miller JM, Horn RC. Significance of mediastinal lymph node metastases in carcinoma of the thyroid. *Am J Surg* 1972;123:702.

Brauer RJ, Silver CE. Needle aspiration biopsy of thyroid nodules. *Laryngoscope* 1984;94:38.

Buckwalter JA, Thomas CG Jr. Selection of surgical treatment for well differentiated thyroid carcinoma. *Ann Surg* 1972;176:565.

Bumstead RM. Thyroid disease: a guide for the head and neck surgeon. *Ann Otol Rhinol Laryngol* Suppl 72 1980;89:1.

Cady B, Ross R. An expanded view of risk group definitions in differentiated thyroid carcinoma. *Surgery* 1988;104:947–953.

Clark OH, Way LH. Total thyroidectomy: the treatment of choice for patients with thyroid cancer. *Ann Surg* 1982;19:362.

Crile G Jr. Survival of patients with papillary carcinoma of the thyroid after conservative operations. *Am J Surg* 1964;108:862.

DeGroot LJ. Thyroid carcinoma. *Med Clin North Am* 1975;59:1233–1246.

Frable WJ. Thin-needle aspiration biopsy. *Am J Clin Pathol* 1976;65:168.

Johns ME, Goldsmith MM. Current management of salivary gland tumors. Part 2. *Oncology* 1989;3:85–99.

Lowhagen T, Granberg P, Lundell G, et al. Aspiration biopsy cytology in nodules of the thyroid gland suspected to be malignant. *Surg Clin North Am* 1979;59:3.

MacDonald J, Kotin P. Surgical management of papillary carcinoma of the thyroid gland—the case for total thyroidectomy. *Ann Surg* 1953;137:156.

Makewari YK, Hill CS Jr, Haynie TP III, et al. I[131] therapy in differentiated thyroid carcinoma. *Cancer* 1981;47:664.

Mazzaferri EL. Impact of initial tumor features and treatment selected on the long-term course of differentiated thyroid cancer. *Thyroid Today* 1995;18(3):1—13.

Mazzaferri EL. Papillary and follicular thyroid cancer: a selective approach to diagnosis and treatment. *Annu Rev Med* 1981;32:73.

Mazzaferri EL, De los Santos, ET, Rofagha-Keyhani S. Solitary thyroid nodules: diagnosis and management. *Med Clin North Am* 1988;72:117.

Mazzaferri EL, Young RL. Papillary thyroid carcinoma: a 10 year follow-up report of the impact of therapy in 576 patients. *Am J Med* 1981;70:511.

McConahey WM, Hay ID, Woolner LB, VanHeerden JA, Taylor W. Papillary thyroid carcinoma treated at the Mayo Clinic, 1946 through 1970: initial manifestations, pathologic findings, therapy and outcome. *Mayo Clin Proc* 1986;61:978–996.

Miller JM, Hamburger J, Kini S. Diagnosis of thyroid nodules: use of fine needle aspiration and needle biopsy. *JAMA* 1979;241:481.

Rose RG, Kelsey MP, Russell WO, et al. Follow-up study of thyroid cancer treated by unilateral lobectomy. *Am J Surg* 1963;106:494.

Russell MA, Glibert EF, Jaeschke WF. Prognostic features of thyroid cancer. *Cancer* 1975;36:553.

Samaan NA, Maheshwari YK, Nader S, et al. Impact of therapy for differentiated carcinoma of the thyroid: an analysis of 706 cases. *J Clin Endocrinol Metab* 1983;56:1131–1138.

Silver CE. Surgical management of well differentiated thyroid carcinoma. *Bull NY Acad Med* 1986;62:854.

Silver CE, Brauer RJ, Schreiber K. Cytologic evaluation of thyroid nodules: new criteria for surgery. *NY State J Med* 1984;84:109.

Silver CE, Stern WB, Kim HH. Thyroid disease and surgery. In: Bailey BJ, ed. *Head and neck surgery—otolaryngology.* Philadelphia: JB Lippincott, 1998.

Simpson WJ, McKinney SE, Carruthers JS, et al. Papillary and follicular thyroid carcinoma: prognostic factors in 1578 patients. *Am J Med* 1987;83:479–488.

Sipple JH. The association of pheochromocytoma with carcinoma of the thyroid gland. *Am J Med* 1961;31:163.

Tollefsen HR, Shah JP, Huvos AG. Papillary carcinoma of the thyroid: recurrence in the thyroid gland after initial treatment. *Am J Surg* 1972;124:97.

Wang C, Vickery A Jr, Maloof F. Needle biopsy of the thyroid. *Surg Gynecol Obstet* 1976;143:365.

Woolner LB, Beahrs OH, Black BM, et al. Thyroid carcinoma: general considerations and follow-up data in 1,181 cases. In: Young S, Imman DR, eds. *Thyroid neoplasia, proceedings of the Second Imperial Cancer Research Fund symposium.* London: Academic Press, 1968;51.

Young RL, Mazzaferri EL, Rahe AJ, et al. Pure follicular thyroid carcinoma: impact of therapy in 214 patients. *J Nucl Med* 1980;21:733.

Salivary Gland

Armstrong JG, Harrison LB, Spiro RH, et al. Malignant tumors of major salivary gland origin: a matched-pair analysis of the role of combined surgery and post-operative radiotherapy. *Arch Otolaryngol Head Neck Surg* 1990;116:290–293.

Armstrong JG, Harrison LB, Thaler HT, et al. The indications for elective treatment of the neck in cancer of the major salivary glands. *Cancer* 1992;69:615–619.

Baker DC, Conley J. Treatment of massive deep lobe parotid tumors. *Am J Surg* 1979;138:572.

Beahrs OH, Chong GC. Management of the facial nerve in parotid gland surgery. *Am J Surg* 1972;124:473.

Blanck C, Eneroth CM, Jakobsson PA. Mucus producing adenopapillary (non-epidermoid) carcinoma of the parotid gland. *Cancer* 1971;28:676.

Blanck C, Eneroth CM, Jakobsson PA. Oncocytoma of the parotid gland: neoplasm or nodular hyperplasia. *Cancer* 1970;25:919.

Conley J. *Salivary glands and the facial nerve.* Stuttgart: Georg Thieme, 1975.

Eneroth CM. Histological and clinical aspects of parotid tumors. *Acta Otolaryngol Suppl (Stockh)* 1964;191:1.

Eneroth CM. Salivary gland tumors in the parotid gland, submandibular gland and the palate region. *Cancer* 1971;27:1415.

Foote FW Jr, Frazell EL. Tumors of the major salivary glands. *Cancer* 1953;6:1065.

Friedman M, Levin B, Gybauskas V, et al. Malignant tumors of the major salivary glands. *Otolaryngol Clin North Am* 1986;19:625–635.

Godwin JT, Foote FW, Frazell EL. Acinic cell adenocarcinoma of the parotid gland. *Am J Pathol* 1954;30:465.

Johns ME, Goldsmith MM. Incidence, diagnosis, and classification of salivary gland tumors. *Oncology* 1989;3:47–62.

Katz AD, Catalano P. The clinical significance of the various anastomotic branches of the facial nerve. *Arch Otolaryngol Head Neck Surg* 1987;113:959–962.

Kim KH, Sung MW, Chung PS, et al. Adenoid cystic carcinoma of the head and neck. *Arch Otolaryngol Head Neck Surg* 1994;120:721–726.

Koka VN, Tiwari RM, van der Waal D, et al. Adenoid cystic carcinoma of the salivary glands: clinicopathological survey of 51 patients. *J Laryngol Otol* 1989;103:675–679.

Krolls SO, Boyers RC. Mixed tumors of salivary glands: long-term follow-up. *Cancer* 1972;30:276–281.

Leegaard T, Lindeman H. Salivary gland tumors: clinical picture and treatment. *Acta Otolaryngol (Stockh)* 1970;263:155.

Maran AG. Sjögren's syndrome. *J Laryngol Otol* 1986;100:1299–1305.

McGurk FM, Main JHP, Orr JA. Adenolymphoma of the parotid gland. *Br J Surg* 1970;57:321.

McNaney D, McNeese MD, Guillamondegi OJ, Fletcher GH, Oswald MJ. Postoperative irradiation in malignant epithelial tumors of the parotid. *Int J Radiat Oncol Biol Phys* 1983;9:1289–1295.

Olsen KD. Tumors and surgery of the parapharyngeal space. *Laryngoscope* 1994;104[suppl]:1.

Rodriguez HP, Silver CE, Moisa II, Chacho MB. Fine needle aspiration of parotid tumors. *Am J Surg* 1989;158:342–344.

Saeed SR, Ramsden RT. Rehabilitation of the paralysed face: results of facial nerve surgery. *J Laryngol Otol* 1996;110:922–925.

Schuller DE, McCabe BF. Salivary gland neoplasms in children. *Otol Clin North Am* 1977;10:39.

Shah JP, Ihde JK. Salivary gland tumors. *Curr Probl Surg* 1990;27:775–843.

Simpson RHW. Classification of tumors of the salivary glands. *Histopathology* 1994;24:187–191.

Spiro RH. Salivary neoplasms: overview of a 35-year experience with 2807 patients. *Head Neck Surg* 1986;177–184.

Spiro RH, Hajdu SL, Strong EW. Tumors of the submaxillary gland. *Am J Surg* 1976;132:463–468.

Spiro RH, Huvos AG, Strong EW. Acinic cell carcinoma of salivary origin—a clinicopathologic study of 67 cases. *Cancer* 1978;41:924.

Spiro RH, Koss LG, Hajdu SI, et al. Tumors of minor salivary origin: a clinicopathologic study of 492 cases. *Cancer* 1973;31:117.

Stern SJ, Suen JY. Salivary gland tumors. *Curr Opin Oncol* 1993;5:518–525.

Tunkel DE, Loury MC, Fox CH, et al. Bilateral parotid enlargement in HIV-seropositive patients. *Laryngoscope* 1989;99:590–595.

Warthin AD. Papillary cystadenoma lymphomatosum. *J Cancer Res* 1929;13:116.

Woods JE. Parotidectomy: points of technique for brief and safe operation. *Am J Surg* 1983;145:678.

Yu GY, Ma DQ. Carcinoma of the salivary gland: a clinicopathologic study of 405 cases. *Semin Surg Oncol* 1987;3:240–244.

20

Thoracic Surgery

Gil Hauer Santos

CHEST WALL

Pectus Excavatum

Pectus excavatum is a congenital malformation that presents as posterior displacement of the sternum distal to the angle of Louis. A large depression on the right side is frequent, and displacement of the heart is variable. Patients with this condition may have frequent respiratory infections and decreased exercise tolerance. These symptoms are usually alleviated after correction. Corrective surgery, done ideally before 7 years of age, consists in removing the deformed cartilages and lifting the sternum, which can be accomplished by performing a posterior osteotomy followed by insertion of a bone wedge at the osteotomy site.

Other sternal defects are rarer. Among them is pectus carinatum, which is forward protrusion of the sternum. Superior, distal, and complete sternal clefts are rare malformations that are often associated with multiple chest wall abnormalities.

Chest Wall Tumors

Primary tumors of the chest wall are rare. They originate equally from the soft tissues and the skeletal struc-tures: bone and cartilage. Metastatic tumors of the chest wall are more common than primary tumors and are frequently multiple. They can result from direct extension of breast, lung, or pleural tumors, although these tumors also metastasize by the usual hematogenous and lymphatic routes. Metastatic chest wall tumors originate from other organs as well, such as the kidney and prostate. An interesting group of tumors originating in the kidneys and thyroid can produce metastasis in the sternum, which presents clinically as a palpable pulsatile mass.

Solitary chest wall tumors can be metastatic or primary with about the same frequency. More than half of the primary tumors are malignant. Usually they are painful, although some small rib tumors are asymptomatic. The anatomic location of the tumor is important when considering a possible preoperative diagnosis; for example, fibrous dysplasia is found in the posterior aspect of the chest wall. Cartilaginous tumors are located anteriorly, at the costal cartilages. Sternal tumors almost always are malignant, particularly if they are more than 4 cm in diameter. A radiographic evaluation of a chest wall tumor is helpful: sharp delineation and intact cortical margins are characteristic of benign tumors. Malignant tumors are poorly defined with frequent cortical disruption, usually with tumor-specific features. Computed tomography (CT) is helpful for defining possible invasion of the pleura, lung, and mediastinum.

Benign Tumors

Benign chest wall tumors are less frequent than malignant tumors. Some of the most frequently seen benign tumors are chondroma, osteochondroma, and fibrous dysplasia. Benign neurogenic tumors such as neurofibroma and neurilemoma (also known as schwannoma) are sometimes seen in the chest wall. Desmoid tumors are rare, and during a 62-year period only 26 were identified at the Mayo Clinic. They arise from intercostal muscles and grow to the surface of the chest wall. Occasionally these tumors grow internally and are detected only with chest radiography. Desmoid tumors are not malignant but locally are highly invasive. Resection should be of a radical nature, avoiding injury to major structures. When local recurrences develop, they should be treated by resection. All benign rib tumors should be excised along with segments of the ribs where they originated. Osteochondromas can be excised flush to the rib, as they present as exostoses.

Primary Malignant Tumors

Soft Tissue Sarcomas

Soft tissue sarcomas comprise 70% of chest wall primary malignant tumors. They are classified as fibrosarcomas, malignant fibrous histiocytomas, rhabdomyosarcomas, angiosarcomas, neurosarcomas, synovial sarcomas, and others.

Chondrosarcoma

Chondrosarcomas constitute 15% of primary malignant tumors of the chest wall. They are found at the costochondral junction or at the sternum, often exceeding 4 cm in size when initially seen. They involve cartilage, ribs, muscle, and pleura; and sometimes when they attain a large size the lung can be invaded. Symptoms are mostly represented by tenderness, redness, and rib fixation. On radiography they appear as a large lobulated mass associated with bone destruction. The treatment should be wide surgical excision, which results in a 70% five-year survival. Inadequate resection often results in early local recurrence.

Osteosarcoma

Osteogenic sarcomas are seen in all age groups and are not as frequent as chondrosarcomas. On radiography they display a typical "sunburst"-like appearance. These tumors tend to produce metastasis early. Treatment consists in wide local surgical excision followed by chemotherapy. When there is ipsilateral pulmonary invasion the affected part of the lung is resected at the time of the initial operation, preferably as a wedge resection. Despite all therapeutic efforts, the 5-year survival with this tumor is only 15%.

Ewing's Sarcoma

The typical onion skin calcifications seen in Ewing's sarcoma are produced by periosteal elevation. These tumors occur more commonly in adolescents. Surgical resection is not sufficient and should be associated with chemotherapy. Sometimes when there is no response to chemotherapy, radiotherapy is considered as well.

Eosinophilic Granulomas

Eosinophilic granulomas are rare and usually multiple. They typically produce fever and leukocytosis.

Before treatment is initiated, a tissue diagnosis is made with a wide, open biopsy to obtain enough tissue for accurate diagnosis, which is often not feasible with a needle biopsy. Radical surgical excision with wide margins of normal tissue (at least 4 cm) is necessary for the treatment of most malignant tumors. Previous biopsy sites should be included. For sternal tumors the uninvolved side may be left in place to preserve the balance of the chest wall. When the tumor is situated in the posterior chest, where the wall is protected by the scapula, three or four ribs may be removed without the need to perform any major reconstruction of the chest wall.

Anteriorly, extensive reconstruction is necessary for large defects. Materials used for reconstruction include Marlex mesh as a composite with methylmethacrylate or solid sheets of Teflon. More recently Gore-Tex has been used successfully for chest wall reconstruction. Autogenous tissues are used when possible as free grafts or transposed grafts, as can be done with the use of skin flaps with muscles attached to it.

Good examples are deltopectoral cutaneous, thoracoabdominal cutaneous, and myocutaneous flaps of latissimus dorsi.

When wide margins are preserved, resection of a primary chest wall tumor can produce 5-year survivals from as low as 15% to as high as 95%, depending on the histology of the tumor.

Thoracic Outlet Syndrome

Thoracic outlet syndrome includes a variety of symptoms resulting from compression of the neurovascular bundle at the thoracic outlet. The brachial plexus, subclavian artery, and subclavian vein are compressed between the first rib and the clavicle. Other components of the compressing structures are the scalenus anterior muscle, situated between the subclavian artery posteriorly and the subclavian vein anterior to it, and the scalenus medius, situated posteriorly and laterally to the neurovascular structures.

Other compressing elements occasionally found are cervical ribs, which are almost always accompanied by congenital fibromuscular bands. These bands can be isolated, not associated with cervical ribs. Thoracic outlet symptoms are produced by compression of the neurovascular structures and depend on which one of these structures is mostly involved by the constricting elements. Ninety percent of patients complain of symptoms related to brachial plexus compression. Pain in the neck spreading to the ear, jaw, forehead, and posterior neck suggests compression of C5 and C6 roots. When lower roots are compressed, pain is experienced as spreading to the scapular area and the ulnar nerve territory. Other neurologic symptoms manifest as paresthesias, motor weakness, and tenderness over the scalenus muscle.

Atrophy of the interosseous muscles in the hand is found in neglected cases. When the subclavian artery is compressed, symptoms of distal ischemia similar to those of Raynaud syndrome may be present, manifested by coldness, claudication, or even necrosis of the digits. When the subclavian vein is compressed it manifests as edema of the extremity, proliferation of collateral veins, and cyanosis. Sometimes subclavian vein thrombosis, or "effort thrombosis," occurs and results in symptoms of acute obstruction to venous return.

Diagnostic Tests

Several tests have been proposed to demonstrate the presence of clinically significant thoracic outlet narrowing. Maneuvers intended to decrease or interrupt the radial pulse were described by Adson and others. These tests are not reliable and may be positive in a large number of normal subjects. Radiography is necessary to diagnose the presence of cervical ribs, elongated cervical vertebral transverse processes, and sometimes the presence of a long-forgotten clavicular fracture. Ulnar nerve conduction velocity across the thoracic outlet is 72 m/sec in normal individuals and less than 57 m/sec in patients who exhibit thoracic outlet syndrome. Not everyone reports reliable information with this test. When there is clinical suggestion of subclavian artery compression, arteriography is useful. Phlebography can be diagnostic when the clinical impression is subclavian vein compression or thrombosis. The clinical picture of nerve compression in thoracic outlet syndrome sometimes makes it difficult to differentiate it clinically from carpal tunnel syndrome and from cervical disc compression.

Treatment

For uncomplicated cases of thoracic outlet syndrome the initial treatment is usually nonsurgical. Early surgery is recommended only when symptoms are persistent, a neurologic deficit is present, or there is a threat of decreased blood supply to the extremity due to subclavian artery compression. The conservative treatment relies on control of posture, avoiding stooping the shoulders, which tends to decrease the space between the clavicle and the first rib, thereby aggravating the compression. It is also recommended that patients avoid carrying loads such as grocery bags. With this basic care, improvement is seen in 50% to 90% of patients.

Patients who do not improve with this treatment must have surgery that increases the space available for the anatomic elements that traverse the thoracic outlet. The most recommended procedure is a first rib resection frequently done through an axillary approach. When the symptoms result from compression of C5 or C6 roots, an anterior scalenectomy is sufficient to obtain proper decompression. Cervical ribs and fibromuscular bands should also be resected when present. Less than good results are obtained when these bands are not recognized and left in place; otherwise, good results are obtained in 95% of patients. Insufficient decompression may also exacerbate the symptoms due to growth of scar tissue.

TRAUMA

Sternal Fractures

Sternal fractures result from severe blunt trauma and are often associated with steering wheel injuries. If displacement with separation of the fragments occurs, reduction or reduction fixation may be required. If no separation occurs, observation alone is sufficient. The patient is carefully evaluated for possible cardiac contusion with serial electrocardiograms and assays for cardiac enzymes. Mortality rates of 20% to 45% are reported, with death almost always due to the severity of the associated injuries.

Isolated Rib Fractures

Isolated rib fractures may be associated with pneumothorax or hemothorax that requires chest tubes for drainage and frequently thoracotomy to control bleeding or repair air leaks. Elderly patients with rib fractures must be given sufficient analgesics to permit them to breathe freely with no splinting to avoid the development of atelectasis.

Flail Chest

Flail chest can occur when several ribs are fractured, especially if there are double fractures on several ribs or the fractures are associated with costochondral separations. The resultant mechanical dysfunction of the chest wall manifests as limited expansion during inspiration and paradoxical movements of parts of the chest wall. It prevents efficient ventilation, producing intrapulmonary shunting of variable degree.

The immediate treatment for patients in respiratory distress who do not improve with face mask oxygen is endotracheal intubation with mechanical ventilation. Some believe that most patients with flail chest also have significant pulmonary contusion and recommend adding fluid restriction and physiotherapy to the venti-

latory support. Endotracheal intubation and mechanical ventilation are indicated in patients with a Po_2 lower than 60 mm Hg on room air or with a Po_2 below 80 mm Hg on oxygen administered by face mask.

Weaning the patient from ventilatory support follows the same guidelines as in other circumstances. If the patient requires prolonged ventilatory support for treatment of flail chest and has no other injuries that require bed rest, internal fixation of the fractured ribs can be considered. This option allows early ambulation by freeing the patient from mechanical ventilation, avoiding the usual complications that result from prolonged bed rest and prolonged artificial ventilation.

MEDIASTINUM

Mediastinal Tumors

Tumors can develop in all mediastinal compartments. A tentative diagnosis, including the probable histologic type of a tumor, can be assigned based on the location of the tumor. For that purpose the mediastinum is divided into anterior, middle, and posterior portions. The superior mediastinum is recognized as the site where tumors arising in the thyroid and parathyroids are most frequently found.

The prevailing nature of tumors varies with the age of the patient. In children 50% of mediastinal tumors are neurogenic, 20% are lymphomas, and 20% are cysts; whereas in adults the tumors are represented equally: 20% neurogenic tumors, 20% thymomas, 20% lymphomas, and 20% cysts.

Neurogenic tumors are mostly found in children less than 4 years of age. Germ cell tumors represented by seminomas, teratomas, choriocarcinomas, embryonal cell carcinomas, and yolk sac tumors found in the anterior mediastinum comprise 10% of mediastinal tumors and are found in adolescents and adults. Thymomas and endocrine tumors are rarely seen on children.

Symptoms are present in 50% of patients with malignant mediastinal tumors and in only 10% of those with the benign variety. The most frequent symptoms are pain, cough, dyspnea, respiratory infections, and dysphagia. Rarely observed are symptoms due to superior vena cava compression or invasion. Horner's syndrome due to involvement of the stellate ganglion is also rare. Even more rare are symptoms due to spinal cord compression. Some mediastinal tumors secrete endocrine substances that are capable of producing metabolic alterations, such as hypercalcemia; they are found in some patients with parathyroid adenomas. Some patients have hypertension due to a neurogenic tumor and some exhibit a clinical picture of thyrotoxicosis due to an intrathoracic goiter. Myasthenia gravis and red blood cell aplasia are associated with thymomas.

The workup of patients with these mediastinal tumors includes routine chest films, followed by computed tomography (CT), in some cases magnetic resonance imaging (MRI), and occasionally angiography. Tissue diagnosis can be obtained by needle biopsy, transcervical standard or extended mediastinoscopy, or anterior mediastinoscopy (Chamberlain procedure). Often specialized studies are indicated. Myelography is useful for clarifying intraspinal extension of neurogenic tumors. Tomography of vertebral bodies or a thin-layer scan is indicated to document increased intervertebral spaces when neurogenic tumor extends into the vertebral canal. Radioisotope scanning is useful for evaluating a possible mediastinal thyroid. MRI is helpful for defining mediastinal masses. It is mostly indicated to evaluate tumors situated in the posterior mediastinum. Anterior mediastinal exploration through a Chamberlain procedure done by resecting the left second costal cartilage is indicated for evaluation and biopsy of a lesion situated in that location. Often light microscopy cannot differentiate between thymomas, lymphomas, and seminomas; the diagnosis is made only by electron microscopy.

Neurogenic Tumors

At least 50% of unilateral paravertebral masses in children are malignant. This is different from the situation in adults where most of the masses in that location are benign. Chest pain produced by bony erosion or nerve root compression is the most frequent symptom. Dyspnea due to tracheal compression is sometimes present. Intraspinal extension of a tumor with compression of the cord produces a resultant neurologic deficit. Hypertension is present when the tumor is a catecholamine-secreting pheochromocytoma. The presence of vanillylmandelic acid, produced by ganglioneuromas and neuroblastomas, manifests clinically as diarrhea, flushing, and diaphoresis.

The most common neurogenic tumor is the neurilemoma (schwannoma) arising from the nerve sheath. It

presents as a well circumscribed lesion that may advance into the intervertebral canal. Less frequently seen are neurofibromas. These poorly circumscribed tumors may be part of generalized neurofibromatosis. It is interesting to note that patients with Von Recklinghausen's disease occasionally have a posterior mediastinal meningocele. Neurilemomas and neurofibromas can undergo malignant degeneration to malignant schwannomas, which are highly invasive tumors. Ganglioneuromas arise from sympathetic ganglia, are well encapsulated, and grow to a large size. Their malignant counterparts, ganglioneuroblastomas, may metastasize widely. Neuroblastoma is the most undifferentiated neurogenic tumor and is extremely malignant. Often when first diagnosed it has already spread to brain, bone, and liver. Fever, cough, and sometimes diarrhea are the presenting symptoms.

Pheochromocytomas are rarely seen. Even more rare are paragangliomas arising from the chemoreceptor tissue located at the aortic arch.

The treatment for neurogenic tumors is surgical resection. When there is intravertebral extension the intravertebral component should be excised synchronously with the intrathoracic tumor. To obtain good exposure for resecting these tumors, the skin is incised with one longitudinal component over the site where laminectomy is to be performed, with a posterolateral thoracic extension for the thoracotomy portion of the operation. Neuroblastomas are not always resectable; and when complete resection is not possible, adjuvant chemotherapy and radiotherapy are added postoperatively to obtain some increase in survival. These tumors have a better prognosis when located in the mediastinum than in other sites.

Thymoma and Parathymic Syndromes

Thymomas are the most common anterior mediastinal tumor in adults over 30 years of age. About 5% of the patients who present with red blood cell aplasia and 10% with myasthenia gravis have associated thymomas. Myasthenia results from the destruction produced by thymic antibodies against acetylcholine receptors located at the neuromuscular endplate.

The malignancy of a thymoma is determined by its clinical behavior and its invasiveness into neighboring tissues. It is therefore relevant to classify them as intracapsular, extracapsular, or invasive. The invasive form can infiltrate the pericardium, heart, pleura, or great vessels. Histologically, thymomas are classified as epidermoid, spindle cell, or mixed. Lymphocytes in these tumors can be found in small or large numbers.

The presence of a thymoma is sufficient indication for surgery. Noninvasive tumors have a good prognosis, with the 10-year survival approaching 90%, whereas the 10-year survival for invasive tumors is only 20%. In the presence of severe myasthenia, plasmapheresis prior to surgery is recommended to remove acetylcholine receptor antibodies from the blood. The perioperative use of steroids has also proved beneficial. Patients with generalized myasthenia without an obvious thymoma should have the thymus removed unless the symptoms can be controlled with immunosuppressive or anticholinergic drugs (or both).

The surgical approach to the thymus is through a median sternotomy. A transcervical incision alone is almost always associated with incomplete removal of the gland. Some claim to have obtained good results with the use of a transcervical incision combined with a thoracoscopic approach to the mediastinum. This approach probably cannot be used for invasive tumors when extensive dissection and resection inclusive of lung, vessels, and pericardium are necessary.

In 50% of patients the symptoms of myasthenia remit during the first year after surgery, and almost 90% of patients improve 4 to 5 years after surgery. When the tumor is invasive, radiotherapy is added to the treatment. Neoadjuvant chemotherapy has improved the resectability rate for some lesions believed to be unresectable.

Lymphoproliferative Diseases

Primary mediastinal lymphomas, observed mostly in young adults, are usually confined to the middle and anterior mediastinal lymph nodes. Hodgkin's disease is the most frequent, representing two-thirds of primary mediastinal lymphomas. Cough, chest pain, and fever are the most common symptoms, as with other mediastinal tumors. When the tumor is bulky it may compress mediastinal structures, including the superior vena cava and trachea; sometimes debulking is required as a life-saving procedure. Otherwise, in most cases the role of surgery is limited to the acquisition of tissue samples for a pathologic diagnosis when a simple needle biopsy is not indicated or was unsuccessful. It can be done through an anterior mediastinotomy as a Chamberlain procedure or through a standard (or if necessary

an extended) cervical mediastinoscopy. The treatment for these tumors is based on radiotherapy and chemotherapy.

Giant lymph node hyperplasia, also known as Castleman's disease or pseudolymphoma, is associated with markedly enlarged lymph nodes in the mediastinum. They have measured up to 700 g.

Germ Cell Tumors

Mediastinal germ cell tumors are found in the anterior mediastinum. Even though rare, this location is second only to the gonads, where 95% of these tumors are found. Similar to other mediastinal tumors, they manifest as cough, pain, and shortness of breath. When invasive they may erode into a bronchus, the pericardium, or the pleural cavity. The most frequently found germ cell tumor is the teratoma, composed of several embryologic layers that may be cystic or solid. They are mostly benign. Often the presence of calcifications inside the tumor mass makes it easy to identify them. These tumors should be resected for diagnosis and treatment when initially demonstrated. Sometimes resection is difficult owing to adhesions and the intimate relationship of the tumor to intrathoracic structures. Teratocarcinomas are their malignant counterparts and are highly invasive, producing metastasis early in the course of the disease.

From therapeutic and prognostic perspectives, mediastinal germ cell tumors can be classified as seminomas and nonseminomatous tumors. Seminomas are an important variety of germ cell tumor, seen almost exclusively in men 20 to 40 years old. Nonseminomatous germ cell tumors are further classified as embryonal cell carcinomas, choriocarcinomas, yolk sac tumors, and mixed forms. These tumors produce increased titers of human chorionic gonadotropins (β-hCG) and α-fetoprotein (AFP). They are highly malignant tumors found in young men, commonly with early metastatic spread. Their course is rapidly fatal.

At the Memorial Sloan–Kettering Hospital (MS-KH) it was shown that seminomas respond well to chemotherapy alone. This is not the case for the nonseminomatous variety. Based in a large experience at MS-KH, it was recommended that after chemotherapy the patient be reevaluated. If residual tumor of more than 3 cm is found, together with a return of the markers to normal titers, surgery is indicated, followed by radiotherapy and chemotherapy. Even with this combination therapy, results for seminomatous germ cell tumors are poor, with 2-year survivals not exceeding 20%.

Benign Tumors

Benign mediastinal tumors are usually asymptomatic when they do not compress a vital structure such as an airway. Superior mediastinal tumors are mostly represented by the thyroid, which may descend into the chest to produce symptoms (depending on its size and occasional compression of vessels and the trachea). An interesting situation occurs when the thyroid pedicle is insinuated between the esophagus and the vertebral bodies, producing dysphagia due to compression of the lumen of the esophagus. When removal of an upper anterior mediastinal thyroid gland is indicated, it can usually be accomplished through a cervical incision by delivering the thyroid from the mediastinum into the neck, where it can be easily removed. When the thyroid is too large to be safely removed from the mediastinum, an upper median sternotomy, created as a trap door, is sometimes necessary.

Otherwise benign mediastinal tumors are found to be comprised of lipomas, fibromas, myomas, or angiomas. When symptoms are present they are usually due to their malignant counterparts (e.g., liposarcomas).

Mediastinal Cysts

Cysts represent 20% of mediastinal tumors in all age groups. They should be excised for the purpose of diagnosis and to avoid future enlargement, infection, or rupture. The most frequently diagnosed cysts are bronchogenic and esophageal cysts, which are malformations derived from the primitive foregut.

Bronchogenic cysts are found close to the tracheal bifurcation and have an inner lining of ciliated respiratory epithelium. Esophageal cysts, also known as enteric or duplication cysts, are situated in close association with the esophagus. They may be found inside the muscular layers of the esophagus. Neuroenteric cysts comprise an interesting group of cysts that are associated with anomalies of the vertebral bodies; they communicate directly with the dural space.

Two frequently diagnosed mesothelial cysts are pericardial and pleural cysts. Pericardial cysts are usually found in the right pericardiophrenic angle. Because of the clear fluid filling them they are known as clear water cysts. Less frequently seen are thymic cysts, found in the anterior mediastinum. These cysts can become acutely symptomatic when they rupture.

Because of the large number of tumors and cysts that can be found in the mediastinum it is important that their diagnosis be established by needle biopsy, mediastinoscopy, or open biopsy so specific treatment can be instituted. Occasionally an isolated lesion can be completely excised without prior diagnosis. AFP and β-hCG assays are important for diagnosing germ cell tumors and are valuable markers for determining the effectiveness of treatment for these tumors.

Pneumomediastinum

The initial approach to clinically finding air in the mediastinum consists in attempts to determine its source. Frequently the diagnosis is made by ruling out possible etiologic factors. The most frequent cause of pneumomediastinum is the forced passage of air alongside pulmonary vascular and bronchial structures toward the hilum of the lung and from there to the mediastinum. This situation is seen sometimes in patients being ventilated with high airway pressures, but it can happen also in seemingly healthy patients. Treatment is usually supportive. In rare cases when excessive air is present and produces discomfort and pressure, an incision may be made above the sternal notch deep to the pretracheal fascia to decompress the air trapped in the mediastinum.

Less frequently air is introduced to the mediastinum when the trachea or bronchus is ruptured due to the deceleration that occurs during a motor vehicle accident. An esophageal spontaneous rupture (Boerhaave syndrome) or a foreign body or iatrogenic perforation also permits air to enter the mediastinum. Rarely, a ruptured posterior wall of the duodenum is responsible for passage of air into the retroperitoneal tissues, from where it insinuates upward, entering the mediastinum. Treatment for these various circumstances must address the initial pathology.

Mediastinitis

Mediastinitis is produced by bacterial contamination of the mediastinum. Proper treatment requires drainage, the use of organism-specific antibiotics, and finding the source of contamination to prevent continuous soiling. When mediastinitis is due to esophageal rupture or perforation, the esophageal opening is closed at the same time the mediastinum is cleaned and drained. Antibiotics are used as necessary.

Mediastinitis occasionally results from extension of a pharyngeal abscess or perforation of the piriform sinus or the hypopharynx proximal to the cricopharyngeus during traumatic intubation. Fibrosing mediastinitis is rare, but when it does occur it may be secondary to *Histoplasma* or tuberculous infection of the mediastinal lymph nodes. Most often, however, it is idiopathic. When advanced, it can result in compression of the superior vena cava, trachea, or esophagus, producing the symptoms and signs, respectively, of superior vena cava syndrome, dyspnea, or dysphagia. Surgery is directed to relieve the constricted structures.

TRACHEA

Tracheal Tumors

Primary tracheal tumors are rare. Sixty percent of these tumors are squamous cell carcinomas and adenoid cystic carcinomas (also known as cylindromas). Tumors less frequently seen in the trachea are sarcomas. Almost half of malignant tracheal tumors when initially seen already have mediastinal or pulmonary metastases. Benign tumors are rare: fibromas, leiomyomas, and chondromas. Secondary tracheal tumors are due to tumors that grow in the vicinity extending into the trachea. Most frequent in this category are esophageal tumors, which may grow through the posterior membranous wall of the trachea. Others that can also invade the trachea are laryngeal, bronchogenic, and thyroid tumors.

Symptoms, which are due to airway obstruction, include shortness of breath, wheezing, and cough. Voice changes and hoarseness are also present when the recurrent nerve is invaded or when the vocal cords are involved.

A physician should be prepared to deal with a patient who comes to the emergency room with tracheal obstruction. A rigid pediatric bronchoscope can be used to provide an interim airway at the same time it is maneuvered to dilate the airway sufficiently to permit intubation with a small-caliber endotracheal tube. After emergency treatment, surgery should be considered. When not resectable, the tumor can be debulked, with the lumen opened endoscopically and biopsy forceps and suction used for the debulking. No advantage is seen with the use of laser. Bleeding is not a critical problem in such cases. The definitive procedure, when feasible, requires resection of the tumor, which can be done through an anterior cervical approach combined (or not) with a median sternotomy. Low, distal tracheal tumors are easier to approach with better exposure through a right thoracotomy. Fifty percent of the tracheal length can be resected. The distal and proximal trachea, after resection, can be approximated by keeping the head flexed during the end-to-end tracheal anastomosis. This flexion should be maintained postoperatively to prevent suture disruption, when necessary by suturing the patient's chin to the chest. Results are satisfactory for benign tumors and for malignant tumors confined to the tracheal wall. Adenoid cystic carcinomas can infiltrate the trachea distant from the area of the original tumor, making complete resection difficult.

Tracheal Stricture

Tracheal stricture results from prolonged endotracheal intubation with trauma to the trachea produced by endotracheal balloon cuffs. Stricture was a major problem in the past due to the early design of endotracheal tubes, but modern low-pressure cuffs have reduced this complication significantly. Another situation responsible for stricture occurs when a tracheostoma heals and contracts after weaning from a tracheostomy. To avoid this complication, the tracheostomy is ideally made with the patient intubated in the operating room (not at bedside). A longitudinal incision is made through the second and third tracheal rings, and the isthmus of the thyroid is divided if necessary for proper exposure. Lower tracheostomies have the potential to injure the innominate artery, producing massive bleeding, which occurs a few days after the initial procedure. Higher tracheostomies may be associated with injuries to the cricoid cartilage with subsequent development of subglottic stenosis. Careful hemostasis is necessary when performing a tracheostomy. The sides of the tracheal wall can be secured with long stitches taped to the skin so as to be able to retrieve the trachea if the tracheostomy tube is inadvertently dislodged during the immediate postoperative period.

Tracheal Disruption

Blunt chest trauma, deceleration injuries, or falls from heights can produce partial or complete tracheal disruption. Few patients with complete tracheal disruption arrive alive in the emergency room. Intubation can be difficult, as a large amount of blood obscures the vision of the endoscopist. If possible, a cervical incision and "fishing" of the distal trachea with a tracheostomy hook may be the only way to direct the endotracheal tube into the disrupted airway. Once the airway is secured, the patient is taken to the operating room for controlled repair of the trachea.

Incomplete disruption of the trachea or the major bronchi is heralded by the patient coughing up blood and by the presence of air in the mediastinum near the site of disruption. Depending on the size of the disruption, treatment may be conservative, or suturing to close the tear may be required.

PLEURA

Pneumothorax

In the absence of adhesions between the visceral and parietal pleura, pneumothorax develops when air enters the pleural cavity. Multiple etiologies are responsible for this situation. Ruptured bullae, damage to the lung by fractured ribs or penetrating injuries, and esophageal perforation or rupture are all capable of producing a pneumothorax.

We address here the spontaneous pneumothoraces that most commonly occur in two distinct groups. One group is composed of tall, slender young men and women in their twenties. The second group comprises mostly elderly patients. In the young adults the pneumothorax is associated with sudden rupture of a congenital pulmonary bulla or a subpleural bleb. In older patients with emphysema, ruptured acquired bullae are usually the cause of pneumothorax.

Symptoms of spontaneous pneumothorax are of variable intensity and consist of sudden chest pain associated with dyspnea and tachypnea of variable intensity. When there is a ball-valve effect at the site where the lung ruptured, it is possible for a large volume of air under pressure to build up inside the pleural space, giving origin to a tension pneumothorax. This dangerous clinical situation manifests as diaphoresis, tachypnea, and shortness of breath associated with decreased breath sounds in the involved hemithorax together with a change in the position of the mediastinum including the cardiac apex and trachea. Imme-

diate relief of the tension is accomplished by draining the hemithorax with a needle or catheter. If not diagnosed and treated, this situation can rapidly evolve to cardiac arrest. There is no place here for radiologic studies. Treatment in all cases of spontaneous pneumothorax is directed to reexpanding the lung, which is accomplished by inserting a small-caliber chest tube connected to a Pleurevac or similar suction system. The chest tube may be introduced into the second interspace at the midclavicular line or at the midaxillary or anterior axillary line where it intersects the xiphoid line. The last approach is preferred in female patients, who may be concerned with scars. During insertion of the chest tube care must be taken to avoid injury to the lung. Unless the lung is detached from the chest wall or totally collapsed as seen on chest films, the pleural space should be identified before inserting the chest tube. If the air leak persists with no decrease in volume after 5 to 6 days of drainage, surgery is indicated. With persistent leak, recurrent pneumothorax, or a patient with previous contralateral lung collapse, the treatment should include (a) bullectomy to close the air leak and (b) abrasion of the parietal pleura (pleurodesis) to create adhesions between the two layers of pleura. The thoracoscopic approach has been associated with only partial success. Some of the difficulties with this method is finding the leak and assessing the size of the bullae. Pleurodesis, undertaken to avoid surgery on patients with spontaneous pneumothorax, is indicated only when surgery is excessively risky and when there is no radiologic evidence of bullae. Attempted pleurodesis fails when the lung becomes only partially attached to the chest wall, thereby creating multiple noncommunicating compartments in the pleural space.

Pleural Tumors

Visceral and parietal pleura are easily invaded by tumors originating in the lung or breast, which are the most frequently found tumors in the pleura. Often major pleural effusions result from these tumors, and supportive treatment that includes drainage and attempted pleurodesis to obliterate the pleural space is indicated. Several substances can be injected into the pleural space for that purpose. Talcum powder, previously used but at times forgotten, is the most effective substance used for pleurodesis, although tetracycline and a few other agents have also been used successfully. Radiotherapy or chemotherapy can also decrease the amount of fluid in the pleural effusion.

The most common primary tumor of the pleura is mesothelioma. The role of asbestos in the genesis of this tumor has been difficult to prove considering that until recently asbestos was used in the production of a large number of items of daily use, including insulating materials, brake linings, and so forth. Despite such widespread use, only 1300 new cases are diagnosed each year in the United States.

Two types of mesothelioma are recognized: the localized benign form, and the diffuse malignant form. The localized form can attain a large size (up to several pounds), is pedunculated, and is treated by resection. The diffuse form can be histologically classified as epithelial, sarcomatous, or mixed.

Once the lesion is diagnosed, the median survival of the patient with the malignant form does not exceed 8 to 12 months. Different from other cancers, mesotheliomas kill by local, uncontrolled growth. Surgical treatment has been discouraging with no significant results. Two surgical treatments are utilized: pleurectomy and extrapleural pneumonectomy. When the pleura is free, with no attachments between the visceral and parietal layers, and the tumor is at the parietal pleura, pleurectomy suffices. When there are attachments with obliteration of the pleural space, an extrapleural pneumonectomy is preferred. Some surgical series report survivals up to 14 to 20 months, but this observed increased survival may be due to patient selection and not to any benefit obtained from surgery. Other series comparing only surgery with chemotherapy or radiotherapy alone do not show any improvement in survival, although minor improvement was noted when a combination of these modalities was used.

The intrapleural injection of various chemotherapeutic agents is an example of new forms of treatment being tested. Photodynamic therapy (PDT), another form of treatment being evaluated, uses the predilection of Photofrin to concentrate selectively in malignant tissues. At 48 hours after injection, the drug present in the tumor can be activated with a laser source, producing tumor necrosis. Other organs including the heart have been damaged with PDT. There is also the danger of sunburn on patients treated with PDT due to accumulation of Photofrin in the skin.

LUNG

Bronchogenic Carcinoma

It was estimated that approximately 170,000 new cases of bronchogenic carcinoma would be diagnosed in 1998. Previously this tumor was rare in women, but now it is the number one cancer in men and women alike. The major carcinogen is cigarette smoking.

Histologically, the largest number of tumors at this time are adenocarcinomas, which account for 45% of cases. Squamous cell carcinoma, which was the most prevalent tumor as little as 10 years ago, is now the second most prevalent, accounting for 35% of cases. Tumors with epidermoid and glandular elements are currently being identified, and these tumors may well prove to be more frequent than we once thought.

Undifferentiated tumors comprise 15% of bronchogenic cancers. They are classified as large-cell and small-cell carcinomas. Small-cell carcinomas are also known as oat cell carcinomas. The oat cell carcinoma is peculiar and different from the other bronchogenic carcinomas in that it behaves more like a systemic disease with a predilection for early spread to other organs. Because of this propensity it must be approached differently than other bronchogenic carcinomas. Removal of a known small-cell carcinoma should not be attempted before an extensive metastatic workup is undertaken.

The remaining 5% of lung tumors, not classified as bronchogenic carcinomas, include such rare tumors as lymphoma, sarcoma, and bronchial adenoma. Bronchial adenomas are slow-growing tumors, mostly represented by carcinoids arising from Kulchitsky cells. Serotonin and other endocrine substances are secreted by these tumors. Other types of adenoma are adenoid cystic carcinomas (originally called cylindromas) and the less frequently found mucoepidermoid adenomas related to salivary glands.

Symptoms

The initial pulmonary intraparenchymal tumor is asymptomatic. It becomes symptomatic when it invades anatomic structures in the chest, including major airways and the chest wall itself. A well defined group of symptoms are related to metastases, and still another less frequent group of symptoms are due to the action of hormonal substances produced by these tumors.

The invasion of intrathoracic structures can give origin to the initial symptoms. In this way tumors that obstruct major airways are frequently associated with clinical episodes of recurrent pneumonia. Various nerves can be invaded by tumor; for example, hoarseness is produced by recurrent nerve invasion. This occurs more frequently on the left side because on this side the recurrent nerve is easily involved near the pulmonary hilum as it loops around the aortic arch where it takes off from the vagus. In this location the recurrent nerve is exposed to invasion by growth of a left hilar tumor. The right recurrent nerve is invaded less frequently because it is positioned around the innominate artery, far from the hilum and therefore less vulnerable to hilar pathology. When the phrenic nerve is compromised, there is paralysis of the respective hemidiaphragm, which becomes elevated, producing basal atelectasis of the lower lobe with symptoms of fever and shortness of breath.

An interesting location of tumors in the apex of the upper lobes was described by Pancoast under the name of superior sulcus tumors. These tumors can invade the structures at the apex of the chest, producing symptoms related to this invasion. Horner's syndrome indicates invasion of the stellate ganglion in the sympathetic chain. The ulnar nerve, which is the lower division of the brachial plexus, can also be invaded as the tumors grow above Sibson's fascia. The invasion of the posterior aspects of the first and second ribs is associated with unrelenting shoulder pain. Chest pain is present in pulmonary cancer patients when the tumor invades the chest wall at any level.

Obstruction of the superior vena cava by a lung tumor manifests as edema of the head, neck, and upper extremities followed by the appearance of collateral veins in the upper chest. The esophagus can also be compressed by a lung tumor or enlarged mediastinal lymph node, causing symptoms of dysphagia even though this situation arises infrequently. Pericardial effusion due to pericardial invasion has been described, and large volumes of fluid may be present inside the pericardium. Differently from acute tamponade, when small amounts of fluid inside the pericardial cavity can prevent diastolic expansion and produce cardiac arrest, the chronicity of the enlargement produced by fluid seeping inside the pericardial space when invaded by tumor permits the pericardium to stretch slowly to accommodate large amounts of fluid. In such cases clinical symptoms of congestive heart failure are evident at presentation.

Another, less frequent group of symptoms results from the production of hormone-like substances by specific histologic types of bronchogenic carcinoma. In this way squamous cell carcinoma produces a parathyroid hormone (PTH)-like substance, whereas adrenocorticotropic hormone (ACTH) and antidiuretic hormone (ADH) are sometimes produced by small-cell carcinoma. Other hormonal substances are responsible for pulmonary osteoarthropathy manifested by clubbing and pretibial pain due to periosteal proliferation.

In some instances the initial symptoms of lung cancer are caused by distant metastases, which frequently are located in the brain or bones. Liver metastases are also frequent, but often they are not symptomatic when the patient is seen initially.

In young patients (less than 30 years of age) solitary pulmonary nodules, formerly known as coin lesions, are rarely malignant (only 1% or 2% of cases). Most of the benign solitary lesions in this age group are hamartomas and granulomas (tuberculosis, histoplasmosis, sarcoid). In older patients, mainly smokers, lung cancer is the most probable diagnosis of a solitary lung lesion.

Workup

When evaluating patients with isolated lung masses the first step should always be a review of previous chest radiographs. When available, they are extremely helpful. If the lesion was present many years before and there has been no growth since then, it can be assumed to be benign. If the tumor was not seen on previous films or if growth is demonstrated, the presumptive diagnosis is malignancy. This important information cannot be obtained when no previous films are available.

The next step for evaluating a lung mass is cytologic examination of the first morning sputum specimen collected on three consecutive mornings. This cytologic examination can be highly informative and requires participation of an experienced cytologist. The next diagnostic step should be bronchoscopy carefully performed in the region where the tumor was detected radiologically. If a lesion is seen, biopsy specimens are obtained; if the lesion is not seen endoscopically, brushings and washings are collected if possible using fluoroscopy to guide passage of the scope and the bronchial brushes toward the site of the lesion.

If the workup to this point has been nondiagnostic, some surgeons and radiologists opt for a percutaneous needle biopsy—more so if the lesion is a peripheral one. Pneumothorax and seeding of tumor in the needle tract in the chest wall are known complications of this procedure. Considering that in the event of positive or negative findings a thoracotomy would be required, I prefer to omit this step and proceed with the thoracotomy. Occasionally a diagnosis is needed on a patient who would not tolerate an open procedure. For those cases I recommend percutaneous biopsy. Recently PET has proved extremely helpful in defining metastatic implants.

Staging

In 1986 an international consensus was adopted for staging lung cancer. The staging is based on the TNM classification, which takes into consideration the size and location of the primary tumor, the presence and location of positive lymph nodes, and the presence or absence of distant metastasis. The following staging was adopted.

Stage	T	N	M
Occult carcinoma	Tx	N0	M0
Stage 0	Tis		
Stage IA	T1	N0	M0
Stage IB	T2	N0	M0
Stage IIA	T1	N1	M0
Stage IIB	T2	N1	M0
Stage IIIA	T3	N0/N1	M0
	T1/T3	N2	M0
Stage IIIB	Any T	N3	M0
	T4	Any N	M0
Stage IV	Any T	Any N	M1

Definitions of the TNM categories are as follows.

Primary tumor (T)

T0 No evidence of primary tumor.

Tx Tumor proved by the presence of malignant cells in bronchopulmonary secretions but not visualized.

Tis Carcinoma *in situ.*

T1 Tumor 3 cm or less in greatest dimension surrounded by lung or visceral pleura, without evidence of invasion proximal to a lobar bronchus at bronchoscopy.

T2 Tumor more than 3 cm in greatest dimension or of any size that either invades the visceral pleura or has associated atelectasis or obstructive pneumonitis extending to the hilar region. At bronchoscopy the proximal extent of the demonstrable tumor must be within a lobar bronchus or at least 2 cm distal to the carina. Any associated atelectasis or obstructive pneumonitis must involve less than one entire lung.

T3 A tumor of any size with direct extension into the chest wall (including a superior sulcus tumor), diaphragm, or the mediastinal pleura or pericardium without involving the heart, great vessels, trachea, esophagus, or vertebral body; or a tumor in the main bronchus within 2 cm of the carina but without involvement of the carina.

T4 Tumor of any size with invasion of the mediastinum or involving the heart, great vessels, trachea, esophagus, vertebral bodies, or carina; or the presence of malignant pleural effusion.

Nodal involvement (N)

N0 No demonstrable metastasis to regional lymph nodes.

N1 Metastasis to lymph nodes in the peribronchial or ipsilateral hilar region (or both) including direct extension.

N2 Metastasis to ipsilateral mediastinal lymph nodes and subcarinal lymph nodes.

N3 Metastasis to contralateral mediastinal lymph nodes, contralateral hilar lymph nodes, ipsilateral or contralateral supraclavicular lymph nodes.

Treatment

In most of the patients who benefit from surgery the tumors are diagnosed at an early stage. By the time symptoms are present, tumors are often in an advanced stage, when cure cannot be obtained with surgery. When a patient is seen with a small lesion (T1 or T2) and negative nodes, the natural course of the disease can be arrested; although 5-year survival is rare with these tumors, when the disease is arrested surgical resection may increase survival in as many as 75% of patients. A complete clinical investigation is necessary prior to surgery, as patients with pulmonary malignancy frequently suffer from chronic obstructive pulmonary disease (COPD) and cardiac conditions. Pulmonary function tests associated with perfusion and ventilation tests permit one to predict pulmonary function after surgery. It also avoids removal of lung tissue essential for gas exchange for a particular patient. Perfusion tests are used to determine the contribution of each lung region for gas exchange. Surgery should be avoided when the predicted postoperative forced expiratory volume in 1 second (FEV_1) is less than 0.8 L.

Because of the high incidence of right-side mediastinal involvement when the tumor is on the left lung, mediastinoscopy to rule out positive mediastinal lymph nodes on the right side is indicated. This seeming paradox is due to the anatomy of the lymphatic pathways, which travel from the left to the right side. The same contralateral spread is not observed for right-side lung tumors.

When the tumor is localized in one lobe, standard lobectomy is advocated. Only when the tumor is hilar or crosses fissures involving all the lobes on one side is a pneumonectomy indicated. The mortality associated with lobectomy is 2%, and that for pneumonectomy is 5%. A lesser resection than lobectomy has been proposed in the form of a segmentectomy or a wedge resection. It is advantageous for patients with limited pulmonary reserve and makes it possible to bring to surgery patients who otherwise would not be considered able to tolerate it. A 5-year survival of 55% has been obtained for patients having this limited resection when the lesion is at stage I.

Patients with more advanced tumors have a much worse prognosis, and even stage IIA patients have a 5-year survival of no more than 40%. Patients with chest wall invasion whose tumor can be resected and who otherwise are good candidates for surgery can be operated. The prognosis for these patients is not related as much to the chest wall invasion but to the N status of the hilar and mediastinal nodes. When the mediastinal nodes are negative, these patients can expect to have a 40% to 50% five-year survival. Locally advanced cancers are best treated initially with multiple-drug chemotherapy. If a response is obtained, surgery is undertaken, followed by resumption of chemotherapy and possibly radiotherapy. If the tumor is completely resected, the 5-year survival is 20%. If incompletely resected there are no long-term survivors.

Trials with brachytherapy have been done in several specialized hospitals with only modest results. Therefore the value of such attempts must be questioned.

Because of the poor results obtained with treatment of advanced carcinomas, screening studies have been undertaken to find these lesions before they become unresectable. One of the first large-scale studies was the Philadelphia Research Project, where a large number of cigarette-smoking men were enrolled. Yearly chest roentgenograms were obtained, and the enlisted subjects were required to report any change in their health status. This study did not improve the results of surgical treatment of tumors detected during the time the studies were conducted. Several reasons were proposed, but it became clear that a regimen of chest films obtained on a yearly basis was not associated with improved survival, probably due to the rapid doubling time of some of these tumors (doubling time ranges from 22 to 400 days).

A multicenter cooperative study was undertaken by the Mayo Clinic, Memorial Sloan-Kettering, and Johns Hopkins Hospital using various protocols, including frequent chest films and frequent sputum cytology, singly or combined. Results from these studies are forthcoming, but at the moment it appears that screening for lung cancer is still awaiting a better, more cost-effective system than is presently available. A difficult situation arises when sputum cytology is positive and chest films and bronchoscopy fail to localize the tumor. These patients know that they have a cancer of the lung but not its location, which requires repeated bronchoscopies and chest films until the tumor is found. Therefore it is the rare patient whose tumor is diagnosed at an early stage, when chest films are obtained for unrelated reasons (while the tumor is still silent inside the lung parenchyma), who can be helped by surgery alone.

Lung Abscesses

The most common sites for lung abscesses are the superior segments of the right and left lower lobes. There is a small preponderance on the right side due to anatomic characteristics, as there is a more direct line between the trachea and the right main bronchus. It is also of note that the main carina is situated more to the left of the midline. Frequently involved (but less often than the superior segments of the lower lobes) is the posterior segment of the right upper lobe.

Lung abscesses may result from aspiration of foreign bodies, including teeth or dental caps. They are also associated with tooth and gum infections. Some alcoholic patients aspirate while intoxicated, and the aspirated material drains into the most depending portions of the airways. Other pulmonary abscesses result from necrotizing pneumonias usually in the basal parts of the lower lobes. Less frequently diagnosed are cavitating carcinomas, which are mostly seen on the upper lobes and obviously have a different clinical presentation. On tomography or CT scans necrotizing carcinomas have a thick, irregular wall. A diagnostic biopsy can be provided by bronchoscopy.

The conservative treatment for abscesses of infectious origin consists in physiotherapy, postural drainage, and broad-spectrum antibiotics. Frequently postaspiration abscesses have a mixed flora including anaerobes. Bronchoscopy is indicated for diagnostic and therapeutic reasons. Sometimes an obstructing foreign body is found that if not removed continues to block drainage of purulent material. Percutaneous drainage of lung abscesses, as described by Monaldi, once abandoned, is again a first-line treatment. When adhesions do not exist between the two pleural layers, the lung may collapse when punctured for drainage, resulting in soiling of the pleural space and giving rise to an empyema. This complication is also possible without the use of the aspirating needle or catheter, as abscesses frequently rupture into the pleural space. A more common complication is soiling of the lung due to drainage of the contents of the abscess into the bronchial tree spilling into other areas including the contralateral lung.

If the abscess is 6 cm or larger and does not respond to conservative treatment, resection is indicated. Preoperatively its contents are emptied percutaneously if possible. A double-lumen endotracheal tube is used by the anesthesiologist to prevent soiling of the dependent lung when the patient is placed in the lateral decubitus position for thoracotomy.

Empyema

Empyema is present when there is pus in the pleural space. It occurs in a number of situations. It may follow an episode of pneumonia, be secondary to a ruptured lung abscess, or result from penetrating trauma produced by stab wounds or gunshot wounds. An infected hemothorax can also be the source of an empyema.

The initial empyema fluid is thin, and there are no adhesions between the two pleural surfaces. At this stage, when it is still uncomplicated, simple chest tube drainage is often all that is needed for treatment. Later, adhesions form and large amounts of fibrin are deposited on the lung surface, preventing reexpansion. The lung becomes immobilized by this fibrinous casing and is virtually trapped, unable to distend when the chest wall expands during inspiration. Treatment with chest tube drainage is then insufficient. At this stage decortication is necessary to free the contracted lung trapped under the fibrinous layer.

If the patient tolerates the lesser lung volume available for gas exchange and there are contraindications for a thoracotomy, an alternative treatment is open drainage, as described by Eloesser. An Eloesser flap requires resection of one or two lower rib segments, followed by suturing a flap of skin based on the upper side of the incision to the parietal pleura. This procedure creates a skin valve that permits the release of purulent material from inside the pleural space. Antibiotics are given according to the results obtained from cultures of the empyema.

In the operated patient, postpneumonectomy empyema can result from a bronchopleural fistula following disruption of the bronchial closure. Muscle-containing pedicle flaps using the intercostals or pectoralis are options for reclosure of the bronchus. Rarely, thoracoplasty is required as a space-reducing procedure for treatment of this surgical complication.

Pulmonary Sequestration

Pulmonary sequestration is a congenital malformation in which the sequestered part of the lung receives its blood supply through an anomalous branch of the aorta that frequently originates below the diaphragm. Sequestrations are located in the basal region of the right or left lower lobe. The artery supplying this anomalous part of the lung is located in the inferior pulmonary ligament and may be of large caliber, making inadvertent injury difficult to repair.

Two types of sequestration are found: The extralobar form is covered by its own visceral pleura and does not communicate with the air spaces in the lung. The intralobar form is not separated and communicates freely with the air spaces in the lung. It does not have a separate visceral pleura layer. Because of this communication with pulmonary air spaces intralobar sequestrations can become infected and develop a clinical picture identical to that of a lung abscess.

The clue to the diagnosis of this entity is the low position of the abscess in the lung, different from other lung abscesses, which are usually in the superior segments of the lower lobes. An aortogram is indicated when a basal segment abscess suggests the possibility of intralobar sequestration. Treatment consists in removing the accessory lung tissue after ligating the arterial branch coming from the aorta.

QUESTIONS

Select one answer.

1. Which predicted FEV_1 value contraindicates pulmonary resection?
   a. Above 0.8 L.
   b. Below 0.8 L.
   c. Above 1.2 L.
   d. Below 1.2 L.
2. Seven days after insertion of a chest tube for a spontaneous pneumothorax several attempts to reposition the chest tube did not decrease the air leak. What is the next step?
   a. Insert a new chest tube.
   b. Reposition the chest tube.
   c. Chemical pleurodesis.
   d. Surgically close the air leak plus pleurodesis.
3. The initial workup of a newly found lung mass in a 30-year-old man does not include:
   a. Sputum cytology.
   b. Bronchoscopy.
   c. Review of old films.
   d. Open lung biopsy.
4. A 50-year-old female cigarette smoker was found to have a 3-cm lung mass not present 1 year before. Cytology and bronchoscopy were negative. The next step should be:
   a. Radiotherapy alone.
   b. Radiotherapy and chemotherapy.
   c. Open lung biopsy.
   d. Follow-up after 3 months.
5. A lung abscess measuring 4 cm in the superior segment of the right lower lobe is best treated with:
   a. Antibiotics and physiotherapy.
   b. Percutaneous drainage.
   c. Resection.
   d. Chest tube drainage.
6. A postpneumonic empyema is best treated with:
   a. Antibiotics and physiotherapy.
   b. Chest tube drainage and antibiotics.
   c. Decortication if more than 7 days old.
   d. Thoracentesis and pleural injection of streptokinase.
7. Oat cell carcinoma is different from other bronchogenic carcinomas in that:
   a. It is always incurable.
   b. It is not seen in female subjects.
   c. It is systemic in early stages.
   d. It is not responsive to chemotherapy.
8. The presence of a thymoma:
   a. Is always associated with myasthenia gravis.
   b. Is never associated with myasthenia gravis.
   c. Is enough indication for resection.
   d. Can be diagnosed by radiographic appearance only.
9. Treatment of an apical tumor with Horner's syndrome is:
   a. Radiotherapy.
   b. Surgery.
   c. Radiotherapy followed by surgery.
   d. Radiotherapy and chemotherapy.
10. The initial treatment for a patient with multiple bilateral rib fractures and flail chest with CO_2 retention is:
    a. Surgical fixation of ribs.
    b. Chest wall immobilization with sand bags.
    c. Endotracheal intubation and positive-pressure ventilation.
    d. Intercostal nerve blocks.

SELECTED REFERENCES

Ferguson MK. Techniques of mediastinal surgery. *Chest Surg Clin N Am* February 1996.
Ginsberg RJ, Faber LP. Current perspectives in thoracic oncology. *Chest Surg Clin N Am* February 1994.
Glenn's thoracic and cardiovascular surgery, 6th ed. Stamford, CT: Appleton & Lange, 1996.

21

Cardiac Surgery

Michael H. Hall and Sheel K. Vatsia

CARDIAC CATHETERIZATION

The development of cardiac surgery has been intimately linked with developments in the cardiac catheterization laboratory. Diagnosis and treatment of cardiac disease have evolved from simple intracardiac pressure measurements to contrast studies of the coronary circulation to catheter intervention treatments such as angioplasty, atherectomy, stenting, and catheter ablation of life-threatening arrhythmias.

Cardiac catheterization is indicated to:

1. Provide information needed to allow decision making concerning therapeutic options for patients (e.g., one with progressive angina)
2. Help plan the operative approach when surgery is clinically indicated
3. Provide a definitive diagnosis when noninvasive techniques are inconclusive
4. Evaluate recurrent symptoms after previous surgery or other intervention
5. Provide a primary therapeutic intervention (e.g., balloon angioplasty of a crititical proximal lesion of the left anterior descending coronary artery)
6. Monitor hemodynamics via right heart catheterization with a Swan-Ganz catheter in the operating room (OR) or intensive care unit (ICU) to allow constant monitoring of cardiac function (e.g., cardiac

output, intracardiac pressures, and mixed venous oxygen as well as provide a means of access for cardiac pacing if needed)
7. Provide electrophysiologic data to assess the need for or efficacy of drug therapy, permanent pacemaker (PPM), or automatic implantable cardioverter-defibrillator (AICD) device for treatment of arrhythmias

Diagnostic information includes hemodynamic data concerning pressure measurements and cardiac output measurement, estimation of left ventricular (LV) function by contrast ventriculography (ejection fraction), detection and quantification of shunts and valve stenosis, and delineation of the coronary circulation.

Hemodynamics

Normal ranges for intracardiac and associated intravascular pressures are shown in Table 21.1. Pressure data are particularly useful when using the Swan-Ganz catheter as a diagnostic and therapeutic tool in the OR and ICU. Low right atrial (RA) and pulmonary artery wedge (PAW) pressures indicate volume depletion or hypovolemia. During the development of LV failure the PAW pressure may rise acutely with a low RA pressure [central venous pressure (CVP)]; thus the RA pressure is not sufficient information in such patients. An elevated right ventricular (RV) pressure is usually related

TABLE 21.1. *Normal adult hemodynamic values*

Site	Systolic (mm Hg)	Diastolic (mm Hg)	Mean (mm Hg)
Right atrium (RA)	—	—	0–8
Right ventricle (RV)	15–30	0–8	—
Pulmonary artery (PA)	15–30	5–15	10–18
Pulmonary artery wedge (PAW)	—	—	1–12
Left ventricle (LV)	90–140	2–12	—
Aorta (Ao)	90–140	60–90	70–105
AV O$_2$ difference		3–5.5 vol%	
%0$_2$ sat-venous (RA, RV, PA)		65–80%	
%0$_2$ sat-arterial (LA, LV, AO)		95–100%	
Cardiac output		3.5–8.5 L/min	
Cardiac index		2.5–4.5 L/min/m^2	

Source: Adapted from Mark (31).

to pulmonary hypertension, although in a child it may be caused by pulmonic valvular stenosis. RV failure is usually associated with an elevated RV end-diastolic pressure (EDP). Elevation and equalization of RA pressure, right ventricular end-diastolic pressure (RVEDP), PAW pressure, and left ventricular end-diastolic pressure (LVEDP) may be seen with cardiac tamponade or constrictive pericarditis. In the absence of increased pulmonary vascular resistance the pulmonary artery diastolic (PAD) pressure is roughly equal to the PAW pressure, which is equal to the left atrial (LA) mean pressure.

In the absence of mitral stenosis, LA mean pressure is approximately the same as the LVEDP. Increased PAW or LA mean pressures is seen with LV failure, mitral valve disease, hypertrophic cardiomyopathy, aortic valve disease, or pericardial constriction or tamponade. Mitral regurgitation may be associated with a late systolic V wave in the PAW tracing.

Cardiac output (CO) refers to the volume of blood ejected from either ventricle over a period of time. In the absence of significant shunting, the output of the two ventricles must be equal. Measurements in the catheterization laboratory include the Fick method, indicator-dilution method, and angiographic method. The most practical technique used in the OR and ICU is the thermodilution technique used in conjunction with a thermistor-tip Swan-Ganz catheter and a computer that integrates the area under the thermodilution curve and calculates CO. Adequate CO is based on body size. Minimal normal cardiac index (CI) = CO/body surface area (BSA) = 2.5 L/min/m^2. This number is a common goal of therapeutic hemodynamic interventions.

Intracardiac shunts are most commonly detected by oxygen analysis or indicator-dilution techniques. Shunts may be left to right, right to left, or bidirectional. They may be located at different levels in the heart depending on the anomaly present, and they must be quantified, usually by comparing pulmonary to systemic blood flow. A left-to-right shunt is characterized by mixing of saturated arterial and desaturated venous blood on the right side of the circulation, which produces an oxygen step-up and increased pulmonary blood flow. Examples include atrial septal defect (ASD), ventricular septal defect (VSD), or patent ductus arteriosus (PDA). A right-to-left shunt involves mixing of desaturated venous blood with saturated arterial blood on the left side of the circulation, producing a decrease in pulmonary blood flow and a decrease in systemic oxygen saturation. The presence of 5 g or more of desaturated hemoglobin results in visible cyanosis. Examples include tetralogy of Fallot or a large VSD with severe pulmonary hypertension and reversal of shunt flow (Eisenmenger syndrome).

Pulmonary vascular resistance (PVR) is useful for determining the operability of certain congenital lesions. When PVR increases to more than 10 Wood units (multiply by 80 to convert to dyne/sec/cm^{-5}) because of increased pulmonary blood flow, it implies that irreversible pulmonary hypertension has developed that cannot be helped by surgical correction of the anomaly involved.

Manipulation of the systemic vascular resistance (SVR) is an important adjunct to therapeutic use of right heart catheterization in the ICU and OR. Because pressure = flow × resistance, one may improve flow

TABLE 21.2. *Adult valve gradients and areas*

Parameter	Normal	Surgery indicated
Gradient (mm Hg)		
Aortic	None	>50
Mitral	None	>15
Area (cm²)		
Aortic	2–3	<1
Mitral	4–6	<1.5

(CO), for instance, by decreasing resistance in a hypertensive patient with a vasodilator drug such as sodium nitroprusside. Conversely, raising pressure with a vasoconstrictor may reduce flow (CO), which may be harmful to renal and other organ perfusion.

Determination of valvular stenosis is based on measurements of pressure and flow across the valve. The valve orifice can be calculated from this information (Table 21.2).

The left ventriculogram is used to estimate the ejection fraction (EF). The end-diastolic volume (EDV) and end-systolic volume (ESV) are determined from the ventriculogram, and EF = (EDV - ESV)/ EDV. The normal range of EF is from 0.50 to 0.75. Although EF is sensitive to changes in volume loading, it has been useful clinically and remains the most important prognostic indicator for chronic coronary disease.

Angiographic assessment of the severity of valvular regurgitation is important when determining optimal timing for valve surgery. Subjective grading is done on a scale of 1 to 4 (Table 21.3).

Coronary angiography provides the basis for coronary risk assessment and interventions such as angioplasty and coronary bypass surgery (Fig. 21.1). Sones and colleagues performed the first selective coronary angiograms in 1958.

The left main coronary artery originates from the left sinus of Valsalva and passes posteriorly between the pulmonary artery and left atrial appendage, where it divides into the left anterior descending (LAD) and the circumflex (CFX) coronary arteries. The LAD continues down the anterior wall along the interventricular septum to the apex of the left ventricle. It has two types of branches: septal branches, which supply the anterior two-thirds of the interventricular septum, and diagonals, which supply the anterolateral free wall of the left ventricle. The CFX runs posteriorly in the atrioventricular (AV) groove, and its branches are called marginals. In about 10% of patients it ends in a posterior descending artery, which supplies the posterior one-third of the interventricular septum and the AV node. This situation is termed a circumflex dominant circulation.

The right coronary arises from the right sinus of Valsalva (the most anterior sinus) and passes along the AV groove between the right atrium and right ventricle. It provides blood supply to the right ventricle and in 85% of patients ends in the posterior descending artery, which supplies the posterior one-third of the inverventricular septum and the AV node. This pattern is termed a right dominant circulation.

A balanced pattern is one in which both the CFX and RCA supply posterior descending branches that supply the posterior septum and AV node. It occurs in about 5% of patients.

Coronary Atherosclerosis and Spasm

The distribution of atheromata in the coronaries is variable, but proximal disease is often worse than distal

TABLE 21.3. *Angiographic evaluation of valvular regurgitation*

Grade	Aortic	Mitral
1+	Small jet of contrast clears with each beat	Small jet of contrast clears with each beat
2+	Contrast fills LV but less dense than Ao, incompletely clears with each beat	Contrast fills LA but less than LV, incompletely clears with each beat
3+	Persistent filling of LV, equal to Ao after several beats	Persistent filling of LA, equal to LV after several beats
4+	Persistent marked filling of LV, density of LV greater than Ao after several beats	Persistent marked filling of LA, greater than LV after several beats with reflux into pulmonary veins

Source: Adapted from Mark (31).
LV, left ventricle; Ao, aorta; LA, left atrium.

CABG indication
① main
3 vessel Δ
2 vessel c̄ symptoms
on med Rx

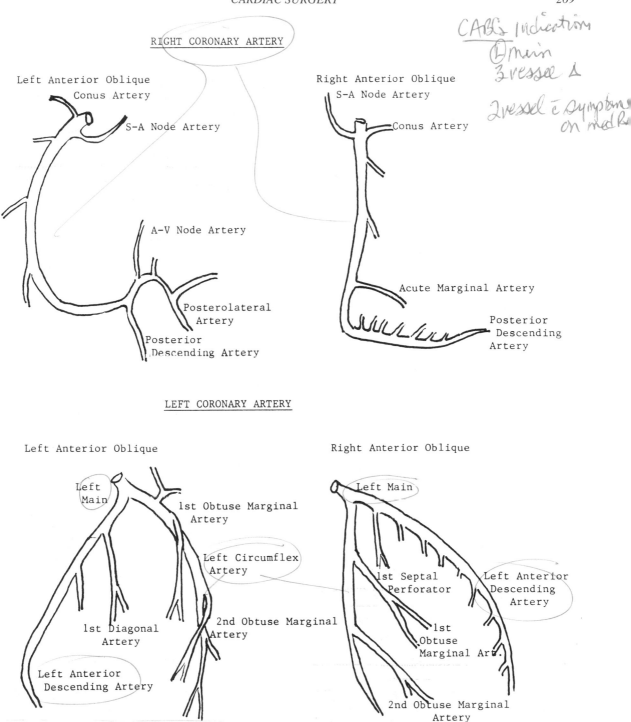

FIG. 21.1. Coronary anatomy.

disease, lesions tend to occur at bifurcations, and lesions are usually seen in epicardial locations, sparing intramyocardial portions of the coronary arteries. Multiple views are obtained because plaques may be eccentric or there may be overlapping of vessels in any one view. A 75% diameter obstruction (which equals a 90% area reduction) is considered significant. A 50% diameter obstruction of the left main artery (75% area reduction) is considered surgically significant because of the poor prognosis of medically treated left main artery disease.

In 1959 Prinzmetal and colleagues described a group of patients with rest angina (nonexertional) who had transient ST segment elevation on electrocardiography (ECG) with no subsequent evidence of myocardial infarction. A small group of patients may have coronary spasm that may or may not be associated with coronary atherosclerosis. It may be demonstrated in the catheterization laboratory by challenge with ergonovine maleate.

CARDIOPULMONARY BYPASS

The first successful open heart operation with an experimental cardiopulmonary bypass machine was performed in 1953 by John Gibbon at Jefferson Medical School in Philadelphia. This successful repair of a secundum ASD in a young woman led to a revolution in the treatment of cardiac disease. The significance of this event over the past 45 years is comparable to the effect of the first successful flight of the Wright brothers on the development of aviation.

The basic components include a venous reservoir that provides storage for blood from the right atrium, which is usually drained by gravity. An oxygenator, preferably membrane, provides oxygenation of the patient's blood and eliminates carbon dioxide. An efficient heat exchanger is used to cool or warm the blood during bypass. The arterial pump may be a roller or centrifugal pump and returns oxygenated blood to the ascending aorta most commonly or the femoral artery in some cases, such as for repair of aortic dissection or aneurysm of the ascending aorta, arch, or descending aorta.

Suction devices return blood to the venous reservoir. In addition, cell-saver devices are commonly used to salvage and concentrate red blood cells from the patient before, during, and after cardiopulmonary bypass to minimize the need for exogenous blood transfusions.

Myocardial protection during cardiac surgery is most commonly obtained by perfusing the coronaries with a hypothermic/hyperkalemic solution, either blood or crystalloid. Although crystalloid is acceptable for most routine situations, considerably more myocardial edema occurs with aortic cross-clamp times of more than 1 hour. Blood cardioplegia provides superior protection for up to 3 hours of aortic cross-clamp time. Cardioplegia may be delivered into the aortic root, directly into the coronary ostia, or into the coronary sinus in a retrograde fashion, or by a combination of the above. Retrograde cardioplegia is particularly effective in improving the distribution to the left ventricle in patients with severe coronary artery obstruction.

CONGENITAL HEART DISEASE

In utero, fetal pulmonary vascular resistance is high, causing blood to shunt right to left through the patent foramen ovale and also from the pulmonary artery into the descending thoracic aorta via the PDA. After birth, pulmonary vascular resistance falls with the initiation of ventilation. By 24 hours the mean pulmonary artery pressure may fall to one-half the systemic pressure. A progressive decrease results in adult levels being reached within 2 to 6 weeks (20). Persistent pulmonary hypertension (persistent fetal circulation) in the newborn may be caused by underdevelopment of the lung and pulmonary bed, perinatal stress such as hemorrhage, hypoglycemia, aspiration, or hypoxia; or it may occur for as yet unknown reasons (38). The pulmonary hypertension that results or that related to congenital heart disease and high-flow systemic-to-pulmonary artery shunting is an important clinical problem. Presently, this is being effectively dealt with by use of inhaled nitric oxide.

Classification of congenital heart disease (CHD) for purposes of this review is based on the clinical features of cyanosis and the appearance on the chest radiograph. Cyanosis is more difficult to assess in neonates than in infants and children, but measurement of arterial Po_2 and hemoglobin and hematocrit values can clarify most problems. It must be remembered that cyanosis can also be caused by noncardiac causes, such as decreased peripheral perfusion or pulmonary conditions such as pneumonia or atelectasis. Four groups exist hemodynamically when the presence or absence of cyanosis is combined with the appearance of the pulmonary vasculature (Fig. 21.2).

Acyanotic with Increased Pulmonary Blood Flow

A combination of the absence of cyanosis and increased pulmonary blood flow indicates a left-to-right shunt. The shunt may occur at the ventricular, great vessel, or atrial level. These anomalies account for about 40% of those diagnosed during the first year of life. These conditions may cause congestive heart failure, failure to thrive, frequent respiratory infections, and ultimately irreversible pulmonary hypertension and death. The goal of surgical therapy is to repair defects with a 2:1 or more left-to-right shunt prior to irreversible changes in the pulmonary vasculature leading to pulmonary hypertension and ultimately to a reversed shunt or Eisenmenger syndrome.

Ventricular Septal Defect

Small VSDs may close spontaneously by the first or second year of life. If the size of the VSD is larger than 80% of the aortic root diameter, there are equal pressures in both ventricles. Isolated VSD is the most common congenital cardiac anomaly and occurs at a rate of 2 : 1,000 live births.

As neonatal pulmonary vascular resistance normally falls, those with a large VSD develop congestive heart failure by the time the shunt reaches 3 : 1 pulmonary/systemic flow. With isolated VSDs this rarely occurs before 6 weeks of age.

Infants with large VSDs and severe, intractable heart failure or respiratory symptoms during the first 3

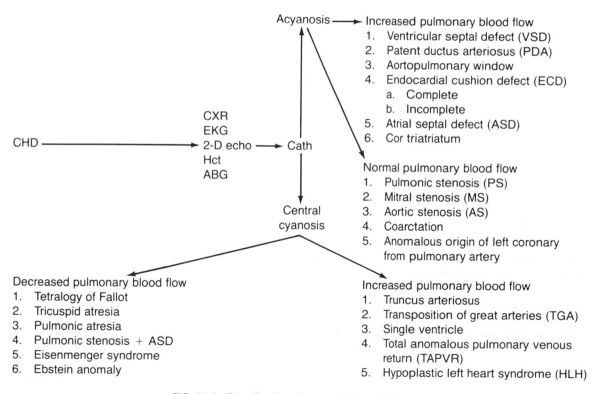

FIG. 21.2. Classification of congenital heart disease.

months should undergo operative repair. Older infants with large VSDs may have repair delayed until 1 year of age if pulmonary vascular resistance is low (less than 4 U/m²), but there is no decrease in operative risk between 6 months and 1 year (24). Generally if pulmonary vascular resistance is elevated but within operable range (5 to 10 U/m²), operation should be done promptly.

Patent Ductus Arteriosus

Patent ductus arteriosus (PDA), a patent communication usually between the descending thoracic aorta and the proximal left pulmonary artery, is the result of a persistently patent fetal ductus. As with large VSDs, large PDAs may result in congestive failure by the fourth to sixth week of life, and by age 2 years irreversible increased pulmonary vascular resistance may be present. During the first month of life, surgical closure is indicated only for heart failure. Otherwise closure can be delayed until 6 months of age. Even small PDAs should be closed to avoid the risk of eventual bacterial endocarditis. Premature infants should have medical therapy, including fluid restriction and indomethacin prior to surgical therapy. Indomethacin works by inhibiting prostaglandin synthesis, and it has been successful in as many as 95% of premature infants.

Closure of PDA in neonates generally is by ligation with heavy suture or hemoclip rather than by division. For infants and older children division is preferred. PDA closure in adults who have developed extensive aortic calcification may require cardiopulmonary bypass and patch closure of the pulmonary end. Closure of the PDA is contraindicated where pulmonary blood flow is dependent on the ductus, as in tricuspid or pulmonary atresia, unless a concomitant shunt is performed.

Presently, PDA closure in patients whose weight is over 5 to 10 kg is being done by coil occlusion and catheter-based technologies in the cardiac catheterization suite. Many PDAs can now be occluded by this methodology. Another innovation is that of minimally invasive video-assisted thoracoscopic surgery. PDAs can be successfully clipped utilizing this technology, but it has been done reliably and in large numbers by only a few surgeons.

Aortopulmonary Window

Aortopulmonary (AP) window, a rare anomaly, involves a large communication between the ascending aorta and main pulmonary artery. A patent ductus may coexist. Operation to repair the AP window is performed through the aortic root because of close proximity to the left coronary ostium.

Endocardial Cushion Defect (Partial or Complete AV Canal)

Endocardial cushion defect (ECD) represents a spectrum of anomalies caused by maldevelopment of structures formed by endocardial cushion tissue, namely, the lower portion of the atrial septum, posteriosuperior portion of the ventricular septum, and septal leaflets of the tricuspid and mitral valves. The more appropriate, and perhaps more contemporary nomenclature, is therefore AV septal defect.

Each of these four structures may be involved alone or in combination. The term partial AV canal has been applied to the ECD with only an atrial left-to-right shunt, also called an ostium primum ASD. This defect involves the lower portion of the atrial septum and commonly is associated with a cleft anterior mitral leaflet with or without mitral regurgitation. Complete AV canal defects involve VSDs and ASDs as well as mitral and triscuspid valve abnormalities. Characteristically, the ECG shows left axis deviation in all of these defects.

Many infants with ECD develop congestive heart failure during the first year of life. At least 50% of patients with complete AV canal die during the first year of life. Complete AV canal is a common cardiac anomaly in children with Down syndrome. Indications for surgery in partial AV canal defects, where pulmonary hypertension is usually absent, are similar to those for any ASD between age 1 and 2 years. When congestive heart failure or severe growth failure occurs earlier in life, repair is indicated at that time. For complete AV canal defects, operation should be done during the first year of life. If an infant with complete AV canal remains well controlled medically, the repair can be done electively by 6 months of age. If congestive failure or failure to thrive supervenes, repair should be done earlier.

Atrial Septal Defects

Atrial septal defects account for 10% to 15% of patients with congenital heart disease. The most common ASD is the fossa ovalis type (or ostium secundum). The ostium primum type was discussed under ECD. The sinus venosus defect is located high in the atrial septum and is almost always associated with partial anomalous pulmonary venous return (PAPVR), usually from the right upper lobe of the lung to the SVC or SVC–RA junction. PAPVR may be found in about 10% of other ASD cases, however. Surgery is indicated when the left-to-right shunt is 1.5 : 1.0 or greater. Usually surgery is planned prior to starting school (by age 5). Age is not a contraindication, but with increasing age the PVR becomes elevated. Premature death with congestive heart failure occurs increasingly after the fifth decade of life. It is rare to see a significant increase in PVR (>4 U/m^2) before age 20 years except when patients reside at high altitudes. The presence of an interatrial communication also exposes one to the small but persistent risk of paradoxical embolism or bacterial endocarditis.

There has been much work with catheter-based technology for occlusion of relatively smaller ostium secundum defects. Soon many of these defects may be routinely closed in the cardiac catheterization suite. New and evolving minimally invasive techniques are being utilized in addition to standard median sternotomy and right thoracotomy approaches, including mini-sternotomy and video-assisted thoracoscopic closure.

Cor Triatriatum

Cor triatriatum is a rare anomaly in which the pulmonary veins enter a common pulmonary venous chamber that is separated from the true left atrium by a restrictive diaphragm. In about 70% of cases a patent foramen ovale or an ASD opens into the pulmonary venous chamber, which results in a left-to-right shunt. The natural history of this lesion depends on the degree of restriction to flow through the membrane separating the pulmonary venous chamber from the left atrium. About 75% of patients die during infancy, so an operation to relieve the obstruction is urgently indicated once the diagnosis is confirmed.

Normal Pulmonary Blood Flow and No Cyanosis

Some patients with normal pulmonary blood flow and no cyanosis still have conditions that cause obstruction to the right or left ventricular outflow. Such conditions include an isolated pulmonary valve stenosis (including infundibular stenosis), mitral stenosis, aortic stenosis,

and coarctation of the aorta. An anomalous coronary artery may cause ischemic LV cardiomyopathy.

Pulmonic Stenosis

In neonates, critical pulmonary stenosis (PS) is usually associated with an enlarged patent foramen ovale resulting in right-to-left shunting and cyanosis (discussed later). After the first year of life the infant may present with dyspnea on exertion and a murmur indicative of PS. Long-neglected PS may result in RV failure, hepatomegaly, and ascites. Sudden death may occur in children and young adults with severe PS, usually with 50 mm Hg or more gradient across the pulmonary valve and severe RV enlargement.

Treatment may involve valvotomy, infundibular resection, or transannular patching in cases with annular hypoplasia. Percutaneous balloon pulmonary valvuloplasty is more frequently being utilized with good immediate relief of obstruction, although long-term efficacy compared to surgical valvotomy remains to be assessed.

Congenital Mitral Stenosis

Isolated congenital mitral disease is rare (less than 0.5% clinical CHD cases). Congenital stenosis may involve any component of the valve apparatus. A supravalvar ring of tough fibrous tissue may be present on the left atrial side of the mitral valve. Usually it coexists with other mitral valve anomalies and may be associated with LV outflow obstruction. The mitral annulus uncommonly is small or atretic but usually in association with severe LV hypoplasia or "single ventricle." There may be a single large papillary muscle with shortened, thickened chordae that restrict the primary valve opening (parachute mitral valve), or the commissures may be absent with leaflet tissue taking the form of an inverted cone, with further obstruction caused by short, thick chordae and abnormal, hypertrophied papillary muscles (hammock valve).

Operation is indicated for severe signs and symptoms of pulmonary venous hypertension. A reparative operation is indicated when feasible. When valve replacement is necessary in infants, children, and young adults, a porcine bioprosthesis is contraindicated because of rapid degeneration when placed in this age group. A St.

Jude valve is the valve of choice universally for this age group.

Congenital Aortic Valve Stenosis

Severe obstruction caused by maldevelopment of cusps with thickened leaflets may result in severe heart failure in neonates. If abnormalities are not severe, symptoms may not develop until calcification occurs, commonly after the fourth decade of life. About 70% of these valves are bicuspid, almost 30% have three leaflets, and less than 1% have a unicusp configuration. In infants this may be associated with hypoplastic aortic annulus, hypoplastic left ventricle, coarctation of the aorta, PDA, and mitral valve disease. The latter is referred to as the Shone syndrome. Less commonly, aortic stenosis is subvalvar or supravalvar.

Treatment for neonatal critical aortic valvar stenosis is usually indicated on an emergency basis. During the first days of life, when the patient has severe metabolic acidosis on admission, prostaglandin E_1 (PGE_1)infusion is begun, which usually opens the ductus arteriosus and improves the systemic circulation, relieving the metabolic acidosis. Percutaneous balloon valvuloplasty is being utilized increasingly to relieve this obstruction. In neonates who are too small for catheter-based intervention or in whom it is unsuccessful, unavailable, or otherwise not appropriate, surgical valvotomy is done. Surgical valvotomy in neonates and infants may be done by closed transventricular valvotomy or more commonly by open valvotomy. It may be done with or without cardiopulmonary bypass.

In older children, the indications for valvotomy are a resting peak systolic gradient greater than 60 mm Hg, ECG changes at rest or after moderate exercise even in the asymptomatic patient, or the presence of any symptoms of aortic stenosis. Premature valvuloplasty or valvotomy for a mild to moderately stenotic valve should be avoided, as important regurgitation may result.

Aortic valve replacement can generally be deferred until later in childhood. It becomes necessary when percutaneous balloon valvuloplasty is unsuccessful or not appropriate. It is often required for important aortic valvar regurgitation secondary to valvuloplasty or valvotomy. In the pediatric age group there are special issues with regard to aortic valve replacement. First, the aortic annulus may be significantly smaller than any available valve prosthesis. Also the chosen prosthesis will almost certainly be "outgrown" with time, necessitating reoperation. Clearly there is significant risk of anticoagulation of a child with warfarin for a mechanical metal prosthesis. Porcine valves are generally not an option in children, as there is accelerated structural valve deterioration at this age. For these reasons, when aortic valve replacement is indicated in children it is best done by replacement with a pulmonary autograft or an aortic homograft/allograft. Homograft valves are not a permanent solution. They do not grow with the child and undergo structural valve deterioration with time. The younger and smaller the child, the sooner a replacement is needed. In an adult-size individual, freedom from reoperation at 20 years is about 20% with an aortic homograft. The use of one's own pulmonary valve (i.e., pulmonary autograft) for aortic valve replacement is named after the British surgeon Donald Ross: the Ross operation. Here it seems that the patient's own pulmonary valve grows with the child and conceivably lasts forever. The pulmonary valve must be replaced with a homograft, however, which may eventually require replacement. Freedom from reoperation at 20 years in the initial series was about 20%.

Coarctation of the Aorta

Coarctation of the aorta refers to obstructive narrowing of the proximal portion of the descending thoracic aorta at the site of the entrance of the ductus arteriosus. The cross-sectional area must be narrowed by at least 50% before a gradient is produced across the narrowing. Rarely, the stenosis is "preductal," which is associated with early death from heart failure if uncorrected. The coarctation in this case separates flow from the left ventricle to the head and arms from flow via the pulmonary artery and a large PDA to the lower body.

More commonly, a "postductal" narrowing is found. Severe coarctation results in proximal hypertension and congestive heart failure and may be recognized by absent or severely diminished lower-extremity pulses. A collateral circulation may develop with time, resulting in classic signs of "rib notching" as a result of enlarged intercostal artery collaterals, which are seen on chest radiographs by age 10 years. A bicuspid aortic valve has been reported to be present in 30% to 45%. Coarctation accounts for 5% to 8% of CHD. About 5% of infants develop intractable congestive heart failure within the first few weeks of life and require urgent surgery. Another 10% develop less severe congestive heart failure and require surgery during the first 6 months of life. The remaining 85% may live into late childhood or young adulthood. Operation is preferably performed at the time of diagnosis to avoid problems with persistent late hypertension. Surgical repair is most often by resection and end-to-end anastomosis. Subclavian-flap aortoplasty is another option, used more commonly with a hypoplastic aortic arch. Patch aortoplasty should be avoided owing to a high incidence of late aneurysms. Recoarctation occurs more commonly after repair in neonates and during early infancy. Recurrence rates in this group are as high as 10% to 25%.

There is increasing use of percutaneous balloon dilatation of coarctation in children weighing over 5–10 kg. Its use for primary coarctation is still considered investigational. Intermediate and long-term outcomes are unknown. The use of balloon dilatation for recoarctation, on the other hand, is becoming fairly well established. The use of intraluminal stents is also being explored for the problem of recoarctation.

Anomalous Origin of Left Coronary Artery from the Pulmonary Artery

Sometimes the left main coronary artery (LCA) arises from the proximal main pulmonary trunk, whereas normally the right coronary artery (RCA) arises from the aorta. Collaterals from the RCA feed the LCA, which drains into the pulmonary artery, creating a coronary arteriovenous (A-V) fistula. This condition is rare (about 0.25% of all CHD). About 65% of infants die within the first year of life from intractable heart failure related to anterolateral myocardial infarction, diffuse LV fibrosis, and usually associated with mitral valve regurgitation because of papillary muscle dysfunction or LV and mitral annular dilatation. If the patient survives the first year of life, it is usually because of extensive collaterals from the RCA. Adults with this anomaly may have angina or dyspnea on exertion, which may result in chronic congestive heart failure or sudden death. Theoretically, the creation of a two-coronary system is ideal and may be accomplished by a "tunnel" procedure using the pulmonary artery to create a channel from the aorta to the orifice of the anomalous left coronary or by reimplantation of the coronary ostium if it can be accomplished without tension or kink-

ing of the left coronary. In critically ill infants the operation of choice is controversial, and some have advocated simple ligation of the anomalous coronary close to the pulmonary artery. In adults, internal thoracic artery (ITA) grafting plus ligation is an acceptable alternative if the size of the ITA is adequate. In this case, probably separate grafts should be placed to the LAD and CFX coronaries to ensure adequate blood supply for the entire left coronary system. Mitral valve repair or replacement may be performed if indicated by the severity of mitral regurgitation. Direct coronary reimplantation is the favored technique. Due to the profound LV dysfunction that may be seen, LV assist devices or external corporeal membrane oxygenation (ECMO) have been found useful during the immediate postoperative recovery of some patients.

Cyanosis with Decreased Pulmonary Blood Flow

Cyanosis with decreased pulmonary blood flow is caused by obstruction to pulmonary blood flow associated with an intracardiac defect at either the atrial or the ventricular level. It creates a right-to-left shunt and subsequent systemic hypoxia.

Tetralogy of Fallot

The most common example of this group is tetralogy of Fallot. Other variants with ventricular septal communication include double-outlet right ventricle with pulmonary stenosis and complete transposition of the great vessels with VSD and pulmonary stenosis, among others.

Tetralogy of Fallot is characterized by underdevelopment of the RV infundibulum with anterior and leftward displacement of the infundibular septum (resulting in so-called dextroposition of the aorta), obstruction of the right ventricular outflow tract (RVOT), large malalignment-type VSD, and RV hypertrophy. The aorta overrides the right ventricle; and if the aorta arises more than 50% from the RV the condition may be termed a double-outlet right ventricle.

Cyanotic spells and failure to thrive are common problems with this anomaly. Progressive polycythemia may lead to pulmonary arterial and cerebral thrombosis. About 25% of unoperated infants die within the first year of life. The few who survive into the fourth and fifth decades may die from chronic congestive heart failure as a result of a secondary cardiomyopathy related to RV failure, chronic hypoxia, and polycythemia. The exact course in any given patient is determined primarily by the degree of RV outflow obstruction.

Palliative surgical treatment was first performed successfully by Blalock in 1945. It consisted of creation of a subclavian artery–pulmonary artery anastomosis (Blalock-Taussig shunt), which is performed on the right side when the arch is left-sided (75%) or the left side when the arch is right-sided. Alternatively a Gore-Tex interposition graft (modified Blalock-Taussig shunt) may be used and may be technically easier in small infants. It is the most commonly employed shunt. Other forms of shunting have been largely abandoned because of subsequent problems with complete repair as a result of distortion or narrowing of the pulmonary arteries, including the Waterston shunt between the ascending aorta and right pulmonary artery and the Potts shunt between the left pulmonary artery and descending thoracic aorta.

Primary repair is desirable if the pulmonary arteries are of acceptable size, although during the first 3 months of life the need for transannular pulmonary patching is high. Shunting has been documented to cause growth of small pulmonary arteries and may make complete repair possible. If a shunt is placed in the infant with tetralogy of Fallot, complete repair is usually performed by age 1 to 2 years, provided pulmonary artery size is adequate. Complete repair involves patch closure of the VSD and relief of RVOT obstruction by pulmonary valvotomy and infundibular resection of hypertrophied muscle. Transannular patching is reserved for those with a hypoplastic annulus and results in pulmonic valve incompetence, which is usually tolerated fairly well, although it may diminish exercise capacity later in life. Occasionally patients with transannular patches develop RV failure later in life. Pulmonary valve homograft placement is useful in the latter circumstance. It is also used in patients with anomalous coronary anatomy, most often when the LAD originates from the RCA. Tetralogy with absent pulmonary valve is repaired with use of a pulmonary homograft as well.

Tricuspid Atresia

Tricuspid atresia is characterized by failure of the right atrium to open into a ventricle through an AV valve. There is almost always a VSD and a hypoplastic right ventricle. The relation of the mitral valve to the left atrium and left ventricle is normal. Tricuspid atresia accounts for 1% to 3% of CHD. The natural history is determined by the severity of the obstruction to pulmonary blood flow. Patients with tricuspid atresia and normal origin of the great arteries normally have important RVOT obstruction and cyanosis at birth; 90% of these infants succumb within the first year of life. In newborns with severe RVOT obstruction, infusion of PGE_1 to maintain patency of the ductus arteriosus stabilizes the patient until a systemic–pulmonary artery shunt can be performed, usually by a Gore-Tex interposition graft between the subclavian and pulmonary arteries. Ultimately a right heart bypass or Fontan-type operation is done. After creation of a modified Blalock-Taussig shunt during the neonatal period, it is taken down at about 6 months of age. A bidirectional cavopulmonary anastomosis is then done, which diverts superior vena caval blood to both right and left pulmonary arteries. Then, by about 4 years of age or when oxygen saturation drops significantly, the inferior vena caval blood is diverted directly into the pulmonary artery. This is presently done most often by creating a lateral tunnel or an extracardiac conduit. This step is referred to as completion of the Fontan operation. It results in all the venous blood flowing directly into the pulmonary arteries. The flow of blood is in a single circuit, in series, having only one ventricle as the pump.

Pulmonic Atresia

Atresia of the pulmonic valve associated with intact ventricular septum presents during the first 24 to 48 hours of life with dyspnea, tachypnea, and cyanosis. Right-to-left shunting occurs through the patent foramen ovale. Pulmonary blood flow is dependent on the PDA, which closes soon after birth. Patency of the PDA with PGE_1 infusion stabilizes the patient for urgently needed surgery. The latter usually consists of a shunt procedure combined with pulmonic valvectomy and transannular patch. The hypoplastic right ventricle may grow after valvectomy and eventually support circulation. A normal biventricular circulation may result. If the right ventricle remains hypoplastic, a right-sided heart bypass (i.e., Fontan-type repair) is commenced.

Pulmonary atresia with VSD is an entirely different entity. The intracardiac anatomy and VSD are similar to tetralogy of Fallot. Variable pulmonary artery blood supply and pulmonary vascular resistance make complete repair challenging.

Eisenmenger Syndrome

Reversal of shunt flow from the left-to-right shunt seen with VSD or ASD may occur with long-standing severe pulmonary hypertension with permanently elevated pulmonary vascular resistance. High-flow systemic-to-pulmonary artery shunts of any kind may induce it. An irreversible histologic picture is seen on microscopic analysis of the lung. The shunt then becomes predominantly right to left, decreasing pulmonary blood flow and causing cyanosis, a contraindication to surgical repair.

Ebstein Anomaly

Ebstein anomaly, a rare tricuspid valve anomaly consists of malformation and downward displacement of the tricuspid valve. Usually a sail-like anterior leaflet is the only functional leaflet; the others are rudimentary. The abnormal chordae divide the RV cavity into an "atrialized" proximal portion, which may become aneurysmal, and a small inefficient distal pumping chamber. There is almost always an associated ASD, which leads to right-to-left shunting, cyanosis, and ultimately congestive heart failure. Polycythemia, arrhythmias, and paradoxical emboli are common clinical manifestations. Repair or replacement of the valve is indicated in symptomatic patients.

Cyanosis with Increased Pulmonary Blood Flow

Certain malformations have been termed "admixture lesions" because both left-to-right and right-to-left shunts are present. They include the following.

1. Truncus arteriosus
2. Transposition of the great arteries
3. Single ventricle
4. Total anomalous pulmonary venous return
5. Hypoplastic left heart syndrome

Congestive failure is common with these lesions because increased pulmonary blood flow leads to ventricular volume overload.

Truncus Arteriosus

Truncus arteriosus is a condition in which a single arterial vessel leaves the heart through a semilunar valve and supplies the systemic, pulmonary, and coronary arterial systems. This vessel overlies a large VSD and receives the entire cardiac output from both ventricles. The anomaly represents about 3% of CHD. Only about 50% of these infants survive beyond the first month of life. Pulmonary artery banding has been associated with high mortality. Ebert and colleagues have had improved success with closure of the VSD and use of a homograft to establish right ventricle–pulmonary artery continuity (14).

Transposition of the Great Arteries

Transposition of the great arteries (TGA) is the most common anomaly producing cyanosis in newborns and represents 8% of CHD. The lesion is characterized by normal venous connections, and the ventricles occupy normal positions; but the aorta arises anteriorly from the right ventricle and the pulmonary artery posteriorly from the left ventricle (D transposition). Successful physiologic correction with an intraatrial baffle was first reported by Mustard in 1964 (34). Senning's modifications allowed intraatrial diversion using atrial tissue instead of a separate baffle (41). Both procedures utilized the right ventricle as the systemic ventricle. Decreased RV ejection fraction with increased end-diastolic pressures during long-term follow-up, as well as occasional late problems with pulmonary or systemic venous obstruction, remain troublesome.

Increasing evidence suggests that the operation of choice is now the arterial switch procedure, which involves switching the great vessels to their normal positions with reimplantation of the coronary arteries. In patients with no VSD, this operation must be done within the first 4 weeks of life before the left ventricle loses its ability to pump in the higher-resistance systemic circuit. Mortality has been lowered to below 10% with this procedure, and midterm follow-up at 10 years has been generally superior to intraatrial repair.

Atrial balloon septostomy (Rashkind procedure) has been successful in stabilizing critically ill neonates prior to definitive surgery. Creation of a surgical atrial septectomy (Blalock-Hanlon procedure) is virtually obsolete.

Single Ventricle

"Single ventricle" represents a diverse group of cardiac malformations characterized by both AV valves or a common AV valve opening into the same ventricle. During the first few months of life pulmonary artery banding may be necessary if congestive failure cannot be controlled by medical therapy. A Fontan-type procedure, with right heart bypass, is possible for various types of single ventricle with low pulmonary resistance. It should usually be delayed if possible to age 2 to 4 years. A septation procedure may be feasible but usually should not be chosen when additional procedures such as AV valve replacement must be done. The Fontan-type procedure should not be chosen when pulmonary vascular resistance is elevated, right and left pulmonary arteries are small, or systolic function of the ventricle is poor.

Total Anomalous Pulmonary Venous Return

Total anomalous pulmonary venous return (TAPVR) is a malformation in which the pulmonary veins do not connect to the left atrium but, rather, to the right atrium or its tributaries. A patent foramen ovale or ASD is present in all neonates who survive beyond birth. In 45% of the cases the connection is supracardiac, usually to a left vertical vein draining into the left innominate vein or superior vena cava. The connection is cardiac in 25% of cases, usually to the coronary sinus. In another 25% the connection is infracardiac, usually into the portal vein, ductus venosus, or inferior vena cava. In 5% the lesion has mixed connections: commonly the left upper lobe drains to a left vertical vein, and the remaining lobes of both lungs drain to the coronary sinus. This anomaly occurs in 1.5% to 3.0% of CHD. Only 50% survive beyond 3 months of age and only about 20% beyond 1 year.

In infants with pulmonary venous obstruction who present during the first few weeks of life with tachypnea, cyanosis, and signs of low cardiac output, operation is urgent. Nonobstructed TAPVR may be managed initially by atrial balloon septostomy and decongestant therapy, but even then operation should be performed by no later than 3 months of age.

Hypoplastic Left Heart Syndrome

Hypoplastic left heart syndrome consists of atresia of the aortic valve and is usually associated with severe LV hypoplasia, intact ventricular septum, and mitral valve atresia or hypoplasia. Newborns with this anomaly usually are of normal size and weight but present with cyanosis, tachypnea, and tachycardia. Usually rapid deterioration occurs with congestive heart failure followed by death within the first few days of life. Two-dimensional echocardiography is diagnostic.

Initial management consists of PGE_1 infusion to maintain patency of the ductus arteriosus. Norwood designed a two-stage procedure to attempt to deal with this problem. Mortality has been high, particularly with the first stage, and efforts to improve the procedure and prognosis continue. Cardiac transplantation has been used to treat this anomaly, but the long-term outlook is unknown.

ACQUIRED HEART DISEASE

Functional classification is helpful when discussing adult cardiac symptoms. Two classification systems are commonly used. The New York Heart Association (NYHA) functional classification is a general subjective classification of symptoms (Table 21.4). The Canadian Cardiovascular Society (CCS) system is used to describe angina symptoms for patients specifically with coronary artery disease (Table 21.5).

Coronary Artery Disease

Coronary artery disease is the leading cause of death in the United States. More than twice as many people die from coronary disease as from all forms of cancer. Risk factors include diet, hypertension, diabetes, smoking cigarettes, lack of exercise, and heredity. Men are more apt to develop symptomatic disease at an earlier age than women until menopause, after which the incidence in women climbs to that in men.

Coronary atherosclerosis progresses from childhood. By 20 years of age, about half the hearts examined at autopsy show signs of atherosclerosis. Studies of the internal thoracic artery (ITA), which is uniquely resistant to atherosclerosis, suggest that deficiencies in the internal elastic lamina of many arteries allow ingrowth of smooth muscle cells, intimal thickening, and later deposition of lipoid material into the intima (42). Early signs of intimal thickening of coronary arteries have been found in about 8% of newborns. The ITA has a particularly completely developed internal elastic lamina,

TABLE 21.4. *New York Heart Association functional classification*

Class I	Patients have anatomic cardiac disease but no limitation of physical activity.
Class II	Patients with cardiac disease having slight limitation of physical activity. Ordinary physical activity causes fatigue, palpitations, dyspnea, or angina. No symptoms at rest.
Class III	Patients with cardiac disease having marked limitation of physical activity. Less than ordinary physical activity results in fatigue, palpitations, dyspnea, or angina. No symptoms at rest.
Class IV	Patients with cardiac disease who are unable to carry on any physical activity without discomfort. Symptoms of cardiac insufficiency or angina may be present even at rest. Any physical activity increases discomfort.

which appears to protect it from the development of atherosclerosis and makes it the ideal graft for coronary artery bypass (27).

The most severe atherosclerotic changes tend to occur in the proximal third or half of coronary arteries. Diffuse disease is often associated with hyperlipidemia and diabetes mellitus.

Clinical manifestations include angina pectoris, myocardial infarction, and sudden death from ventricular arrhythmias. Unfortunately, not all severe coronary disease is found in symptomatic patients. About half of fatal heart attacks are not preceded by symptoms of angina. Identification of asymptomatic patients at high risk for cardiac events is currently made possible by use of stress ECGs and thallium tests, stress echocardiography, and intravenous dipyridamole thallium-201 scintigraphy (DTS). The latter test is most useful for patients with peripheral vascular disease or who, for other reasons, cannot perform the exercise required by a standard stress test.

This ability to identify patients at high risk is particularly pertinent to the practice of surgery, as the leading cause of death after surgery and anesthesia is cardiac. It has been estimated that about 3 million of the 25 million who annually undergo surgical procedures are at risk for coronary disease, and about 2% to 15% of these patients have significant cardiac morbidity (29). Of all groups particularly prone to cardiac morbidity, the patients undergoing surgery for peripheral vascular disease are particularly at risk.

The magnitude of the problem of serious coronary disease in peripheral vascular patients was perhaps best defined by Hertzer, who reported in 1984 on 1,000 patients at the Cleveland Clinic who had undergone coronary angiography prior to peripheral vascular surgery (19). Severe correctable coronary artery disease was identified in 25% of the entire series, including 31% with abdominal aortic aneurysms (AAAs), 26% with cerebrovascular disease (CVD), and 21% who had lower extremity ischemia (LEI). An additional 5% of the series were thought to have severe inoperable coronary disease. Thus, almost one-third of the series had potentially fatal coronary artery disease.

Intravenous DTS appears to have the best sensitivity and specificity of the noninvasive screening tests (32,33). It is also the most practical for the peripheral vascular patients who cannot exercise under a standard treadmill protocol for vascular, orthopedic, neurologic, or other medical reasons. A negative DTS is associated with a low (4%) risk of perioperative cardiac events (unstable angina, myocardial infarction, or death). If positive, DTS should be followed by coronary angiography so appropriate therapy, whether medical or surgical, can be determined. A positive DTS usually means that a myocardial perfusion defect exists initially, but there is delayed reperfusion 4 hours later. However, McEnroe et al. (32) found that patients with a fixed thallium defect (thought by some to represent prior infarction with low risk) were found to have 46% of all the postoperative cardiac complications in a group of abdominal aortic

TABLE 21.5. *Canadian Cardiovascular Society functional classification*

Class I	Ordinary physical activity does not cause angina. Angina may occur with strenuous or prolonged exertion.
Class II	Slight limitation of ordinary activity. Angina may occur with walking or climbing stairs rapidly; walking uphill; walking or stair climbing after meals or in the cold, in the wind, or under emotional stress; walking more than two blocks on the level; climbing more than one flight of stairs under normal conditions at a normal pace.
Class III	Marked limitation of ordinary physical activity. Angina may occur after walking one or two blocks on level ground or climbing one flight of stairs under normal conditions at a normal pace.
Class IV	Inability to carry out any physical activity without anginal discomfort; angina may be present at rest.

aneurysm patients. Other investigators (15,46), using a more sensitive imaging method, single photon emission computed tomography (SPECT), have found late reversibility in 53% of patients undergoing exercise thallium-201 scintigraphy. This correlates with results of positive emission tomography (PET), in which viable myocardium has been detected in 47% of "fixed" defects on exercise thallium-201 scans (3). Leppo et al. (25) found a predictive probability of postoperative ischemic cardiac events when redistribution is seen on DTS is 33% ±7% by stepwise logistic regression analysis.

Clinical risk variables associated with higher risk of significant coronary disease include a history of angina, the presence of Q waves on the ECG, age over 70 years, ventricular ectopy requiring medical therapy, diabetes mellitus, and clinical evidence of LV failure (13). Patients with none of the clinical variables were found to have a 3% incidence of cardiac events versus a 50% incidence with three or more clinical risk variables. Use of DTS was most helpful with patients at intermediate risk, who had one or two clinical variables. Patients without redistribution on DTS had a low risk (3%), but the risk increased to 30% in patients with redistribution.

Guidelines for risk assessment are suggested in the flow sheet in Fig. 21.3 and were originally devised for patients with peripheral vascular disease. Other patients with any of the clinical risk variables mentioned may benefit from similar screening.

Indications for Revascularization

Guidelines for referring patients for coronary revascularization, whether by coronary bypass or balloon angioplasty, have been developed by a task force of the American College of Cardiology and American Heart Association (23). Generally revascularization is indicated because of intractable symptoms, to prevent myocardial damage in high-risk patients, or to prolong life.

Intractability is a subjective term and may relate to the inability of a patient to tolerate the side effects of medical therapy, which may include βblockers, calcium channel blockers, or nitrates. A patient with minimal symptoms who does not have evidence of life-threatening coronary disease and who has normal LV function may be treated medically until symptoms become unmanageable.

Patients with progressive or unstable symptoms despite maximum medical therapy frequently have significant amounts of myocardium at risk and are candidates for revascularization. Angioplasty is frequently chosen for single- or double-vessel disease because 20% to 30% of initially successful angioplasties result in restenosis within the first 6 to 12 months after the procedure (21). The use of stents has reduced restenosis to only 10% to 15% within the same time period. Potentially life-threatening anatomy includes more than 50% left main disease (especially dangerous if the RCA is closed), triple-vessel disease with more than 70% proximal obstruction of three main coronaries, or double-vessel disease that includes severe obstruction of the LAD proximal to the first septal perforator. This group also includes patients with postinfarction angina who are at great risk of infarct extension.

Life has been shown to be prolonged in patients who undergo surgery for significant (more than 50%) left main artery disease, severe triple-vessel disease, or double-vessel disease where the LAD has a severe (more than 70%) obstruction proximal to the first septal perforator. Survival is especially enhanced by surgery if the patient has CCS class III or IV angina (35). If there is LV dysfunction (ejection fraction over 0.20 but less than 0.50), life is prolonged after surgery for left main artery or severe triple-vessel disease.

The long-term benefits of coronary artery bypass graft (CABG) tend to decrease with time primarily because of the development of vein graft disease. At 10 years after CABG, only 50% to 60% of saphenous vein grafts remain patent. This poor record has prompted great interest in use of the ITA, which has more than 95% patency at 20 years post-CABG. Other arterial grafts, such as the right gastroepiploic artery and inferior epigastric artery free grafts, have been used, but their long-term fate is unknown. Although initial data appeared adequate to show that the radial artery is not an acceptable long-term graft substitute, the technique of radial artery harvest appears to be crucial to its long-term patency (16). Caution should be used when adopting the use of ITA substitutes, particularly when the LAD is grafted. Data indicate significant improvement in long-term survival and freedom from cardiac "events" when the LAD receives an ITA graft (27). Use of both ITAs may well improve survival and freedom from reoperation, but this judgment awaits long-term studies.

FIG. 21.3. Guidelines for cardiac risk assessment prior to peripheral vascular surgery. *AAA,* abdominal aortic aneurysm; *CVD,* cerebrovascular disease (e.g., carotid endarterectomy); *LEI,* lower extremity ischemia surgery. **A:** Evaluation and treatment of class III or IV patients. **B:** Evaluation of class I or II patients. **C:** Management of class I or II patients after coronary angiography.

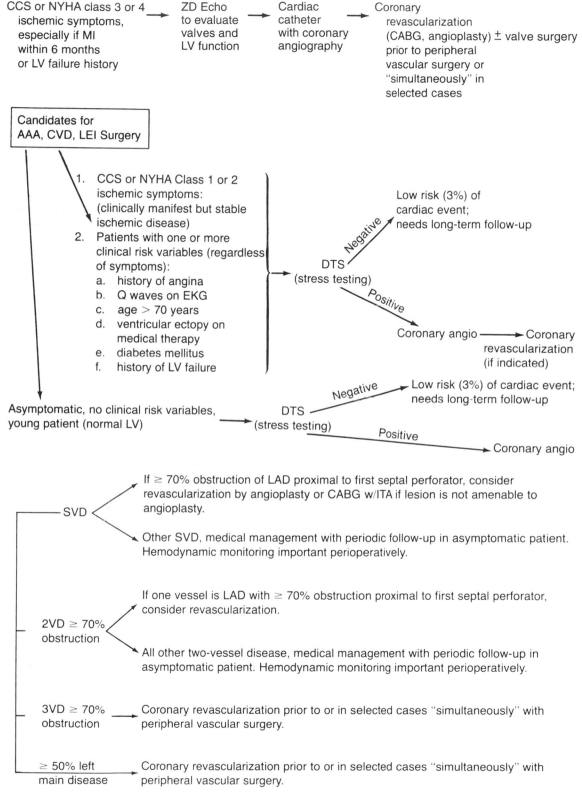

A

CCS or NYHA class 3 or 4 ischemic symptoms, especially if MI within 6 months or LV failure history → ZD Echo to evaluate valves and LV function → Cardiac catheter with coronary angiography → Coronary revascularization (CABG, angioplasty) ± valve surgery prior to peripheral vascular surgery or "simultaneously" in selected cases

B

Candidates for AAA, CVD, LEI Surgery

1. CCS or NYHA Class 1 or 2 ischemic symptoms: (clinically manifest but stable ischemic disease)
2. Patients with one or more clinical risk variables (regardless of symptoms):
   a. history of angina
   b. Q waves on EKG
   c. age > 70 years
   d. ventricular ectopy on medical therapy
   e. diabetes mellitus
   f. history of LV failure

DTS (stress testing)

Negative → Low risk (3%) of cardiac event; needs long-term follow-up

Positive → Coronary angio → Coronary revascularization (if indicated)

Asymptomatic, no clinical risk variables, young patient (normal LV) → DTS (stress testing)

Negative → Low risk (3%) of cardiac event; needs long-term follow-up

Positive → Coronary angio

C

SVD

If ≥ 70% obstruction of LAD proximal to first septal perforator, consider revascularization by angioplasty or CABG w/ITA if lesion is not amenable to angioplasty.

Other SVD, medical management with periodic follow-up in asymptomatic patient. Hemodynamic monitoring important perioperatively.

2VD ≥ 70% obstruction

If one vessel is LAD with ≥ 70% obstruction proximal to first septal perforator, consider revascularization.

All other two-vessel disease, medical management with periodic follow-up in asymptomatic patient. Hemodynamic monitoring important perioperatively.

3VD ≥ 70% obstruction → Coronary revascularization prior to or in selected cases "simultaneously" with peripheral vascular surgery.

≥ 50% left main disease → Coronary revascularization prior to or in selected cases "simultaneously" with peripheral vascular surgery.

Progression of disease in the native vessels is a factor in limiting the long-term benefit of CABG. This underscores the continued need for medical management postoperatively in terms of diet control, cholesterol-lowering medications when needed, exercise, avoidance of cigarette smoking, and control of hypertension.

Acute Evolving Myocardial Infarction

Emphasis has been placed on early reperfusion in acute evolving infarction within the first 3 to 6 hours after onset of infarction. Thrombolytic therapy is unsuccessful in about one-third of cases and is contraindicated in many patients because of previous bleeding or other medical problems.

If a 24-hour a day cardiac catheterization team is available, angioplasty of the infarct vessel is successful in about 95% of cases. Surgical intervention is generally reserved for patients with residual multivessel disease (2).

Surgical Complications of Myocardial Infarction

Acute mitral regurgitation, VSD, and LV aneurysm may be the result of myocardial infarction. Papillary muscle infarction or rupture may require mitral valve replacement. VSD usually results in a large left-to-right shunt and a rapidly deteriorating course without surgical therapy. LV aneurysms, a late development of myocardial infarction, are operated on for congestive heart failure, embolism, or recurrent ventricular tachyarrhythmias. Use of the intraaortic balloon pump (IABP) is frequently helpful for preoperative and postoperative stabilization.

Acquired Valve Disease

Aortic Stenosis

Etiology

Most commonly in the United States one finds degenerative calcification in the elderly in which the commissures do not become fused, but the leaflets calcify and become immobile. Acquired calcification of a congenitally deformed, usually bicuspid valve commonly occurs by the fourth or fifth decade of life. Rheumatic

fever during childhood may result in an ongoing process of fibrosis, commissural fusion, and calcification. Symptomatic aortic stenosis usually occurs long before irreversible LV damage occurs.

Symptoms and Indications for Surgery

The development of angina, syncope, or dyspnea on exertion or frank congestive heart failure are indications for surgery. Usually the aortic valve area is less than 1 cm^2 in the adult, and the gradient between the LV systolic pressure and systemic pressure is at least 50 mm Hg. The gradient may be less in patients with decreased cardiac output. Generally, even severe LV hypertrophy and elevated LVEDP improves or resolves after aortic valve replacement.

Aortic Insufficiency

Etiology

Aortic insufficiency is commonly caused by myxoid degeneration. It may be seen in younger patients with rheumatic valvulitis but is no longer common in the United States. Patients with annuloaortic ectasia from cystic medial necrosis, which may be a manifestation of Marfan syndrome, may develop significant aortic insufficiency. Similarly, ascending aortic aneurysmal disease caused by atherosclerosis or rarely syphilitic aortitis may result in annular dilatation and aortic insufficiency. Endocarditis is a common cause in the urban intravenous drug abuser. Blunt chest injury has been reported to cause traumatic aortic insufficiency.

Clinical Manifestations

Patients with severe aortic insufficiency may develop angina or congestive heart failure (or both). Angina develops because of decreasing diastolic pressure with increasing leakage of the aortic valve. Because about 80% of coronary blood flow occurs during diastole, this drop in diastolic pressure can significantly reduce coronary artery filling and thus myocardial blood flow. As the volume-overloaded ventricle dilates with increasing aortic insufficiency, the LV volume increases. LVEDP rises, and congestive heart failure ensues.

Surgical Indications

Patients with angina or congestive heart failure have clinical indications for aortic valve replacement: The problem that arises is that patients who have minimal symptoms may develop irreversible LV dysfunction prior to developing significant symptoms. Therefore valve replacement is recommended when there is a progressive increase in heart size or LV dimensions as determined by echocardiography. The finding of decreased LVEF or increased LVEDP at rest indicates the need for valve replacement in this group of patients.

Mitral Stenosis

Etiology

The most common cause of mitral stenosis (MS) remains rheumatic fever. A relation between an antecedent bout of group A streptococcal pharyngitis is usually documented. The exact mechanism is unclear, but patients who develop rheumatic fever tend to have strong antistreptolysin O (ASO) titers, and it is believed that rheumatic valve disease is in essence an acquired immune disease. Mitral stenosis may also be caused by degenerative calcification in the elderly, although it appears to be much less common than with aortic stenosis. Rare causes include malignant carcinoid, systemic lupus erythematosus, and rheumatoid arthritis.

Clinical Manifestations

Although it takes at least 2 years after rheumatic fever for severe MS to develop, it is much more common for an asymptomatic latent period of at least two decades to pass. The most prominent symptom is dyspnea, which initially occurs with exertion and then progresses to occur at rest, often at night when lying flat (orthopnea). Awaking at night from sleep because of severe shortness of breath is termed paroxysmal nocturnal dyspnea (PND). These symptoms are caused by severe elevation of pulmonary venous pressure which is exacerbated by lying flat. Pulmonary hypertension develops from a reactive elevation in pulmonary vascular resistance, which may reach systemic pressures and may become irreversible. In severe cases, RV enlargement and eventually failure results, with subsequent tricuspid annular dilatation and insufficiency. This state is followed by peripheral edema, pulsatile hepatic enlargement and ascites, and eventually cardiac cirrhosis, anasarca, and renal failure. Development of atrial fibrillation and possible systemic embolization are further dangers of MS.

Indications for Surgery

The normal mitral valve area is 4 to 6 cm² in the adult. Patients with valve area of 1.5 to 2.0 cm² have mild stenosis with minimal symptoms. An area of 0.5 to 1.0 cm² usually causes symptoms at rest (NYHA class IV). Usually a valve area of about 1.5 cm² or less in a symptomatic patient is an indication for surgery.

The natural history of MS is poor, ranking second only to AS in terms of mortality. When hemodynamically significant valve obstruction exists, firm indications for surgery include NYHA class III or IV, onset of atrial fibrillation regardless of symptoms, increasing pulmonary hypertension, an episode of systemic embolization, and infective endocarditis. Patients who have experienced atrial fibrillation for less than 1 year frequently can be reverted to sinus rhythm with cardioversion, quinidine or other drug therapy, or both. Surgery is recommended to class II patients over age 40 years who have a severe reduction in valve area demonstrated at catheterization or who experience undesirable limitation in exercise capacity or life style. The availability of open commissurotomy, which has substantial long-term benefits, and more complex valve repair techniques makes early repair attractive prior to the onset of atrial fibrillation. Asymptomatic patients can be carefully followed with Doppler echocardiography.

Mitral Regurgitation

The competence of the mitral valve depends on the unified function of the various components, including the annulus, leaflets, chordae tendineae, papillary muscles, and ventricular wall. Rheumatic valve disease still accounts for almost half of the cases of mitral insufficiency. Fibrosis and retraction of the leaflet cusps and fusion and shortening of the chordae may result in mitral regurgitation (MR), which may be associated with MS. The next most common cause is myxomatous degeneration, which produces thinning, elongation, and redundancy of the valve cusps and choradae tendineae. Mitral valve prolapse is present in 3% to 4% of the general population and may be associated with a midsystolic click and late systolic murmur. About 5% of these patients eventually develop clinically significant MR.

Isolated rupture of the chordae due to myxomatous degeneration may cause severe acute MR with pulmonary edema, sometimes requiring emergency surgical therapy. Leaflet or chordal rupture may also occur after blunt chest trauma or bacterial endocarditis.

Ischemic heart disease can cause severe mitral regurgitation. It may present as an intermittent event associated with acute ischemia, or it may be the result of myocardial infarction.

Clinical Manifestations

As in patients with MS, left atrial hypertension is transmitted to the pulmonary bed, resulting in dyspnea, pulmonary hypertension, and eventually RV failure and functional tricuspid incompetence. Unlike MS, the left ventricle is subjected to chronic volume overload, which ultimately leads to LV dilatation, increased LVEDP, decreased ejection fraction (EF), and failure. Symptoms usually begin about the time the MR represents 50% of the stroke volume.

Indications for Surgery

As seen with aortic insufficiency, patients may be relatively symptom-free for long periods. However, irreversible LV dysfunction may develop if symptoms alone are used as the indication for surgery. Surgical therapy is certainly indicated for patients whose symptoms compromise their life style or for those with NYHA class III or IV symptoms. In NYHA class I or II patients, operation is recommended for progression of pulmonary hypertension, onset of atrial fibrillation, or if the left ventricle is shown to be dilating. Data from the VA Cooperative Study on Valvular Heart Disease (9) suggest that three important variables predict normal LV size and function after mitral valve surgery: EF over 0.50, end-systolic volume less than 50 mL/m^2, and mean pulmonary artery pressure under 20 mm Hg. All three variables can be measured noninvasively by echocardiography. The failure of the EF to increase with exercise also suggests abnormal systolic function, which indicates the need for surgery.

As previously mentioned, acute MR secondary to ruptured chords or head of a papillary muscle may require urgent surgery. Typically a large V wave is seen in the pulmonary wedge trace after placement of a Swan-Ganz catheter. If the V wave is caused by myocardial infarction, the prognosis is determined by the extent of damage to the left ventricle.

Tricuspid and Pulmonary Valves

Acquired disease is most often due to dilatation and functional incompetence of the tricuspid valve. Rheumatic involvement more commonly causes stenosis, which may be associated with insufficiency. Tricuspid endocarditis is common among intravenous drug abusers.

Acquired pulmonary valve disease is unusual, although rheumatic involvement can occur. Carcinoid syndrome may be associated with fibrosis and stenosis, most commonly of the right-side heart valves.

Idiopathic Hypertrophic Subaortic Stenosis

Idiopathic hypertrophic subaortic stenosis (IHSS) is a form of asymmetric obstructive hypertrophic cardiomyopathy. A pull-back measurement at cardiac catheterization can demonstrate a subvalvular gradient in the LVOT secondary to muscular obstruction. The obstruction is dynamic, increasing with factors that reduce ventricular volume, such as inotropes, decreased afterload, or decreased venous return. Medical therapy with β blockers or verapamil usually relieves symptoms. Sudden death is common and does not correlate with hemodynamics and is not ameliorated by relief of obstruction. If disabling symptoms of dyspnea, angina, dizzy spells, and syncope persist despite appropriate medical therapy, surgical relief of obstruction may be performed by Morrow's technique of removing a longitudinal furrow of muscle from the LVOT. In certain special cases, mitral valve replacement is indicated for MR with IHSS, and this alone can relieve the obstruction. Operative mortality is about 8%, and sudden postoperative death continues to occur at a rate of 2% to 3% per year.

Current Valve Prostheses

Three general types of valve are used for valve replacement: tissue heterograft valves (primarily glutaraldehyde-fixed porcine or bovine pericardial valves), mechanical valves (including tilting-disk and ball-and-cage varieties) and aortic valve homografts (obtained from human hearts that are then cryopreserved). Valve comparisons are primarily made by comparing hemodynamics, durability, and the risk of thromboembolism or the need for anticoagulation with attendant risk of hemorrhage.

Hemodynamics

All prosthetic valves are stenotic in relation to normal heart valves. Most currently available prostheses are adequate in sizes equivalent to 23 mm aortic or 27 mm mitral, depending on body size. For 19- to 21-mm aortic valves, the St. Jude prosthesis, a low-profile bileaflet design, appears to be superior to other mechanical prostheses and at least equal to if not better than the best tissue valves. Among commonly available tissue valves, the Hancock modified orifice valve (which replaces the muscular shelf with the leaflet from another valve) and the Carpentier-Edwards bovine pericardial valve significantly improve the hemodynamics of small-orifice valves. The original Carpentier-Edwards porcine valve was introduced in 1969.

Durability

The durability of currently available mechanical valves is similar and superior to that of biologic valves. In adults, porcine valves tend to calcify over time, and about 30% of them require replacement within 10 years. These valves rapidly calcify in children and are contraindicated. Early data from several centers suggests improved longevity of bovine pericardial valves in adults with 93% to 95% freedom from reoperation for structural failure at 14 years. Homograft cryopreserved valves are particularly useful in children, where they are often used as valve conduits in repairs of complex congenital lesions. Homograft valves appear to be more durable than porcine valves but are not as readily available. Long-term follow-up of cryopreserved homograft series are limited, but preliminary data suggest excellent durability 15 years after implantation.

Thromboembolism and Anticoagulation-Related Hemorrhage

All mechanical valves require anticoagulation to prevent thromboembolism. This complication is more likely with mitral valve prostheses and particularly so when the patient is in chronic atrial fibrillation. Mortality or major morbidity occurs in about 1% to 2% of patients per year taking oral anticoagulants (coumadin). Patients in normal sinus rhythm who have a bioprosthesis placed, whether porcine, bovine pericardial, or homograft, do not require long-term anticoagulation.

Valve Selection

Currently it is recommended that porcine heterografts be reserved for patients with a limited life expectancy, those over the age of 70 years, and those who may have contraindications to permanent anticoagulation. The same may be said of the bovine pericardial valve, although somewhat younger patients (in their sixth decade) may be candidates because of apparently greater valve longevity. The St. Jude mechanical valve is preferred for replacement when necessary in children and young adults because of superior hemodynamics and long-term durability. Cryopreserved homograft valve conduits are frequently used to repair complex congenital problems with good results. A homograft valve is probably the best choice for aortic valve replacement in a young woman of childbearing age who wishes to have children.

The Ross procedure is a complex operation involving substitution of the patient's pulmonary valve for the diseased aortic valve, with reimplantation of the coronary ostia in the new aortic root and replacement of the pulmonary valve with a homograft. This procedure was originally designed to address the problem of aortic valve disease in children and was useful because the pulmonary (now aortic) valve can grow with the child. Unfortunately, it requires removal of a perfectly normal valve (pulmonary) and replacement with a homograft, which is likely eventually to require reoperation. This procedure has been used in selected young adults with good immediate results in experienced hands. Ultimately, the indication for this procedure in adults depends on the long-term fate of homografts in the pulmonary position and comparisons of morbidity, mortality, and the need for reoperation when the Ross procedure is used versus more traditional valve replacement procedures.

Patients who are in chronic atrial fibrillation and require mitral valve replacement gain no particular benefit from heterograft valve replacement because permanent anticoagulation is recommended in this situation. Therefore a mechanical valve should be chosen.

Prosthetic Valve Endocarditis

Endocarditis is virtually unknown with homograft valves but occurs with equal frequency whether mechanical valves or porcine heterografts are used. The incidence of prosthetic valve endocarditis (PVE) in valves containing prosthetic material is similar and related more to patient-determined factors such as poor dental hygiene than to the prostheses themselves. Antibiotic coverage for dental procedures, including routine tooth cleaning and invasive (diagnostic or surgical) procedures is mandatory to offset bacteremia. Antibiotic regimens vary, and the American Heart Association guidelines should be followed.

Advantages of Valve Repair

More emphasis has been placed in recent years on valve repair than on replacement. Repair has been successful primarily when dealing with mitral and tricuspid valves. Débridement of the calcified aortic valve has generally been disappointing, as has balloon valvuloplasty of that valve.

Carpentier et al. (5) opened the modern era of valve repair by reporting the use of a rigid annuloplasty ring that was designed to approximate the shape of the mitral annulus during systole, maintain the size and the mobility of the anterior leaflet, and perform a segmental plication of the posterior portion of the mitral annulus. A similar ring was developed for the tricuspid valve. Further refinements were developed in the reconstruction of regurgitant valves and reported by Carpentier et al. (6). Duran and Ubago (12) proposed use of a flexible annuloplasty ring to allow the annular shape to change during the cardiac cycle.

Several studies have now demonstrated that valve repair is associated with lower mortality than replacement. This occurs paradoxically despite the fact that repair may take considerably more time than replacement, probably because of improved LV function after repair when compared to replacement. Rushmer in 1956 first suggested that continuity of the mitral valve and LV wall via the chordae tendineae and papillary muscles plays an important role during the isometric contraction phase and increases stroke volume (40). Lillehei et al.

(26) were the first to apply this concept to mitral valve replacement by saving the posterior leaflet during mitral valve replacement.

Although patients in chronic atrial fibrillation generally require coumadin whether repair or replacement is performed, the ability to repair has prompted earlier referrals for surgery, which results in better long-term results. This is because problems of thromboembolism and endocarditis are rare after repair. Long-term results show repairs by Carpentier's techniques to be durable. Perier et al. (37) in 1984 reported a series of 400 patients who had mitral valve surgery, with 100 in each group: porcine valve, tilting disk valve, ball-and-cage valve, or valve repair. Initially the repair group had significantly lower mortality and, at 10 years, fewer thromboembolic events and a higher survival rate. The reoperation rate was no higher than with the mechanical valve groups and superior to that in the porcine valve group. Long-term results of repair for myxomatous degenerative disease have been superior to those for rheumatic valve disease, apparently because of a tendency for gradual disease progression with rheumatic valves.

Intraoperative Doppler echocardiography, by transesophageal or epicardial technique, has improved results of repairs by supplying instant accurate feedback in the operating room so any major problems can be corrected at the first operation (44). This has been useful in shortening the surgeon's learning curve when valve repair techniques have been introduced.

Minimally Invasive Cardiac Surgery

There has been an explosion in interest in minimally invasive cardiac surgical techniques. Efforts have involved CABG with and without cardiopulmonary bypass (CPB) and aortic and mitral valve operations as well as a number of new approaches to the repair of congenital heart problems. Several paths have been taken and this is still clearly a "work in progress."

Approaches to CABG procedures have been both with and without CPB. Robinson et al. (39) described an approach for bypassing the LAD with the left ITA (LITA) through a small left thoracotomy incision. Subramanian et al. (45) reported preliminary data from a multiinstitutional study using this approach without the use of CPB. Benetti et al. (1) reported the use of video-assisted LITA takedown for these procedures. The RCA has also been approached successfully through a small thoracotomy using the right ITA (RITA) radial artery, and saphenous vein grafts, and the posterior descending branch (PDA) of the RCA has been bypassed successfully through a minilaparotomy using the right gastroepiploic artery (RGEA). The off-pump procedures have been made much easier by coronary stabilization devices and have the advantage of avoiding the many potential problems associated with CPB, including stroke, coagulopathy, hemodilution with associated increased need for transfusions, renal failure (particularly in patients with severe preoperative renal impairment), and neuropsychological impairment. Additionally, off-pump procedures through small incisions are associated with decreased recuperation time, faster return to work, and shorter length of stay in the hospital, resulting in lower costs. Unfortunately, only about 5% of the CABG population are candidates for CABG off-pump procedures, as this is not applicable to the CFX system and most patients referred for CABG have multivessel disease. Furthermore, most patients currently referred for surgery are catheter intervention (e.g., angioplasty, stent) failures, as patients are still referred to surgeons by invasive cardiologists.

The development of a CPB approach by Stevens et al. (43) in conjunction with Heartport (Redwood City, CA), involves peripheral CPB based on femoral artery and vein cannulation, the use of both arterial and venous pumps, and an endoaortic balloon occlusion catheter designed to deliver antegrade cardioplegia without opening the chest. Jugular vein directed retrograde cardioplegia and pulmonary artery vent catheters are now also available. This system was designed to allow cardiac surgery through small incisions while providing the advantages of CPB bypass, namely a still, bloodless field with excellent myocardial protection. It was further designed to allow a minimally invasive approach to valve replacement or repair, which is not possible without CPB. Several problems have limited its general acceptance, however. The technique has been used most successfully for mitral valve procedures and CABG to the LAD with a LITA. The endoaortic balloon concept has not been as useful for aortic valve procedures because of difficulties keeping the balloon in place and out of the way. Furthermore, the use of expensive disposable equipment for a single bypass to the LAD seems excessive when CPB is not usually needed to bypass this artery. Efforts to perform multiple bypasses to the left coronary system have thus far been limited to basing all of the inflow on the LITA by creating one or

two proximal anastomoses to the LITA using radial artery or saphenous vein grafts. The possibility of jeopardizing the blood supply to the LAD or having inadequate total blood flow through the LITA to multiple vessels is a disturbing possibility that needs to be evaluated. Finally, several initial series have reported a 1% to 3% incidence of retrograde dissection even in a carefully selected patient population without peripheral vascular disease. The presence of peripheral vascular disease, seen in about 20% to 25% of CABG patients, contraindicates the Heartport port-access approach.

In an effort to overcome some of these problems, Cosgrove developed an alternate technique for aortic and mitral valve procedures using small incisions and chest cannulation for CPB. He reported the first 100 cases of aortic and mitral valve operations and performed two "live" procedures during a video teleconference from the Cleveland Clinic in September 1996. This approach can be used with partial sternotomy, right parasternal incision, or a short transsternal incision for the aortic valve (all with about 8-cm skin incisions). Mitral valve procedures can be accomplished through partial sternotomy or right parasternal incisions as well. Applying 10 to 40 mm Hg suction to the adult hard shell oxygenator reservoir allows one to use half the size of the usual venous cannulas, which vastly improves exposure through the small incisions used. The ascending aorta can be directly palpated and is available for intraoperative epiaortic echocardiography prior to cannulation, which should decrease the risk of embolism from manipulation of the ascending aorta. Chest cannulation completely eliminates the problem of retrograde dissection of the femoral artery and makes the minimally invasive surgery that requires CPB feasible for patients with peripheral vascular disease.

Hall and Vatsia (18) reported a successful triple CABG procedure through two small parasternal incisions with chest cannulation for CPB with all-arterial grafts (LITA, RITA, and radial artery) to the LAD, RCA, and CFX. Burke (4) described his experience with a video-assisted approach to PDA ligation and other conditions. Minimally invasive approaches are being used successfully for ASD and VSD repair by us and others.

Pace Sense Inhibit (Regans)

Arrhythmia Surgery and Pacemakers

Surgical procedures have been developed to treat medically refractory supraventricular tachycardia. Al-

For surgery
Set VVI → VOO

VOO = pace Vent
& sense
Rx

though atrial flutter, atrial fibrillation, junctional tachycardia, chaotic atrial tachycardia, and most sick sinus syndrome cases can be diagnosed by routine ECG, other conditions require electrophysiologic study. When supraventricular tachycardia is caused by an accessory AV connection [Wolff-Parkinson-White (WPW) syndrome], enhanced AV node conduction, AV node reentry, Mahaim fibers, or concealed accessory connections with retrograde conduction, endocardial catheter ablation or surgical ablation may be required.

Most ventricular arrhythmias occur in association with ischemic heart disease. Surgical intervention is indicated in cases that are refractory to medical treatment, where patient tolerance to medication is poor, or where patient compliance is poor. Patients who have intractable angina pectoris and associated ventricular tachycardia or who have congestive heart failure related to an LV aneurysm with associated ventricular tachycardia require a procedure directed at the arrhythmia. Patients with poor LV function who do not have discrete aneurysms but who have recurrent ventricular tachycardia may be candidates for an automatic internal cardioverter/defibrillator (AICD) device. These can now be placed transvenously in the electrophysiology laboratory.

In patients with bradyarrhythmias, permanent pacemaker insertion may be indicated. Commonly accepted indications for permanent pacing are listed in Table 21.6.

Pacing systems have become complex, but most commonly VVI and DDD systems are used. VVI refers to ventricular demand pacing in which only the ventricle is paced and sensed. This form of pacing lacks AV synchrony, which is not feasible in patients with slow atrial fibrillation. VVI pacing is unable to respond to increased physiologic stress by increasing the heart rate. DDD systems sense and can pace both chambers, which maintains AV synchrony and allows the heart rate to increase when physiologically needed. The AV synchrony can increase cardiac output by 20% to 25% and may be important in certain patients, especially those with impaired LV function.

Cardiac Neoplasms

About 80% of cardiac neoplasms are benign, 50% of which are myxomas. About 75% of myxomas occur in the left atrium, 20% in the right atrium, and 5% in more than one chamber. Ventricular myxomas are rare. They characteristically grow from the area of the fossa ovalis, do not extend deeper than the endocardium, but form a large, friable, multilobulated mass on a stalk that causes intermittent mitral valve obstruction and may present as a systemic embolus. Surgery is indicated when the diagnosis is confirmed. Echocardiographic findings are usually adequate to make the diagnosis.

Rhabdomyomas account for about 20% of benign cardiac tumors. They are congenital hamartomas and are the most common cardiac tumor of childhood. The lesions usually present as multicentric ventricular masses with poor encapsulation and may not be surgically resectable. Malignant tumors account for about 20% of all primary cardiac neoplasms and are almost always sarcomas. The most common is angiosarcoma. They tend to grow rapidly and have already metastasized in about 80% of cases by the time the diagnosis is made. These tumors typically present with rapidly progressive congestive heart failure. Cardiac metastases can occur with lung and breast carcinoma as well as leukemia, lymphoma, and melanoma. *most common tumors*

Intraaortic Balloon Pump

The intraaortic balloon (IABP) is positioned just below the left subclavian artery in the descending thoracic aorta. It inflates during cardiac diastole, improving coronary perfusion, and deflates during cardiac systole, reducing afterload, which reduces myocardial oxygen consumption. Indications for use include the following:

TABLE 21.6. *Indications for permanent pacemaker*

Sick sinus syndrome and bradytachyarrhythmia syndrome
Mobitz type II AV block (symptomatic)
Complete AV block
Symptomatic bilateral bundle branch block
Bifascicular or incomplete trifascicular block with intermittent complete AV block following acute myocardial infarction
Carotid sinus syncope (selected patients)
Recurrent drug-resistant tachyarrhythmias improved by temporary overdrive pacing
Intractable low cardiac output syndrome benefited by temporary pacing

Source: Adapted from Lowe (28).
AV, atrioventricular.

1. Refractory unstable angina (including postinfarct angina)
2. Complications of myocardial infarction
   a. Mitral regurgitation
   b. Ventricular septal defect
   c. Refractory arrhythmias
   d. Ventricular aneurysm
   e. Cardiogenic shock prior to planned revascularization
3. Preoperatively for severe left main coronary disease with unstable symptoms
4. Intractable failure following cardiac surgery
5. High-risk noncardiac surgery (rarely used)
6. Septic shock (selected cases)

Contraindications include aortic insufficiency, acute aortic dissection, and cardiomyopathy. Relative contraindications include severe peripheral vascular disease or the presence of a thoracic or abdominal aortic aneurysm.

Ventricular Assist and Total Artificial Heart

Various devices have been utilized to provide left heart assist, right heart assist, and biventricular assistance after failure to wean from cardiopulmonary bypass despite IABP and inotropic support. This was done in the hope that reversible myocardial injury would improve over the course of a few days. Long-term survival with these techniques has been disappointing, with survivors in reported series usually numbering fewer than 20%. Development of the total artificial heart, most recently the Jarvik-7, which was designed by Robert K. Jarvik at the University of Utah, continues with the hope that eventually a totally implantable pump and power source may be available. Currently, these techniques are most often effective as a bridge to cardiac transplantation rather than as a final therapy.

Cardiac Transplantation

With the development of the new cyclosporin-based, steroid sparing immunosuppression regimens, cardiac and lung transplantation must be considered in the armamentarium of therapies for congestive heart failure and end-stage lung disease. The nationwide 1-year survival for patients receiving cardiac transplantation now

exceeds 80%. When the total artificial heart is used as a bridge to transplant, survival at 1 year exceeds 50%. Advances developed by the Toronto Lung Transplant Group, along with immunosuppressive advances, have allowed prolonged survival after single-lung transplantation (7). This technique is currently the procedure of choice for end-stage fibrotic lung disease with restrictive physiology.

Indications for cardiac transplantation include disabling, irreversible cardiac disease that has a limited prognosis. Absolute contraindications include the presence of an active malignancy, elevated pulmonary vascular resistance, active infection, severe hepatic or renal dysfunction, and positive human immunodeficiency virus (HIV) antibody. Relative contraindications include age over 55 years, insulin-dependent diabetes mellitus, psychological instability, and economic factors. Donor availability remains the greatest hurdle the transplant candidate must face. About 30% of transplant candidates die while waiting for a donor organ.

Cardiovascular Trauma

Penetrating Cardiac Injury

Studies suggest that 50% to 80% of patients sustaining penetrating cardiac injuries do not survive to reach the emergency room. Mortality is higher for patients with gunshot wounds than for those with stab wounds. A review of 1,802 patients with penetrating cardiac injuries revealed 43% involved the right ventricle, 33% the left ventricle, 14% the right atrium, and 5% the left atrium (22). About 5% involved the intrapericardial SVC, IVC, or great vessels. This preponderance of RV injuries provides some justification for left anterolateral thoracotomy as a resuscitative measure when required in the emergency room. In patients with additional intraabdominal injury, cardiac repair precedes laparotomy. Injuries to major coronary arteries may be repaired on cardiopulmonary bypass. Injuries to the distal third of the LAD may be treated by suture-ligation. Valve injuries or VSD may become apparent later, depending on the degree of functional significance. A VSD with a left-to-right shunt of more than 2 : 1 requires surgery. Stabilization with IABP is required in some patients prior to surgery.

Cardiac tamponade may be produced by a penetrating injury or by blunt trauma. The patient presents with hypotension, distended neck veins, and a narrow pulse pressure. Pericardiocentesis with removal of only 20 cc of blood from the pericardium may be enough to stabilize the patient until emergency thoracotomy can be performed for definitive treatment of the injury. Pericardiocentesis is performed with a long large-bore (16 or 18 gauge needle placed at the left costoxiphoid angle and directed superiorly and posteriorly toward the left shoulder. If possible, an ECG V lead can be attached to the needle, and an injury current is evident on ECG if the myocardium is entered. Intrapericardial blood should not clot, and removal of small amounts of fluid usually results in dramatic hemodynamic improvement.

Blunt Cardiovascular Trauma

A variety of blunt injuries can lead to severe cardiovascular trauma. Automobile accidents provide the most common source of blunt trauma. Cardiac contusion may occur, which may resolve or may result in myocardial infarction. Patients with myocardial contusions generally have ECG findings that may include ventricular arrhythmias, supraventricular tachyarrhythmias such as atrial flutter or fibrillation, new bundle branch block, new Q waves or ST elevation, varying degrees of heart block, or cardiac standstill. Valve injuries are more common after blunt trauma than after penetrating injuries and should be sought by careful examination. Echocardiography is particularly helpful for visualizing LV segmental contractility, assessing valve function, and ruling out pericardial effusion. Patients with suspected myocardial contusion should be monitored for 24 to 48 hours while cardiac enzymes and serial ECGs are obtained.

Blunt trauma to the chest may result in severe stress to the thoracic aorta. The most common site of rupture is the area of the ligamentum arteriosum followed by the pericardial reflection on the ascending aorta. Patients with frank rupture usually die at the scene of the accident; 15% to 20% survive to reach the hospital. Widening of the mediastinum on chest radiographs, which may be associated with rib or sternal fractures, may be seen. Aortogram should be performed as soon as the patient is stabilized. Usually there are multiple injuries, and if the patient is actively bleeding intraabdominally it may have to be addressed prior to angiography, especially if there is no evidence of blood in the left chest on the chest radiograph. In this situation there may be containment of the aortic blood by aortic adventitia despite rupture of the intima and media. Of 275 persons with aortic rupture reported by Parmley, 237 died immediately at the scene of the injury (36). Of the 38 who reached the hospital, about one-third were dead within 24 hours and two-thirds within the first week after the accident.

The repair generally requires replacement of a segment of aorta with a graft. Controversy remains about spinal cord protection during repair, but most cardiovascular surgeons are more comfortable with a bypass technique, whether by partial cardiopulmonary bypass or by use of a heparin-bonded shunt, than with the clamp-and-sew technique, which allows a maximum of 20 to 30 minutes of safe spinal cord ischemia time. No technique, including the use of sensory evoked potential monitoring, which is becoming more popular, allows the surgeon to completely protect the patient from paraplegia (10). The latter remains a greater risk after traumatic aortic rupture of a normal descending thoracic aorta than it does after repair of an atherosclerotic aneurysm in the same region because of the absence of collaterals in the normal aorta.

Aortic Dissection

Aortic dissection is characterized by the development of hematoma within the middle to outer third of the aortic media. The separation begins at the site of a tear in the intima and media in about 95% of cases. The dissecting hematoma may extend around the circumference of the aorta but also extends distally parallel to the flow of blood.

Laennec described this condition as a "dissecting aneurysm," but this term is misleading. It is neither a true nor a false aneurysm. With a true aneurysm all layers of the vessel wall are included in the dilatation, and with a false aneurysm a paravascular encapsulated hematoma communicates with the lumen of the blood vessel wall, and the wall of the structure is not composed of elements of the blood vessel wall. The etiology most commonly is cystic medial necrosis, a tissue factor defect seen with Marfan syndrome and in many patients without the stigmata of Marfan syndrome. It may be associated with aortic stenosis, especially a bicuspid aortic valve, and is usually associated with a history of hypertension.

An aortic dissection is classified by duration and anatomy (Fig. 21.4). An acute dissection is less than 2

*TA indications to operate
>6cm, Aortic valve replacement, ascending (will break into pericardium)*

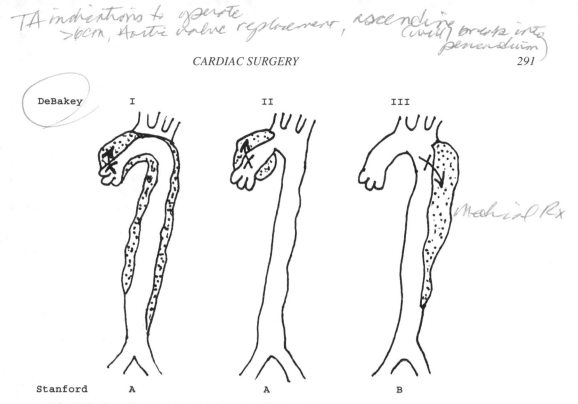

DeBakey I   II   III

Medical Rx

Stanford   A   A   B

FIG. 21.4. Classification of aortic dissection. [Adapted from Doroghagi et al., (11).]

weeks old and chronic dissection older than 2 weeks. Anatomic classifications include the DeBakey system, which classifies a dissection as type I, II, or III depending on the location of the original intimal tear. Types I and II involve the ascending aorta, but only type I extends beyond the ascending aorta for a variable distance; type II is confined to the ascending aorta. Type III originates below the left subclavian artery but may extend distally or proximally. The Stanford classification is used more commonly now. Type A involves the ascending aorta, and type B does not. This is done because the therapy generally involves emergent surgery for an acute type A dissection versus medical therapy for acute type B. About 80% of acute dissections cause demise within the first 24 hours as a result of rupture and pericardial tamponade, myocardial infarction from extension to the coronaries, or massive aortic insufficiency and congestive heart failure.

More than 90% of patients have severe, excruciating pain in the back. Loss of pulses may be present because of occlusion of individual arteries by the dissecting hematoma, which may result in stroke or limb ischemia.

Type A acute dissections are surgical emergencies except in cases where it is possible to demonstrate thrombosis of the false lumen. The operative mortality

of acute type A dissections is 8% to 10%. Type B acute dissections generally are successfully treated medically unless the aorta leaks or ruptures into the left chest or signs of severe major organ or limb ischemia occur. Operative mortality with acute type B dissection is generally no better than with medical therapy aimed at reducing blood pressure and force of contractility of the left ventricle (with βblockers). In addition, the significant risk of paraplegia with operative treatment of acute dissection of the descending thoracic aorta deters most surgeons from routinely operating on these patients.

Chronic dissections are operated on for specific indications. Chronic type A usually requires surgery for the late development of aortic insufficiency and congestive heart failure or a documented enlarging aneurysmal dilatation of the ascending aorta more than 5 cm in diameter. Chronic type B dissections may require surgery for documented enlarging aneurysmal dilatation over 8 cm (18).

Operative repair primarily attempts to replace the segment of aorta that contains the intimal tear with a Dacron graft. In the case of an acute type A dissection, the graft may be limited to the ascending aorta, even when the dissection progresses far beyond this area. This procedure is designed to prevent the causes of death attributed to ascending aortic dissection without subjecting the patient to the risk of replacing the entire aorta. Lifetime follow-up is necessary to identify the 5% to 10% of patients who develop aneurysmal dilatations of their aorta at other locations as a late complication of multiple reentry points distal to the original intimal tear. This can easily be seen on MRI or CT scans of the thorax and abdomen, and yearly studies are recommended after the first one, which is done 6 months postoperatively.

Central Aortic Disease

Ascending and Arch Aneurysms

Aneurysms of the ascending aorta or arch are dealt with on cardiopulmonary bypass. The etiology includes atherosclerosis, chronic dissection with aneurysm formation, and aneurysmal dilatation with annuloaortic ectasia caused by cystic medial necrosis, which involves dilatation of the sinuses of Valsalva with displacement of the coronary ostia away from the annulus. In the latter situation, a valve conduit is employed with reimplantation of the coronary ostia into the graft. Arch aneurysms are generally repaired with a period of total circulatory arrest under profound hypothermia (rectal temperature of 14° to 15°C). This procedure has greatly improved results, with mortality of about 10%. The approach is through a median sternotomy incision.

Descending Thoracic and Thoracoabdominal Aneurysms

The etiology of thoracic and thoracoabdominal aneurysms includes atherosclerosis or aortic dissection in 97% of cases. Trauma may result in the development of descending thoracic aortic aneurysms, as previously discussed. Prognosis without resection is poor in both situations.

Size indications for surgery are somewhat controversial, but asymptomatic patients with documented enlargement of a descending thoracic aneurysm or with an aneurysm over 8 cm in diameter but who is otherwise a reasonable surgical candidate should have surgery (17). A symptomatic aneurysm should be resected regardless of size.

For descending thoracic aortic aneurysms some method of distal perfusion is preferred. They may be managed with a left atrial to femoral artery bypass using a roller pump or centrifugal pump with or without an oxygenator or with a heparin-bonded shunt from the as-

cending aorta to the distal thoracic aorta or femoral artery. Ischemia during aortic repair may cause spinal cord injury and may produce paraplegia. The arteria magna, which provides most of the blood to the spinal cord, arises variably between the T4 and L4 vertebral bodies. Attempts should be made to preserve all large intercostals not involved in the aneurysm. Resection of acute traumatic aneurysms is more hazardous than resection of chronic atherosclerotic aneurysms, where adequate collateral circulation to the spinal cord has usually developed. Use of the clamp-and-sew technique has been associated with an increasing incidence of paraplegia in most series as the aortic clamp time increases beyond about 30 minutes. Operative mortality varies by etiology, age, and associated disease but averages 5% to 10%. Although measurement of somatosensory or motor evoked potentials has been useful for intraoperative spinal cord monitoring, no technique has been successful in eliminating the risk of paraplegia (30).

Thoracoabdominal aortic aneurysms have been most successfully repaired by the graft inclusion technique with direct branch vessel reattachment to openings made in the graft. Crawford et al. (8) reported a series of 605 patients with a 30-day mortality of about 9%; paraplegia or paraparesis occurred in 11%.

QUESTIONS

Select all correct answers.

1. Cardiac tamponade is characterized by:
   a. Low cardiac output.
   b. Hypotension.
   c. Elevation and equalization of CVP, RVEDP, PAD, and PAW.
   d. Removal of a small amount of fluid dramatically improves hemodynamics.
   e. Hypertension.
2. With regard to patent ductus arteriosus:
   a. Indomethacin may be useful for neonates.
   b. During the first months of life surgical closure done only for heart failure.
   c. Should eventually be closed regardless of size.
   d. May result in irreversibly elevated pulmonary vascular resistance.
   e. Can result in bacterial endocarditis.
3. Coronary artery bypass may be indicated for the following reasons:
   a. Intractable symptoms.

b. Single vessel disease that is asymptomatic.

c. 50% or more stenosis of the left main coronary.

d. 70% or more obstruction of three main coronaries with an EF of 30%.

e. Postinfarct angina.

4. The following are characteristic of ventricular septal defects:

a. May close spontaneously.

b. Most common isolated congenital cardiac anomaly.

c. Right-to-left shunt.

d. Left-to-right shunt.

e. Should be repaired if shunt is 2 : 1 or more.

5. Indications for aortic valve replacement:

a. Mild aortic insufficiency.

b. Moderate aortic insufficiency with LV enlargement.

c. Severe aortic insufficiency with decreased ejection fraction.

d. Asymptomatic child with 50 mm gradient.

e. Symptomatic adult with 30 mm gradient and low cardiac output.

6. Indications for mitral valve replacement/repair:

a. NYHA class III symptoms.

b. New-onset atrial fibrillation.

c. Echocardiographic demonstration of mitral regurgitation with normal LV and LA dimensions.

d. Asymptomatic mitral regurgitation with decreased ejection fraction.

e. NYHA class II patients over age 40 with reduced exercise capacity.

7. The intraaortic balloon pump (IABP):

a. Reduces diastolic pressure.

b. Increases diastolic pressure.

c. Reduces systolic pressure.

d. Increases systolic pressure.

e. Improves coronary blood flow.

8. Myocardial contusion:

a. Most often associated with blunt trauma.

b. May be associated with ventricular arrhythmias.

c. May be associated with new bundle branch block.

d. May be confirmed by serial cardiac enzyme determinations.

e. Requires no monitoring until the diagnosis is proved.

9. Management of aortic dissection includes the following:

a. Medical stabilization with β blockers and antihypertensives.

b. Immediate surgery for all dissections.

c. Surgery only for chronic stable dissections.

d. Surgery for acute dissections involving the ascending aorta.

e. Surgery for uncomplicated descending dissections.

10. Characteristics of descending thoracic aneurysms:

a. Should be resected regardless of size if symptomatic.

b. Should be resected if documented enlargement even if asymptomatic.

c. Should be resected if more than 8 cm if patient is otherwise a reasonable candidate.

d. Resection may result in paraplegia regardless of technique used.

e. Somatosensory evoked potential monitoring prevents paraplegia.

REFERENCES

1. Benetti FJ, Ballester C, Sani G, et al. Video assisted coronary bypass surgery. *J Card Surg* 1995;10:620–625.
2. Birnbaum PL, Weisel RD, Goldman BS. Acute evolving myocardial infarction: medical or surgical reperfusion? *Card Surg Rev* 1988;2:241–256.
3. Brunken RC, Kotton S, Nienaber CA, et al. PET detection of viable tissue in myocardial segments with persistent defects at Tl-201 SPECT. *Radiology* 1989;172:65–73.
4. Burke RP. Minimally invasive techniques for congenital heart surgery. *Semin Thorac Cardiovasc Surg* 1997;9:337–344.
5. Carpentier A, Deloche A, Dauptain J. A new reconstructive operation for correction of mitral and tricuspid insufficiency. *J Thorac Cardiovasc Surg* 1971;61:1–13.
6. Carpentier A, Relland J, Deloche A, et al. Conservative management of the prolapsed mitral valve. *Ann Thorac Surg* 1978;26;294–302.
7. Cooper JD, Pearson FG, Patterson GA, et al. Technique of successful lung transplantation in humans. *J Thorac Cardiovasc Surg* 1987;93:173–181.
8. Crawford ES, Crawford JL, Safi HJ, et al. Thoracoabdominal aortic aneurysms: preoperative and intraoperative factors determining immediate and long-term results of operations in 605 patients. *J Vasc Surg* 1986;3:389–404.
9. Crawford MH, Oprian C, Miller DC, et al. Determinants of left ventricular size and function following mitral valve replacement. *J Am Coll Cardiol* 1989;13:148A.
10. Cunningham JN, Laschinger JC, Merkin HA, et al. Measurement of spinal cord ischemia during operations upon the thoracic aorta—initial clinical experience. *Ann Surg* 1982;196:285–296.
11. Doroghagi R, Slater EE, DeSanctis RW. Medical therapy for aortic dissections. *J Cardiovasc Med* 1981;6: 187.
12. Duran CG, Ubago JL. Clinical and hemodynamic perfor-

mance of a totally flexible prosthetic ring for atrioventricular valve reconstruction. *Ann Thorac Surg* 1976;22:458–463.

13. Eagle KA, Coley CM, Newell JB, et al. Combining clinical and thallium data optimized preoperative assessment of cardiac risk before major vascular surgery. *Ann Intern Med* 1989;110:859–866.

14. Ebert PA, Turley K, Stanger P, et al. Surgical treatment of truncus arteriosus in the first 6 months of life. *Ann Surg* 1984;200:451.

15. Fintel DJ, Links JM, Brinker JA, et al. Improved diagnostic performance of exercise thallium-201 single photon emission computed tomography over planar imaging in the diagnosis of coronary artery disease: a receiver operating characteristic analysis. *J Am Coll Cardiol* 1990;15:334–340.

16. Fremes SE, Christakis GT, Del Rizzo DF, et al. The technique of radial artery bypass grafting and early clinical results. *J Card Surg* 1995;10:537–544.

17. Griepp RB, Ergin MA, Lansman SL, et al. The natural history of thoracic aortic aneurysms. *Semin Thorac Cardiovasc Surg* 1991;3:258–265.

18. Hall MH, Vatsia SK. Successful minimally invasive triple coronary bypass through bilateral parasternal incisions. *Ann Thorac Surg* 1997;64:1484–1486.

19. Hertzer NR, Beven EG, Young JR, et al. Coronary artery disease in peripheral vascular patients: a classification of 1000 coronary angiograms and results of surgical management. *Ann Surg* 1984;199:223–233.

20. Heymann MA. In *Moss' heart disease in infants, children and adolescents,* 4th ed. Baltimore: Williams & Wilkins, 1989;24–35.

21. Hochberg MS, Gielchinsky I, Parsonnet V, et al. Coronary angioplasty versus coronary bypass: three year follow-up of a matched series of 250 patients. *J Thorac Cardiovasc Surg* 1989;97:496–503.

22. Karrel R, Shaffer MA, Franaszek JB. Emergency diagnosis, resuscitation and treatment of acute penetrating cardiac trauma. *Ann Emerg Med* 1982;11:504.

23. Kirklin JW, Akins CW, Blackstone EH, et al. ACC/AHA Task Force report: guidelines and indications for coronary bypass graft surgery. *J Am Coll Cardiol* 1991;17:543–589.

24. Kirklin JW, Barratt-Boyes BG. *Cardiac surgery.* New York: John Wiley & Sons, 1986;599–664.

25. Leppo J, Plaja J, Gionet M, et al. Noninvasive evaluation of cardiac risk before elective vascular surgery. *J Am Coll Cardiol* 1987;9:269–276.

26. Lillehei CW, Levy MJ, Bonnabean RC. Mitral valve replacement with preservation of papillary muscles and chordae tendineae. *J Thorac Cardiovasc Surg* 1964;47:532–543.

27. Loop FD, Lythe BW, Cosgrove DM, et al. Influence of the internal mammary artery graft on 10 year survival and other cardiac events. *N Engl J Med* 1986;314:1–6.

28. Lowe JE. Cardiac pacemakers. In: Sabiston DC Jr, ed. *Sabiston's textbook of surgery.* Philadelphia: WB Saunders, 1986;2413–2443.

29. Mangano DT, Hollenberg M, Fogert G, et al. Perioperative myocardial ischemia in patients undergoing noncardiac surgery. I. Incidence and severity during the 4 day perioperative period. *J Am Coll Cardiol* 1991;17:843–850.

30. Marini CP, Cunningham JN. Evoked potentials: ten-year experience with a valuable research and clinical tool. *Semin Thorac Cardiovasc Surg* 1991;3:286–292.

31. Mark DB. Cardiac catheterization. In: Sabiston DC Jr, ed. *Sabiston's textbook of surgery.* Philadelphia: WB Saunders, 1986.

32. McEnroe CS, O'Donnell TF, Yeager A, et al. Comparison of ejection fraction and Goldman risk factor analysis to dipyridamole thallium 201 studies in the evaluation of cardiac morbidity after aortic aneurysm surgery. *J Vasc Surg* 1990;11:492–504.

33. McPhail NV, Ruddy TD, Calvin JE, et al. A comparison of dipyridamole-thallium imaging and exercise testing in the prediction of postoperative cardiac complications in patients requiring arterial reconstruction. *J Vasc Surg* 1989;10:51–56.

34. Mustard WT. Successful two-stage correction of transposition of the great vessels. *Surgery* 1964;55:469.

35. Myers WO, Schaff HV, Gersh BJ, et al. Improved survival of surgically treated patients with triple vessel coronary artery disease and severe angina pectoris. *J Thorac Cardiovasc Surg* 1989;97:487–495.

36. Parmley LF. Nonpenetrating traumatic injury of the aorta. *Circulation* 1958;17:1086.

37. Perier P, DeLoche A, Charwand S, et al. Comparative evaluation of mitral valve repair and replacement with Starr, Bjork, and porcine valve prostheses. *Circulation* 1984;70[suppl I]:187–192.

38. Riemenschneider TA, Emmanouilides GC. In: *Moss' heart disease in infants, children, and adolescents.* 4th ed. Baltimore: Williams & Wilkins, 1989;837–841.

39. Robinson MC, Gross DR, Zeman W, Stedje-Larsen E. Minimally invasive coronary artery bypass grafting: a new method using an anterior mediastinotomy. *J Card Surg* 1995;10:529–536.

40. Rushmer RF. Initial phase of ventricular systole: asynchronous contraction. *Am J Physiol* 1956;184:188–194.

41. Senning A. Surgical correction of transposition of the great vessels. *Surgery* 1959;45:966.

42. Sims FH. In: Green GE, ed. *Surgical revascularization of the heart: the internal thoracic arteries.* New York: Igaku-Shoin, 1991;18–62.

43. Stevens JH, Burdon TA, Siegel LC, et al. Port-access coronary artery bypass with cardioplegic arrest: acute and chronic canine studies. *Ann Thorac Surg* 1996;62:435–441.

44. Stewart JS, Currie PJ, Salcedo EE, et al. Intraoperative Doppler color flow mapping for decision making in valve repair for mitral regurgitation: technique and results in 100 patients. *Circulation* 1990;81:556–566.

45. Subramanian VA, Sani G, Benetti FJ, Calafiore AM. Minimally invasive coronary artery bypass surgery: a multicenter report of preliminary clinical experience. *Circulation* 1995;92[suppl I]:645.

46. Young LD, Berman DS, Kiat H, et al. The frequency of late reversibility in SPECT thallium-201 stress-redistribution studies. *J Am Coll Cardiol* 1990;15:334–340.

22

Management of Burns

Steven A. Blau

The knowledge needed to care for burn patients is increasingly recognized as important in the education of general surgeons, especially as an adjunct to their experience in a surgical intensive care unit (SICU). This chapter is intended simply to help the examinee pass that portion of the American Board of Surgery's examination. It is clearly not a substitute for a multiauthored treatise on burn management or for the experience gained while serving as a house officer on a good burn service. The content of this chapter has been deliberately slanted toward issues with which a general surgeon must deal; topics such as rehabilitation and physical therapy, for instance, have been given relatively little attention. Basic physiology and biochemistry have been included when they elucidate the problem, but the newest advances are deliberately not discussed. Similarly, areas of controversy in the management of burn patients are largely avoided, the text emphasizing the current or most widely accepted ideas. The reader must be wary of denigrating the value of this knowledge or relegating it to the purview of the plastic surgeons.

Mortality associated with burn injury (Table 22.1) has decreased over the years as a direct consequence of our understanding of basic science and its application at the bedside. Burn surgeons introduced (or sometimes reintroduced) to their general surgical colleagues such novel ideas as hypertonic fluid resuscitation, aggressive nutritional support, and bacterial translocation. When

confronted by questions beyond one's experience, it is probably safe to consider the burn-injured patient as a trauma patient, using your knowledge of the trauma process.

INITIAL MANAGEMENT

At the Scene

Unlike the victim of an automobile accident or a shooting, the burn patient is undergoing continuing trauma at the scene of the accident. If the victim of a flame burn, the patient should be removed from the place of injury, the flames extinguished, and burning or smoldering clothing removed. If possible, the wounds are cooled immediately to decrease the extent of burn injury and to relieve pain, but with care to avoid hypothermia. The wound is covered with clean sheets or a blanket if available. For chemical burns, copious irrigation or lavage with water is started at once. If the injury is related to an electric current, the patient is carefully moved away from the current source without additional trauma to the patient or injury to the respondent.

Adherence to the ABCs of trauma as taught by the American College of Surgeons' Advanced Trauma Life Support (ATLS) Course is indicated for the burn patient. Obvious immediate respiratory distress, although rare,

TABLE 22.1. *Burn size associated with 50% mortality*

Study	No. of pts.	% TBSA, by age group (0 to >65 years)			
		0–14	15–44	45–64	>65
Bull & Fisher (1942–1952	2807	49 ($n = 1366$)	46 ($n = 967$)	27 ($n = 1330$)	10 ($n = 144$)
Bull (1967–1970)	1917	64 ($n = 962$)	56 ($n = 565$)	40 ($n = 246$)	17 ($n = 144$)
Curreri & Abston (1975–1979)	1508	77 ($n = 803$)	63 ($n = 413$)	38 ($n = 178$)	23 ($n = 114$)
SBI/UTMB (1980–1994)	2164	98 ($n = 1524$)	70 ($n = 450$)	46 ($n = 127$)	19 ($n = 63$)

Source: Rose et al. (1997), with permission.
TBSA, total body surface area; *SBI,* Shriners Burn Institute; *UTMB,* University of Texas Medical Branch.

must be dealt with promptly. Circulatory collapse is uncommon immediately (that is, within 30 minutes) after a burn injury; but if it has occurred, it should be treated appropriately, initially with isotonic intravenous hydration. The patient is transported as quickly as possible to an appropriate facility. As the patient is already at a high risk of infection, routine placement of intravenous lines in the field is considered both unwise and unnecessary.

Triage

Burn injuries affect some 2 million persons a year; but with the increased use of inexpensive devices such as smoke detectors and preventive measures such as flame-retardant children's sleepwear, the number of burned patients may be decreasing. Although only about 5% of these patients require hospitalization, some 30% are cared for at specialized centers and units. The burn-injured patient should be transferred to the most appropriate facility as determined by the criteria recognized by the American Burn Association (Table 22.2).

Emergency Room

As discussed above, the burn patient in the emergency room is still undergoing a traumatic process. Hot grease or oil adherent to the skin, for instance, continues to cause a burn injury, and smoldering fabric creates noxious vapors that are being inhaled by the patient. The initial therapy, then, for the burn patient is to stop the burning process. This requires, first, removal of all clothing, which allows complete examination and assessment of other injuries. The skin should be bathed with cool, not cold, sterile saline. Although experimental data suggest that early application of cold may decrease the size of the burn injury, it is questionable

whether this is clinically relevant by the time the burn patient has been brought to the emergency room. Cold solutions, moreover, especially if applied to a large area, may result in hypothermia. Children and the elderly may be more sensitive to this induction of hypothermia. Chemical burns must be copiously irrigated with saline or water, avoiding the tendency to try to neutralize the offending agent. Dilute acid, for instance, should not be applied to an alkali burn or vice versa, because it only increases the exothermic chemical reaction. Because of the nature of the chemical injury, at least 1 hour of irrigation is recommended for acid burns and 3 hours for alkali burns. Burns to the eyes should be treated with this same lavage regimen. Until irrigated away, these chemicals continue their exothermic chemical reactions. Some chemical burns require specific chemical antidotes (see Special Burn Problems, below).

A brief history can usually be obtained from the patient. The circumstances of the burn injury are critical. Knowing that the fire was in a closed space is important, for instance, for assessing both the risk of serious inhalation injury and the management of it. The history of an explosion alerts the staff to the possibility of extremity, head, or abdominal trauma. Unconsciousness at the scene is another vital bit of information. Critical at this point is the patient's previous medical condition, especially the presence of cardiopulmonary or renal disease or diabetes mellitus. Current medications and allergies must be described. Tetanus immunization status must be confirmed. If the patient is within 10 years of his last tetanus immunization, 0.5 ml of tetanus toxoid is recommended. If the interval is greater or if the patient was never properly immunized, 250 U of Hypertet is added. Assessment and management of the airway are discussed below.

Injury to the eyes must be suspected in all patients with facial burns and all patients who are unconscious.

TABLE 22.2. *Criteria for triaging burn-injured patients*

Severity	Facility
Major Burns	Burn unit or burn center
2° > 25% BSA, adult	
2° > 20% BSA, child	
3° > 10% BSA, adult or child	
All burns of face, hand, eyes, feet, perineum	
Inhalation injury	
Chemical burns	
Electrical burns	
Burns associated with other trauma	
Poor-risk patients (diabetics, elderly, heart disease)	
Moderate uncomplicated burns	Hospital with burn experience
2° 15–25% BSA, adults	
2° 10–20% BSA, children	
3° < 10% BSA, adults and children	
Not involving critical areas	
No associated injuries	
No serious illnesses	
Minor burns	
2° < 15% BSA, adults	
2° < 10% BSA, children	
3° < 2% BSA, adults and children	

2°, second-degree burn; 3°, third-degree burn; BSA, body surface area.

Fluorescein is applied to evaluate corneal injuries, a technique that does *not* require an ophthalmologic consultant. At our institution, frequent application of topical antibiotics, rather than patching, is recommended for corneal abrasions. Chemicals in the eye must be copiously irrigated with sterile saline.

The skin is covered with a sterile sheet until the extent of injury has been evaluated by the team that will care for the patient. Several studies have demonstrated the unreliability of surface area assessments in the field and even in the emergency room. The patient should not be left on wet sheets because they predispose to hypothermia. Although dramatic and sometimes horrific to those passing by, the burn wound is almost the last part of the patient that needs to be addressed. Focusing on the cutaneous manifestations of the burn injury may lead the team to overlook other, more significant problems.

Pain control is a problem in burn patients, and the problem begins as early as in the emergency room. Although circulating endorphins have been described following burn injury and may explain the brief period of lucidity commonly seen in the burn patient, the patient is usually in severe pain in the emergency room. For small burns that require neither hospitalization nor aggressive fluid therapy, analgesia requires little constraint other than common sense. Patients with large burns, however, should not receive intramuscular medication because of their decreased cardiac output and consequent reduction in muscle blood. Initially, the medication is not carried into the central circulation. Restoration of circulation with fluid therapy, however, leads to absorption of all of the administered drug. Therapy consists, instead, of small, frequent intravenous doses of morphine or another opiate analgesic. The patient is likely to be scared and apprehensive, and maintenance of good communication regarding his or her care may decrease the need for pain medication. There must always be a concern, too, that the patient flailing around in the emergency room stretcher is manifesting not pain but hypoxia.

Throat cultures should be obtained from all patients in the emergency room, looking specifically for the presence of β-hemolytic streptococcus, which must be treated with the appropriate antibiotics if cultured. This practice has largely superceded the empiric penicillin therapy previously advocated, although some centers hold to this practice in children.

Any patient with burns covering more than 20% of the body surface area (BSA) will probably develop a gastric ileus, and a nasogastric tube is therefore indicated to prevent aspiration and the complications of aspiration pneumonitis. Aggressive fluid therapy leading to peripheral edema and hypoalbuminemia may also result in an increase in small bowel edema and a subsequent small bowel ileus.

INHALATION INJURY

The respiratory consequences of the burn injury may be divided into three distinct pathophysiologic entities that may be present singly or in combination: upper airway injury, lower tract injury, and carbon monoxide poisoning.

Upper Airway Injury

The upper airway is defined anatomically as the nasopharynx, the oropharynx, and the airway extending down to and including the vocal cords. This injury in the burn patient is a heat injury due to direct thermal injury to the mucosa. The physiologic consequence of this injury is edema, and the clinical consequence of this edema is upper airway obstruction. The development of this edema represents a dynamic process, increasing over the first 24 to 36 hours and then resolving slowly.

Which patients are at risk of an upper airway injury? Clearly, patients who present with facial burns are at obvious risk. They may present with singed eyebrows and eyelashes or singed nasal vibrissae or mustache hairs. They may have obvious cutaneous burns of the face. Unfortunately, some patients, especially those with steam injuries, have less obvious facial burns and still develop upper airway edema. One child recently admitted to our facility had aspirated a burning ember from a campfire and presented in unexplained but florid respiratory distress. The patient may be producing carbonaceous sputum. In the presence of stridor or obvious respiratory distress, the patient must be intubated immediately to protect the airway and to maintain ventilation.

Not every patient with a facial burn needs to be intubated. The patient without obvious distress should be assessed carefully recognizing that the responsibility of the airway falls on the shoulders of the caring physicians and that continuous assessment of the airway may not be possible when the patient is in transit to another facility. A chest radiograph is a poor diagnostic test for upper airway injury, as it is nearly always normal. The same can

be said for arterial blood gases, which usually demonstrate both normal oxygenation and normal or even low P_{CO_2}. Before patients develop chemical evidence of hypercarbia, their clinical condition should have alerted the staff to the problem. Airway injury can be diagnosed by endoscopy, either fiberoptic (bronchoscope or nasopharyngoscope) or simple direct laryngoscopy. Recognizing the progressive nature of the process, management is prompt intubation if the patient shows signs of erythema and edema. Patients who have no evidence of airway injury should be reexamined at 2- to 4-hour intervals. Some physicians treat these patients with racemic epinephrine to reduce the edema, but this is not done at all burn centers. Corticosteroids to reduce edema, although attractive physiologically, are generally condemned in the burn patient because they further increase the risk of infection. Pending endoscopy, a useful provocative test is forced rapid exhalation by the patient. The guiding principle, though, should be that, when in doubt, intubate the patient because the consequences of an incorrect assessment are probably more severe than the consequences of an "unnecessary" intubation. Always intubate a patient who is to be transported to another facility because the patient probably cannot be assessed during transit. Nasotracheal intubation is preferred at some centers because it is regarded as less uncomfortable for the patient, but the physician must feel secure in using endotracheal intubation if he or she is more comfortable with this technique.

Patients with isolated upper airway injury should remain intubated for at least 2 to 3 days and, after extubation, should be followed closely for signs of upper airway obstruction. An overly awake patient flailing around in bed and pulling on the endotracheal tube may produce further airway injury, which would prolong resolution of the edema. Appropriate sedation is therefore recommended. Few patients require long-term intubation for isolated upper airway injuries. Prolonged upper airway difficulties should alert the clinician to consider mechanical injury either from the initial trauma or as a complication of intubation in the field, the emergency room, or the burn unit.

Lower Tract Injury

The pathophysiology of a lower tract injury is completely different and reflects, in part, anatomic considerations. The naso- and oropharynx are efficient air conditioners, warming inhaled cold air on a wintry day and dissipating hot air in a flaming building. Consequently, the lower tract injury is rarely caused by heat (unless the patient inhales superheated steam) but, rather, is caused by the chemical products of combustion. Smoke from burning wood or natural substances such as cotton or wool contains some 200 distinct chemical products that can irritate the respiratory mucosa. Synthetic materials contribute their own collection of noxious gases. These substances cause a chemical pneumonitis with the elaboration of interstitial edema and a progressive barrier to gaseous diffusion.

Clinically, the patient does not usually manifest much in the way of respiratory distress when first seen. Suspicion is raised when there is a history that the patient was in a confined-space fire (e.g., a burning stove in a house trailer) because of the consequent high smoke concentration. Unconsciousness at the scene is another important historical consideration. Initially, the chest radiograph is clear and the arterial blood gases are either normal or reflective of hyperventilation and a consequent respiratory alkalosis. The most useful early clinical adjuvant is the demonstration of significant carboxyhemoglobin levels (see Carbon Monoxide Poisoning, below) because the amount of inhaled smoke frequently correlates with the amount of inhaled carbon monoxide.

The best early diagnostic test of lower tract injury is available, unfortunately, at only a few hospitals. A ^{133}Xe ventilation scan is frequently positive early in the process, demonstrating areas of ventilation–perfusion mismatch. In hospitals without this technology, the routine technetium perfusion scan is not an effective diagnostic substitute. The principal diagnostic tool available to most clinicians is fiberoptic bronchoscopy, which allows a direct view of the tracheobronchial tree but may underestimate the injury because the small airways are not examined. Significant findings include erythema, edema, and loss of definition of the septa dividing the bronchial orifices. If these characteristics are demonstrated, the patient should be intubated. For this reason, the author advances the fiberoptic bronchoscope over an endotracheal tube. If the patient requires intubation, the endotracheal tube is advanced over the bronchoscope into the trachea without additional trauma.

Again, the pathologic process is progressive but usually self-limited, resolving in about a week in most cases. The sloughing of cells lining the tracheobronchial tree along with transudation of plasma is usually seen during the first 24 to 48 hours. The release of thromboxane and vasoconstrictors leading to increases in pulmonary vasculature resistance and subsequent pulmonary edema occurs with the initial insult, but the edema is not usually clinically relevant until several days later. The initial management is oxygen, and the patient requires sufficient oxygen enrichment to allow maintenance of an arterial Po_2 of 90% saturation. The alveolar–arterial gradient in these patients is usually large. Aggressive and appropriate use of positive end-expiratory pressure (PEEP) tends to maintain aeration of a sufficient number of alveoli to allow use of a lower Fio_2. I begin with 5 cm H_2O PEEP and increase it as needed and as tolerated by the patient. Although the use of pulmonary artery catheters is controversial in the burn patient, we continue to recommend it in patients requiring high positive-pressure ventilation (i.e., PEEP of more than 12 cm H_2O). We are less adamant about recommending prophylactic chest tubes (to avoid tension pneumothoraces) in patients who require PEEP in excess of 15 cm H_2O. The patient should be suctioned frequently, and routine sputum Gram stains and cultures must be obtained. The fluid therapy the patient is receiving is adjusted downward if possible to decrease the hydrostatic driving force of fluid into the lungs. Pulmonary compliance is recorded, especially in patients receiving high PEEP therapy.

Like the patient with adult respiratory distress syndrome (ARDS) in the SICU, other modalities of ventilatory assistance are appropriate in these patients. The combination of an enriched oxygen atmosphere and the need for high pressures to overcome poor compliance result in secondary injury to the lung due to oxygen toxicity and barotrauma. This has opened a role for pressure control ventilation (to prevent the highest peak inspiratory pressures), permissive hypercapnia (accepting a higher than normal Pco_2 by decreasing the alveolar ventilation and thereby decreasing the pressures necessary to inflate the alveolus), and high-frequency jet ventilation. These modalities are discussed at greater length in Chapter 23. Their clinical utility remains somewhat controversial, as improvements in pulmonary management have not always been associated with a lower mortality rate.

Pharmacologic interventions are few. Steroids are not indicated and, frankly, are condemned. Although some animal studies have shown an improvement in airway function after steroid use, bacterial challenge confirmed the consequences of the drugs' immunosuppression.

Prophylactic antibiotics should be similarly avoided, as they merely predispose the patient to infection, selecting out another, more virulent organism. The throat culture obtained in the emergency room should guide the choice of antibiotics if no other data are available and the patient develops fever and pneumonia. Serial sputum cultures and Gram-stained material are better guides to the antibiotic therapy required, making empiric therapy unnecessary. Despite the burn patient's immunosuppression, the respiratory infection is likely to be caused by the same gram-negative bacteria that afflict other ventilated patients in SICUs.

Of greater interest, though, are drugs that interfere directly with the two sides of the problem: (1) thromboxane inhibitors to decrease the vasoconstriction that may initiate pulmonary edema and (2) oxygen free radical scavengers to address toxic metabolites of oxygen. In addition to the usual cast of characters, vitamin E (which must be given enterally), vitamin C, dimethyl-sulfoxide (DMSO), and n-acetylcysteine have been investigated. These chemicals have been effective in some cases when administered by aerosol.

Carbon Monoxide Poisoning

Carbon monoxide (CO) poisoning, frequently associated with smoke inhalation, represents a distinct biologic process. The clinical effect comes from the ability of CO to displace oxygen from the hemoglobin molecule. Although the process is reversible, the affinity of hemoglobin for CO is more than 2,000-fold greater than its affinity for oxygen. As a result, the patient's blood is able to carry less oxygen to the tissues, which then suffer from hypoxia, anoxia, and tissue death.

The classic clinical picture of a patient with CO poisoning includes cherry-red lips and unconsciousness, but this picture is more likely to be seen in the morgue than in the emergency room, where subtle neurologic complaints are more important, including confusion, lightheadedness, nausea, and headache. The classic findings are commonly associated with carboxyhemoglobin levels of 60% or higher, explaining the consequent mortality of these patients. Diagnosis of CO poisoning requires detection of carboxyhemoglobin on a CO oximeter. The "normal" level is less than 3% to 5% in nonsmokers and up to 7% to 10% in smokers. With aggressive care, levels of 40% to 50% are commonly recorded in survivors.

The therapy for CO poisoning is dictated by a principle learned in high school chemistry—the law of mass action. The CO is simply displaced by an excess of oxygen. The half-life of carboxyhemoglobin is about 5 hours in room air at normal pressure and falls to approximately 60 minutes with 100% oxygen, 45 minutes with forced ventilation at 100% oxygen, and approximately 25 minutes with hyperbaric oxygen (100% oxygen at 2.5 atmospheres). Patients need not be intubated to receive oxygen therapy, although intubation is necessary for the patient with upper or lower airway injuries.

Although the hypoxia secondary to CO poisoning may be self-limited, the neurologic sequelae of CO poisoning may persist. Early descriptions of CO poisoning included patients whose hypoxia was corrected and who left the hospital or emergency room only to develop delayed neurologic injuries. More recent reports have suggested a CO-specific computed tomography (CT) scan appearance of the brain in these patients. Hyperbaric oxygen treatment, because it rapidly decreases the half-life of CO–hemoglobin, has been advocated as the best management for CO poisoning, but definitive demonstration of its benefit has been lacking, even in large-scale studies. Moreover, relatively few data have accumulated regarding the long-term neurologic sequelae in CO poisoning managed by various treatment modalities. The decision to use hyperbaric oxygen therapy is largely moot, though, because few hospitals have the necessary equipment; 100% humidified oxygen then becomes the treatment of choice.

Management of the patient in the hyperbaric chamber requires some basic recollection of physics. Gas occupies a smaller volume when subjected to increased pressure. An air-filled endotracheal tube balloon, for instance, might not occlude the hypopharynx when the chamber is pressurized. The cuff is usually filled with water, which is less compressible. A pneumothorax increases in size as the chamber is depressurized. The major complication of hyperbaric therapy is barotrauma to the ear, and a few patients require myringotomy.

BURN SHOCK AND FLUID RESUSCITATION

Burn shock represents a physiologic nightmare, the details of which have still not been completely elucidated. Burn shock is principally a problem of the loss of intravascular volume. The burned tissue is characterized by edema; capillaries are injured and become "leaky." The vapor barrier of intact skin is lost in the burned areas, and fluid is lost into the room air. The intubated patient, furthermore, loses fluid into the ventilator circuit. Early, there is apparently a global change in capillary permeability leading to a movement of fluid out of undamaged capillaries into the interstitial space. There are changes in the electrical charge of the ground substance, which tends to result in a net movement of water into the tissue space. In addition to the volume losses, there is increasing evidence that the burn injury produces toxins that may lead to myocardial depression.

Clinical data from humans and data from animal experiments have confirmed that the patient who presents with 50% BSA burn has had a reduction of cardiac output of nearly that amount. This patient is in shock, and management must reflect this understanding.

The patient has lost the ability to thermoregulate in part because the damaged capillaries do not respond to the usual neurohumoral controls. Hence hypothermia must not be allowed in the emergency room. The management of the patient's burn (see below) must not jeopardize body temperature. Hypermetabolic elevation of the core temperature is not seen until later, usually about a week after injury.

The most commonly used formula for fluid resuscitation in the burn patient is the Parkland or Baxter formula. As with most resuscitation schedules in current use, this one avoids colloid infusion during the first 24 hours of therapy because of the aforementioned loss of vascular integrity. The volumes infused tend to be enormous. The estimated infusate for the first 24 hours is calculated according to the following formula:

$$\text{24-Hour infusion} = 4 \text{ ml/kg} \times \% \text{ BSA burn} \times \text{body weight (kg)}$$

For the purposes of this formula, only second and third degree burns are included in the calculation of BSA. One-half of the total volume is infused during the first 8 hours, and the other half over the next 16 hours. For a 70-kg man with a 50% BSA second and third degree burn, the formula works out to: $4 \times 50 \times 70 = 14,000$ mL, or approximately 1,000 mL/hr for the first 8 hours. This formula markedly underestimates the needs of children, whose weight–surface area relation is much different from that of adults. Most pediatric formulas use BSA, not weight, for this reason.

Remember that this formula is empirically derived, and therapy must be individualized for each patient. Patients with inhalation injuries frequently have increased fluid requirements (estimated to be as high as 2 mL per percent burn per kilogram body weight in 24 hours). Because the goal is normalization of a satisfactory cardiac output, one could measure cardiac output directly as a guide to fluid therapy. In most patients, the urine output is measured more easily and serves as a guide to cardiac output because it correlates with the glomerular filtration rate. A goal of a 50 mL/hr is sought in adults and 0.5 to 1.0 mL/kg/hr in children. The fluid infusion rate is adjusted hourly to maintain this urine output goal. Failure to monitor the patient continuously, following the formula blindly, usually leads to an unsatisfactory outcome.

Most patients can be managed without intensive monitoring of their intravascular status, but should they be? If the patient is not responding to the fluid management as expected or if the patient is elderly or has preexisting cardiac, pulmonary, or renal disease, conservatism probably has no place. A central venous pressure catheter, at least, or a Swan-Ganz catheter may improve the results of fluid resuscitation. The goal of the initial fluid therapy is a cardiovascularly intact patient 24 hours after the burn. During the second 24 hours fluid therapy is marked by restriction of the sodium intake, addition of colloid, and induction of brisk diuresis.

Management of the patient who does not respond with satisfactory urine output or adequate cardiac output is complicated. Inotropic drugs are probably indicated, but they do not always work. Several investigators have pursued the concept of circulating toxins and have employed plasmapheresis in patients whose response to fluid is markedly abnormal. Some patients have survived the period of burn shock when this technique was used. Unfortunately, some patients simply cannot be resuscitated.

Further problems of resuscitation arise in small children whose needs for glucose and calcium are not met by infusion of Ringer's lactate solution. Supplemental glucose must be provided. For those with small burns, the glucose can be given by mouth.

The consequence of this initial 24-hour volume of fluid therapy is usually gross peripheral edema. Damaged capillaries have leaked. Some of the fluid has been lost because of evaporation, but most has been translocated to the interstitial space. If the patient had significant pulmonary injury, some of this fluid may have produced pulmonary edema. Management over the next 24 hours, then, attempts to mobilize this fluid. Little addi-

TABLE 22.3. *Representative fluid resuscitation regimens*

Formula	First 24 hours		Second 24 hours	
	Electrolyte solution	Colloid component	Electrolyte solution	Colloid component
Evans	Normal saline: 1.0 ml/kg/% burn 2,000 ml D5W	1.0 ml/kg/% burn	1/2 of first 24 hr 2,000 ml D5W	1/2 of first 24 hr
F.D. Moore burn budget	Ringer's lactate: 1,000–4,000 ml 0.5 NS: 1,200 ml 1,500–5,000 ml D5W	7.5% body weight	Ringer's lactate: 1,000–4,000 ml 0.5 NS: 1,200 ml 1,500–5,000 ml D5W	2.5% body weight
Brooke	Ringer's lactate: 1.5 ml/kg/% burn 2,000 ml D5W	0.5 ml/kg/% burn	1/2 to 3/4 of first 24 hr +2000 ml D5W	1/2 to 3/4 of first 24 hr
Modified Brooke	Ringer's lactate: 2.0 ml/kg/% burn No glucose	None	D5W as necessary for urine output	0.3–0.5 ml/kg/% burn
Parkland or Baxter	Ringer's lactate: 4 ml/kg/% burn No glucose	None	D5W as necessary for urine output	20–60% of plasma volume
Hypertonic	250 mEq Na⁺liter Volume titrated to urine output	None		
Jelenko HALFD	240 mEq Na⁺/L 120 mEq lactate/L Volume titrated to urine output	12.5 g albumin/L	No additional salt	As needed

D5W, 5% dextrose in water; NS, normal saline.

tional salt or sodium is provided, and patients frequently receive colloid (human serum albumin) infusions. Diuretics are used as needed. Mannitol is usually considered a better choice than furosemide.

Although popular today, the Parkland formula is not without its detractors. Early fluid regimens (Table 22.3) that included colloid still have their adherents. Other investigators have focused on fluid management schedules to decrease the net fluid balance in burn patients. Some have advocated decreasing the amount of Ringer's lactate solution by using 3 mL/kg instead of 4 mL/kg. Others have suggested "capping" the body surface area at 50%. Still others have advocated hypertonic fluid resuscitation with a Na^+content of 200 to 300 mEq/L instead of the 130 mEq/L found in Ringer's lactate solution. Clinicians using these schedules, titrating their infusions based on urine outputs of only 30 mL/hr and carefully monitoring serum electrolytes and osmolarity, report markedly decreased fluid needs with less edema and fewer pulmonary complications. These solutions have been efficacious for both children and the elderly. One variant on hypertonic fluid resuscitation calls for the early addition of albumin (the Jelenko, or hypertonic albuminated lactate fluid demand, regimen). In comparison to the Parkland regimen, however, these hypertonic regimens probably require increased vigilance for maintaining acceptable levels of electrolytes. Severe hypernatremia can occur with these fluids, and the serum sodium must be kept below 160 to 165 mEq/L to avoid central nervous system (CNS) complications and the possible cellular injury due to dehydration. The tendency of patients resuscitated with Ringer's lactate solution to develop hyponatremia is well known, but the commonly observed serum sodium level of 130 to 135 mEq/L is higher than that usually associated with CNS disturbances.

The markedly hypertonic fluid regimens advocated recently for trauma patients (7.5% NaCl in 6% dextran) have also been applied to burn injury, but only in experimental animal models. Small-volume resuscitation with these solutions produced increased survival compared to survival after large volumes of hypotonic fluids.

Comparison of these various formulas has been difficult. Randomized trials in a single center are easily criticized because the investigators are likely to be less familiar with one or another solution. Multicenter trials require investigators to abandon what they believe is the best solution and accept the choice of management of physicians in another center. Finally, there are just so

many patients with severe burns. Prospective randomized comparisons with hypertonic resuscitation, for instance, suggested excessive morbidity due to renal failure, a complication rarely reported by the advocates of this resuscitation technique.

Pharmacologic fluid schedules have been tested in animals combining known free radical scavengers to decrease the possible role of free radical injury in decreasing myocardial performance and producing capillary leak distant from the burn injury. These trials have usually used superoxide dismutase. Other free radical scavengers have been advocated as adjuncts to management of burn shock, but free radical scavenger therapy today is still outside the mainstream of burn resuscitation. Mega-doses of vitamin C and high doses of vitamin E, though, are considered standard interventions and may be efficacious because of their free radical scavenging.

BURN INJURY

Mortality due to burns is a function of a number of factors including the age of the patient, the extent of the burn, and the depth of the burn injury. Mortality for a given size burn is highest in older patients and small children. Older patients are adversely affected by coexisting cardiopulmonary and renal disease, for instance. Children have increased mortality because of their diminished metabolic reserve. Respiratory tract injury also increases the mortality of a given size burn.

An understanding of the burn injury requires a brief description of skin anatomy (Fig. 22.1). The most superficial layer is a dead keratinized layer, or stratum corneum. It is biologically inactive except for functioning as a barrier to retain water vapor. Underneath it is the epidermis. All growth of the epidermis takes place at the basal cell layer. This layer extends down around hair follicles and sweat glands and rises and falls over the dermis so a straight tangential cut across the skin would reveal dermis covered with epidermis in places and exposed in others. Underneath the epidermis is the delicate dermis, wherein are found sweat glands, hair follicles, and some capillaries. This dermis is fragile and easily injured after it is denuded of the overlying epidermis. Underneath is the subcutaneous fat, fascia, and muscle.

With a first degree burn (Table 22.4) only the epidermis is damaged, and the injury is confined to that layer. The skin appears reddened, and the patient complains

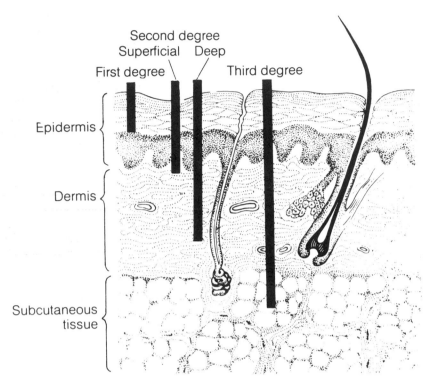

FIG. 22.1. Relation of the depth of the burn to the location of adnexal structures in skin and subcutaneous tissue. A partial-thickness or second-degree burn, if protected from infection, desiccation, and subsequent ischemia, heals spontaneously as epithelial cells migrate from residual viable hair follicles and sweat glands. Because all adnexa are destroyed in full-thickness or third-degree burns, such wounds do not reepithelize and must be closed by skin grafting.

of warmth and superficial pain. The injury frequently results from sunburn or a hot-water scald. It is a self-limited process, with complete healing in 5 to 7 days. The patient needs some protection from trauma, which would cause pain. Antihistamines may decrease the erythema. Nonsteroidal antiinflammatory agents may de-crease the associated inflammation and are effective as analgesics. Healing depends on an increase in the mitotic activity of the basal epidermal layer with repopulation of the defect.

Deeper trauma results in extending the injury into the dermis. Two distinct clinical entities are described that

TABLE 22.4. *Characteristics of skin burns*

Characteristic	First degree	Second degree	Third degree
Color	Pink or red	Pink or red	Brown and leathery or white
Surface	Usually dry	Superficial: bullae intact or ruptured Deep: generally moist	Dry
Sensation	Painful and warm to touch	Generally painful Deep: frequently anesthetic early	Anesthetic
Healing	3–7 days	Superficial: 10–21 days Deep: >14 days	Does not heal Wound may contract

depend on the depth of the injury: a superficial second degree burn and a deep second degree burn. The former manifests as blister formation, which represents fluid accumulation between dead epidermis and damaged dermis. This injury, again, is a self-limited process that heals entirely if it is not traumatized or infected. The management of intact blisters, which contain myriad vasoactive substances, has become controversial. Left intact, the blisters provide an effective biologic dressing of the tissues below. In some cases, however, an intact blister prevents the clinician from recognizing the depth of the burn injury underlying it. At our institution, intact blisters are left intact. Obviously, broken blisters should be débrided and dressed similarly. The underlying dermis appears somewhat shiny and reddened. If healing takes place normally, it becomes covered by epidermis migrating from the sides and the basal epidermis along the depths of the hair follicles. The healing wound appears pink, but less shiny, as the epidermis covers the dermis. Small burns normally heal in 7 to 14 days. Larger surface area burns take longer.

Healing of the dermis involves a second process, namely, ingrowth of fibroblasts with deposition of collagen. The extent of this scar formation correlates with the depth of the initial injury. For this reason care must be taken to avoid infection, which would further damage the dermis. The use of topical antimicrobial preparations is advised for this purpose, and they are dis-

cussed in detail below (Table 22.5). Deep second degree burns, because of their tendency to heal with significant scarring, constitute an area of surgical decision making. In anatomic areas where such scarring would result in marked functional impairment, such as the hands and over joint surfaces, many surgeons recommend excision and skin grafting instead of allowing the area to heal spontaneously. This controversy is discussed more fully below (see Surgical Management).

First and second degree burns are partial-thickness injuries that can and usually do heal. A full-thickness, or third degree, burn by definition does not. Here the epidermis and the entire dermis have been destroyed. The third degree burn can "heal" only by wound contraction. The clinical appearance of this burn varies with the status of the hemoglobin contained in the capillaries at the time of injury. It appears waxy white (if there was no extravasated hemoglobin) or dark brown (because of fixed hemoglobin). The sine qua non of the third degree burn is the anesthesia that appears because of the extensive nerve destruction. It is sometimes difficult to differentiate early between deep second degree and third degree burns, but this distinction is not critical during the early hours after the burn. Initial assessments of burn injury are frequently incorrect and are changed by the patient's course with burns that are usually deeper than they initially appear but cover less surface

TABLE 22.5. *Topical antimicrobial agents*

Generic name	Proprietary name	Advantages	Disadvantages	Side effects
Silver sulfadiazene	Silvadene	Painless, well tolerated Minimal staining	Poor eschar penetration Minimally effective against *Pseudomonas* Ineffective against *Enterobacter*	Sulfa allergies Hemolytic anemia in G6PD-deficient patients Reversible leukopenia
Mafenide acetate	Sulfamylon	Excellent eschar penetration	Painful	Carbonic anhydrase inhibitor Sulfa allergies Hemolytic anemia in G6PD-deficient patients
Povidone–iodine	Betadine	Better eschar penetration than Silvadene Free of sulfa allergies Desiccates the wound	Desiccates the wound May not be available any more	Risk of iodine toxicity in large, open areas
0.5% Silver nitrate		Wide microbial spectrum	Requires wet dressings	Stains everything Produces hyponatremia and hypochloremia

area. Infection plays a major role in this transformation, converting a partial-thickness injury to a full-thickness one. Young children and the elderly most often have burns that are deeper than they appear on initial examination. Vital stains, ultrasonography, thermography, and laser Doppler flowmetry have been suggested as means of determining burn depth more accurately, but these procedures have generally not replaced clinical judgment.

There are several useful rubrics for evaluating the extent of a burn injury. The most popular technique is the "rule of 9s." Here the upper extremities, anterior chest, posterior chest, anterior abdomen, posterior abdomen, and head are each assumed to comprise 9% of the BSA in the adult. The lower extremities are each 2 ×9%. The perineum covers 1% of the BSA. In children, proportionally more surface area is assigned to the head, so here the rule of 9s breaks down. Another useful technique is to assume that the patient's hand is equal to 1% of the body surface area. If the assessment of the burned area is to be more exact, though, examiners are urged to use the Lund-Browder or similar chart (Fig. 22.2) and to describe the findings completely with the diagram in view while examining the patient.

SPECIAL BURN PROBLEMS

Electrical Burns

Unlike flame burns or contact burns in which heat is applied to the surface of the skin, the electrical burn produces its injury by the production of heat, and this heat is a function of the resistance of the various tissues through which the current passes. Because the skin has relatively low resistance, the cutaneous portion of the electrical injury is marked by a point of entrance and a point of exit. This initial evaluation, however, tends to minimize the extent of the burn because the underlying muscle, bone, arteries, and nerves between are frequently damaged. The picture is a bit more complicated in high voltage electrical injuries, where the body acts as a volume conductor and the injury produced is a function of the current density per cross-sectional area. This accounts for the predilection of high voltage injuries to injure the extremities more seriously.

In contrast to the more typical presentation, the patient with an electrical burn is frequently in shock when seen and severely acidotic and hyperkalemic because of the mass of dead and damaged tissue. Cardiac

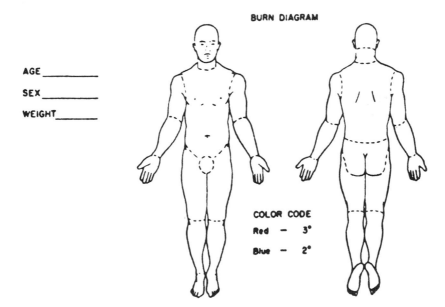

BURN DIAGRAM

AGE_____

SEX_____

WEIGHT_____

COLOR CODE

Red — 3°

Blue — 2°

FIG. 22.2. Burn diagram and table used to estimate the extent of the burn. Note that the fractions of total body surface represented by the head and lower limbs change with age and assume constant proportions after age 15.

arrest may have occurred at the scene and electrocardiographic (ECG) monitoring is mandatory even if the current path is not through the chest. Such monitoring should be continued until days after any arrhythmias have resolved. Fluid therapy must be started quickly and be sufficient to produce not merely the 50 mL/hr an adult should be expected to produce but a brisk diuresis. Damaged muscle releases free myoglobin, which leads to myoglobinuria. The myoglobin can, in turn, precipitate in the renal tubule, leading to acute renal failure. Although detectable spectrophotometrically, myoglobin (or hemoglobin) is detected by examining the supernatant of the centrifuged urine sample. A positive test for blood with the appropriate urine test paper establishes the diagnosis. The serum, similarly centrifuged, is red in patients with hemoglobinemia (also seen in extensively burned and electrically injured patients) and clear with myoglobinemia. The adult patient must produce a urine output in excess of 100 mL/hr. Mannitol infusion (up to 300 g in 24 hours) may be a necessary adjunct to this fluid management by adding an osmotic diuresis. Alkalinization of urine can also improve the patient's chance of avoiding renal failure by keeping the myoglobin or hemoglobin in solution rather than allowing it to precipitate in the renal tubules.

The damaged muscle tends to swell in the patient with electrical injury. The patient may develop a compartment syndrome identical to that of a patient with vascular trauma or ischemia. Clinically, the patient manifests the five Ps: pain, paresthesia, pallor, pulselessness, and poikilothermia. However, the limb's functional survival is dependent on acting before the onset of pallor and pulselessness. Laboratory tests, including Doppler ultrasonography, are usually not necessary. Clinical signs alone should lead to prompt fasciotomy.

The nature of the heat injury leads to what is occasionally described as fourth and fifth degree burns because muscle and bone are involved. Obviously, dead tissue requires aggressive amputation surgery. Delayed injury such as arterial bleeding is not uncommon. Sometimes the extent of muscle necrosis is not readily apparent, and such modalities as arteriography and technetium-99m pyrophosphate scanning have not been universally helpful for establishing the extent of the injury.

In the patient with an electrical injury, one must search for associated orthopedic injuries. Extremity fractures are common, reflecting the effects of simultaneously contracting the muscles of extension and flexion. Vertebral body fractures are also seen with electrical injury.

Neurologic injuries are problematic, and the clinician may be unable to distinguish a reversible neuropractic injury from a permanent nerve injury. In general, motor nerves tend to be involved more often than sensory nerves. Early cord neuropathies tend to be transient, and delayed onset of neurologic compromise is a serious sign suggesting that the defect may be permanent.

The most common electrical injury in children occurs when toddlers bite through electrical line cords. The patient is usually admitted, monitored for a few days, treated with topical therapy, and discharged. Reconstruction of the commissure is indicated for cosmetic needs 6 to 9 months later. If the patient develops problems with feeding, reconstruction or a dental appliance is indicated early. Injuries caused by lightning are an uncommon form of electrical injury and are dramatic but associated with 70% survival in many series.

Frostbite

Frostbite, although usually cared for on a burn service, is a pathophysiologically different process. With freezing, intracellular water crystallizes to ice and disrupts the cell membrane, leading to cell death. At less severe temperatures, cell water may extravasate into the interstitium, resulting in a sublethal injury in which tissue can be salvaged. Frostbite injuries tend to be well demarcated.

Initial management of frostbitten tissue includes local warming of the tissue and systemic warming of the patient. Marked tissue edema is common with warming, reflecting the extravasation of plasma-rich fluid into the interstitium. Sympathectomy and regional anesthetic nerve blocks have been advocated for relief of symptoms, and they may play a role in healing. Topical antimicrobial therapy for frostbite is the same as it is for thermal burns. Surgical management of frostbite is generally expectant, and the nonviable mummified tissue is thought to be protective of the underlying healing injury. Radionuclide studies and arteriography have been advocated as adjuncts to the management of these injuries, but time is probably the most effective test of long-term viability.

Chemical Burns

The general principles of management for the patient with chemical burns were discussed above. These chemicals commonly cause injury by producing an exothermic chemical reaction in the skin or by dehydrating the tissue, leading to cell death. Alkali and acid burns from household products (e.g., drain cleaners) are the most common reported in civilian (nonindustrial) practice. Chemical injury from the inadvertent addition of ammonia and hypochlorite (bleach) is usually pulmonary and responds to nonspecific management. Some specific remedies must be discussed, though.

Hydrofluoric acid burns used to be confined to professionals who used the acid for glass etching, but the agent has become a general hazard recently. It is available in combination with other acids as a home cleaning agent, the introduction of which may keep injury lawyers in business for the foreseeable future. Hydrofluoric acid produces its injury by complexing with calcium. Clinically, the patient presents with a history of painlessness followed by intense pain and pallor. Topical therapy with calcium chloride or calcium gluconate gel is usually the initial therapy, although calcium may be injected directly into the wound using a 27-gauge needle and restricting the volume to decrease the risk of adding pressure necrosis. Our own experience suggests that arterial infusion of dilute calcium is superior for decreasing pain and limiting the extent of necrosis. Most of these patients, however, must undergo surgery for at least some débridement of damaged tissue. Systemic hypocalcemia, sometimes seen in these patients, responds to intravenous calcium infusions.

Phenol burns necessitate the use of a lipophilic solvent to remove residual phenol, which is not particularly water-soluble. Products such as polyethylene glycol and glycerol have been used to achieve this end.

Dry alkali or anhydrous ammonia may cause damage. It should be brushed off the wound before the wound is lavaged for the obvious reason of limiting the injury.

White phosphorus injuries are almost always consequent to military exposure. The risk to the patient and the care-giving medical staff is explosion of residual powder. Hence the patient's wounds and any particles removed must be kept moist or under water.

Tar burns should be treated with cool water, which allows the tar to harden. It can then be peeled off the wound.

SURGICAL MANAGEMENT

Nonburn Surgery

Because burn patients may be traumatized in other ways as well, the first operation performed may be for a nonburn condition. For example, the victim of an explosion may have suffered a ruptured spleen in addition to his 50% BSA burn. Although laparotomy increases the mortality risk for the patient, not performing the operation increases it to 100% The burn victim must always be viewed as a whole patient, considering the possibility of additional trauma and underlying surgical problems. A complete history and a complete physical examination must be performed early in the patient's course.

Escharotomy

The first operation for a burn indication is escharotomy. A full-thickness burn is covered by an eschar, a nonviable mass of dead and dying cells and denatured protein that has lost the elastic properties of unburned skin. As the interstitial space fills with fluid and expands, the eschar acts as a tourniquet, increasing pressures in the deeper spaces. In a manner analogous to the development of a compartment syndrome, the pressure increases to the point of interfering with venous outflow and arterial inflow and compromises the viability of the deeper tissues. Although one could measure subcutaneous pressures as one measures compartment pressure, clinical considerations are used for the decision making in most cases. I look for signs of decreased capillary refill on the fingertips and for paresthesia of the fingers and decreased active range of motion of the metacarpophalangeal joints on the hands. Some advocate Doppler ultrasonography to detect decreased or absent pulses, but this loss of pulse may be a late sign in the development of the syndrome.

An escharotomy is not removal of the eschar but an incision into it, allowing the edges to separate and thus relieve the pressure. The incisions must be made along anatomically appropriate lines. These incisions are designed to avoid the major subcutaneous sensory nerves, thereby not predisposing the patient to further injury. I recommend biaxial incisions of the upper and lower extremities and uniaxial incisions on the fingers, avoiding the major sensory aspects of the hand (the ulnar side of the small finger and the radial aspect of the index finger where it meets the thumb). If these finger incisions are inadequate, of course biaxial incisions are made. Incisions must be carried across joints in most situations. The intrinsic space of the dorsum of the hand is opened with two or three incisions.

An eschar of the chest wall acts as a corset, making ventilation of the patient difficult or impossible. A burn patient should never be placed on a pressure-cycled ventilator for just this reason. As the compliance of the chest wall/lung unit decreases, the ventilator delivers less and less volume until the patient's ventilation is adequate for his or her physiologic needs. Peak pressures of 90 to 100 cm H_2O are not uncommon on a volume-controlled ventilator. I place escharotomy incisions along both midaxillary lines, across the chest just below the clavicles to the neck, and along the base of the chest to join the two axillary incisions. Many others include an incision along the sternum, but it rarely relaxes the chest wall. Escharotomy usually results in a dramatic decrease in peak pressures (30 to 40 cm H_2O) and a patient who can suddenly be ventilated.

The eschar is not viable and is insensate, so additional anesthesia is not necessary. A scalpel is an appropriate instrument provided the surgeon does not try to incise the unburned subcutaneous tissue below. It must be remembered that the blood vessels may not bleed simply because the patient is still deep in shock. (Some years ago I admitted a patient being transferred from another institution, status post escharotomy with blood-soaked dressings and a hematocrit of 8%.) Escharotomy by electrocautery is certainly safer. I perform escharotomies in the emergency room or at the bedside using sterile technique. The procedure does not require a trip to the operating room unless the patient requires additional procedures best performed there.

Escharotomies are performed when they are perceived to be needed. This need may arise early, when the patient is seen in the emergency room, or up to two or more days later in the burn unit. Physicians should not be so embarrassed by "missing" the procedure initially that they avoid doing it later. Dependent edema has been suggested as a mechanism for delayed need for escharotomy and demonstrates the need for the physician to place the patient in the correct position, usually with the burned extremities elevated. Once an escharotomy is performed, the wound must be dressed with the same topical agent as the burn wounds. The escharotomy defect is closed with an autograft when the burn wound is grafted. Occasionally, I have performed escharotomies on deep second degree burns and watched the defect contract and be epithelialized weeks later. Fasciotomies as an additional procedure are usually required only in patients with electrical burns and are performed with the standard fasciotomy technique used for compartment syndrome.

Chemical eschar removal is possible, but the agents are rarely substitutes for surgical escharotomy. Some clinicians report that their use decreases the amount of nonviable tissue that must be excised in the operating room. Travase ointment is an example of such an agent. The active ingredient, sutalains, removes the denatured protein when used with good wet-to-dry dressing technique. The wounds are cleansed, any topical agent is removed (heavy metals destroy the enzyme), and the wounds are dressed with Travase and moistened fine-mesh gauze. The technique works well on burned hands and in children. The agents are neither bacteriostatic nor bactericidal; hence a large surface area burn cannot be covered with them as it would expose the patient to a serious risk of infection. Many believe that collagenase is not an acceptable enzyme for removing eschar because it irritates undamaged tissue, but the agent is undergoing further study in this regard.

Excision and Grafting

Classic burn care called for expectant management of the burn wound: allowing the eschar to separate, the wounds to declare themselves, and only third degree burns to be skin grafted. Unfortunately, the same bacteria that caused the eschar to separate (the bacteria underneath produce collagenases and hyaluronidase) infected the patient and resulted in high mortality rates on burn services. A more "modern" approach to the care of the burn wound recognizes that the patient must have the wounds covered, and dead eschar is simply not coverage.

Patients are taken to the operating room as soon as they are cardiovascularly stable for burn wound excision. Some centers operate on patients during their shock phase, especially those that care for large numbers of pediatric patients. In most centers the first operation is performed within 2 to 4 days of the burn injury. Patients with isolated small area burns can usually undergo surgery earlier, as they do not require the massive fluid resuscitation patients with larger burns receive, nor do they develop the consequent edema that necessitates diuresis. I try to limit excision and grafting to 10% to 15% of the BSA with 1 to 2 hours of operating time at a session. These limitations are based on recognition of the physiologic stress of surgery and the major fluid shifts that occur during the procedure (sometimes the anesthesiologist is simply not able to keep up with the patient's needs). Blood loss can be as great as 4 units during just 30 minutes of excision. The common rubric estimates blood loss to be as much as 0.5 unit per percent body surface area. Many have advocated the use of tourniquets when excising extremity burns to decrease the blood loss. Although this is an effective adjunct to reducing blood loss, it may make the amount of excision required less obvious.

Because the initial operative procedures may be lifesaving, I have elected to excise a large surface area burn (e.g., the back) before a smaller but more complicated area (e.g., a hand). Functional considerations therefore take second place to those preserving life. The tangential excision of the wound is usually performed using Goullian knives, which carry guards to limit the depth of the excision, or the Humby knife. Excision is carried down to bleeding tissue: the punctate bleeding of viable dermis or the bleeding of viable fat. The excision can also be performed completely freehand by surgeons who enjoy the challenge of using a dermatome. Bleeding may be controlled with topical thrombin or gauze soaked in low concentrations of epinephrine. Use of epinephrine to control capillary bleeding in the operating room should be with the knowledge of the anesthesiologist, and it should be restricted to small areas because of possible absorption into the circulation.

The wound, now excised and clean, must be covered. The best coverage is obviously an autograft, but homografts, xenografts, and artificial temporary skin substitutes (e.g., Biobrane) have a role to play. The decision making is not standardized, but one must consider (a) the availability of the patient's own skin; (b) the cosmetic results of excising skin (the donor site); (c) the infectious status of the patient; (d) the remaining operations; and (e) the anatomy in question. It would be incorrect, for instance, to cover the back with unmeshed sheets of skin when the patient still had significant hand and forearm burns. The skin graft is usually harvested with a mechanical dermatome, although the most adroit sometimes use a freehand knife. The Padgett electrodermatome is favored at our institution. The skin graft varies from 0.010 to 0.016 in., with thicker skin usually

being placed on the dorsum of the hand and the soles of the feet. The observation that thinner skin "takes" better is probably valid, as epidermolysis is more common in the thicker skin grafts.

The autograft may be placed as it is removed, or it may be meshed with a Tanner mesher to expand the surface area covered. Expansion varies from 1.5 : 1.0 to as much as 9 : 1. This expansion is provided by changing the carriers in the mesher or, more recently, using different blades on the mesher. Incidentally, the Tanner mesher was developed not to "expand" the area that could be covered but to prevent the accumulation of serum and hematoma underneath, which leads to graft loss.

Unmeshed autograft is placed where the burn wound is most visible to provide the best cosmetic effect. I use it on the face and frequently on the dorsum of the hand. Because subgraft hematomas interfere with graft take (the graft initially living on oxygen and nutrients that diffuse from the bed underneath), the unmeshed graft is almost always "pie-crusted." Most of my grafts are meshed 1.0 : 1.5, which provides a satisfactory cosmetic result that can be improved by not pulling the interstices fully open. I use a Tanner mesher for expanding autografts. Expansions of 3 : 1 and larger are employed principally when satisfactory skin is not available.

Excisions are carried down into bleeding tissue, as discussed above. For classic tangential excision and grafting, this practice takes one down to dermis, which can always support a skin graft. If no bleeding is encountered prior to reaching the fat or subcutaneous tissue, care must be taken to excise the nonviable fat, which frequently appears gray or brown in contradistinction to the healthy yellow fat. Thrombosed blood vessels must be excised completely. I have no difficulty placing meshed autograft directly on fat, which has good graft take, but some others believe that fat is a poor recipient and so carry their excision down to fascia or muscle, which are generally considered better recipient sites. For large surface area burns, excision to fascia rather than to fat is faster and generally leads to diminished blood loss. The cosmetic consequence of removing the layer of fat is minimal in most patients. Autograft also takes on periosteum or peritenon. Graft does not adhere or take on bone (without periosteum) or on tendon. In places where the excision is down to bone, the cortex of the bone may be removed or small holes drilled into it to encourage growth of granulation tissue, which can take a graft. On the skull it may be necessary to remove a portion of the outer table and place the graft directly on the diploë.

The graft must be immobilized early to allow its early nutrition and to encourage collagen bundles and blood vessels to grow into it. On a convex surface this poses little difficulty. On concave or complicated surfaces, I frequently use a tie-over bolster. Few areas of contention are quite as fierce as placing grafts on the dorsum of the hand of burn victims. Some authors are adamant that the metacarpophalangeal joints must be pinned in 70 to 90 degrees of flexion to lengthen the extensor mechanism and to immobilize the graft. Although I frequently place these pins or K-wires, the same graft success has been achieved with the application of bulky dressings. Either technique is probably adequate.

There are circumstances where a skin graft should not be placed after an excision. If the patient has an untreated bacteremia, placing an autograft may be an invitation to failure. A heavily colonized bed of granulation tissue might not support a graft. A burn excised because of documented invasive burn wound sepsis is similarly a poor candidate for definitive grafting. Heterografts and allografts (homografts) are placed to buy time and as biologic predictors of subsequent graft success. Early "take" is achieved with blood vessels growing into the graft before the body's immune system recognizes them as foreign. Because of the extensive immunosuppression seen in burn patients, homografts may take and remain for weeks to months. A colony count of more than 10^5 organisms per gram of net weight tissue precludes graft healing. Conversely, the take of a homograft ensures that the colony count is less than 10^5 organisms. Covering a wound with such a biologic dressing increases the number of leukocytes in the wound, thereby clearing the local wound of bacteria. Care must be taken when using a homograft in female patients of childbearing years, as a "taking" graft exposes her to HLA-mismatched antigens, which could lead to later fetal loss. Concerns have been raised about the role of banked human homograft in the transmission of human immunodeficiency (HIV) infection and hepatitis, but the skin bank centers that provide the material are scrupulous in protecting their reputations.

The skin graft is not the final decision when managing the burn wound—the dressing is. A meshed autograft must have its interstices protected. The healing of a meshed autograft is marked by tiny areas of wound

contracture followed by epithelial migration from the areas of autograft that have taken. Sheets of Vaseline gauze may cover the interstices to maintain the proper moist microenvironment. The interstices may be left completely open and sterile saline sprayed on the wound hourly. Larger expanded grafts (1 : 3 or more) benefit from sandwich techniques, covering the wound with meshed allograft or with synthetic material such as Biobrane.

The goal of the skin graft is not so much coverage as function. This is why I excises and skin-graft burns on the dorsum of the hand that are only deep second degree. To maintain function, the skin grafting must be recognized during the course of rehabilitation. Joints must not be allowed to stiffen prior to definitive autografting. Pins that are impediments to dynamic positioning and movement must be removed expeditiously. A fully grafted but dysfunctional patient benefits no one. Early coverage, moreover, need not be final coverage.

A word on donor sites is in order. Preferred sites for the skin include the anterior and posterior thighs and buttocks. In women I consciously avoid the calves and legs if possible. Grafts from dependent sites (e.g., the back) do not do well usually. The scalp is an excellent site for skin grafts. The graft should be taken no deeper than necessary and the site allowed to heal. It can usually be reharvested in about 3 weeks—somewhat earlier on scalp because of its more abundant blood supply. Reharvested skin is not as flexible as that initially taken, which should be considered when planning the patient's operation. Unused skin can be placed back on the donor site or "banked" for subsequent application. Preservation with tissue culture fluid has extended the shelf life of refrigerated banked skin to nearly 4 weeks.

The discussion on skin grafting so far has dealt only with split-thickness skin grafts, which although the most common grafts performed are not the only ones. Split-thickness grafts provide only a relatively thin covering of the tissue below and despite our best efforts are prone to contract. Full-thickness grafts provide more bulk, do not contract, and are used principally in areas where additional padding is required or where contraction must be prevented. Their most common use is for grafting eyelids, correcting the ectropion that occurs when the full-thickness defect contracts. They are sometimes used as well for closing hand burns in children. Taking a full-thickness graft produces a full-thickness defect at the donor site, and so sites are carefully chosen to allow primary closure rather than grafting. These areas include the groin creases and the posterior auricular spaces.

Adjuncts to traditional grafting have not always produced the intended benefits. Recombinant human growth hormone increased the rate of healing of the donor site but not the rate of healing of the grafted areas. As patients with large surface burns require reharvest of these limited donor sites, this is of clinical utility.

Cultured human skin grown from the individual patient has been used in many patients but its use was generally reserved to centers that specialize in this work. Commercial laboratories can now grow cultured epidermis but at an almost prohibitive cost and with a minimum delay of about 2 to 3 weeks before enough tissue is available for grafting. The initial take of this "graft" is good, especially on dermis and muscle; but long-term cosmetic results are poor, the tissue being prone to break down and result in unfortunate scarring. Cultured skin is indicated today only in patients who have no recourse to skin grafts because of the limited surface area available. "Artificial" skin, which is really a bilaminate tissue composite that resembles dermis, has also been used to close burn wounds.

More interesting, perhaps, has been the use of cadaveric human dermis, depleted of much of its antigenity (which resides in Langherhans cells) by the application of ultraviolet light. This tissue seems not be rejected and can be covered with cultured epidermal cells or extremely thin skin grafts.

PHARMACOLOGY

Physicians caring for the burn patient must be aware of the changes in the patient's metabolism and physiology, which affect the use of medications. The need for frequent intravenous analgesics, in contrast to large intramuscular injections, was discussed earlier in the chapter, relative to the early decrease in cardiac output after burn injury. With resuscitation, the patient's cardiac output increases to supranormal levels and he is both hyperdynamic and hypermetabolic.

Aminoglycosides, commonly used for management of infection in these patients, are excreted by the kidneys. Because burn patients have increased cardiac output during the hospital course, they also have an increased glomerular filtration rate (GFR). Burn patients, managed with the usual doses of antibiotic (3 to 5 mg of gentamicin per kilogram, for instance) do not achieve satisfactory serum or tissue levels. Such patients commonly receive 50% to 100% more drug than would be deduced from their weight or from nomograms. Because they require more drug, the physician must be even more careful to monitor drug levels. The major cost of aminoglycosides at most hospitals is not for the drugs but for the laboratory tests to determine drug levels, which are obtained at least every third day. The same need for increased drug administration applies to vancomycin.

The neuromuscular blockading agents are of critical importance in burn patients. Not immediately after the burn, but certainly by 1 week afterward, the patient is highly sensitive to the effects of succinylcholine. Administration of succinylcholine can lead to massive hyperkalemia and even death by cardiac arrest. The mechanism is not clear. How long it lasts is also unclear, but most anesthesiologists shy away from using the drug in that patient for some years after the burn injury. On the other hand, the nonpolarizing agents exhibit the opposite picture. The burn patient is less responsive to these agents, and so the drugs must be given in larger quantities to achieve the same physiologic result. The mechanisms suggested here is that there is an induction of receptors at the neuromuscular junction. The effect increases with the surface area of the burn and reaches its peak after a few weeks. This increased need persists but is less marked. Remember as well that aminoglycosides can prolong the effectiveness of neuromuscular blockade.

Morphine and the other opiate agonists are usually required in increased doses in the burn patient. Whether this represents an increase in hepatic clearance of the agent or an up-regulation of receptors in response to frequent administration is unclear.

Cimetidine, used in these patients as an adjunct to gastric acid control, must also be used carefully. With the increased GFR during the "flow" phase, dosages may have to be increased to about twice normal in adults and even more in children. Of course, the use of H_2 blockers in burn patients is as controversial as it is in SICU patients in general. The use of sucralfate has become more common, but acid control may be unnecessary provided the patient is fed enterally.

NUTRITION

Malnutrition is a major factor in the mortality of burn patients. Anyone who has cared for burn patients realizes the pronounced need to repair tissue, lay down new tissue, and maintain defenses against infection. In the burn patient the provision of calories is relatively simple, as most patients can be fed enterally. Few patients require parenteral nutrition, and its associated infectious complications argue strongly against it. Anergy developing in a burn patient consequent to malnutrition markedly increases the risk of death. Moreover, correcting anergy by the appropriate nutritional interventions reverses that increase.

The problems of nutrition in the burn patient stem from determining how to evaluate the patient's nutritional status and the difficulty of maintaining enteral nutrition with recurrent trips to the operating room.

The burn patient can be weighed on admission to the burn unit, but subsequent weights determine less the loss of lean body weight than the fluid shifts associated with resuscitation, diuresis, and bulky dressings. Bioimpedance has been suggested as a means of determining lean body mass in these patients, but this technique is largely unworkable with large surface area burns. Nitrogen balance would be a useful means of determining the efficacy of protein intake, but few centers can weigh the dressings to determine the nitrogen losses from the wound, which can be prodigious. Measurement of oxygen consumption by indirect calorimetry can be a useful tool for determining caloric needs, but consumption varies during the day and is markedly affected by pain, bedside procedures, and aggressive physical therapy.

The currently favored method for estimating caloric needs in the adult patient is the Curreri formula, which estimates caloric needs at 25 kcal/kg body weight plus 40 kcal for each percent body surface area burned. This calculation is probably better than the modified Harris-Benedict equation, which has frequently led to overfeeding, and it correlates well with measured energy expenditure. In children this formula produces useless recommendations. The "junior" formula suggests a daily requirement as a function of the patient's age, where BMR is the basal metabolic rate.

0–1 year	BMR + 15 kcal/% burn
1–3 years	BMR + 25 kcal/% burn
4–15 years	BMR + 40 kcal/% burn

Nitrogen needs are more difficult to measure, and we currently estimate needs in adults at 3 g of nitrogen per kilogram body weight. Overfeeding with nitrogen is probably uncommon, so this formulation is probably safe. Furthermore, we look for changes in serum transferrin, prealbumin, and albumin as guides to the success of protein intake.

Some investigators have developed nutritional support that includes supplemental arginine (an immunoadjuvant that increases T cell function and a secretagogue for growth hormone), RNA, and ω-3 fatty acids. This formulation is commercially available and does seem to have attenuated some of the infectious complications seen in burn patients. It has spawned a series of tube feedings and a specialty called immunonutrition.

The major problem of feeding these patients is commonly the dictum of the anesthesiologist that the patient be NPO for at least 8 hours prior to the induction of general anesthesia. This is sometimes difficult when the patient is having the operation done emergently. Sometimes this rule is stretched to allow more time to feed the patient, with the anesthesiologist having to rely on the efficacy of the nasogastric tube to decompress the stomach prior to operation. Sometimes an empty stomach is a high price to be paid. Use of promotility agents has been advocated as a useful adjunct in these patients.

COMPLICATIONS OF BURN INJURY

Infection

With the successful resuscitation of the burned patient and a knowledge of airway problems, infection has been recognized as a major source of patient morbidity and mortality. The reasons are multifactorial, but current research has demonstrated major defects of the immune system in burn patients and in experimental animals subjected to burn injury.

The first part of the immune system of the burn patient that fails is the cutaneous barrier, which protects against bacterial invasion. Levels of opsonic proteins, which are cofactors for neutrophilic phagocytosis, decrease early in burn patients, recover over the next few days, and decrease again with episodes of sepsis. Early there may be defects in neutrophil migration and chemotaxis. T cell lymphocyte function is depressed, apparently consequent to an increase in the number of suppressor T cells (CD4) and a decrease in the number of T-helper cells (CD8). B-cell function and consequently circulating immunoglobulin levels decrease early and remain low, especially if the patient's nutritional status is not adequate. Complement levels fall, as complement seems to be "used up" by heat-damaged tissue. The fixed reticuloendothelial system functions poorly because of the loss of circulating fibronectin and other opsonic proteins.

How does this polyfactorial problem affect clinical care?

1. All personnel who have contact with the patient must practice strict, aseptic, sterile technique.
2. Infection must be suspected early and diligently sought if the patient deteriorates.
3. Prophylactic antibiotics are usually not indicated because, as indicated earlier, they lead to the selection of more virulent bacteria.

A significant advance in the prevention of infection in the burn patient has been the appropriate use of logically developed topical agents. These agents are applied to the burn wound initially and reapplied frequently. Each has its own peculiar advantages and disadvantages (Table 22.5).

Silvadene (1% silver sulfadiazine) is probably the most commonly used product. This white cream, developed by Dr. Charles Fox, is available in both proprietary (Hoechst-Marion Roussel) form and generic forms. Its bacteriologic activity comes from both the Ag$^+$ion and the polymerized sulfa compound. It is less effective against some *Pseudomonas* strains and most Enterobacteriaceae. It is well tolerated by patient and staff and is not painful when applied to the wound. Its major shortcoming is that is does not penetrate the eschar adequately. Many patients also develop a little-understood leukopenia after a few days' therapy. It is usually a self-limited process, and the patient's leukocyte count returns after the drug is discontinued. In some patients the drug is continued because of the absence of a therapeutic substitute, and the white blood cell count usually recovers as well.

Betadine Helafoam is a topical form of povidone-iodine and offers the advantage of increased penetration into the eschar. It is somewhat more painful on application but does not cause the bone marrow suppression seen with Silvadene. Frequent application over large areas may subject the patient to iodinism, though this occurs rarely if at all. At present, this formulation is an "orphan," having being abandoned by its previous manufacturer.

Sulfamylon (11% mafenide acetate) offers the deepest penetration into the eschar but is the most painful of the commonly used agents. The increased penetration makes this agent a common choice when other topical therapy has failed. It has a unique side effect, however,

which is secondary to its status as a carbonic anhydrase inhibitor. Patients treated with this agent may develop a metabolic acidosis and attempt to compensate by hyperventilating. Mafenide has been found useful for preventing chondritis in patients with ear burns. Like Silvadene, Sulfamylon is a sulfa compound and should be avoided in patients with allergies to sulfas or with glucose-6-phosphate dehydrogenase (G6PD) deficiency.

Silver nitrate (0.5%) is less commonly used now than in the past. Its use necessitates very wet dressings and predisposes the patient to major electrolyte disturbances, especially hyponatremia and hypochloremia. It is a difficult preparation with which to work because it stains everything black with which it has contact: patient, bedsheets, floor, and nursing and medical staff alike. It is, however, an effective agent for sterilizing a wound, and its electrolyte composition has been of value in patients managed with a hypertonic resuscitation regimen.

Antibiotic preparations are available but should be condemned because they combine the twin disadvantages of sensitizing the patient to the antibiotic and inducing the development of resistant strains of bacteria. The only single antibiotic agent commonly employed today is bacitracin, which is commonly applied on the face because of the possible eye and conjunctival irritation caused by other preparations. Bacitracin and Silvadene are commonly used for outpatient burn therapy.

The value of topical antifungal agents has been demonstrated in several centers, nystatin powder being mixed with Silvadene and other topical agents. The incidence of systemic candidiasis was markedly reduced by this regimen as was the incidence of recovering *Candida* from the burn wound. Many centers previously used nystatin (Mycostatin) orally to decrease the incidence of systemic candidiasis. Our practice is to use Silvadene and Sulfamylon at alternate dressing changes and to add nystatin powder for patients with large surface area burns.

The patient is at risk of infection from a variety of sources. Respiratory tract infections have already been alluded to and defy prophylactic therapy. Intravenous lines must be changed frequently, certainly every 48 hours. Central venous catheters and especially Swan-Ganz catheters are removed as expeditiously as possible. Routine over wire changes remain controversial and have been abandoned in the typical SICU patient. Patients managed with a Swan-Ganz catheter appear to be at increased risk of developing endocarditis, which is most often caused by *Staphylococcus aureus*.

The risk of a wound infection is a peculiar problem in the burn patient, and the wound must be assessed frequently, at least daily. Signs of infection include cellulitis at the border of the wound, conversion of partial-thickness to full-thickness burns, and the development of hemorrhagic changes in the wound. A burn wound infection is definitively diagnosed by burn wound biopsy. A colony count of more than 10^5 organisms per gram of wet tissue is an indication of a burn wound infection. In some hospitals a frozen section of the burn wound can be obtained and read by the pathologist. The presence of invasive microorganisms establishes the diagnosis.

Therapy of this infection is determined by the patient's clinical status. The topical agent is usually changed to one with increased eschar penetration. If this management is unsuccessful in decreasing the colony count, subeschar clysis injection of an appropriate antibiotic may be considered. The patient probably needs parenteral therapy, and an infected burn wound frequently requires prompt excision.

The clinical correlates of burn wound sepsis must be mentioned. The traditional markers of infection—increased white blood cell count and fever—are not always reliable. The patient may have a fever or be hypothermic. Leukocyte counts may be increased or extremely low. The patient commonly manifests mental confusion, develops an ileus, and demonstrates a decreased platelet count. Burn wound sepsis is not merely a complication; it can prove fatal.

The most common infection in the burn patient continues to be pneumonia; although it is seen much more often in the intubated patient, it also occurs in the nonintubated patient. Similar to the pattern seen in the burn wound, early pneumonias are commonly caused by gram-positive organisms such as *Steptococcus* and *Staphylococcus aureus* (which is often methicillin-resistant). The later pneumonias (more than 7 days after hospitalization) are caused by gram-negative organisms.

Curling's Ulcer

Acute upper gastrointestinal bleeding in the burn patient from Curling's ulcer was once fairly common, analogous to the incidence of Cushing's ulcer in patients in the SICU. This complication has been largely eliminated, largely due to three improvements in our knowledge and care of the patient. First, our increased ability to resuscitate the patient prevents shock and decreases gastric perfusion. Second, our ability to alkalinize the stomach with antacids or to inhibit acid production with H_2 blockers decreases gastric acid secretion and lessens the risk of mucosal injury and bleeding. Finally, we have learned the importance of feeding the patient, a process that effectively buffers gastric acid in the stomach and provides nutrition, thereby allowing repair of injury.

Other Gastrointestinal Complications

Acalculous cholecystitis can occur in any critically ill patient, especially those who have been deprived of enteral nutrition. Although reported in burn patients, this complication is relatively uncommon today. It is seen primarily in patients who are septic and whose concomitant ileus makes enteral feeding impossible. Patients with extreme weight loss in the burn unit are candidates for duodenal obstruction from an superior mesenteric artery (SMA) syndrome, although it is uncommon today. Acute colon dilatation has been seen in septic burn patients probably as a consequence of a low-flow state. It has been known to progress to transmural necrosis, and a few patients have required emergency colonic resection.

Marjolin's Ulcer

Marjolin's ulcer is a complication unique to burn patients in which a squamous cell carcinoma develops in an unstable burn scar consequent to a full-thickness burn injury. These aggressive tumors develop late after injury and are thought to be secondary to the chronic injury in the wound with a continuing stimulus to healing. They should be of historical significance only, as few surgeons would observe a wound in this state for long.

QUESTIONS

1. A 40-year-old 60-kg woman is admitted with second and third degree flame burns to 40% of her body. What is her estimated fluid needs according to the Parkland formula?
   a. 4,800 ml.
   b. 6,400 ml.
   c. 9,600 ml.
   d. 14,000 ml.

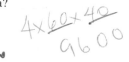

2. Resuscitation with hypertonic fluids usually requires:
   a. Less fluid than the Parkland formula.
   b. More fluid than the Parkland formula.
   c. As much fluid as the Parkland formula.

3. Which of the following topical agents penetrates the eschar best?
   a. Silvadene.
   b. Sulfamylon.
   c. Betadine.
   d. Dakin's solution.

4. The risk of renal failure in patients with electrical injuries can be decreased with:
   a. Induction of diuresis with mannitol.
   b. Alkalinization of urine.
   c. Prompt excision of necrotic tissue.
   d. All of the above.

5. By the Curreri formula, the estimated daily caloric needs of an 80-kg burn patient with burns to 50% of his body is:
   a. 4,000 kcal.
   b. 6,000 kcal.
   c. 3,000 kcal.
   d. 5,500 kcal.

6. Silver nitrate used as a topical agent is associated with:
   a. Hypochloremia and hyponatremia.
   b. Hypochloremia and hypernatremia.
   c. Hyperchloremia and hypernatremia.
   d. Hyperchloremia and hyponatremia.

7. The half-life of carboxyhemoglobin in patients treated with 100% oxygen at one atmosphere pressure is:
   a. 4 Hours.
   b. 2 Hours.
   c. 1 Hour.
   d. 15 Minutes.

8. Burn patients should be treated with succinylcholine:
   a. Never.

b. Not after the first week following the burn injury.
c. Whenever clinically indicated (e.g., for intubation).

9. Specific therapy for a patient with hydrofluoric acid injury includes:
   a. Magnesium.
   b. Topical Sulfamylon.
   c. Calcium.
   d. Potassium.

10. Escharotomy requires:
    a. Operating room and general anesthesia.
    b. Operating room but no anesthesia.
    c. Neither operating room nor anesthesia.
    d. Anesthesia but not the operating room.

SELECTED REFERENCES

Artz CP, Moncrief JA, Pruitt BA Jr. *Burns—a team approach.* Philadelphia: WB Saunders, 1979;4–5.

Barlow Y. T lymphocytes and immunosuppression in the burned patient: a review. *Burns* 1994;20:487–490.

Nguyen TT, Gilpin DA, Meyer NA, Herndon DN. Current treatment of severely burned patients. *Ann Surg* 1996;223: 14–25.

Pruitt BA Jr. The burn patient. I. Initial care. II. Later care and complications of thermal injury. *Curr Probl Surg* 1979;16. (An excellent monograph not diminished by the years since its publication.)

Pruitt BA Jr, ed. Progress symposium—progress in burn care. *World J Surg* 1992;16:1–96. (An up-to-date review of many of the major problem areas in burn care today. Not recommended for neophytes.)

Pruitt BA Jr, Goodwin CA Jr, Pruitt SK. Burns, including cold, chemical and electric injuries. *In:* Sabiston DC Jr, ed. *Textbook of surgery,* 15th ed. Philadelphia: WB Saunders, 1997; 221–252. (A good review covering many aspects of contemporary burn management.)

Purdue GF, Hunt JL. Inhalation injuries and burns in the inner city. *Surg Clin North Am* 1991;71:385–397.

Rose JK, Barrow RE, Desair MH, Herndon DN. Advances in burn care. In: *Advances in surgery,* vol 30, St. Louis: Mosby-Year Book, 1997.

23

Surgical Critical Care

Steven A. Blau

The American Board of Surgery has placed increasing emphasis on the role of critical care in the education of the general surgeon. This emphasis has meant a recommendation of increased experience in the surgical intensive care unit (SICU) by residents and an increased emphasis on critical care issues both on the annual in-service examination and on the "Boards." The Board has offered, starting in 1987, a certificate of "Added Qualification in Surgical Critical Care" as recognition of the increased education many have acquired. The above notwithstanding, the surgeon is even less involved in the care of his or her patients than ever. Most SICUs in the United States are being run by internists and anesthesiologists, many of whom are certified in pulmonary medicine or intensive care. The picture in "combined" units is even bleaker.

It is obvious that with a large amount of material germane to critical care, this chapter must be considerably less than complete. The explosion of important material in this area makes a truly up-to-date summary of care even more difficult. This chapter could not possibly substitute for the material gained during months of caring for patients in the SICU and using departmental libraries and the wealth of clinical consultants as educational sources. It is designed, instead, to stress those concepts with which the reader is probably already familiar and to reinforce the reader's bedside experiences.

In the years between the second and third editions of this book, a number of important new innovations have become popular in critical care, and many more ideas are moving from the laboratory to clinical application in controlled populations. The greatest activity seems to have been, though, deep introspection and an attempt to "prove" the validity of a large number of concepts, interventions, and management schemes that were generally assumed to be valid and correct. In this regard, we intensivists lack the authority of our colleagues in surgical oncology, for instance, in not having conducted our own large-scale, multicenter, doubled-blind clinical studies.

SHOCK

It has been more than a century since Samuel Gross defined shock as the "rude unhinging of the machinery of life." This Victorian concept, although obviously imprecise and often repeated in derision, is interesting in that it views shock as a process. The "modern" definition—that shock represents a point where tissue perfusion is inadequate for the needs of the cell or the point at which inadequate oxygen is provided the cell—may be a bit more precise, but it is certainly drier. These modern definitions fail to consider shock as a dynamic state where there is an insult to the organ, tissue, or organism and a physiologic response to that insult. They are helpful, though, for focusing the initial discussion of shock on events that occur at the cellular level. In the simplest terms, the cell requires perfusion to deliver to it supplies of oxygen and energy substrate (to metabolize to produce energy) and as a means of ridding itself of waste products.

Cells exist bathed in interstitial fluids whose electrolytic constitution resembles that of plasma. Whereas the "outside" of the cell is characterized by high sodium (130 to 140 mEq/L) and low potassium (4 to 5 mEq/L) concentrations, the relation of the two cations is reversed within the cell. Intracellular sodium is low (only about 10 to 15 mEq/L) and potassium high (about 100 mEq/L). This difference creates an electrical potential across the cell membrane. Cellular integrity is dependent on the exclusion of sodium and water from the cell, and it is maintained by the membrane-bound, ATP-dependent, magnesium-requiring sodium/potassium pump.

To maintain the electrical potential of the cell membrane and to "drive" the pump, the cell must produce energy. Normally, this energy is produced by the aerobic metabolism of glucose, which is converted to carbon dioxide and water. The metabolic pathways traversed include the Embden-Meyeroff glycolytic pathway (in which glucose is cleaved into two three-carbon fragments) and the Kreb's tricarboxylic cycle. The net yield of this aerobic glycolysis of 1 mol of glucose is 38 mol of ATP (18 mol of ATP per three-carbon fragment in the Krebs cycle plus 2 mol of ATP for the production of pyruvate).

In shock, adequate oxygen is not provided to the cell, which must then metabolize glucose by an alternative pathway, namely anaerobic glycolysis. The end-product of this metabolic pathway is lactate and the yield a paltry 2 mol of ATP per mole of glucose. This deficiency of energy production leads directly to failure of the pump, with inflow of sodium and water and a decrease in the electrical potential across the cell membrane. Prolonged dysfunction of the "pump" leads to cell death, either immediately or upon reconstitution of effective perfusion. At a biochemical level, then, shock results in lactic acidosis.

Lactic acidosis as a marker of shock entered the clinical world with the observations of the American physiologist Walter B. Cannon in the fields of France during World War I. The lactate level is predictive of the risk of death in some series and has been used as a guide for resuscitation of patients by many clinicians, especially those who advocate resuscitation to "supranormal" endpoints of cardiac output. Lactate can be cleared more rapidly by the infusion of dichloroacetate, but this measure has not been associated with any meaningful reduction in mortality. An additional caveat to the emphasis on lactate as a marker of ischemia is that it may alternatively be produced by inhibition of pyruvate dehydrogenase, leading to the accumulation of pyruvate outside the mitochondria and thus production of lactate, a condition seen in experimental endotoxemia. Finally, lactate must be remembered as a cellular substrate that can be utilized by such tissues as heart (where it may be a preferred fuel) and brain.

Moving from shock at the cellular level to shock at the organism level, the clinician recognizes a number of shock states. Indeed, clinicians have become taxonomists of shock. The following two-compartment model of shock is a simplification of Blalock's schema and serves to describe all clinically relevant forms of shock. Shock may be categorized as a defect in a pump (the heart) or in a fluid-filled container (the intravascular space and fluid within it).

Cardiogenic shock, then, may be defined as an isolated pump defect. Clinically, this state may occur in a patient with an acute myocardial infarction who cannot adequately contract the left ventricle, in a patient with acute pulmonary embolism whose right ventricle cannot empty against the increased pulmonary vascular resistance, or in a patient with cardiac tamponade who cannot fill the chambers of the heart.

Surgeons must deal with the events that usually affect the second compartment of the model. Conditions where the volume in the container decreases include hypovolemic and hemorrhagic shock. Conditions where the container becomes larger (and therefore "less full") include septic shock (in which endotoxemia causes relaxation of precapillary arteriolar sphincter tone) and neurogenic or spinal shock (in which vascular tone is decreased). In anaphylactic shock there is a similar effective expansion of the vascular space.

Two clinical conditions exhibit properties suggesting that these forms of shock occur secondary to defects in both compartments. The burn patient, for one, has a marked fall in intravascular volume secondary to fluid losses into the atmosphere, the burn wound, and cells. Some investigators believe that there is also a defect in myocardial performance. This was first ascribed to ill-defined circulating burn toxins, then to a specific myocardial depressant factor, and now to some oxygen-derived free radical. In experimental models, ventricular performance can be improved by free radical scavengers such as superoxide dismutase. The second condition is acute pancreatitis, in which fluid losses are consequent to peritonitis and retroperitoneal weeping. These patients also exhibit a similar pump defect that is thought to be secondary to a myocardial depression factor elaborated in this condition. This myocardial depressant factor is better described in animal experiments than in the human condition.

Hemorrhagic Shock

Hemorrhagic shock may be subclassified into four states based on the degree of blood loss in a schema derived from the American College of Surgeon's Advanced Trauma Life Support (ATLS) Course. This description also demonstrates the graded physiologic responses of the patient. The reader must note as well that these physiologic observations are consistent with those seen in otherwise healthy young adults, and that a less healthy or older patient may be unable to maintain an adequate blood pressure in the face of less severe blood loss. Concomitant organ dysfunction or concurrent medications may further blunt these homeostatic physiologic responses.

The patient with a class I hemorrhage has suffered a loss of about 10% of the intravascular volume (for a 70-kg man that is about 1 unit of whole blood). The patient is alert but may be a bit lightheaded. The blood pressure is normal, and the major organs are satisfactorily perfused as seen by a normal urine output. Less important vascular beds such as the skin have not been sacrificed.

The patient has compensated for the blood loss by a tachycardia, that is, by increasing the heart rate. Physiologically, this response is effected by secretion of catecholamines and an increase in sympathetic tone. The impetus to this catecholamine response is probably a transient decrease in pressure as recognized by aortic arch baroreceptors. Catecholamines also produce vasoconstriction as less important vascular beds are "closed," but this situation is not usually perceived with such a relatively minor blood loss. This change in vascular resistance is described as a change in afterload.

In the language of the model, the body adjusts to the decreased vascular content by making the container smaller and increasing the work of the pump. It is important to realize that the intravascular space is repleted over the ensuing hours with the movement of fluid from the interstitial space to the vascular space. This movement follows the Starling relation and is discussed in greater detail later in the chapter.

As the blood loss increases to about 20% to 25% of the blood volume the patient develops a class II hemorrhage. He or she is likely to be confused and combative. Although the mean arterial blood pressure is normal, the pulse pressure (systolic minus diastolic pressure) has narrowed. Urine output has decreased. The skin is cool and moist. The patient is manifesting further effects of catecholamine release along with some degree of decreased perfusion. The mental status reflects in part the "flight or fight" reaction to sympathetic discharge and some degree of cerebral hypoxemia. The change in pulse pressure is consistent with increased vasoconstriction, as with shunting of the available circulatory output from less critical vascular beds such as the skin.

The patient with a class III hemorrhage has lost about 35% to 40% of the blood volume and can no longer maintain his blood pressure. He has sought to maintain cardiac output by increasing the heart rate and increasing afterload. The mental examination demonstrates stupor. Urine output has decreased further. Additional bleeding brings the patient to a class IV hemorrhage, with coma and blood pressure incompatible with life. This patient requires prompt therapeutic intervention for survival.

Hemodynamic Monitoring

The goal of therapy for hemorrhagic or hypovolemic shock is restoration of cardiac output by replacing the volume losses from the vascular tree. Physiologically, one must measure the preload. The filling pressure of the heart can be assessed by a variety of increasingly invasive maneuvers: visual inspection of the neck veins, placement of a central venous line, and placement of a pulmonary artery or Swan-Ganz catheter.

Bedside inspection and examination of neck veins is simply not reliable enough in the setting of acute care and was long ago replaced by direct measurement of the central venous pressure (CVP). It cannot be stated too often that central lines are introduced for the purpose of *monitoring,* not for *treating,* the patient in shock. Their small caliber and relatively long length make them generally inadequate for infusion of large quantities of fluid, where resistance varies with the fourth power of the radius. The CVP directly measures the filling pressure of the right heart and does not specifically indicate anything about the intravascular volume status. A patient with continued blood loss may have a high CVP because the cardiac mechanism is incapable of pumping the little intravascular volume available.

The "gold standard" for measuring the filling pressure of the heart is to measure the preload presented not to the right ventricle but to the left ventricle. Although in otherwise healthy patients without cardiopulmonary disease the two filling pressures are nearly identical, the same cannot be said for patients with previous cardiac or pulmonary disease. Ventricular dysfunction secondary to myocardial infarction, for instance, may produce ventricles of different mechanical efficiency. Severe pulmonary disease with chronic cor pulmonale renders the right ventricle filling pressures (as determined by the CVP) of little value for assessing the filling of the less damaged left ventricle. The Swan-Ganz catheter allows direct determination of this filling pressure and the cardiac output.

The Swan-Ganz catheter is usually introduced via the subclavian vein into the right atrium of the heart and passed through the tricuspid valve into the right ventricle. It can be advanced safely via the internal jugular vein, but this approach makes a stable dressing more difficult and increases the risk of an infected line. It can also be advanced via the femoral vein, but this method seems more difficult and some clinicians have reported an increase in arrhythmias acutely and an increase in infection using this approach. The casual observations by surgeons are apparently correct as lines placed by anesthesiologists are associated with a marked increase in the incidence of infection. Proper placement of the catheter is usually achieved by observing the pressure waves measured at its tip as it traverses the chambers of the heart. The chest radiograph obtained after placement is usually performed to determine the presence of a pneumothorax or to determine which pulmonary vasculature has been entered (important if the patient is to be placed in a lateral decubitus position in the operating room) The reader is referred to standard texts for a description of the waveforms encountered as the catheter is placed. The "balloon" is inflated with the catheter in the right ventricle, and the tip of the catheter is carried downstream along the pulmonary outflow track into the pulmonary artery. The balloon is deflated to confirm a satisfactory pulmonary artery pressure tracing, and the catheter is secured in position if reinflation produces the expected dampened tracing of the "wedged" pulmonary artery. The "wedge" pressure (technically, the pulmonary artery capillary wedge pressure or the pulmonary artery occlusion pressure) is usually greater than the pulmonary artery diastolic pressure (except with a pulmonary embolism, where the pulmonary artery diastolic pressure is increased in response to the augmentation of pulmonary vascular resistance).

Swan-Ganz catheters are indicated for the sicker patient in whom preexisting conditions render the CVP reading inaccurate. Numerous studies have shown that patients managed pre- and intraoperatively with Swan-Ganz catheters do better than those managed without them, especially if there is adequate time to optimize cardiac function. Their efficacy when placed postoperatively is more difficult to confirm. The decision to place a Swan-Ganz catheter should not be considered lightly, however. The risk of complications is greater with these than with CVP catheters. Neglecting the risks attendant on subclavian venous puncture (which are common to both), the patient has a markedly increased risk of cardiac arrhythmias during both placement and manipulation and so long as the catheter traverses two cardiac chambers. Valvular lesions have been reported with catheters that have been maintained for long periods. Catheters that have been wedged for long periods may produce pulmonary infarctions. The balloon may even tear the pulmonary artery and cause fatal bleeding. This problem is demonstrated clinically by the acute onset of hemoptysis after balloon inflation; emergency surgery can sometimes be avoided by retracting the catheter and inflating the balloon to tamponade the bleeding site. The infectious risks of Swan-Ganz catheters may be greater than for CVP catheters (possibly because of their longer length), but the incidence of left-sided endocarditis is definitely increased. Swan-Ganz catheters do not by themselves improve patient outcome. Misinterpretation of the data obtained and therapeutic misadventures in response to that data outweigh any potential benefits. Retrospective studies to assess the role of the Swan-Ganz catheter in clinical practice have suggested that these catheters, in use since the early 1970s, are not panaceas.

Cardiac output may be measured directly with the Swan-Ganz catheter in place by the dye dilution technique using the Fick principle or by thermodilution. The latter is performed far more commonly. Although accuracy is increased with higher-volume, lower-temperature injectates, even room temperature injections are reproducible and adequate in clinical practice. Errors are less associated with warmer temperatures than with incorrect assumptions of the volume and temperature of the injectate. Injecting 10 ml of saline when the cardiac output computer "anticipates" 2 ml, results in a falsely low cardiac output. Low cardiac output can result when the patient has tricuspid insufficiency. With this measurement, "optimum" filling pressure may be determined. The Frank-Starling relation between end-diastolic fiber length and muscle contraction can be converted to the relation between the pulmonary artery capillary wedge pressure and the cardiac output. This point is illustrated in Fig. 23.1. The normal response demonstrates that increased wedge pressure increases cardiac output only to a point, beyond which increases in filling pressure produce virtually no augmentation of the cardiac output. The second curve illustrates the failing myocardium. Two salient points are demonstrated here: (a) for a given wedge pressure the cardiac output is lower in the failing myocardium; and (b) there is a maximum wedge pressure beyond which cardiac output decreases.

It is possible (and necessary in elective circumstances) to generate a curve such as this to determine the optimum filling pressure of the heart. It is a mistake to assume that a given patient needs a certain filling pressure; it is individualized for each patient. Moreover, cardiac outputs should be determined at least in triplicate to avoid error. The physiologic distinction between these two curves is the fourth factor by which the cardiac output is controlled, contractility. The four factors, then, are contractility, rate, afterload, and preload. These compensatory homeostatic mechanisms are, in reality, two-

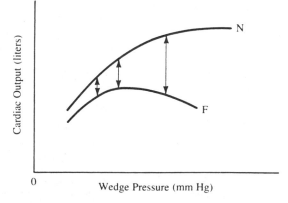

FIG. 23.1. Frank-Starling law of the heart. *F*, response with failing myocardium; *N*, normal response.

edged swords. The adverse effects of these intrinsic and therapeutic maneuvers are discussed further below.

Pulmonary Artery Catheter Controversy

Despite its clinical use for nearly 30 years and the annual insertion of more than 1.5 million catheters, the Swan-Ganz catheter's use continues to be controversial, with an increasing number of papers questioning its ultimate value in medical and surgical patients. It is generally agreed that the filling pressures determined by these catheters provide information at odds with that attained by the bedside clinician. It is also accepted that the data obtained using these catheters can precipitate a change in clinical management. Not everyone is convinced that those changes are appropriate or that the numbers are always valid. Incorrect filling pressures can be attributed to mis-zeroed pressure transducers, incorrect interpretation of the pressure waveform, malposition and inconsistent positioning of the patient, misplacement of the catheter, errors in inflating the balloon, and so on. The gold standard for generating a wedge pressure remains a flat patient, a "hard copy" rather than a quick view on a monitor screen, and always using the pressure at the end of exhalation. Examples of catheter waveforms are included in Fig. 23.2. Clinical controversy extends to the determination of cardiac output as well.

The major problem, though, is that Swan-Ganz catheters do not cure patients by themselves. They are not antibiotics or vaccines. Once the proper data are obtained, what to you do with it? If the goal is to "normalize" cardiac output and filling pressures, we are not asking a lot of the device and are probably being rewarded. Not every patient can evidence a "normal" output at a "normal" filling pressure. Most of the clinical studies with this endpoint have failed to prove the value of the pulmonary artery catheter. Some studies, striving for "hyperdynamic" indices, have shown benefit, although mostly in the hands of a few investigators. Other studies have demonstrated that many patients, especially the elderly, cannot reach these cardiac milestones. Here the clinical failure is not the catheter's fault, although it takes the blame.

Septic Shock

Septic shock represents another form of shock where the fluid-filled container of the model is the source of the disturbance. Here endotoxins elaborated by gram-

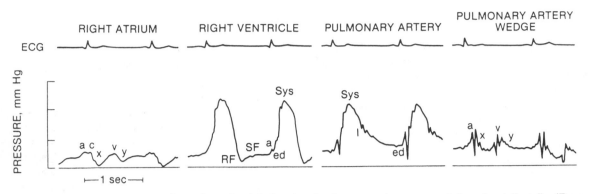

FIG. 23.2. Normal-pressure waveforms from the right heart and pulmonary artery. *sys,* systolic; ed, ed-diastolic. (From Grossman W, Barry WH. Cardiac catheterization. In: Braunwald E, ed. *Heart disease: a textbook of cardiovascular medicine.* Philadelphia. WB Saunders, 1988;250.)

negative bacteria "turn on" a cascade of intrinsic mediators that ultimately affect the precapillary arteriolar sphincters, relaxing them and causing an increase of the intravascular space. In the language of the model, the container is now larger and therefore less full. Importantly, the increased vascular space results in pooling, not in an increase in the delivery of circulation to the tissues that require it. The effective perfusion, in fact, decreases. The clinical clue that the patient is in septic shock is a reflection of this change in vascular status: The skin is usually warm to the touch, not cold and clammy as is the skin of the patient in hypovolemic or hemorrhagic shock.

The therapy of septic shock must include elimination of the source of sepsis as the initial goal. In reality, however, this step takes a back seat to dealing with the expanded vascular space. Therapy here is directed toward filling the container by increasing the volume in the vascular space. The role of corticosteroids is controversial, with the current literature demonstrating little benefit. More interesting and perhaps of much greater clinical benefit are monoclonal antibodies directed against endotoxin (see Pharmacologic Interventions, below).

More Hemodynamic Monitoring

The Swan-Ganz catheter allows one to demonstrate the change in vascular dynamics by a number of means. The vascular resistance can be calculated in both halves of the circulatory circuit: the systemic vascular resistance (SVR) for the peripheral circulation and the pulmonary vascular resistance (PVR) for the pulmonary circulation (Fig. 23.3). The equation used is analogous to the familiar Ohm's law equations, where R (resistance) is a function of change in pressure (or voltage) divided by cardiac output (or current).

$$SVR = 80 \times (MAP - CVP)/CO$$
$$PVR = 80 \times (mean\ PA - wedge)/CO$$

where MAP is the mean arterial pressure; mean PA is the mean pulmonary artery pressure; wedge is the wedge pressure; and CO is cardiac output.

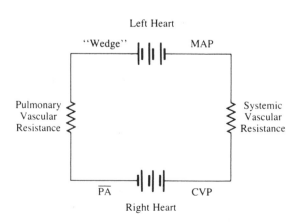

FIG. 23.3. Cardiac circuit diagram. *Wedge,* wedge pressure; *MAP,* mean arterial pressure; *PA,* mean pulmonary artery pressure; *CVP,* central venous pressure.

Care must be taken in these and subsequent calculations that the user remembers whether the cardiac output or the cardiac index (which normalizes cardiac output for surface area) is used. Although either number may be used, interpretations of the data are predicated on using the proper normals. SVR, for instance, is normally 1,200 to 1,400 dynes/sec/cm^{-5}, or 1,800 to 3,000 dynes/sec/cm^{-5}/M^2.

Systemic vascular resistance is increased in conditions in which the vascular resistance would be expected to increase, that is, hypovolemic or hemorrhagic shock. It is decreased in septic shock and can be decreased in cirrhosis (where arteriovenous shunts are open in the liver) and with aggressive overhydration where capacitance vessels are open to allow the increased fluid load. The SVR must be remembered as a construct that reflects an arbitrary model. It does not indicate where the vascular resistance is decreased or increased. The body, it must be recalled, attempts to maintain circulation to the most critical of organs (brain and heart) while depriving less important tissues (e.g., skin and the splanchnic circulation).

The opening of these sphincters in septic shock results in shunting blood away from the arterial system and into the venous system without feeding a nutrient vessel. This shunting is also reflected in another Swan-Ganz parameter, the arteriovenous (A-V) oxygen difference. The oxygen content of the radial artery is a measure of the most saturated blood in the body. With the catheter in the pulmonary artery one can calculate the oxygen content of the desaturated blood, which reflects the net effect of all tissues extracting oxygen from the blood. Measurements obtained by substituting central venous blood for mixed venous are not absolutely correct, but the differences are not sufficient to obscure the clinical picture. It should be remembered, incidentally, that mixed venous blood is not the most desaturated blood available, a status accorded to blood in the coronary sinus where oxygen has been extracted by the functioning heart muscle. Thus

Arterial oxygen content = saturation × 1.34 × hemoglobin (g/dL)

Mixed venous oxygen content = saturation × 1.34 × hemoglobin (g/dL)

A-V oxygen difference = arterial − mixed venous oxygen content

where saturation is the fractional saturation of the blood gas, 1.34 is a coefficient reflecting the oxygen-carrying

capacity of 1 g of hemoglobin, and the hemoglobin is expressed in grams per deciliter. The A-V oxygen difference is normally 3 to 5 mL/dL.

The difference between the content of the arterial and venous bloods is, as mentioned above, a measure of both A-V shunting and the metabolic activity of the body. The A-V oxygen difference is increased in conditions of inadequate tissue perfusion, wherein the tissue tries to extract as much oxygen as it can. It is decreased in patients in septic shock and somewhat in patients with cirrhosis and portal hypertension.

The product of the A-V oxygen difference and the cardiac output (or cardiac index) is a reflection of net oxygen utilization by the body and is the most direct measure of the "hypermetabolic" state. This number can also be generated by bedside indirect calorimetry as described in Chapter 31.

One cannot introduce the matter of oxygen consumption without discussing oxygen extraction. Most of the oxygen transported by the blood is attached to hemoglobin. The classic S-shaped oxyhemoglobin dissociation curve illustrates the binding of oxygen to the carrier molecule (Fig. 23.4). The right side of the curve demonstrates that increases in the partial pressure of oxygen at high levels do not significantly increase oxygen saturation. Therefore there is no reason to keep a patient's P_{O_2} higher than that which produces more than 90% saturation. The left side of the curve indicates that

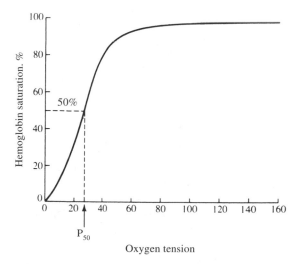

FIG. 23.4. Oxyhemoglobin dissociation curve.

the unloading of oxygen from hemoglobin becomes progressively more difficult at lower saturations. The increased A-V oxygen difference observed in a patient in cardiogenic shock may not reflect the physiologic needs of the tissues.

The factors that affect the dissociation of oxygen from hemoglobin are all clinically relevant. High temperatures, high partial pressures of carbon dioxide, and acidosis aid in oxygen extraction. This is teleologically understandable because there are the local conditions one would expect to find in the neighborhood of an exercising muscle. Clinically, this is a caveat against the overuse of sodium bicarbonate in shock states because it would tend to decrease the available oxygen to the tissues in need.

More important, perhaps, is the role of 2,3-diphosphoglycerate (2,3-DPG) in oxygen transport. 2,3-DPG is a product of red blood cell glycolysis. As the stored erythrocytes in the blood bank exhaust their supply of glucose, their intracellular content of 2,3-DPG decreases. The low levels of 2,3-DPG cause an increased affinity for oxygen by the hemoglobin molecule, rendering it less able to release oxygen to the tissues. This clinical problem is posed to the physician by the blood bank anxious to release the oldest blood from the backmost shelves of its refrigerator. This blood is relatively easy to oxygenate but holds onto its oxygen tightly and may further embarrass cellular respiration.

The classic teaching of septic shock as a hyperdynamic state with elevated cardiac output, decreased SVR, and decreased A-V oxygen difference is attainable only with optimum fluid replacement therapy and with a sound cardiac mechanism. The patient early in septic shock who has not yet received adequate fluids may not demonstrate a hyperdynamic state. Similarly, the patient in septic shock whose heart cannot meet the increased demand placed on it does not demonstrate the classic picture.

Although oxygen consumption (discussed above) can be determined from the A-V oxygen difference, this equation does not describe the reason for the value. The question to the surgeon must be whether a oxygen consumption is dependent on the oxygen delivered to the tissue or is independent of it. As seen in Fig. 23.5, oxygen consumption is *dependent* on oxygen delivery at low deliveries and independent at higher deliveries. Just as one must generate a family of curves at different filling pressures to determine optimum cardiac output, one should prove that a patient's oxygen consumption is flow-independent of delivery. This determination is

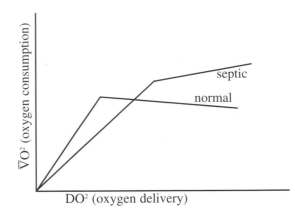

FIG. 23.5. Relation of oxygen consumption to oxygen delivery.

increasingly recognized as critical for care of the seriously ill. The combination of lactic acidosis with being at the "left" of the curve is associated with increased mortality.

The relation between oxygen delivery and consumption can be expressed as an "extraction," where extraction is oxygen consumption/oxygen delivery. Normal extraction is 25% to 35%. What can the surgeon do when the patient is extracting a higher percentage, especially if the consumption seems to be limited by oxygen delivery? To increase oxygen delivery, the physician can increase saturation, cardiac output, or hemoglobin. Increasingly, the dictum that the optimum hematocrit is 28% in the ICU patient is coming under attack and probably can be retired. For some patients, especially those in whom cardiac output cannot be increased, higher hematocrits are not only indicated they are efficacious. Hematocrits as high as the mid-30s are acceptable. The previous reticence to transfuse beyond the 10g limit was an erroneous assumption regarding the viscosity of blood. It is today bolstered by concerns about the transmission of blood-borne infections and the documented immunosuppression associated with autologous blood transfusions that has been demonstrated in the surgical oncology literature and almost as well in the trauma literature.

Regional Hemodynamics

At its best, the Swan-Ganz catheter measures global perfusion, but events may be occurring in one or another regional circulation that have clinical import but cannot be detected by this device. Global acidosis or lactic acidosis is a poor prognostic sign, but it may be observed too late to allow clinical manipulation of the patient and decrease the mortality associated with elevated lactate levels, for instance. The regional circulation of greatest concern at present is the splanchnic circulation because of the obvious concern for bacterial translocation. If acidosis or hypoperfusion in this region could be determined early, appropriate clinical intervention could be effected.

Gastric tonometry attempts to demonstrate this problem, and some investigators regard it as a remarkably useful tool. Others counter that the device measures something other than what it purports to and does not improve patient survival. First the physiology: Carbon dioxide production correlates with oxygen utilization. A carbon dioxide-permeable silicone balloon is introduced into the stomach and filled with saline. Abutting the gastric mucosa, the carbon dioxide content within the balloon equilibrates with that of the gastric wall. After 30 to 90 minutes of dwell time, the fluid is aspirated and the P_{CO_2} determined. The arterial bicarbonate is then determined from a simultaneously obtained arterial blood specimen, and this figure is used in the Henderson-Hasselbach equation to determine the "intramucosal" pH.

Patients with low intramucosal pH_i values have a higher mortality rate than those with normal pH, as do those who become acidotic. The advocates of this technique claim that the hypoperfusion demonstrated by this method precedes any evidence of hypoperfusion revealed by other means and demonstrates a need for more timely resuscitation or a trip back to the operating room. Reproducibility is a problem; and a decision based on a low pH_i on one determination may be obviated by a normal pH_i with the next determination. The patient cannot be fed intragastrically with the gastric tonometer in place, and gastric acid must be controlled with H_2 blockers or antacids.

Physiologic Responses

As alluded to above, the physiologic responses to maintain cardiac output are not without their drawbacks. The interventions that physicians add in attempts to control cardiac output are similarly problematic and must be used with as thorough an understanding as possible.

The increase in cardiac rate to compensate for decreased intravascular volume seems initially innocuous.

To achieve the increase in rate, the systolic time remains the same, but the diastolic time is shortened. Two important events occur during diastole: filling of the ventricles and perfusion of the heart via the coronary arteries. As the heart rate increases, the time available for filling the pumping chambers may shorten to the point that the effective stroke volume is reduced. This reduction may be sufficient to result in a net decrease in cardiac output, even as the heart rate is increasing.

The problems with coronary perfusion are even greater. As the heart rate increases, the mechanical work of the heart increases, and its consumption of oxygen increases. Yet the heart may be working so fast the coronary arteries are unable to meet that oxygen demand. Uncontrolled tachycardia, then, may lead to myocardial ischemia and infarction. The physiologic response of the heart is appropriate, but, if prolonged, the heart can literally beat itself to death.

The goal of optimizing cardiac output is reached by pushing the wedge pressure to the appropriate level dictated by the Frank-Starling relation. This preload, though, is the hydrostatic force of the other Starling equation, which describes the movement of fluid across the capillary membrane.

$$\text{Flow} = \text{capillary pressure difference} - (\rho \times \text{oncotic pressure difference})$$

where ρ is the variable indicating the permeability of the cell membrane. This driving force can lead to the accumulation of fluid in the lungs known as pulmonary edema. The problem is worsened if the fluid replacement effectively decreases the colloid oncotic properties of the intravascular space (as would be the case with massive infusions of crystalloid solutions, such as Ringer's lactate). Although the lung has the advantage of a dual blood supply and a rich network of lymphatics, their capacity to return interstitial fluid is not infinite. Increasing the wedge pressure, then, may increase cardiac output but may also embarrass oxygenation and ultimately worsen the patient's shock.

Cardiac contractility is amenable to improvement by the action of a number of pharmacologic agents. Unfortunately, with the possible exception of digoxin, these agents also increase myocardial oxygen consumption. Because of the aforementioned problem with cardiac perfusion, increasing oxygen consumption may result in myocardial ischemia.

Finally, the fourth component in the control of cardiac output, afterload, is a source of potential problems. Vasodilation may improve the performance of the heart but perhaps at the expense of tissue perfusion. On the other hand, pharmacologic intervention with vasopressors may maintain blood pressure but at the expense of increased cardiac work function.

NEUROENDOCRINE RESPONSES

In addition to the physiologic responses to shock that serve to return the cardiac output to normal and the cellular perfusion to a satisfactory level, there are a number of neuroendocrine changes elicited by the shock state. They are both beneficial and harmful to the patient.

Trauma results directly in increased levels of adrenocorticotropic hormone (ACTH) and subsequently in increased levels of the glucocorticoids. Elevated cortisol results in an increase in circulating glucose and free fatty acids, thereby increasing the availability of energy substrate to the cells. Prolonged stimulation by ACTH can result in adrenocortical hyperplasia and persistence of these metabolic changes for weeks to months.

A decrease in renal blood flow stimulates the production of angiotensin, which acts directly on the adrenal cortex to cause the production of aldosterone. ACTH is a cofactor in this aldosterone production. Aldosterone then acts on the kidney to increase sodium reabsorption (and along with it water) and potassium excretion. The water retention favors amelioration of the cardiac output deficit. The body also produces an increase in antidiuretic hormone (ADH) secretion to further decease net water losses from the kidney.

Catecholamines are elaborated as described earlier to increase vasoconstriction and tachycardia. Metabolically, the catecholamines inhibit the release of insulin and oppose the effects of circulating insulin. This decreases the availability of glucose at the cellular level and favors the burning of fatty acids. It also forces an increase in muscle protein catabolism. Simultaneously, glucagon levels increase, further diverting energy utilization away from glucose. The catecholamine response seems beneficial to the patient when it is brief and progressively detrimental if catecholamine release is prolonged.

Pharmacologic Interventions

As stated earlier, the basic pharmacologic intervention for shock states involving the fluid-filled compart-

ment is fluid. The choices for fluid include electrolyte solutions (sometimes referred to as crystalloid), colloid protein solutions, and blood. Fluid volume expansion with dextrans has been considered problematic with a significant risk of coagulopathy. When colloid and electrolyte solutions have been compared, colloid has generally failed to justify its increased cost, and some investigators have found that it causes additional problems. The optimum solution regimen probably includes a combination of the two with crystalloid infusions of the initial measure. The ultimate role of hypertonic solutions, with or without dextran or colloid, is unclear.

Blood transfusions are usually not indicated for class I and II hemorrhage unless the patient had a decreased red blood cell mass before the onset of shock. Experimental animal models have demonstrated the adverse effects of full replacement of shed blood with reinfused blood. Because of the redistribution of fluid (discussed below), the replacement for each milliliter of blood lost is 2.5 to 3.0 ml of crystalloid. Of course, smaller volumes are appropriate when the blood loss is early and the temporal physiology has not yet developed.

Pressors are usually inappropriate as first-line drugs for shock because they improve the blood pressure at the expense of further decreasing perfusion of capillary beds. However, while the patient is being resuscitated with fluids for volume expansion, pressors may be useful to support some regional vascular beds. Although autoregulation maintains cerebral perfusion as cardiac output declines because of vasodilatation consequent to increases in Pco_2, the cerebral circulation benefits from increases in blood pressure produced by pressors. Renal perfusion does not benefit from pressor-induced increases in blood pressure nor does perfusion of the mesenteric circulation. Renal-dose dopamine (see below) probably offers some protection for the patient treated with pressors by preserving renal artery flow. Norepinephrine (Levophed) is usually prepared at a concentration of 4 μg/mL by adding 4 mg to a liter of solution. Higher concentrations are useful when using high doses to avoid the large volumes of salt or sugar water. Drug administration is defined in micrograms per minute and doses of 5 to 10 μg are common. There are no maximal doses reported in the literature, and patients frequently require increased doses over time to maintain the same degree of vasoconstriction or to overcome the vasodilatation of sepsis. Neo-Synephrine is an alternative to norepinephrine.

Dopamine is commonly used as an adjunct for management of shock. Dosages of this drug are always given in micrograms per kilogram body weight per minute. The drug has three broadly different effects depending upon the dose given. At low doses (less than 3 to 5 μg/kg/min), the effect is stimulation of dopamine receptors along with some β-adrenergic activity. The cardiac rate is mildly increased, and there may be some augmentation of contractility. Splanchnic flow is maintained. Renal blood flow seems to be increased, and a net natriuresis ensues. As the dose of dopamine is increased, there is an increase in α-adrenergic effect but β-adrenergic activity predominates until the dose reaches about 10 to 15 μg/kg/min. Beyond that, the effect is nearly pure α-adrenergic, and dopamine offers little more than Levophed. It is important to note that the effectiveness of the drug is decreased by acidosis. Renal-dose dopamine is administered in many units with an unbridled enthusiasm, treating the drug as akin to mother's milk. Although safe, some patients, especially those with decreased intravascular volumes, exhibit a profound tachycardia even at low doses. Patients in atrial fibrillation seem especially sensitive to dopamine, and increasing the ventricular rate may be dangerous.

Dobutamine seems to have greater effect on cardiac contractility than does dopamine, and this effect is maintained even in the face of acidosis. The improved cardiac function, unfortunately, is associated with increased oxygen consumption by the myocardium. Initially the dose is 2.5 to 5.0 μg/kg/min, and it may be increased to 15 to 20 μg/kg/min.

Amrinone, a phosphodiesterase inhibitor, has come into increased use in the SICU. Like dobutamine, it increases cardiac output and is indicated in patients who already have an increased filling pressure. Initially, it was reserved until the patient was receiving a dose of dobutamine, but the combination of the two drugs seems better than either alone, and it is commonly used in this fashion. Milranone came into clinical practice later and avoids the antiplatelet problems of the earlier drug; it has largely displaced the earlier version from hospital formularies.

Isoproterenol may be used to increase the heart rate, but its effect on the peripheral circulation (vasoconstriction) is adverse to the needs of the patient. β-Dose dopamine is probably more useful for achieving this end, especially in patients whose normal chronotropic response is blocked by β-antagonists and calcium channel blockers.

Epinephrine also exhibits a two-phase response according to the infused dose, with β-adrenergic activity predominating at lower doses and α-adrenergic activity at higher doses. Although it enjoys fairly widespread use in children in ICUs, the arrhythmogenic potential decreases its value in adults. I have used it occasionally as a pressor in concert with other agents, such as norepinephrine and Neo-Synephrine.

Vasodilators may improve cardiac performance by decreasing cardiac work function. Most of these drugs (which includes nitroglycerin and topical nitrates) are means of administering nitric oxide.

Digoxin seems to improve cardiac contractility without significantly increasing the oxygen consumption of the heart. Its use for clinical shock states is equivocal because of questions about its rapidity of action. Although I was trained in an era where it was almost routine to digitalize the elderly patient in shock or suffering burns, unequivocal benefit was never demonstrated. The drug is indicated in patients with obvious congestive heart failure, and a surprising number of patients have never taken this agent before coming to the SICU. Moreover, digitalizing the patient forces the clinician to be even more vigilant regarding electrolyte abnormalities. Rapid-acting cardiac glycosides are being developed, and they may have a role here.

Steroids in septic shock have a checkered history. The older literature suggested a definite benefit, probably because of the effect of the steroid on stabilizing cell membranes. Clinical studies, although flawed, have failed to show the drug's benefit. It is unclear whether this represents poor methodology in the study or the ineffectiveness of the drug. As a last effort, when all else has failed, I have been tempted to resort to methylprednisolone at a dose of 30 mg/kg body weight. The dose is administered early along with antibiotics, fluid, and drainage of infected collections. Remember, though, that this intervention is not standard and has been frequently condemned. It is defensible, though, in patients who have been treated with steroids in the past who may still have a depressed pituitary–adrenal response, in those with documented adrenal failure (or after adrenalectomy), and in those who have pituitary failure.

Equally problematic has been the experience regarding the use of naloxone and other experimental opiate antagonists for septic shock. Researchers have demonstrated the role of endogenous endorphins in the vascular collapse of shock, suggested that blocking these substances with naloxone would improve survival. The experience in experimental animals is mixed, at best. The human data are nearly all anecdotal and reflect interventions in the preterminal setting. For today, though, they represent a failed intervention.

The experience with monoclonal antibodies directed against endotoxin and tumor necrosis factors represents another failure, to the investors and the companies that developed them and to the patients who could have used a novel innovation. The initial salutory clinical data for HA-1A (Centocor), for instance, which demonstrated decreased mortality in septic patients after treatment with this agent compared to placebo, was followed by a larger study that doomed the agent. Readers searching for innovative ways to treat septic shock should look to recent work on the extraction of circulating endotoxin by polymyxin-charged columns and work on free radical scavengers.

RESPIRATORY PHYSIOLOGY AND CARE

Basic Physiology

The basic principles of oxygen transport were described in some detail above. It is important to remember that at normal atmospheric pressure nearly all oxygen is transported coupled to the hemoglobin molecule. Carbon dioxide, on the other hand, is transported dissolved in plasma. Oxygen affinity for the carrier molecule is dictated by the oxyhemoglobin dissociated curve (Fig. 23.4).

Respiration is a property of all cells. Ventilation is a mechanical process designed to move gas through the lungs. Ventilation is maintained under close neurologic control and is modified as a consequence of acidosis and hypercapnia.

The patient's normal breathing produces a "tidal volume." The mathematic product of rate and tidal volume yields "minute ventilation." Maximum inspiratory effort produces a volume termed the "inspiratory capacity," which is the sum of the tidal volume and the inspiratory reserve (Fig. 23.6). This inspiratory reserve demonstrates the fact that most patients are breathing at less than maximum volumes. Similarly, with maximal exhalation patients are able to empty their "expiratory reserve volume." The patient is unable to empty the lungs of gas completely so there is always a "residual volume." It represents a physiologic deadspace. The ex-

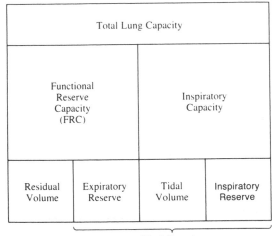

FIG. 23.6. Pulmonary volume spaces.

piratory reserve volume and the residual volume constitute the function residual capacity.

Ventilation and perfusion are closely linked in the intact patient. Blood is rapidly shunted away from areas of the lung that are not adequately ventilated. Similarly, interruption of blood flow soon results in collapse of the alveoli. This association is destroyed in conditions of ventilation–perfusion mismatch. Anatomically, there normally exists some mismatch, with three "zones" identified within the lung that were apparently consequent to humans attaining an erect posture millions of years ago. The upper lung fields are somewhat better ventilated than the perfused fields (zone I), and the lower (zone III) fields are better perfused than ventilated fields.

Alveoli remain distended because of the effects of pulmonary surfactant, a detergent produced by alveolar cells that serves to lower the surface tension. The absence of this substance in premature infants produces progressive alveolar collapse and a clinical condition known as hyaline membrane disease. Surfactant production is inhibited by high oxygen concentrations and in adults the respiratory distress syndrome (ARDS).

The goal of oxygenation of the patient is a partial pressure of oxygen sufficient to maintain arterial saturations in excess of 90%. Oxygen is administered to patients at a given Fio_2, and blood gases are expressed as the partial pressure of the gas, Po_2.

Breathing and Ventilation

Breathing is a mechanical process unconsciously performed by patients outside the hospital. The diaphragm and intercostal musculature work in tandem to produce a negative pressure, and the tidal volume is inhaled. Exhalation is effected by elastic recoil of the lungs and chest wall. Difficulties with breathing (in contrast to oxygenation) may be caused by problems with neuromuscular control and coordination or mechanical factors.

Patients with CNS depression, whether intrinsic or secondary to the effects of sedation, may lose control of their breathing. This may occur because of destructive lesions in the brain stem but is more commonly an effect of narcosis, with the result that hypercapnia does not trigger increased ventilation.

More important clinically is the loss of motor control produced by neuromuscular blocking agents. Here the "perception" of not breathing may be intact, but the patient cannot make the muscles do the work required. This is almost a mechanical factor in that the diaphragm and intercostal musculature are mechanically unable to do what is required of them. It is important to note that although the patient may be exposed to these agents in the operating room by the anesthesiologist the surgeon's simultaneous use of aminoglycosides may augment neuromuscular blockade.

The absence of medications may also serve to decrease breathing. Patients in pain soon "recognize" pleuritic components of pain or the effect of breathing deeply on peritoneal pain. This situation is seen in patients postoperatively and, along with the excessive sedation, is the principal cause of postoperative atelectasis.

Chest wall pain may also decrease the effectiveness of breathing in the presence of such conditions as chest wall contusion or rib fracture. Here the patient splints the ribs by the action of the intercostals and therefore decreases the effective depth of ventilation. It also leads to some degree of ventilation–perfusion mismatch. Flail chest represents an even worse case in which ventilatory volumes are decreased as the patient breathes in and are increased with exhalation. A pneumothorax also decreases the effective volume for ventilation.

Airway problems should not be overlooked as causes of inadequate breathing. Unconscious patients may occlude their airways with their tongue. Patients with facial or neck trauma have upper airway obstruction from debris or laryngeal injury.

In general, changes in the partial pressure of carbon dioxide (Pco_2) represent changes in ventilation. Changes in the partial pressure of oxygen (Po_2) reflect changes in V/Q mismatch or reflect barriers to the movement of oxygen from the alveolar space to the arterial space; they include such conditions as ARDS and pulmonary edema. Although elevations in Pco_2 can occur with increased production of carbon dioxide, it is more likely to represent a decrease in minute ventilation. The difference between the partial pressure of oxygen in the alveolar and arterial spaces yields the A-a gradient, where

$$P_AO_2 \text{ (alveolar partial pressure)} = Fio_2 \times \text{atmospheric pressure} - PH_2O - Pco_2/\text{respiratory quotient}$$

and P_aO_2 is directly measured.

$$\text{A-a gradient} = P_AO_2 - P_aO_2$$

The partial pressures of all the gases in the alveolus must total the atmospheric pressure. Two gases are present in the alveolus that are not present in inspired dry gas: water and carbon dioxide. The partial pressure of water at 37°C and one atmosphere is 47 mm Hg. Therefore the alveolar partial pressure of oxygen is 713 × Fio_2 less the partial pressure of carbon dioxide divided by the respiratory quotient. Normally, the A-a gradient is 5 to 10 mm Hg. In the supine, intubated patient, the "best" A-a gradient is about 100 mm Hg.

Therapeutic Interventions

Management of the patient with inadequate ventilation requires first the physician's assumption of responsibility for breathing the patient and the prompt recognition of problems that have led to the situation. As indicated above, sedation should be discontinued if indicated, neuromuscular blockade should be reversed, pneumothoraces should be aspirated, and so on. To ventilate the patient adequately, the physician must control the airway. Mechanical obstructions must be removed. The tracheobronchial tree may be approached emergently with cricothyrotomy (which has largely replaced tracheostomy as an emergency procedure in the field or in the emergency room).

More commonly the patient is intubated. Endotracheal intubation is easier, but nasotracheal intubation may be better tolerated by the patient. Although low-pressure, low-volume endotracheal tubes can allegedly be maintained for 3 to 4 weeks without adverse sequelae, tracheostomy is usually considered if the patient continues to require intubation at 10 to 14 days. The timing of tracheostomy, however, continues to be controversial. Some studies have demonstrated a significant reduction in nosocomial pneumonia when tracheostomy is performed within the first 5 days of admission. Unfortunately, it is not always easy to predict which patients will need ventilatory support days in advance. Determination of "work-of-breathing," by analysis of pressure–volume curves or measurement of oxygen consumption by indirect calorimetry, may aid in deciding when to perform tracheostomy. The availability of bedside percutaneous tracheostomy may decrease the interval between the patient's needing the procedure and the surgeon performing it.

Preoperative Assessment and Management

Many patients admitted to the hospital already have preexisting pulmonary insufficiency. Patients with chronic obstructive lung diseases have an increased functional deadspace. A portion of their tidal volume does not participate in gas exchange. They are therefore less able to increase oxygen delivery during periods of increased stress. As they exhale, small airways collapse, leaving alveolar spaces that are not adequately ventilated. These areas may easily become infected.

Patients with advanced chronic obstructive pulmonary disease are poor surgical risks if they are admitted for emergent procedures. With an aggressive program of preoperative respiratory support and good pulmonary toilet, however, they may be better prepared for elective operations. Such remedies include the judicious use of bronchodilators and the appropriate use of antibiotics. These patients are also candidates for intermittent positive pressure breathing therapy.

Preoperative pulmonary function tests are useful for predicting patients at definite risk of postoperative pulmonary insufficiency. However, many patients with acceptable preoperative tests experience difficulty after their operations.

Mechanical Ventilation

Modern mechanical ventilators have been designed to offer increased flexibility to the clinician over the previous generation of machines. Microcomputer circuitry exposes the internal workings of the ventilator, so the physician caring for the patient can see just what the machine is doing.

Machines are designated as volume-control and pressure-control ventilators. The older generation of pressure-cycled ventilators has little place in critical care today, except perhaps as sources of oxygen. The pressure-regulated machines deliver a flow of gas with the patient defining the volume of breathing. The machine continues to offer a flow of gas until the pressure in the circuit reaches some previously set maximum. The patient may initially be adequately ventilated; but as the patient's compliance and level of consciousness change, the machine fails to deliver an adequate tidal volume.

Most of the machines now in widespread clinical use are volume-control ventilators. With these, the physician sets the tidal volume (or minute ventilation and rate) and a pressure alarm limit. The machine then ventilates the patient with that preset volume up to the point where the pressure limit is exceeded. If the patient's compliance worsens, the tidal volume may not be given, but the clinician is apprised of the problem by the ringing of the appropriate alarm.

Technical Terms and Concepts

The machine allows a number of "modes" of ventilation. Effective use of the machine requires understanding these terms. In the control or assist/control mode of ventilation, the patient receives the tidal volume set by the physician at the rate set by the physician. When the patient attempts to take a breath and develops a sufficiently negative pressure to trip a valve on the machine, the ventilator delivers the preset volume of gas. The advantage of this mode of ventilation is that it requires no mechanical activity on the part of the patient, who need not attempt to breathe at all.

An awake patient, however, may be hyperventilated because every potentially small breath becomes a large breath. Anxious patients who are not adequately sedated frequently develop respiratory alkalosis. Management decisions to correct respiratory difficulties in a patient in this condition are choices of sedating patients so they cannot pull the increased minute ventilation or modifying the mode of ventilation.

The other side of the ventilatory spectrum exists when the patient essentially bypasses the ventilator, and the endotracheal tube is attached directly to humidified wall oxygen, usually via a T-piece. Here the tidal volume and rate of ventilation are entirely under the control of the patient. This is not normal breathing, however, because the patient still has a narrow-lumen tube (instead of a relatively large trachea and hypopharynx), and there is no resistance to exhalation. This lack of resistance frequently results in progressive alveolar collapse. Consequently, patients who are candidates for extubation are weaned to T-piece oxygen for brief periods, if at all.

Midway between controlled ventilation and no machine ventilation is intermittent mandatory ventilation (IMV). Here the clinician sets the tidal volume and the rate of ventilation. When the patient tries to breathe the machine is bypassed and the tidal volume is dictated only by the patient's own respiratory function. In other words, if the patient can only move 200 cm^3 of air by himself, that is all he receives when breathing on his own. The machines are now designed to compensate for any differences between the patient's intentions and those of the machine by not forcing a breath while the patient is exhaling.

The major advantage of IMV is as an adjunct to weaning. The rate set on the machine may be gradually decreased as the patient assumes increasing responsibility for his own breathing. This is a marked improvement over the weaning machinations of 10 years ago when the patient would be taken off the ventilator for a few minutes an hour and carefully watched by an anxious intern. Today the patient's progress is followed with arterial blood gas assays; if these levels are adequately maintained at an acceptable rate of ventilation, the IMV rate may be decreased. There are theoretic benefits from the patient controlling his own breathing. Most importantly, patients who are rapidly moved from assist/control ventilation to IMV may not lose the mechanical coordination of breathing. In clinical trials, though, IMV does not usually live up to its billing as a useful mode for weaning and allowing timely extubation.

Patients on IMV ventilation may not be able to overcome the mechanical problems posed by the small lumen of the endotracheal tube. Many machines now offer augmentation of the flow when the patient breathes on his own. This is usually referred to as pressure support. In this mode, the flow of gas into the patient is increased, so a small mechanical effort may produce a better tidal volume. The patient who is tachypneic,

breathing 30 times a minute with a 300 cc tidal volume, is not being benefited.

Increasingly, our practice has been to abandon the IMV mode almost completely and move patients immediately from controlled ventilation to pressure support. If the patient's mechanical effort is insufficient to maintain an acceptable tidal volume, the pressure support is increased (we usually have to use about 20 to 30 cm H_2O) until one is achieved. This phase is usually followed by a decreased ventilatory rate as the patient's minute ventilation can be met by this augmented volume at a lower rate. Compliance is a measure of the distensibility of the lungs and the chest and is calculated from the pressures developed as the patient receives a given volume. For a patient receiving a set volume, changes in compliance are reflected in serial changes in peak pulmonary pressure.

The patient's tidal volume is usually set at 10 to 12 cm^3/kg body weight, but it may be decreased or increased as necessary to maintain adequate blood gases. Inadequate minute ventilation is usually reflected in an elevated arterial carbon dioxide partial pressure. These goals for tidal volume may not be appropriate in conditions where compliance is seriously compromised. The volumes may be associated with severe barotrauma, and the machine attempts to move this volume of gas through noncompliant lungs. To avoid this situation, lower volumes (as low as 5 cc/kg) are chosen and the consequent increase in carbon dioxide accepted. This is "permissive" hypercapnia and is acceptable, provided renal compensation for the respiratory acidosis is still available.

Patients breathing through closed mouth and nares are breathing normally against resistance. It is possible to emulate this condition by adding positive end-expiratory pressure (PEEP) to the regimen. This resistance increases the chance that the patient's alveoli will not progressively collapse. A PEEP of 5 cm H_2O is physiologic in that it mimics the normal condition (0 cm PEEP is defined by the endotracheal tube alone); 5 cm is usually tolerated, but increasing amounts of PEEP may embarrass the cardiac output by interfering with the heart filling because of the transmission of intrathoracic pressures. Generally, I recommend placing of a Swan-Ganz catheter with pressures approaching 15 cm H_2O. This level allows maintenance of cardiac output (with fluids or inotropes) before hypotension becomes the first manifestation of cardiac failure. When more than 15 cm H_2O of PEEP is indicated, I previously recommended prophylactic chest tubes because of the risk of pneumothorax and, more importantly, tension pneumothorax. Reducing barotrauma and peak airway pressures may have decreased the incidence of pneumothorax. Today I believe that acute decompensation in a patient on high PEEP prompts consideration of a tube thoracostomy even before a chest radiograph demonstrates the pneumothorax. Another theoretic contraindication to PEEP is its deleterious effect on transdiaphragmatic lymph flow.

The action of PEEP is not to decrease lung water. The pressure does not "squeeze" out the pulmonary edema; rather, PEEP maintains the number of alveoli that are distended and can maintain gas exchange, and it recruits additional alveoli into effective gas exchange. The maximum pressure developed is maintained for only a brief period. To enjoy the benefits of this pressure, it is possible to prolong the peak pressure by converting the patient's breathing from a biphasic process to a triphasic one. Using a "plateau," or "inspiratory pause," the pressure is maintained and more alveoli are brought into the gas exchange. The cardiac consequences of high PEEP with a pause, or plateau, may be greater than those of PEEP alone, and close cardiac monitoring is necessary.

Continuous positive airway pressure (CPAP) differs minimally from PEEP. CPAP is the preferred term when patients are breathing on their own. With a tight-fitting mask, it is possible for the patient to maintain 10 cm H_2O resistance. Many patients cannot tolerate this feeling of breathing against resistance and so cannot tolerate this therapy.

Some machines allow the physician to change the inspiratory/expiratory relation. Usually 25% to 33% of the respiratory cycle is devoted to inspiration. With stiff lungs it may not be possible to ventilate the patient during this time, and so the time for inspiration may be increased. The peak pressure developed during ventilation is usually lower when additional time is provided for inspiration.

Some machines allow modification of the waveform of the pressure cycle from the standard square wave to a modified sawtooth wave. This change may be of value in patients with borderline compliance.

Finally, the most recent changes in ventilatory management are a throwback to the practices of a generation ago, namely a control for pressure-control ventilation. With this mode (fortunately available on only a few machines), the physician selects the maximum pressure the ventilator can develop, and the patient's compliance determines the tidal volume. This process generally results in lower mean airway pressure because (a) the pressure chosen by the physician, and (b) the inspiratory time is markedly prolonged. Again, the cardiac effects of this mode of ventilation may limit its use to patients without intrinsic preexisting cardiac disease.

The goal of ventilatory support is eventually to remove patients from their need for mechanical ventilation. The decision to separate patients from the machine requires that they be able to deal with the mechanical aspects of breathing and oxygenation. The patient must be able to maintain satisfactory blood gases on an FiO_2 easily administered by mask without marked tachypnea, manifesting a forced vital capacity of 10 to 12 cm^3/kg body weight. They should be able to generate a negative inspiratory pressure of 25 cm H_2O (as an adjunct to subsequent coughing).

Adult Respiratory Distress Syndrome

Adult respiratory distress syndrome justifies the early observation that something referred to as a syndrome is likely to be poorly understood. Briefly, ARDS is a clinical condition characterized by profound hypoxemia, increased lung water, increased functional residual capacity, and decreased pulmonary compliance; the reported mortality rate ranges from 60% to 100%. ARDS is associated with a number of synonyms that commonly reflect its associated conditions (e.g., shock lung, posttraumatic pulmonary insufficiency), its historic trappings (DaNang lung), or the diseases it resembles (adult hyaline membrane disease). It is reproducible in experimental models as a consequence of the infusion of fatty acids or microaggregates or even trauma, and these experiments have helped to explain it somewhat.

The primary pathway of injury involves activation of the C5 fragment of complement. Activated C5, cleared in the pulmonary circulation, is a chemotactic factor for neutrophils attracted to the pulmonary microcirculation. Anthropomorphically, these white blood cells arrive prepared to engulf bacteria, find nothing, but discharge their proteolytic enzymes nonetheless. The oxygen free radicals damage the integrity of the endothelial–alveolar interface, which results in increased interstitial fluid and movement of proteinaceous fluid into the alveolus. The alveolar spaces fill and collapse. If the patient or animal survives long enough, it becomes the lattice for ingrowth of fibroblasts and deposition of collagen, resulting in pulmonary fibrosis. The above pathway seems to explain most of the experimental animal evidence and reflects much of the clinical picture. Unfortunately, it is probably incomplete. Neutropenia does not protect against ARDS.

Although this scheme also describes clinical pharmacologic interventions, they must be regarded today as only potential interventions. Research is ongoing regarding the role of oxygen free radical scavengers and prostaglandins in this condition. The bulk of effective therapy is designed to deal with injury already present.

The clinical picture begins with the increasingly hypoxic patient who manifests the tachycardia, tachypnea, anxiety, and restlessness observed with hypoxemia. The patient finally reaches the point where satisfactory blood gases cannot be maintained without intubation and ventilatory support, and he is intubated. Chest radiography may be normal at this point but invariably shows the effects of increased total lung water shortly.

The patient's hypoxia must be reversed as rapidly as possible. The Fio_2 is increased progressively and usually reaches 1.0 without significant improvement because gas diffusion is markedly decreased. The patient requires increasing application of PEEP, which is usually increased in 2- to 5-cm H_2O increments per half-hour. The PEEP is increased until the oxygenation improves or the cardiac output falls. Swan-Ganz catheters are indicated for patients who require more than 12 cm H_2O PEEP. If the patient cannot tolerate the high levels of PEEP because of the interference with cardiac filling, the PEEP is dropped to previously tolerated levels, the intravascular volume is increased, and the PEEP then is increased again.

The Swan-Ganz catheter also helps confirm the diagnosis of ARDS versus pulmonary edema from other causes. The latter is associated with increased wedge pressure, with that being the stimulus to the transudation of fluid into the interstitium. The patient with ARDS has pulmonary edema because the permeability coefficient in the Starling equation has changed.

Patients are followed with repeated calculations of their A-a gradient, which is a measure of the difference between alveolar (A) oxygen tension and arterial (a) oxygen tension and is a measure of the diffusion barrier. The A-a gradients are normally about 10 mm Hg; with severe ARDS the gradient may exceed 600 mm Hg.

The patient's calculated shunt fraction may also be followed as a guide to the use of PEEP. The shunt is equal to the alveolar oxygen content minus the arterial oxygen content, divided by the alveolar oxygen content minus the mixed venous oxygen content.

Prophylactic chest tubes remain controversial with PEEP levels in excess of 15 cm H_2O, especially with decreased pulmonary compliance. Many of the newer ventilators demonstrate directly the peak pressures in the ventilatory circuit.

In my patients the PEEP is increased up to the point that the Fio_2 can be decreased. Once that point is reached the patient often begins to recover, allowing a progressive decrease in the oxygen concentrations. The goal is to decrease the oxygen concentration to 0.5 or less. At this point the oxygen toxicity seems to be tolerable.

Other adjuncts in the management of the patient have been alluded to, but the general dictum is to avoid further injury. Oxygen toxicity is real and can be controlled with the appropriate use of PEEP. Barotrauma is also probably real and is managed with a decrease in the minute ventilation, permissive hypercapnia, and even pressure control ventilation. The ratio between inspiratory time (I) and expiratory time (E) can also be manipulated to decrease barotrauma. The normal ratio of 1 : 4 means that the lungs must be inflated with the set tidal volume relatively rapidly, leading to increased pressures. Lengthening the time of inspiration decreases the pressure generated for a given compliance. Care must be taken not to shorten the expiratory time to the point that the alveolus cannot empty before the next inspiration.

The cardiovascular system in my patients is supported with the appropriate pharmacologic agents, commonly including digitalization. The patient receives whatever nutritional support can be tolerated. Supplemental vitamin E is added to the diet for its role as an antioxidant. Prophylactic antibiotics are not indicated, but close bacterial surveillance is needed because the proteinaceous secretions provide an excellent culture medium.

During the acute phase of manipulation the patient is sedated or paralyzed, and the mode of ventilation is control or assist/control. This decision is made because the patient's bucking the ventilator only increases the barotrauma involved. Moreover, the risk of a rambunctious patient extubating himself is high. After the patient has reached that turning point, the mode of ventilation is returned to IMV if the patient can tolerate it.

With aggressive pulmonary manipulation, as described above, the diagnosis of ARDS does not seem equivalent to a death sentence. Moreover, the physician who can successfully care for a patient with ARDS proves his or her understanding of cardiopulmonary disease and the whole gamut of the ICU armamentarium.

Another technique for managing the patient with ARDS is jet ventilation. With this device the normal volumes of breathing are obviated; the lungs are inflated with gas, and tiny volumes are inhaled and exhaled at rates of several hundred "breaths" per minute. This process markedly reduces barotrauma and is especially useful in patients with severe air leaks or bronchopleural fistulas. Like many modalities, it is probably more effective in children. Removing the injured lungs entirely from breathing can be accomplished with extracorporeal membrane oxygenation (ECMO) a technique with a considerable track record in children and neonates. Finally, we can turn the concept of gas exchange on its head with liquid ventilation, using perfluorocarbons as a means of ventilating the patient. Another novel strategy, reported to have been used with surprising success, is to place the patient in the prone position to better utilize functional lung segments.

Exogenous surfactant is now available and has been shown to improve the course in pediatric but not adult patients. Inhaled nitric oxide, which results in improved perfusion to the lung segments ventilated, should have solved the clinical problems of ARDS by abolishing the V/Q mismatch. Although effective in decreasing this mismatch, the studies have not yet demonstrated a consistent benefit in terms of patient survival.

FLUIDS AND ELECTROLYTES

Body Compartments

Water constitutes approximately 60% of the total body weight in young healthy men and about 55% of the weight in young women (consequent to their increased total body fat content). The average 70-kg man therefore contains about 40 L of fluid. This fluid is divided into three distinct compartments: intracellular, interstitial, and intravascular.

Intracellular fluid exists within the cells of the body and constitutes about two-thirds of the total body water. Interstitial fluid exists outside of both the cells and the intravascular space and includes such fluids as cerebrospinal fluid, lymph, and tissue fluids. Interstitial fluid represents about two-thirds of the extracellular fluid or about 20% of total body water (TBW). The smallest space is the intravascular fluid, which represents about one-ninth of TBW and about 7% of body weight. This space is filled with plasma and the formed elements of the blood.

Fluid movement between these compartments is dictated by a number of principles, all of which are clinically relevant. Fluid shifts between the intracellular space and the interstitial space are dictated by the electrical potential across the cell membrane. A charged ion moving into the cell is balanced by a similarly charged ion moving out of the cell. This movement principle is valid only so long as the cell membrane retains its semipermeable integrity.

Movement of fluid between the intravascular and interstitial fluid spaces is dictated by the Starling relation, which states that the hydrostatic forces moving fluid out of the capillary are opposed by oncotic and osmotic forces. The latter forces depend on a structurally intact semipermeable membrane; hence the variable ρ below:

$$Q_c = (P_c - P_i) - \rho(\pi_c - \pi_i)$$

where Q_c = flow; P_c and P_i are hydrostatic pressure in capillary and interstitial space, respectively; π_c and π_i are colloid oncotic pressure in capillary and interstitial spaces; and ρ is permeability.

Water Balance

In addition to the movement of water between these body compartments, water moves into and out of the body. Intake is usually oral and averages about 2 L a day for the average adult. This figure includes not only fluids drunk but the water absorbed from foodstuffs. The kidneys excrete most of the body's water (about 1.0 to 1.5 L), with additional water lost from the skin (as insensible loss) and in the stool (as rarely measured loss). The net water balance is usually zero because the patient neither gains nor loses water weight. Water intake is necessitated by the kidney's need to eliminate nitrogenous waste.

An increase in water balance is usually the product of injudicious physician intervention. It may also occur as a consequence of chronic malnutrition with the loss of visceral protein mass or acute or chronic renal failure.

The clinical problems with water balance are usually secondary to excessive losses. Insensible losses increase as a function of the increase in the body's temperature. Vasodilation of cutaneous capillaries increases the rate at which water may be lost from the patient. Direct access to the tracheobronchial tree opens another surface for water exchange, and intubated patients who do not receive satisfactory humidification from a nebulizer experience drying of their respiratory epithelium and so lose fluid. The protective barrier of the keratinized layer of the skin protects against fluid loss; and the destruction of this layer with a burn injury, especially if the burn is moderate to deep second degree, is another area of fluid loss (areas of third degree burns lose less fluid because of the reconstitution of a vapor barrier by the eschar formed).

Polyuria and diarrhea are other common sources of fluid loss that can be measured. Fluid may be lost directly from the intravascular space because of bleeding. Blood collected for diagnostic tests is another major source of water loss in the SICU. Loss of other body secretions such as nasogastric or ileostomy losses may decrease the fluid volume status. Note that these lost fluids are associated with the loss of other specific electrolytes and protein.

In addition to the fluid losses due to renal failure, there are a number of other neuroendocrine responses that affect water balance. Antidiuretic hormone (ADH) is released by the posterior pituitary in response to hypothalamic stimulation. It acts on the kidney's distal tubule to increase water reabsorption. Patients with head injury may manifest inappropriate ADH levels and become progressively water-intoxicated and hyponatremic. Water balance is also affected by sodium reabsorption and excretion. Clinically, this becomes important in conditions such as cirrhosis, where high levels of aldosterone favor both sodium and water retention. The body's response to loss of fluid from one compartment results in redistribution of fluids to compensate. Loss of fluid from the intravascular space, for instance, is followed by slow movement of fluid from the interstitial space into the vascular space. This movement is seen clinically as a consequence of blood loss, where the hematocrit is initially stable following the loss of volume and then decreases as the plasma space increases. This equilibration is not rapid; it takes about 4 to 8 hours for the hematocrit to stabilize. Severe constriction of the interstitial space may result in cellular dehydration, but it is uncommon.

Expansion of the intravascular space produces changes within the space and in the other spaces. The vascular tree initially distends to carry the fluid, principally by opening capacitance vessels. The cardiac output is augmented, which increases the glomerular filtration rate in the kidney. The kidney then excretes urine until the intravascular space is normalized. At the same time, the pressure relation of the Starling relation have changed, and fluid is moved into the interstitium. This situation is especially a factor during fluid resuscitation with noncolloid, hypotonic fluids, where the oncotic forces that normally move fluid back into the vascular space are reduced. In the presence of microvascular injury the coefficient of permeability is additionally changed, rendering the vascular space leakier and pushing more fluid into the interstitium.

The intracellular space rarely increases as a consequence of overloading the intravascular space. This situation usually arises only if the fluid expansion is secondary to the treatment of shock, where, as described above, the intracellular space expands because of failure of the sodium–potassium pump.

Therapeutic Interventions

The therapy for intravascular fluid loss is replacement of that loss in quantities sufficient to expand the space, using urine output and the filling pressures of the heart as guides. For blood loss due to trauma, the volumes of crystalloid infusion are usually 2.5 to 3.0 times the volume of shed blood. This increased replacement is a consequence of the movement of fluid out of the vascular space to compensate for contraction of the interstitial volume and to meet the fluid demands of the cells that have swollen. Cardiac output is restored and cellular integrity is reconstituted; and the body usually eliminates the excess load.

Specific pharmacologic intervention is indicated for conditions in which specific mediators are at fault. In cirrhotics, for instance, spironolactone is indicated as an adjunct for patients excreting excess water and sodium.

Cation Imbalances

Sodium

Sodium is the principal cation of the extracellular fluid space, and changes in sodium content usually follow logically from changes in water content. Hypernatremia usually occurs as a consequence of water excess. The latter is generally iatrogenic, although abnormally high circulating ADH is responsible in a few patients.

Clinical evaluation of the patient usually demonstrates the water problem directly, with dry mucous membranes and signs of hypovolemia in the patient who is hypernatremic. The hyponatremic patient appears wet. Central nervous system changes are demonstrable. The water-intoxicated patient is progressively hyperactive, even to the point of convulsions. These changes are usually encountered when the serum sodium has fallen to about 120 mEq/L. Similar neurologic signs of restlessness and delirium occur with hypernatremia but are probably secondary to volume contraction and the catecholamine responses.

Hypernatremia may also develop as a consequence of the use of hypertonic fluid regimens employed at some centers for the treatment of burn shock. Therapy is as indicated below for other causes of hypernatremia.

Hyponatremia is usually a preventable condition that should not occur. If it occurs, it should not be treated with infusions of isotonic or hypotonic fluids but with fluid restriction. Hypernatremia requires appropriate reexpansion of the vascular space with hypotonic fluids. It may also be seen in hyperglycemic states, although the measured sodium level does not demonstrate it. For every 100 mg/dL increase in glucose, plasma sodium falls about 2 mEq.

Potassium

Sodium is the major extracellular cation, and potassium is the major intracellular cation. Whereas the body can conserve sodium if required, it cannot compensate for hypokalemia by decreasing its urinary losses. The major route of potassium excretion is the kidney, and most of the abnormalities associated with this ion impinge on renal sufficiency. The ion's most important function is to regulate the electrical potential across cell membranes, especially for controlling the automaticity of the pacemaker of the heart.

Hyperkalemia sufficient to cause electrical problems of the heart begins as early as a serum K^+ level of 6.0 mEq/L. The condition usually occurs in patients with renal failure but is also seen in patients with normal renal function who have increased tissue destruction, releasing potassium into the intravascular space. It is possible to kill a burn patient by the injudicious use of succinylcholine, which causes muscle cells to release a huge dose of potassium into the blood. Potassium may also be elevated as a consequence of excessive treatment with

spironolactone to compensate for aldosterone excess because the body loses sodium in the urine and reabsorbs potassium. Electrocardiographic signs of hyperkalemia include high peaked T waves, widened QRS complexes, and eventually disappearance of T waves.

Hypokalemia is usually a consequence of body depletion of the ion. Diarrhea results in a large loss of circulating potassium, which is eventually replaced up to a point by movement of potassium out of cells. Large losses of gastric juice via a nasogastric tube may also produce hypokalemia, even though the potassium content of gastric juice is minimal. Here the loss of potassium is secondary to the loss of chloride. The kidney, without adequate chloride, cannot reabsorb sodium. To compensate for the sodium loss, the aldosterone system secretes potassium as the sodium is reclaimed. Another clinical condition of hypokalemia is caused by the injudicious use of diuretics. Inadequate replacement of potassium during hyperalimentation may also produce hypokalemia.

High levels of potassium may be life-threatening. The solution is to eliminate the potassium ion from the intravascular space, which can be done by moving the ion into the cells or eliminating it entirely from the body. Potassium is a cofactor in the transport of glucose, and giving the patient a large glucose infusion along with insulin moves the ion into cells. Alkalosis also moves potassium into cells. Kayexalate is a cation-exchange resin that can bind potassium and carry it out of the gastrointestinal tract. Kayexalate may be introduced per rectum or via a nasogastric tube along with sorbitol.

The clinical problem posed by hypokalemia is the rate at which potassium can be replaced. The limit seems to be somewhat shy of 40 mEq/hr, under close ECG scrutiny.

Calcium

Calcium is principally found in bone in association with phosphate and carbonate. In serum only about half of the calcium is ionized, and it is important for neuromuscular control. This ionized faction is a function of the protein level and the pH (acidosis increases ionization).

Hypercalcemia results from two relatively uncommon conditions: hyperparathyroidism and widespread osseous metastases. Clinical signs and symptoms of hypercalcemia are largely vague and include the classic complaint of "groans, moans, and stones" along with weakness and stupor.

Hypocalcemia presents as marked hyperactivity, a positive Chvostek's sign, tetany, and carpopedal spasm. Clinically it is commonly associated with acute pancreatitis and renal insufficiency. Questionably, it may occur in a consequence of massive infusion of large amounts of citrated blood.

ACID–BASE BALANCE

Hydrogen ion concentration is usually defined in terms of pH (the negative logarithm). In the intact patient its concentration is maintained within fairly tight limits by a combination of respiratory and metabolic compensatory mechanisms. Acid added to the extracellular fluid is buffered by a number of systems, especially the bicarbonate–carbonic acid system, with excretion of the acid effected by the lungs or the kidneys.

The bicarbonate buffer system is described by the Henderson-Hasselbach equation, which states that

$$pH = 6.1 + \log [bicarbonate/(0.03 \times P_{CO_2})]$$

So long as the ratio between bicarbonate and carbonic acid remains 20 : 1, the pH remains normal. When the system is working properly, adding acid decreases serum bicarbonate. Ventilation is increased to eliminate carbon dioxide and reestablish the 20 : 1 ratio. More slowly, the kidney eliminates the acid and reabsorbs additional bicarbonate.

Four nonnormal states are recognized: respiratory acidosis, respiratory alkalosis, metabolic acidosis, and metabolic alkalosis. Each state may be associated with some degree of appropriate compensation. The diagnosis of acidosis is made with a pH less than 7.40. Elevated P_{CO_2} produces a diagnosis of respiratory acidosis, and the reverse is found with respiratory alkalosis. Similarly, the metabolic component is deduced from the level of the serum bicarbonate.

Respiratory acidosis is a common clinical result of inadequate alveolar ventilation with an elevated P_{CO_2}. If it persists, the patient attempts to compensate by retaining bicarbonate and excreting acid in the urine. Therapy must obviously be directed toward improving ventilation.

Metabolic acidosis is usually a consequence of the accumulation of acid, commonly lactic acid, and usually reflects tissue hypoperfusion. Measurement of the anion gap usually points to elevated lactate levels even if they are not measured directly. Nonanionic gap acidosis includes hyperchloremic metabolic acidosis. Acidosis may result from the kidneys' inability to excrete acid. Therapy again is directed against the underlying causes. Correction of metabolic acidosis with exogenous bicarbonate must not overcorrect the problem. The usual replacement is calculated from the difference between the patient's bicarbonate and the standard bicarbonate multiplied by 0.25 times the patient's weight in kilograms.

Respiratory alkalosis is commonly seen in overventilated, anxious, tachypneic patients. The alkalosis forces a movement of potassium into cells and forces the kidney to retain acid.

Metabolic alkalosis is commonly seen in association with hypovolemia in a state known as contraction alkalosis, which is usually a result of excessive loss of gastric secretions as seen in patients with pyloric outlet obstruction. Chloride is lost in large quantities into the nasogastric fluid. The kidneys are unable to absorb sodium without the anion, and sodium and water are lost. The kidney attempts to correct this imbalance by exchanging potassium and hydrogen ions for sodium. The alkalotic patient thus produces a paradoxical aciduria. Therapy requires reexpansion of the vascular space with isotonic saline along with appropriate infusions of potassium chloride. Severe alkalosis may require infusion of hydrochloric acid.

BLOOD AND BLOOD COMPONENT THERAPY

Blood Banking

Today's blood bank represents a compromise between the surgeon's impression of the needs of the patient and the hospital's need for efficiency and cost containment. When blood bank technology was in its infancy, blood banks were run by surgeons. Now we merely wait in line, frequently behind internists, oncologists, and obstetricians. Fresh whole blood is virtually impossible to obtain in any hospital today, the technology of component therapy having evolved to the point that a given unit of donated blood is divided and redistributed to a number of patients. The red blood cells may be centrifuged and infused into one patient, the plasma frozen and available for another, and the platelets given to a third.

The problem today is less with the uses of blood than with the increased attention to the risk of infection consequent to the administration of blood and blood components. The risk of acquired immunodeficiency syndrome (AIDS) joins the various forms of hepatitis as risk factors the physician and patient want to avoid. The increase in the use of freely donated blood and the availability of hepatitis B and C antibody testing has decreased the overall risk of acquiring hepatitis. It is hoped that the same is occurring with AIDS as a consequence of anti-HIV antibody assays. On the other hand, products such as γ-globulin, which require large donor pools, may increase the damage caused by contamination of a single unit or by a single donor. In an era of medical litigation, good sense dictates that the therapy selected for the patient be both necessary and appropriate.

Red Blood Cells

Erythrocytes are indicated for the replacement of lost blood, but only to the point that the patient's hemoglobin content is adequate for the needs of oxygen transport. There is no need to transfuse the patient back to a premorbid hematocrit of 45% when a hematocrit of 30% can suffice. Remember, too, that fully saturating these 10 g of hemoglobin provides better tissue oxygen delivery than poorly saturating a large mass of hemoglobin. Increased viscosity is a potential problem when increasing the hematocrit much above 30% because there may be a decrease in the efficiency of the microcirculation.

Red blood cells (RBCs) infused for this purpose are commonly packaged as packed RBCs. These cells are stored in the refrigerator of the blood bank in citrate-phosphate-dextrose (CPD), and the shelf life (defined as 70% of infused cells surviving 24 hours after transfusion) is about 28 to 35 days. In the refrigerator the cells metabolize the glucose to lactate. Older units of blood contain increased amounts of extracellular potassium and decreased amounts of intracellular 2,3-DPG (see Shock, above).

Blood is usually crossmatched prior to transfusion, but in urgent situations type-specific blood (matching only ABO group and Rh factor) may be employed. In emergency situations the infusion of type O negative blood may be lifesaving. Even the most careful crossmatching may miss some of the minor histocompatibility antigens and produce a mild hemolytic reaction. Reactions to mismatched blood may be dramatic, with fever and chills, tachycardia, hypotension, and brisk intravascular hemolysis. The patient under general anesthesia may not manifest these signs, but the surgeon can diagnose the hemolytic reaction by the diffuse oozing in the operative field.

Therapy for transfusion reactions must include immediate cessation of the infusion, returning the infusate and a sample of the patient's blood to the blood bank. The released hemoglobin may precipitate in the renal tubules and lead to acute renal failure. This situation is best prevented by alkalinizing of the urine and inducing a brisk diuresis. Other causes of fever, chills, and hypotension (e.g., bacterial contamination of the line) should also be considered and sought.

Blood transfusions are also infusions of extracellular fluid. As stated above, old blood may have high levels of potassium, which could be a problem in patients with renal insufficiency. Ammonia tends to accumulate as well. Rapid infusion of cold blood may lead to hypothermia. Citrate accumulation and consequent hypocalcemia is probably rare, but the risks increase with massive transfusion and in patients with poor hepatic function due to drugs or toxic injury or because of immaturity, as in neonates. The addition of intravenous calcium is therefore somewhat controversial. I arbitrarily infuse 1 ampul (10 ml) of calcium chloride for every 4 units of blood or blood products, and I have never noted the effects of either hypo- or hypercalcemia.

Micropore filters are probably indicated during massive transfusions to decrease the infusion of RBC aggregates and cellular debris. These particles, if infused, are capable of producing pulmonary insufficiency. Blood should not be infused through small-caliber needles and probably should not be administered through narrow cannulas such as those in Swan-Ganz catheters. Blood warmers should be employed whenever available.

Clotting Factors

Patients who have bled and been transfused with significant volumes are at risk of developing a washout coagulopathy because the transfused blood contains neither clotting factors nor platelets. I routinely transfuse fresh frozen plasma into patients who have received massive amounts of RBCs and add platelets when the shed (and replaced) blood volume reaches 10 units. These criteria are, admittedly, arbitrary.

Clotting factors are also indicated in patients with coagulopathies who have not bled. Factors VII, IX, X, and XI may be found in pooled plasma. Factor V replacement requires the use of fresh frozen plasma. Factor VIII is available in fresh frozen plasma or in factor VIII concentrates. Cryoprecipitate contains not only coagulation factors but the circulating opsonic protein fibronectin. Theoretic use of cryoprecipitate to replace the opsonin factors lost during and after trauma and with sepsis have not been borne out in clinical trials, however.

Platelets

Platelet deficiency is rarely the cause of clinical bleeding unless the platelet count is less than 30,000/mm³. Prophylactic platelet transfusion is indicated with that count. Care must be taken not to filter the platelet preparation because the platelets then end up in the filter, not in the patient.

Acute Renal Failure

Acute renal insufficiency, whether a decrease in urine volume (oliguria), an increased in blood urea nitrogen (BUN), or a decrease in serum creatinine or creatinine clearance is a common observation in the surgical patient in the ICU. Fortunately, most of these patients do not require the services of the nephrologist (though many are called in for consultation) or need hemodialysis. These patients do require, however, an early diagnosis and appropriate management. The patient with decreased urine volumes may be suffering from a prerenal, renal or postrenal problem. Remember, an occluded Foley catheter should be the first diagnosis ruled out.

Prerenal oliguria is consequent to a decrease in renal perfusion. Cardiac output is directly related to renal blood flow, as the renal arteriolar system cannot change its vascular resistance, so prerenal oliguria is usually associated with any conditions that decrease cardiac output, especially hypovolemia. It is also associated with drugs that increase vascular resistance, either globally (e.g., norepinephrine) or locally (e.g., ACE inhibitors). Patients with prerenal disease usually have an elevated BUN/creatinine ratio (more than 20 : 1) and

restrict excretion of sodium to compensate for the real or apparent decrease in intravascular volume. Spot urine electrolyte assays usually demonstrate a sodium level of less than 30 mEq/L. Fractional excretion of sodium (FE$_{Na}$), as described below, is usually less than 1%.

$$FE_{Na} = (\text{urine Na}^+/\text{plasma Na}^+)/(\text{urine creatinine/plasma creatinine}) \times 100$$

Therapy is relatively straightforward and includes reduction of hypovolemia and maintenance of cardiac output.

Intrinsic causes of acute renal failure are most often acute tubular necrosis (ATN) and nephritis, the latter being drug-related. The urinary sodium concentration is increased in these conditions because of tubular injury and consequent leak of sodium into the urine beyond that which the body would otherwise excrete. The urinary sodium level is higher than 50 mEq/L in most conditions. Fractional excretion of sodium is more than 2%, as the body is better able to control creatinine excretion than sodium. The cause of ATN is often hypoperfusion, which usually indicates intraoperative hypovolemia in major cases or decreases in cardiac output from other causes. Initial management is correction of cardiac output. Management of drug-induced nephritis is removal of the drug. Examination of the urinary sediment, a process virtually unknown to house officers today, frequently demonstrates white blood cell casts in drug-induced nephritis.

A more controversial management practice for the patient with ATN is increasing the urine output to convert an anuric or markedly oliguric picture to a less oliguric one. The data suggest that patients whose urine output is 30 mL/hr or more do better, which suggests a role for pharmacologic intervention to achieve the higher urine output and the better clinical outcome. These data are scarce. The initial therapies advanced to produce this end include diuretics (usually furosemide) at increasing doses and then other agents such as bumetanide (Bumex), diuretic drips, and finally renal-dose dopamine. Furosemide (Lasix) drips increase urine output better than bolus therapy in some but not all patients. Dopamine, because of its effect on renal blood flow, increases urine output and produces a natriuresis, but it has not been shown to improve outcome. In the setting of decreased cardiac output, it must be used carefully because of its arrhythmia potential and the risk of worsening tachycardia.

Additional support for the patient must include antic-ipation of the need for hemodialysis and the need to prevent further injury. Acidosis should be avoided. Potassium should be removed from all intravenous flu-ids and the serum potassium carefully observed. Water balance must be maintained as tightly as possible, as the excess water infused today must disappear tomorrow. Excessive nutritional support must be abandoned, an-ticipating a problem in urea excretion; and the adminis-tration of other nitrogen compounds must be limited, especially in the patient with acute liver injury. Boluses of glucose, insulin, and bicarbonate can transiently lower the serum potassium by moving potassium into cells. Kayexelate enemas or per nasogastric tube de-crease the potassium load rather than merely moving it around. As the patient develops profound renal insuffi-ciency, other adjuncts include erythropoietin to main-tain erythrocyte mass, DDAVP to treat the coagulopa-thy associated with uremia, and appropriate nutritional support (see Chapter 31).

Indications for hemodialysis include severe water in-toxication (worsening congestive heart failure), hyper-kalemia, acidosis, and severe azotemia (BUN over 100 mg/dL). The newer machines and increased experience of the nephrologists have decreased the acute hemody-namic consequences of hemodialysis (which is avail-able even on Sundays and holidays now). Moreover, ar-teriovenous hemofiltration and venovenohemofiltration are adjuncts that aid in water balance and azotemia.

Myoglobinemia is seen in patients with severe rhab-domyolysis, commonly after lengthy vascular proce-dures with inadequate peripheral perfusion. The diag-nosis requires spectrochemical demonstration of myoglobin, but the test is rarely performed in the hospi-tal, must be sent to an outside laboratory, costs too much, and takes too long. A useful alternative is a sim-ple urine dipstick for blood. A positive test indicates erythrocytes, hemoglobin, or myoglobin. A positive test on the supernatant of a centrifuged urine specimen sug-gests one of the latter. Acute muscle damage leading to myoglobin is usually associated with a markedly ele-vated serum creatine phosphokinase (CPK) level. Treatment for both myoglobin and hemoglobin excess is the same. First, anticipate further production of the chemical if the underlying cause is hypoperfusion (myoglobin) or hemolysis (hemoglobin). Second, in-duce prompt diuresis in an attempt to clear the material before it precipitates in the urine. Mannitol or a similar osmotic diuretic is generally used here along with vol-ume infusion. Alkalinization of urine with sodium bi-carbonate may decrease the precipitation of these chro-magens, but this point remains controversial.

Postrenal causes of acute renal failure include ob-struction to urine flow from the kidney. Serum creati-nine is used as marker of renal function. It can distin-guish prerenal from renal causes because of the increased BUN/creatinine ratio in the former. The serum creatinine level must be used with caution in the elderly and in those with extensive muscle wasting (as creatinine is derived from muscle). Serum creatinine declines normally with age, as reflected in the formulas below for estimating creatinine clearance.

Creatinine clearance (males) = [(140 − age in years)
$\times$ weight (kg)]/72 $\times$ serum creatinine (mg/dL)
Creatinine clearance (females) = 0.85 $\times$ above

In ill patients, creatinine clearance is better determined directly, most accurately with a 24-hour urine sample and less so with a 2- or 6-hour specimen.

Infectious Problems in the SICU

The infectious disease problems seen in the SICU would fill up another chapter by themselves. Some of these issues are addressed in Chapter 32. Three areas of interest have arisen during the past few years, and ques-tions in these areas are likely to appear on the Board ex-amination.

Nosocomial pneumonia is a major problem in the critically ill, and it may lead directly to pulmonary in-sufficiency. Temporally, the lung is usually the first or-gan to succumb to multiple organ failure. Although the incidence of nosocomial pneumonia is increased in the most seriously ill patients (those with the highest APACHE II scores) and in patients who are intubated, it occurs in less sick, nonintubated patients as well. Nu-merous articles have appeared that demonstrate a corre-lation between stress ulcer prophylaxis and the inci-dence of pneumonia. The risk is increased in patients receiving antacids and those managed with a variety of H_2 blockers; the incidence is decreased in patients man-aged with sucralfate (Carafate). The suggested explana-tion is that in the presence of an elevated, less acidic pH there is overgrowth of bacteria, which the patient aspi-rates, producing pneumonia. Some investigators have gone so far as to suggest that gastric acid exists in hu-mans predominantly as a means of sterilizing the gut and not to improve the efficacy of gastric proteases. In some studies sucralfate was found to be as effective as antacids for preventing the complication for which they are usually administered, namely stress-induced gastritis and acute gastrointestinal tract bleeding. Other studies have produced results that question this therapeutic equivalence. Finally, in at least one published study the incidence of stress gastritis in intubated, mechanically ventilated patients on total parenteral nutrition (TPN) was not decreased by *any* prophylactic regimen, as the control group did not experience the complication.

The evidence favoring sucralfate has not been completely accepted, and the extensive experience with antacids and H_2 blockers documenting an association between high acid levels and gastric bleeding has not resulted in their disappearance from the SICU pharmacopeia. On the other hand, improved resuscitation, the early and aggressive use of enteral nutrition, or some new knowledge of the critically ill has resulted in a marked decrease in acute gastric bleeding. The use of enteral feeding especially has made this question moot, as food is as effective a buffer as antacids for gastric acid. A final point about nosocomial pneumonia: Its occurrence may increase the length of SICU care but does not independently increase mortality in many studies.

Translocation of intestinal bacteria has been suggested as another mechanism to explain both the nosocomial pneumonia and the presence of gram-negative bacteria in infections that develop in the critically ill patient. The bacteria in the gut (both luminal and those attached to the mucosal wall) do not usually enter the patient and prove pathogenic. In a variety of experimental situations including shock, hemorrhage, starvation, endotoxemia, and burns, these bacteria and their products including endotoxin translocate to mesenteric lymph nodes and even to the portal and systemic circulations. The barrier loss can be viewed as either a mechanical one (intestinal mucus and cells) or a functional one (local immunoglobulins and lymphatic protection).

This concept has prompted a renewed interest in prophylactic antibiotics and is frequently cited as a further indication for early enteral nutrition. Appropriate enteral feeds (those including fiber or those with a less elemental configuration) change the intestinal microflora back to a more normal one and have been shown to reverse atrophy of gut microvilli. Glutamine, usually supplied from the breakdown of muscle protein and the most common circulating amino acid in the amino acid pool, appears to be a specific fuel required for gut mucosal integrity. High circulating levels of glutamine are found following stress or injury. In animals with little intestinal mass the apparent efflux from muscle cells is attenuated. If glutamine is important to intestinal barrier integrity, it reveals an important flaw in parenteral hyperalimentation because none of the commercially available preparations contains glutamine. Glutamine is (or, rather, was) not considered an essential amino acid and in the original mixtures was found to be associated with neurologic complaints in patients; it was thought to be unstable in acidic solutions. Experimental glutamyl dipeptides are available in Europe and are part of ongoing trials. Pending the arrival of these products in the United States we must rely on enteral glutamine to support the gut. The manufacturers of tube feedings have been only too willing to add enriched concentrations of glutamine to, and increase their prices of, the preparations. Some of this enthusiasm may have been pointless, as clinical studies of benefit are inconsistent at best.

Indeed, the major amino acid considered today as a useful adjunct to infection control is arginine, and its presence along with ω-three fatty acids and ribonucleoprotein has led to concoctions grouped together under the term "immunonutrition." This subject is discussed at greater length in Chapter 31. Arginine is a precursor for nitric oxide, and several studies have suggested a major role for nitric oxide in the killing of bacteria in mesenteric lymph nodes. These data suggest that even when the gut barrier fails and bacteria do arrive at mesenteric lymph nodes their killing may proceed as normal, provided nitric oxide production in unimpeded.

If the gut is the site of bacterial translocation and maybe even of the hypermetabolic responses we see in the critically ill (secondary to the effects of absorbed endotoxin, for instance), perhaps we can help patients by decreasing the population of intestinal bacteria. Selective decontamination of the gut has been reported in numerous studies, most of which have come from Europe. A variety of regimens have been employed, but in general they employ a nonabsorbable antibiotic directed against the common intestinal gram-negative bacteria and a topical antifungal given by mouth or used as a mouthwash. In a few studies an intravenous cephalosporin was given for a brief period early in the patient's course. These studies have not demonstrated a significant overgrowth of pathogenic bacteria in the gut. In fact, the patients who were followed serially by pharyngeal, gastric, and rectal swab cultures demonstrated a progressive decrease in the number of gram-negative rods found. The physiologic benefit of this intervention, however, has not been universally demonstrated. Most studies have failed to demonstrate a significant decrease in mortality or length of SICU stay for patients so managed, although one did demonstrate just that in a subset of trauma patients. Nearly all the studies, though, including those performed in the United States, demonstrated a decrease in the incidence of nosocomial pneumonia. Again, it was not associated with any survival benefit and brings into question the biologic significance and importance of this infection.

Prevention of infection in the SICU is more likely to derive from better designed invasive devices and even more so by the prudent use of the devices we already have. Closed urine collection systems decreased the incidence of urinary tract infections. Today we have silver-impregnated and antibiotic-coated catheters, which may help decrease the problem further. Similar coatings on central venous catheters have not always decreased the incidence of infection, which may be better prevented by judicious aseptic technique. The length-of-stay issue for central lines has been resolved in favor of not removing them routinely at a certain time after insertion. Swan-Ganz catheters, though, clearly must be removed in a timely fashion or replaced. The large, flexible, more frequently manipulated introducers must be removed as well. Finally, arterial catheters, for which there are no guidelines for length of use, must be remembered as possible sources of bloodstream infection.

Neurosurgical Critical Care

Probably no aspect of surgical critical care has undergone as abrupt a change as has that of the head-injured or general neurosurgical patient. Concepts, biases, and manipulations that seemed so logical in the past are being abandoned and replaced with new ideas, some of which remain untested.

The physiology of the head-injured patient rested on the concept that there were three volumes held together within a rigid barrier called the skull: brain, blood, and the cerebrospinal fluid (CSF) space. Increases in intracranial pressure (ICP) were not tolerated well by the brain, and all interventions were predicated upon reducing this pressure. The brain's autoregulation, a system that allows the brain to increase its "share" of the cardiac output as the latter fails, had to be managed to decrease

this perfusion because cerebral edema had to be prevented. The cornerstone of management, then, after placing a ventriculostomy or an ICP bolt, was hyperventilation to decrease the vasodilatation so as to prevent edema. There were two problems with this concept. First, it would not work for long because the difference in carbon dioxide tension between blood and tissue would soon disappear, and it suggested that depriving the brain of oxygen and perfusion were the keys to its repair. This would be analogous to treating the edema consequent to a fractured femur by ligating the femoral artery.

As a clinical intervention it seemed to work, but only because there was nothing with which to compare it. Hyperventilation did decrease ICP, at least transiently, so the theory seemed sound; but the patients did not necessarily wake up, either in the SICU or afterward. The classic Cushing phenomenon (hypertension and bradycardia), which was observed in patients with malignant increases in their ICP was seen as representing an appeal by the brain to generate perfusion.

Replace it now is the current concept of maintaining cerebral perfusion, thereby maximizing delivery of blood, oxygen, and nutrients to the brain. Cerebral blood flow is difficult to measure, either clinically or experimentally. Flow probes can be placed on the inflow vessels, but in an intact human that means two carotid arteries and two vertebral arteries. This is not clinically feasible. Xenon-CT scanning allows quantification of both total and regional blood flow, but this technique is not yet universally available. Alternatively, one can determine the adequacy of perfusion by measuring the decrease in oxygen content across the brain, which can be done by placing an oxygen sensor in the jugular bulb. Some clinical centers do use this technique, but it remains controversial and the data are questionable because of the alternative venous channels. Moreover, the A-V oxygen difference reflects a global picture, and the regional perfusion of the brain remains indeterminate.

Current clinical practice focuses on cerebral perfusion pressure rather than blood flow. The difference between mean arterial pressure (MAP) and ICP is the cerebral perfusion pressure (CPP). It must be kept above 70 mm Hg, and the critical level is 50 mm Hg. To maintain this pressure most patients require healthy doses of pressors. Because perfusion is not really a pressure, cardiac output is maintained, if not maximized, by the use of fluids and inotropes.

The third arm of what is now hyperdynamic, hypertensive therapy is hemodilution. The idea now is to maintain blood flow at almost all cost. Mean arterial pressures above 130 mm Hg have been reported as a way to control intracranial hypertension. As perfusion is maintained, the ICP frequently decreases, consequent to the collapse of venous capacitance vessels. Hyperventilation is still effective as a last means of controlling malignant ICP, as is drainage of fluid via a ventriculostomy. The proof of the pudding is that many of the patients managed with these newer techniques recover a higher neurologic level than did historical controls managed using the previous techniques.

Decreasing oxygen demand by inducing coma, as can be done with barbiturates and thiopental, is still sometimes used. Its clinical value remains unclear. Other adjunctive measures for modern management of the head-injured patient include avoidance of hypoglycemia (glucose being the predominant metabolic fuel of the brain) and hyperglycemia (the brain apparently producing increased lactate and further vasodilating). Oxygenation is obviously also maintained.

QUESTIONS:

1. The net result of aerobic metabolism of 1 mol of glucose is:
   a. ATP, (18 mol), lactate.
   b. ATP, (38 mol), carbon dioxide, and water
   c. ATP, (38 mol), lactate.
   d. ATP, (2 mol), lactate.

2. An estimated blood loss of 35% of blood volume reflects:
   a. Class I hemorrhage.
   b. Class II hemorrhage.
   c. Class III hemorrhage.
   d. Class IV hemorrhage.

3. Swan-Ganz parameters include a PACWP of 12 mm Hg and a cardiac index of 2.7 L/min/m. The patient is:
   a. Normal.
   b. Hyperdynamic.
   c. Hypodynamic.
   d. Requires more information to determine.

4. A 70-kg man receives dopamine at a dose of 700 μg/min. This drug effect is best described as:
   a. Dopaminergic.
   b. β-Adrenergic.
   c. α-Adrenergic.

5. An arteriovenous difference of 2.0 ml is most consistent with:
   a. Septic shock.
   b. Cardiogenic shock.
   c. Hemorrhagic shock.
   d. Spinal shock.

6. A patient in being mechanically ventilated on assist/control mode. His arterial blood gases are: pH 7.55, P_{CO_2} 24, P_{O_2} 79, saturation 92%. The set rate is 12 breaths per minute; the patient is breathing 20 times per minute. What should be done?
   a. Increase the F_{IO_2}.
   b. Sedate the patient.
   c. Add deadspace to the circuit.
   d. Increase the rate of ventilation.

7. Low levels of erythrocyte 2,3-DPG:
   a. Increase oxygen affinity.
   b. Decrease oxygen affinity.
   c. Increase acidosis.
   d. Increase alkalosis.

8. A patient with a known blood loss of 1,500 ml probably requires how much crystalloid?
   a. 1,500 ml.
   b. 3,000 ml.
   c. 4,500 ml.
   d. 6,000 ml.

9. A patient has ARDS. On an F_{IO_2} of 75% on 10 cm H_2O PEEP, the P_{O_2} is only 50 mm Hg, P_{CO_2} is 39 mm Hg, and pH is 7.28. What would you do?
   a. Increase the F_{IO_2} to 100%.
   b. Increase the PEEP.
   c. Increase the ventilatory rate.
   d. Give bicarbonate.

10. A postoperative patient has a platelet count of 50,000/mm^3 and no clinically apparent bleeding. You would:
   a. Transfuse 6 units HLA-matched platelets.
   b. Transfuse 6 units of banked platelets.
   c. Do not transfuse unless the platelet count falls to 30,000/mm^3.
   d. Administer cryoprecipitate.

SELECTED REFERENCES

Fulkerson WJ, MacIntyre N, Stamler J, Crapo JD. Pathogenesis and treatment of the adult respiratory distress syndrome. *Arch Int Med* 1996;156:29–38.
Leibowitz, ed. Controversies in critical care medicine. *Crit*

Care Clin 1996;12(3). (Whole issue describes a number of important issues.)

Marino PL. *The ICU book,* 2nd ed. Baltimore: Williams & Wilkins, 1998. (Despite the provocative title, this volume continues to be a most readable critical care book. The cover is still blue but lighter and the weight of the tome heavier. My residents discovered the book first. I still wish I had written it.)

Moore FA, Haenel JB. Ventilatory strategies for acute respiratory failure. *Amer J Surg* 1997;173:53–56.

Sachdeva RC, Guntupalli. Acute respiratory distress syndrome. *Crit Care Clin* 1997;13:503–521.

Thadhani R, Pascual M, Bonventre JV. Acute renal failure. *N Engl J Med* 1996;334:1448–1460.

Wilmore DW, Brennan MF, Harken AH, Holcroft JW, Meakins JL. *Care of the surgical patient,* Vol. I. *Critical care,* New York: Scientific American, 1988. (The whole section on critical care is excellent, the graphics, in color, superb, and the algorithms useful.)

24

Radiology of the Liver, Biliary Tract, and Pancreas

Shelley Nan Weiner

Diagnostic imaging is essential for the evaluation and management of many surgical problems. It is not practical to discuss all of the surgical applications of radiology in the context of a surgical review book. The following is a review of the use of some of the imaging modalities available for evaluating the liver, biliary tract, and pancreas. The information was compiled from many of the references included at the end of the section. A more complete discussion can be obtained by consulting the sources listed.

LIVER

The major imaging modalities used to evaluate the liver are (a) ultrasonography; (b) computed tomography (CT) with and without the use of intravenous iodinated contrast; (c) magnetic resonance imaging (MRI); (d) scintigraphy; and (e) angiography.

Benign Space-Occupying Lesions of the Liver

The most common benign neoplasm of the liver is a cavernous hemangioma. It is usually an incidental finding in a patient being evaluated for another problem. Often a hepatic mass is detected on a sonogram or a CT scan of the abdomen, which can be compatible with many types of space-occupying masses of the liver, including cavernous hemangioma, hepatic cyst, hepatic adenoma, hemangioendothelioma, abscess, and primary or secondary carcinomas of the liver.

The typical sonographic appearance of a hepatic hemangioma is a well defined, homogeneous echogenic mass (Fig. 24.1), a pattern seen in about 70% to 80% of the cases. A hypoechoic center is occasionally seen. On a contrast-enhanced CT examination not directed specifically at the diagnosis of hemangioma, an area of diminished attenuation with or without an enhancing rim may be seen. To use CT to help identify a hemangioma, a problem-directed scan must be performed at another time. This study consists of a noncontrast scan of the liver to identify the lesion followed by dynamic scanning over the lesion during a bolus injection of iodinated contrast material. A pattern of early peripheral enhancement of the mass followed over time by extension of enhancement toward the center until the entire lesion enhances is seen in 54% to 79% of the cases (Fig 24.2).

Because neither CT nor sonography is definitive, a confirmatory test is recommended. The procedure of choice is a technetium-99m (^{99m}Tc) red blood cell scan with single photon emission computed tomography (SPECT) imaging if the lesion is more than 2.0 to 2.5 cm in diameter. On this examination a hemangioma is seen as a photon-deficient area in the early dynamic

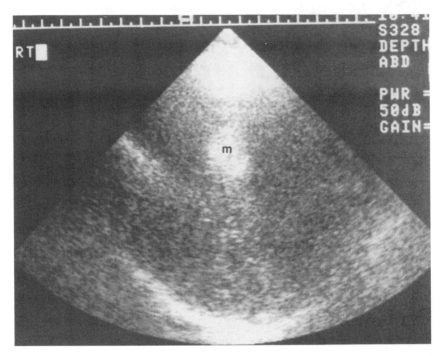

FIG. 24.1. Hemangioma. Transverse sonogram of the liver demonstrating a highly echogenic mass (*m*) in the right lobe of the liver consistent with a hemangioma.

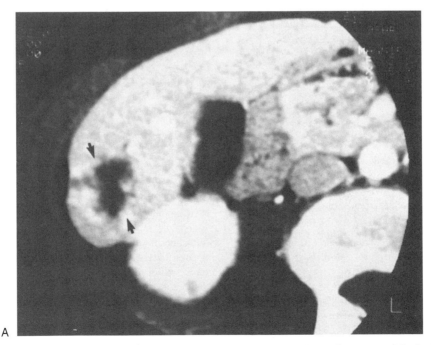

A

FIG. 24.2. Hemangioma. Dynamic CT scan of a cavernous hemangioma. **A:** Immediate scan of the lesion following the rapid bolus injection of iodinated contrast material demonstrating an area of diminished attenuation in the right lobe of the liver with a thin area of peripheral enhancement (*arrows*).

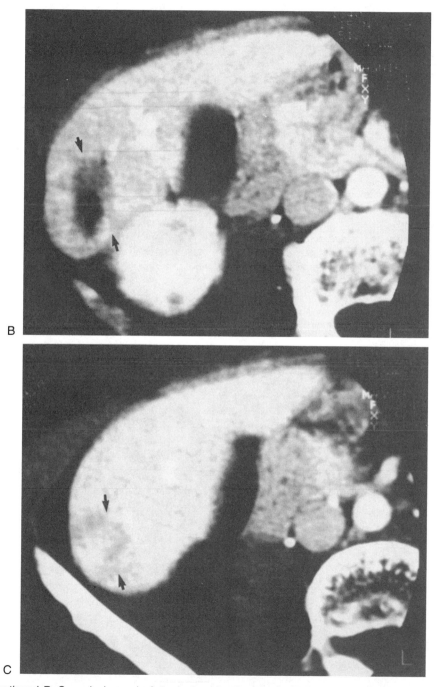

FIG. 24.2. *Continued.* **B:** Same lesion as in **A** 5 minutes after the injection demonstrates extension of the enhancement toward the center of the lesion (*arrows*). **C:** Same lesion as in **A** and **B** 15 minutes after the injection with essentially complete enhancement of the lesion (*arrows*).

phase scan with persistent accumulation of the isotope on the delayed SPECT images. The diagnostic specificity and sensitivity of this examination approaches 100% if the lesion is 2 cm or larger (Fig. 24.3). For lesions less than 2 cm in diameter the imaging examination of choice to confirm the presence of a hemangioma is MRI. On an MRI examination hemangiomas tend to be hypointense on T1-weighted images and hyperintense on T2-weighted images with a long second echo (Fig. 24.4).

The distinction between hepatic adenoma and focal nodular hyperplasia is difficult. Sonography is not helpful for differentiating between these two entities, which both tend to be discrete hepatic masses of variable echogenicity. These lesions appear as areas of decreased attenuation on a nonenhanced CT scan, and they rapidly enhance after intravenous injection of a bolus of iodinated contrast material. On delayed postcon-

trast scans these lesions appear to have the same attenuation coefficients as normal liver. MRI of these lesions is also nonspecific.

At times scintigraphy is helpful for differentiating between the two lesions. Hepatic adenomas are photon-deficient areas on ^{99m}Tc-sulfur colloid scans. However, masses secondary to focal nodular hyperplasia often take up the isotope because these lesions contain Kupffer cells.

Hepatic cysts, which are common, may be congenital or acquired and are often an incidental finding. Sonographically, a cyst is a well demarcated sonolucent area with posterior acoustic enhancement (Fig. 24.5). On CT examination a hepatic cyst appears as a well marginated lesion of diminished attenuation compared to normal liver, with no evidence of significant enhancement following intravenous administration of iodinated contrast material. Attenuation coefficients are consistent with those of fluid.

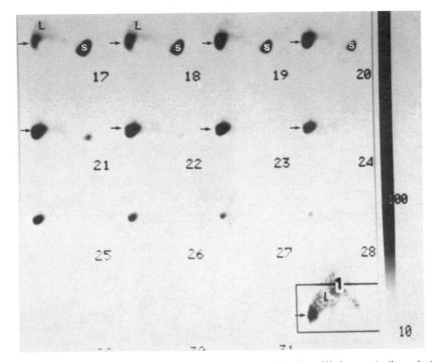

FIG. 24.3. Hemangioma. ^{99m}Tc-labeled RBC coronal SPECT images of the liver (*L*) demonstrating a hot area in the right lobe of the liver (*arrows*) compatible with a hemangioma. *S*, spleen.

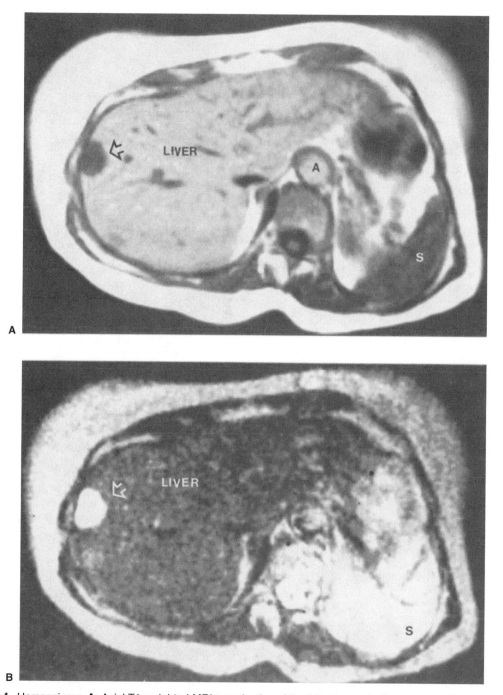

FIG. 24.4. Hemangioma. **A:** Axial T1-weighted MRI examination of the liver demonstrating an area of decreased signal intensity in the right lobe of the liver (*arrow*). **B:** Axial T2-weighted MRI with a long second echo of the same lesion as in **A** demonstrates the area to be hyperintense. These findings are compatible with a hemangioma. *S,* spleen; *A,* aorta.

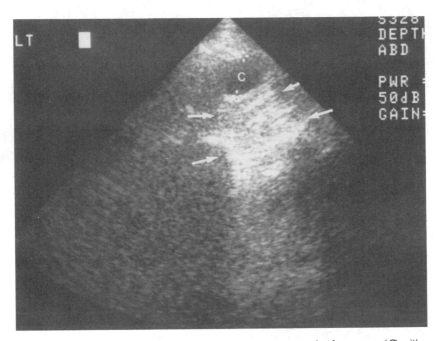

FIG. 24.5. Hepatic cyst. Transverse sonogram of the liver demonstrates an echo-free mass (*C*) with posterior acoustic enhancement (*arrows*) consistent with a hepatic cyst.

Hepatic Abscess

The preoperative diagnosis of a liver abscess can usually be established by the available imaging modalities. Plain films of the abdomen may be normal or may demonstrate elevation of the right hemidiaphragm, a right subpulmonic effusion, hepatomegaly, or rarely gas within the liver.

Ultrasonography and CT scans are the modalities of choice to establish the diagnosis of a suspected liver abscess. The sonographic appearance of an abscess can be variable, but generally an inhomogeneous mass with areas of sonolucency (fluid) and thick, irregular walls is demonstrated (Fig. 24.6A). If gas is present within an abscess it produces bright central echoes. CT performed after intravenous contrast demonstrates an area of diminished attenuation that may contain air–fluid levels and may have an enhancing rim. This imaging appearance by itself, without the presence of air-fluid levels, may be nonspecific but in the proper clinical setting is compatible with the presence of an abscess (Fig. 24.6B). Computed tomography, ultrasonography (US), or both can be used as a guide for aspiration and drainage of a pyogenic liver abscess.

Amebic abscesses and echinococcal cysts can also be imaged by CT and US. Echinococcal cysts (Fig. 24.7) may contain calcifications and often appear as multiloculated cystic areas with multiple daughter cysts.

With the increased use of cross-sectional imaging techniques, fatty infiltration (focal, geographic, and diffuse) of the liver has been observed. It is a benign process and must be differentiated from primary or secondary neoplasms of the liver. Sonographically, focal fatty lesions appear as homogeneous hyperechoic masses. On CT these focal fatty lesions are well defined masses with diminished attenuation coefficients consistent with those of fat. When diffuse fatty infiltration of the liver is present (Fig. 24.8) the area of involvement has attenuation numbers equal to or less than those of the spleen on a noncontrast scan. Following an intravenous bolus injection of contrast material, the area of fatty infiltration enhances less than the normal hepatic parenchyma and significantly less than the spleen. The presence of diffuse fatty infiltration of the liver can be

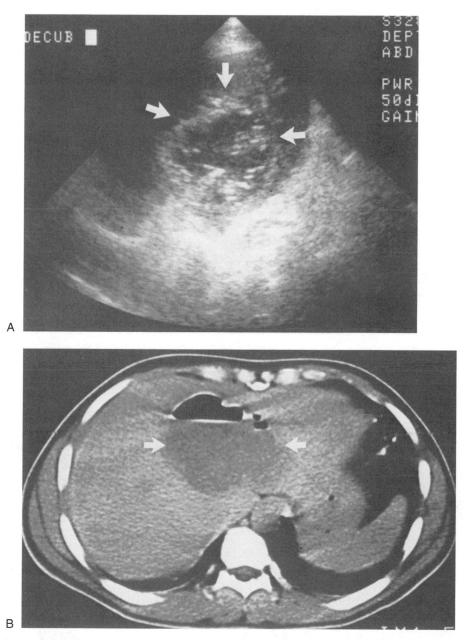

FIG. 24.6. Intrahepatic abscess. **A:** Longitudinal sonogram of the liver demonstrating a heterogeneous mass (*arrows*) with irregular margins. There are hypoechoic and hyperechoic areas. **B:** CT scan of the same patient demonstrating an irregular mass (*arrows*) with an air–fluid level.

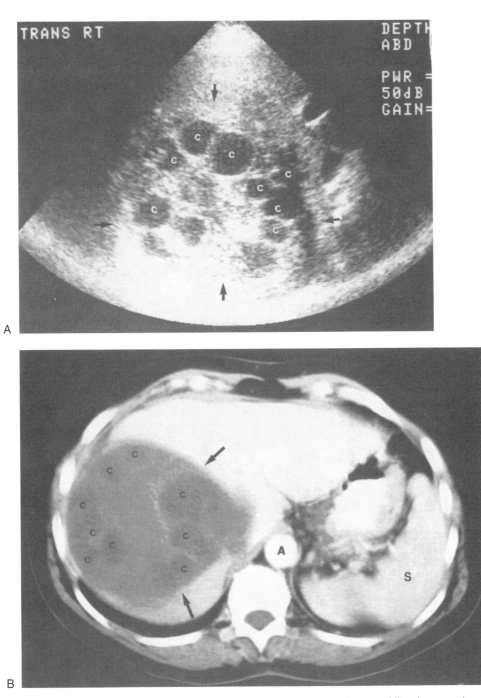

FIG. 24.7. Echinococcal cyst. **A:** Longitudinal sonogram of the liver demonstrating a multilocular mass (*arrows*) containing many small cysts (*c*). **B:** CT scan of the same patient also demonstrating a multilocular cystic mass (*arrows*) containing many smaller daughter cysts (*c*) in the liver. *A,* aorta; *S,* spleen.

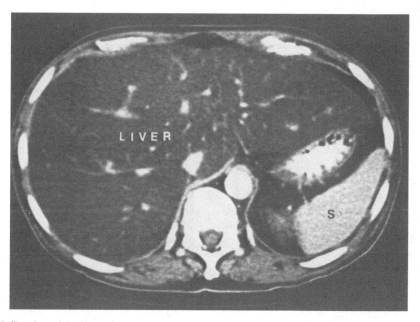

FIG. 24.8. Fatty infiltration of the liver. Contrast-enhanced CT scan of the liver demonstrating diminished attenuation of the liver compared to that of the spleen (*S*).

confirmed with a 99mTc-sulfur colloid liver scan. If the area of abnormal attenuation on the CT scan represents fatty infiltration, the sulfur colloid scan is normal, as the Kupffer cells that take up this isotope have been neither displaced nor destroyed. If the lesion seen on CT does not represent fatty infiltration, however, the sulfur colloid scan shows a photon-deficient area that corresponds to the abnormality on the CT scan.

Malignant Space-Occupying Lesions of the Liver

Primary Malignant Neoplasms

Hepatoma is the most common primary malignant neoplasm of the liver. A space-occupying mass within the liver is seen on ultrasonography. The lesion may be solitary, multiple, or infiltrating. The echo pattern of hepatoma is variable. Occasionally a hypoechoic band or rim surround the tumor is seen, which is thought to be related to a fibrous capsule that surrounds some hepatomas. Ultrasonography is valuable for evaluating this neoplasm because of it ability to image the portal vein.

Invasion of this vascular structure by a hepatic neoplasm is strong evidence for hepatoma.

The appearance of a hepatoma on CT scans is also variable. On a scan performed after intravenous administration of a bolus of iodinated contrast material, an inhomogeneous mass with areas of enhancement and nonenhancement is seen. An enhancing rim is occasionally present. Tumor thrombus in the portal vein may also be detected.

Cross-sectional imaging (US or CT) can be used to direct an aspiration biopsy of a space-occupying mass in the liver. It can also be used to document its histology.

Arteriography is no longer the procedure of choice for evaluating the resectability of a hepatoma. Several studies have shown that dynamic CT and CT with arterial portography can reliably determine the number and size of lesions, their segmental location, and the relation of these lesions to the hepatic vasculature; and it can identify any extrahepatic disease. This increasingly important use of CT for the surgeon is too complex to discuss in detail here. The reader is referred to the references at the end of the chapter for a complete discussion of this technique.

Metastatic Neoplasms of the Liver

Ultrasonography, CT, and MRI are acceptable, reliable methods for evaluating the liver for metastases. Scintigraphy is rarely used at this time.

Normal liver parenchyma is sonographically homogeneous. Metastases appear as multiple areas of increased or decreased echogenicity (Fig. 24.9A,B). Sometimes these lesions demonstrate areas of liquefaction secondary to tumor necrosis. Intraoperative sonography can be used to assist in the identification of metastases during surgical exploration.

Spiral CT with two- to three-phase (noncontrast, arterial phase, and portal venous phase) imaging is the most sophisticated CT technique available today. If spiral CT is not available, the liver should always be examined by CT for metastatic disease after contrast enhancement. Most metastatic lesions appear as areas of diminished attenuation (Fig. 24.9D,F). Occasionally they are of increased attenuation or exhibit an enhancing rim. Vascular metastases may have the same attenuation as normal liver following intravenous administration of a bolus of iodinated contrast material and therefore may be difficult to detect. Patients with known vascular primary tumors, such as islet cell carcinomas of the pancreas, should undergo noncontrast scanning as well. Mucin-producing tumors of the colon, ovary, stomach, and breast and islet cell adenocarcinomas of the pancreas frequently contain punctate calcifications that can be detected by CT (Fig. 24.9C,D) or US (Fig. 24.9B).

Cirrhosis and Portal Hypertension

Portal hypertension may be pre- or postsinusoidal. Presinusoidal obstruction is related to tumors of the reticuloendothelial system, viral hepatitis, schistosomiasis, congenital hepatic fibrosis, chronic biliary tract obstruction, and cavernous transformation of the portal vein. The most common cause of postsinusoidal portal hypertension is alcoholic cirrhosis, but it can also be seen with congestive heart failure, postnecrotic cirrhosis, and the Budd-Chiari syndrome. Occasionally, portal hypertension is secondary to a visceral arteriovenous fistula.

Plain films of the abdomen in a patient with portal hypertension may be normal or may demonstrate hepatosplenomegaly or increased density secondary to ascites. An upper gastrointestinal (GI) series may reveal serpiginous filling defects (varices) in the distal esophagus and fundus of the stomach (Fig. 24.10).

Hepatic scintigraphy with ^{99m}Tc-sulfur colloid is nonspecific in the presence of cirrhosis. Often an inhomogeneous liver with increased uptake by the spleen and bone marrow is demonstrated (Fig. 24.11).

Sonography and CT can detect small amounts of ascites and the presence of varices. In addition, morphologic changes of the liver, such as a decrease in the size of the right lobe with enlargement of the caudate lobe or left lobe (or both) and nodularity of the liver surface, can be seen. A diffuse decrease in attenuation of the liver on CT (which is more pronounced after contrast enhancement), characteristic of fatty infiltration of the liver (Fig. 24.8), can be seen.

The most widely accepted methods for imaging the portal venous system are a combination of arterial portography (selective celiac and superior mesenteric arteriography) and hepatic venography or transhepatic portal venography. The latter procedure is more complex and has a higher complication rate, especially in the presence of ascites.

In patients with cirrhosis, arterial portography may demonstrate the following.

1. *Dilatation of the hepatic artery.* A normal liver receives 75% to 80% of its blood supply from the portal vein. When portal hypertension is present, flow in the portal vein is reduced, resulting in a reciprocal increase in hepatic artery blood flow.
2. *Tortuosity and elongation of the intrahepatic arteries* is a small, shrunken liver. This picture is often referred to as a "corkscrew" appearance of the intrahepatic arteries.
3. *Varices.* Esophageal, mesenteric, and retroperitoneal varices may be demonstrated by arterial portography.
4. *Reverse flow* in the inferior mesenteric vein, dilatation of the umbilical vein, or splenorenal shunts.

Hepatic venography is performed when a portosystemic shunt is contemplated. The hepatic veins are catheterized via a transfemoral or transjugular approach. Pressures are obtained in two or three hepatic veins. These pressures should be similar to that in the inferior vena cava. Free hepatic venography is then performed. Normally, fourth- to fifth-order branching is

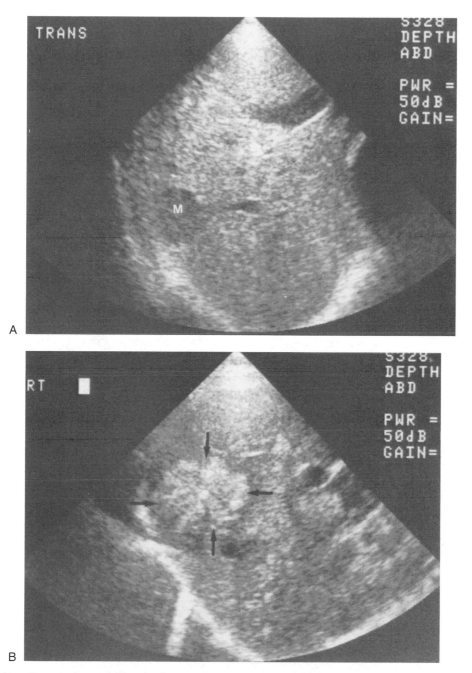

FIG. 24.9. Hepatic metastases. **A:** Longitudinal sonogram of the liver demonstrating a hypoechoic mass (*M*) in the right lobe of the liver. This lesion is metastatic from a renal cell carcinoma. **B:** Longitudinal sonogram of the liver demonstrating a large hyperechoic mass (*arrows*) in the right lobe of the liver. The marked increased echogenicity suggests psammomatous calcifications in this patient with metastatic colon carcinoma.

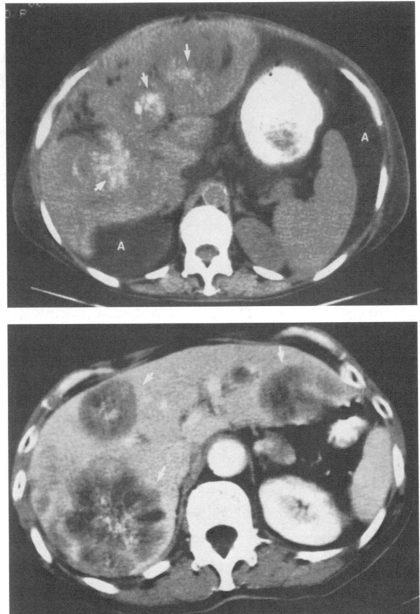

FIG. 24.9. *Continued* **C:** Non-contrast-enhanced CT scan of the same patient as in **B** demonstrating multiple areas of diminished attenuation in the liver consistent with metastases. Fine calcifications are seen within the masses (*arrows*). Ascites (*A*) is present. **D:** Contrast-enhanced CT scan in another patient with metastatic colon carcinoma demonstrating
multiple areas of decreased attenuation that also contain calcification (*arrows*).

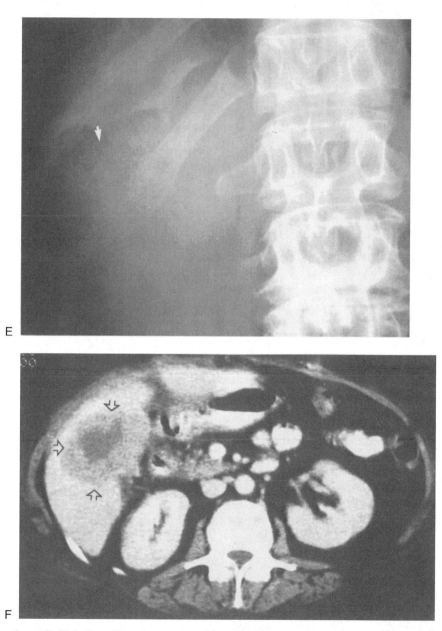

FIG. 24.9. *Continued* **E:** Plain film of the abdomen in same patient as in **D** with metastatic colon carcinoma demonstrating the fine calcifications in the liver (*arrows*) that can be seen in metastatic mucinous carcinomas. **F:** Contrast-enhanced CT scan demonstrating a single heterogeneous metastatic lesion in the liver (*arrows*). This patient had metastatic gallbladder carcinoma.

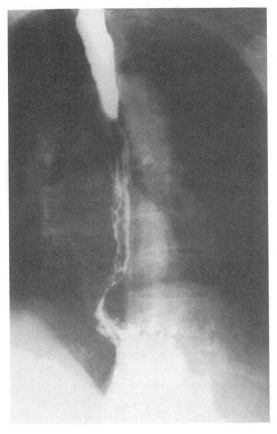

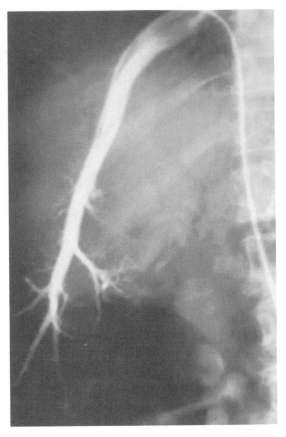

FIG. 24.10. Varices. Varices are seen as serpiginous filling defects in the distal esophagus on this upper gastrointestinal series in a cirrhotic patient.

FIG. 24.11. Free hepatic venogram. Free hepatic venogram demonstrates decreased arborization and irregularity of the hepatic veins in a patient with Laennec's cirrhosis.

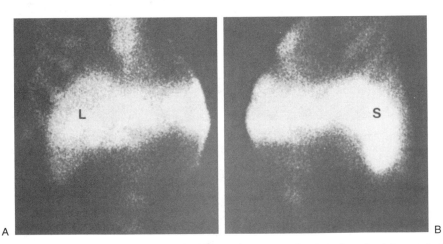

FIG. 24.12. Colloid shift. **A:** Anterior ^{99m}Tc-sulfur colloid liver spleen scan of a cirrhotic patient demonstrating decreased uptake of the isotope in the liver (*L*). **B:** Anterior ^{99m}Tc-sulfur colloid scan from the same patient as in **A** demonstrating a shift of the colloid to the spleen (*S*) and bone marrow of the spine and ribs.

seen. With postsinusoidal cirrhosis there is decreased arborization of the hepatic veins with evidence of venous stenoses and occlusions (Fig. 24.12). The catheter is then wedged into at least two hepatic veins, and pressures are recorded. The corrected sinusoidal pressure, or that part of the pressure due to intrahepatic obstruction, is equal to the wedged hepatic venous pressure minus the free hepatic venous pressure. The corrected sinusoidal pressure should be 100 mm of saline or less. Varices develop at pressures higher than 200 mm of saline. A wedged hepatic venogram is then obtained. Normally there is a homogeneous parenchymal stain with filling of hepatic veins and small portal radicals (Fig.

24.13), and there is hepatopedal flow of contrast. With postsinusoidal portal hypertension the parenchymal stain is inhomogeneous, and hepatofugal flow in the portal vein may be seen. Inferior venocavagraphy is also performed to demonstrate any anatomic variants prior to shunt surgery.

Transjugular intrahepatic portosystemic shunt (TIPS) can be performed in the radiology department in patients with intractable variceal bleeding who may be too sick to go to the operating room for surgical shunt.

BILIARY TRACT

The biliary tract may be evaluated by plain films, oral cholecystography, US, CT, cholescintigraphy, endoscopic retrograde cholangiopancreatography (ERCP), and percutaneous transhepatic cholangiography.

Plain Films

For evaluating a patient with normal liver function tests and intermittent right upper quadrant pain, plain films are occasionally helpful. Calcified gallstones are found in 10% to 15% of patients with stones. Milk of calcium bile (calcium carbonate, calcium phosphate, or calcium bilirubinate) may also be detected (Fig. 24.14) and is often associated with chronic cholecystitis. Calcification of the gallbladder wall (porcelain gallbladder) is also associated with both chronic cholecystitis and an increased incidence of gallbladder carcinoma (Fig. 24.15). Emphysematous cholecystitis (air in the gallbladder) is uncommon but may be detected on plain films.

Cholelithiasis and Cholecystoses

The evaluation of a patient with chronic right upper quadrant pain and normal liver function tests should begin with US. The advantage of this examination over oral cholecystography is its relative ease of performance, the absence of ionizing radiation, completion at a single examination, and the fact that normal liver and gallbladder function is not required. Biliary calculi are highly echogenic and are usually associated with acoustic shadowing (Fig. 24.16A). Echoes within the

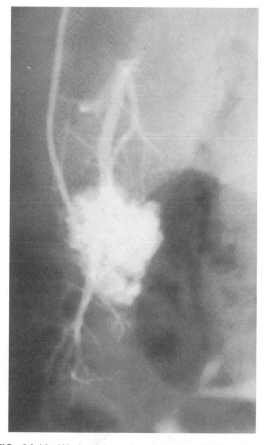

FIG. 24.13. Wedged hepatic venogram. Wedged hepatic venogram of the same patient as in Fig. 24.12 demonstrates inhomogeneous parenchymal staining.

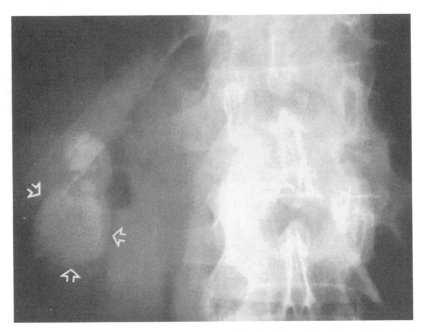

FIG. 24.14. Plain film of the abdomen demonstrates milk of calcium bile in the gallbladder (*arrows*).

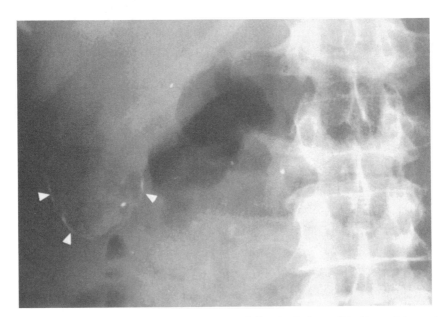

FIG. 24.15. Plain film of the abdomen demonstrates calcification in the gallbladder wall (*arrowheads*).

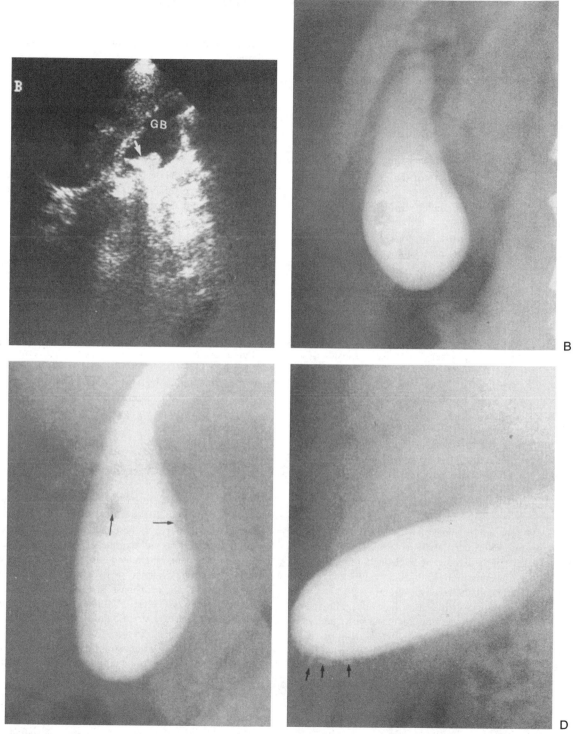

FIG. 24.16. Cholelithiasis. **A:** Decubitus sonogram of the gallbladder (*GB*) demonstrates a dense echo (*arrow*) with posterior acoustic shadowing diagnostic of cholelithiasis. **B:** Oral cholecystogram demonstrating multiple filling defects compatible with cholelithiasis. **C:** Oral cholecystogram demonstrating two fixed filling defects (*arrows*) compatible with cholesterol polyps in a patient with cholesterolosis. **D:** Oral cholecystogram in a patient with adenomyomatosis. Rokitansky-Aschoff sinuses (*arrows*) are seen at the fundus of the gallbladder.

gallbladder that do not shadow may be related to sludge, polyps, gallbladder carcinoma, and occasionally stones.

If the US examination of gallbladder is inadequate or equivocal, oral cholecystography can be performed. Up to 30% of patients require a 2-day study (which is done routinely at some institutions). The most commonly used contrast agent is iopanoic acid tablets, but others are available. Nonvisualization of the gallbladder may be related to failure of the patient to take the contrast or nonabsorption of the contrast (gastric or esophageal obstruction, malabsorption, liver disease, acute pancreatitis).

In addition to demonstrating stones (Fig. 24.16B), an oral cholecystogram can detect hyperplastic cholecystosis (cholesterolosis and adenomyomatosis). The presence of fixed filling defects (cholesterol polyps) within the gallbladder (Fig. 24.16C) is compatible with cholesterolosis. With adenomyomatosis, multiple outpouchings or Rokitansky-Aschoff sinuses are present (Fig. 24.16D). With both of these conditions there is hyperconcentration and hyperexcretion of the contrast.

Cholecystitis

Cholescintigraphy is the modality of choice for evaluating a patient with suspected acute cholecystitis because it is a specific test for cystic duct patency. This examination has a sensitivity of more than 90% and a specificity over 90%. A patient must be fasting for at least 2 hours prior to the examination. A ^{99m}Tc-labeled iminodiacetic acid derivative (Tc-IDA) is injected intravenously. It is rapidly taken up by the liver and excreted into the bile. Normally, there is symmetric homogeneous uptake of the isotope by the liver 15 minutes after injection. The common bile duct, gallbladder, and bowel should be visualized by 1 hour (Fig. 24.17A).

With acute cholecystitis, at 1 hour the gallbladder fails to visualize, but the bile ducts and bowl are well seen. With chronic cholecystitis, there is delayed visualization of the gallbladder; it is usually detected by 4 hours, although visualization may be delayed up to 24 hours.

This examination may not be reliable in the population of extremely ill patients, who may be receiving hyperalimentation. There is a significant false-positive rate among these individuals. To avoid this problem

(and to speed up the examination in all other patients, eliminating the need for 4- and 24-hour scans) many centers are using morphine-augmentation cholescintigraphy. The morphine is given 40 to 60 minutes after the isotope if there is no visualization of the gallbladder but the common duct and small bowel are seen. The morphine causes spasm of the sphincter of Oddi, resulting in increased pressure in the common bile duct, which in turn causes reflux of contrast into the cystic duct filling the gallbladder if the cystic duct is patent. This maneuver improves the reliability of the examination in the severely ill population and may decrease the time of diagnosis in the rest of the population from 4 hours to 90 minutes (Fig. 24.17B–E). It should be noted that some controversy still exists about this technique.

In patients with early extrahepatic obstruction there is poor hepatic uptake of the isotope, with visualization of the bile ducts but not the bowel. With long-standing biliary tract obstruction or hepatocellular disease there is poor hepatic uptake of the radioisotope, and no excretion is detected.

Percutaneous cholecystostomy can be performed at the bedside with sonographic guidance or in the radiology department in patients with acute cholecystitis who are deemed too ill for surgery. This measure often palliates the situation until the patient can tolerate a more definitive procedure.

Biliary Tract Obstruction

Cross-sectional imaging (US and CT) is an essential part of evaluating patients with suspected biliary tract obstruction. Not only can these modalities document dilatation of the intra- and extrahepatic bile ducts, often they can document the site and etiology of the obstruction. In addition, evidence of liver metastases, an intraabdominal mass, or a mass in the porta hepatis or gallbladder may be detected. CT and US are not reliable for diagnosing early obstruction of the bile ducts before dilatation has occurred. In this situation cholescintigraphy can be helpful by demonstrating normal hepatic uptake and excretion into the common bile duct and gallbladder but no filling of the duodenum.

Sonography, because of its lower cost and lack of ionizing radiation, should be the initial examination in a patient in whom obstruction of the biliary tree is clinically suspected, especially if the patient is jaundiced.

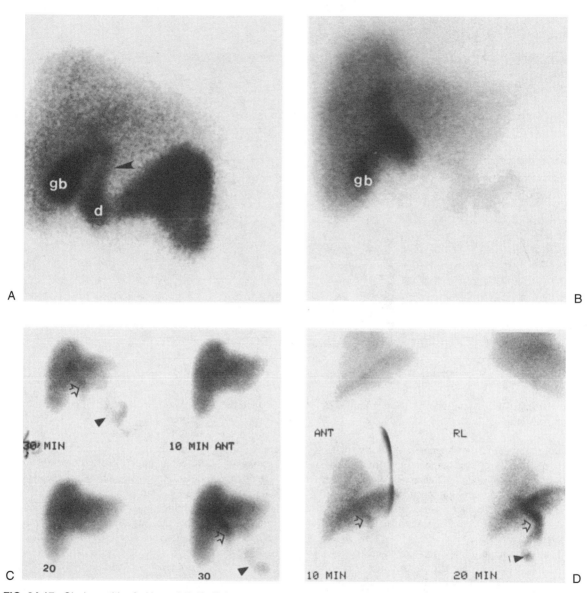

FIG. 24.17. Cholecystitis. **A:** Normal 99mTc-IDA scan 30 minutes after injection of the isotope demonstrates prompt filling of the gallbladder (*gb*), duodenum (*d*), and common bile duct (*arrowhead.*) **B:** 99mTc-IDA scan at 10, 20, 30, and 40 minutes after injection of the isotope demonstrates filling of the common bile duct (*arrowheads*) and small bowel but not the gallbladder. **C:** Same patient as in **B** 30 minutes after intravenous administration of morphine sulfate demonstrates the gallbladder (*gb*). This patient did not have cystic duct obstruction. **D:** 99mTc-IDA scan in a different patient demonstrates filling of the common bile duct 10 minutes after injection of the isotope (*arrow*) and the small bowel 20 minutes after the injection (*arrowhead*) but no filling of the gallbladder.

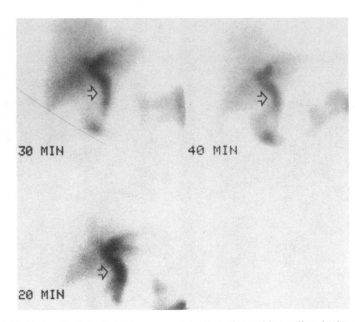

FIG. 24.17. *Continued.* **E:** Forty minutes after intravenous injection of morphine sulfate in the same patient as in **D** the gallbladder fails to visualize. The common bile duct (*arrows*) is well seen. This patient had cystic duct obstruction and acute cholecystitis.

CT can be used when sonography is equivocal or fails to demonstrate clearly the site and etiology of the obstruction.

Sonographyically, the diagnosis of biliary tract obstruction depends on the demonstration of dilated intra- or extrahepatic ducts, which appear as tubular structures with increased through transmission (Fig. 24.18A). The common hepatic duct is anterior and lateral to the portal vein and should not be more than 6 to 8 mm in diameter.

Dilated intrahepatic bile ducts are branching, linear, or circular structures that do not enhance after intravenous contrast on CT. Dilated extrahepatic ducts are seen as a series of circles coursing toward the ampulla of Vater. The CT scan or US should always include the entire liver, gallbladder, and pancreas because these organs often give a clue as to the cause of the obstruction. If a mass is identified by CT (or US) a percutaneous aspiration biopsy can be performed. Distal common bile duct calculi can also be detected by both CT and US if the studies are directed to this area. US is less reliable than CT because of the problem of overlying bowel gas (Fig. 24.19A).

Once the diagnosis of obstructive jaundice has been established, an attempt is made to establish the etiology of the obstruction. Obstruction at the level of the pancreas is most commonly due to pancreatic carcinoma, although the differential diagnosis of obstruction at this level also includes strictures, cholelithiasis, metastases, sclerosing cholangitis, and cholangiocarcinoma. Obstruction of the common hepatic duct is usually due to cholangiocarcinoma, but carcinoma of the gallbladder, sclerosing cholangitis, and metastases must also be considered. Obstruction at the porta hepatis is most commonly due to cholangiocarcinoma (Klatzkin's tumor), but sclerosing cholangitis and metastases must be excluded.

Once the diagnosis of obstructive jaundice has been established and the etiology is determined, there are several nonoperative techniques that can be employed for management of these patients if surgery is not indicated or possible. Endoscopic sphincterotomy can be used for treatment of common bile duct stones prior to laparoscopic cholecystectomy or in postcholecystectomy patients (Fig. 24.20). In the presence of a malignant obstruction of the bile duct a stent can be placed

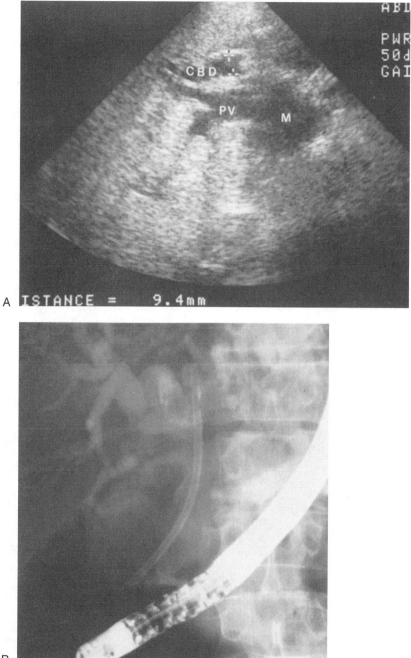

FIG. 24.18. Biliary obstruction. **A:** Transverse sonogram of the liver demonstrates dilatation of the common bile duct (*CBD*), which is anterior to the portal vein. A mass (*M*) is seen in the head of the pancreas. This mass is obstructing the bile duct. **B:** ERCP examination in the same patient demonstrates obstruction of the common bile duct. A stent has been placed endoscopically to relieve the obstruction.

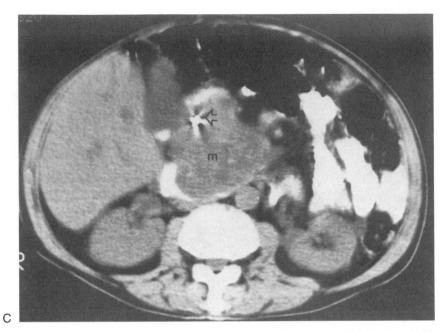

FIG. 24.18. *Continued.* **C:** CT scan in the same patient demonstrates a large mass (*M*) in the head of the pancreas. The stent (*arrow*) is seen as well.

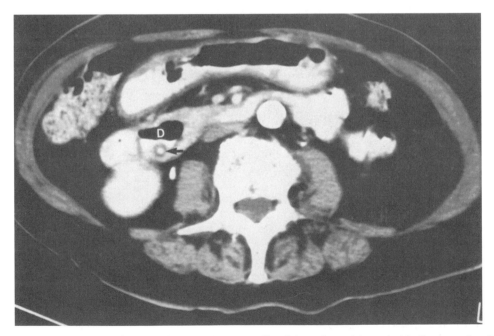

FIG. 24.19. Contrast-enhanced CT scan demonstrates a small gallstone (*arrow*) impacted in the ampulla of Vater. *D,* duodenum.

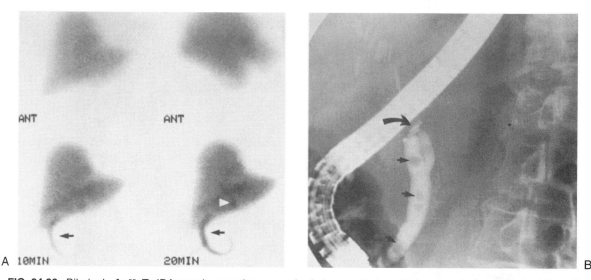

FIG. 24.20. Bile leak. **A:** 99mTc-IDA scan in a postlaparoscopic cholecystectomy patient demonstrating a bile leak from the common hepatic duct. There is rapid filling of the subhepatic drain (*arrows*) and no filling of the distal bile duct or small bowel. The proximal common hepatic duct is filled (*arrowhead*) at 20 minutes. **B:** ERCP in the same patient demonstrates retained common bile duct calculi (*small arrows*) and complete obstruction of the common bile duct at the level of the cystic duct (*curved arrow*) The common duct was transected at surgery. The retained calculi were removed via a sphincterotomy.

across the obstruction endoscopically or percutaneously (Fig. 24.18B).

Bile Leaks

Biliary tract leaks may be the result of hepatic trauma, or they may be iatrogenic. In the case of acute trauma CT is the procedure of choice. Cholescintigraphy is the procedure of choice for evaluating surgical anastomotic leaks or patency (Fig. 24.20A).

Bilomas can usually easily by imaged by US. They usually appear as well defined, anechoic collections with posterior wall acoustic enhancement, and they may be loculated. Bilomas may be intrahepatic, subcapsular, or extrahepatic. If they become infected, internal echoes may be seen. CT also can detect bilomas.

Bile leaks from the cystic duct after laparoscopic cholecystectomy can frequently be managed by endoscopic placement of a common bile duct stent.

PANCREAS

The best imaging modalities for the pancreas are CT and US.

Acute Pancreatitis

Plain film findings in patients with acute pancreatitis must be interpreted in conjunction with the clinical setting and laboratory findings. A localized, gas-filled, dilated loop of small bowel in the left upper quadrant (sentinel loop) is seen in fewer than 10% of patients with acute pancreatitis. Distension of the colon with an abrupt change of caliber at the splenic flexure is called the "colon cutoff sign." Both of these findings are due to a localized ileus.

Bolus-enhanced dynamic CT is the examination of choice for evaluating patients with suspected acute pancreatitis. It permits visualization not only of the pancreas but of the entire retroperitoneum. The CT findings with acute pancreatitis are (a) diffuse enlargement of the pancreas with areas of decreased attenuation; (b) focal enlargement; (c) irregular and indistinct margins of the gland; (d) areas of increased attenuation in the peripancreatic tissues; and (e) pancreatic and extrapancreatic fluid collections. Most pancreatic fluid collections are in the left anterior pararenal space and lesser sac. Less frequently, they occur in the perirenal space, posterior pararenal space, left lobe of the liver, transverse mesocolon, root of the small bowel mesentery, and me-

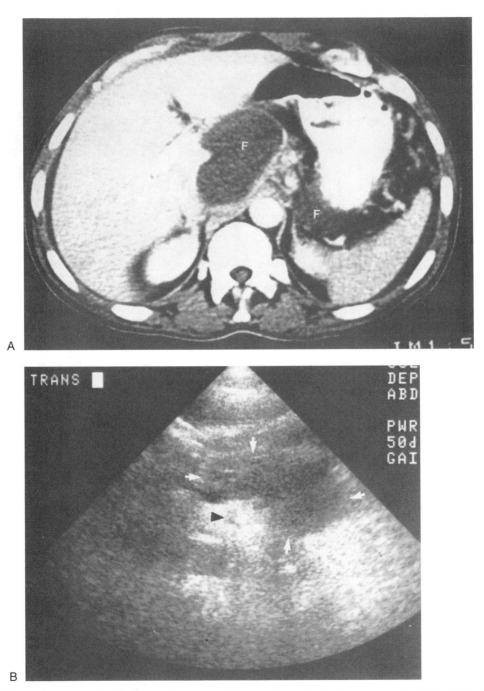

FIG. 24.21. Acute pancreatitis. **A:** Contrast-enhanced CT scan demonstrates two pancreatic fluid collections (*F*) in this patient with acute pancreatitis. **B:** Transverse sonogram of the same patient as in **A** demonstrating enlargement of the body and tail of the pancreas (*arrows*). The superior mesenteric artery (*arrowhead*) is identified.

diastinum (Fig. 24.21A). Pleural effusions may be detected, and in severe cases pancreatic ascites is present.

Computed tomography of a pancreatic phlegmon demonstrates a poorly defined mass with attenuation values greater than those for fluid but less than those for soft tissue. The presence of gas within a pancreatic fluid collection or a phlegmon is consistent with an abscess.

Ultrasonographic evaluation of the abdomen in a patient with acute pancreatitis may be limited by the presence of small bowel gas secondary to an ileus. It is useful, however, in patients in whom the clinical course is mild, in whom biliary pancreatitis is suspected, and for following the course of pancreatic fluid collections or phlegmon. The US findings associated with acute pancreatitis are similar to those on CT: Diffuse or focal areas of enlargement may be seen, low-level echoes consistent with edema of the gland are present (Fig. 24.21B), and peripancreatic fluid collections may be detected.

Chronic Pancreatitis

With chronic pancreatitis US or CT may demonstrate a normal or shrunken gland that possibly contains calci-

fications (Fig. 24.22). Focal enlargement of the gland can also be seen. Dilatation of the pancreatic duct to more than 4 mm or a pseudocyst may be present. On CT, pseudocysts have a thick wall with central attenuation values close to those of fluid. Sonographically, a pseudocyst often contains central echoes, probably related to debris, in the center of a sonolucent mass.

Adenocarcinoma of the Pancreas

Ultrasonography or CT should be the first imaging examinations in a patient with a suspected pancreatic carcinoma. These examinations are valuable because they can detect a pancreatic mass and demonstrate the extent of disease (liver metastases, dilatation of the bile ducts, and lymphadenopathy).

Bolus dynamic CT of the pancreas should reveal generally soft tissue masses that alter the normal contour of the gland. A dilated pancreatic duct may be demonstrated. Needle biopsy can establish the histologic diagnosis (Fig. 24.18C, 24.23). Obliteration of the fat surrounding the celiac and superior mesenteric arteries can be seen with both adenocarcinoma of the pancreas and

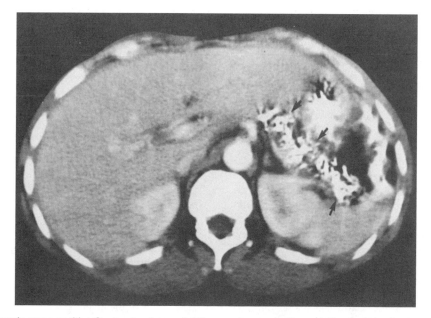

FIG. 24.22. Chronic pancreatitis. Contrast-enhanced CT scan demonstrating calcifications in the body and tail of the pancreas (*arrows*).

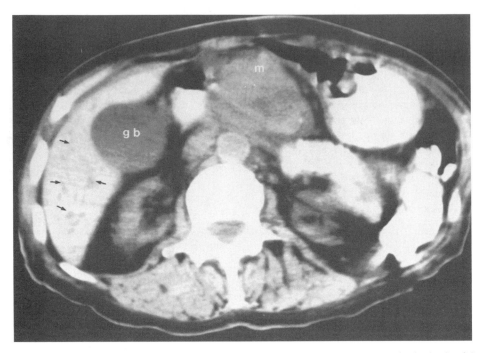

FIG. 24.23. Pancreatic carcinoma. Contrast-enhanced CT scan demonstrates a large mass in the body of the pancreas (*M*) distorting the normal contour of the gland. The gallbladder (*gb*) is distended, and there is dilatation of the intrahepatic ducts (*arrows*).

acute pancreatitis. It may also be observed in other neoplasms in or around the pancreas and cannot be used to determine the resectability of tumors of the pancreas.

For a pancreatic mass to be considered resectable the CT scan must demonstrate: (a) the absence of hepatic or nodal metastases; (b) no evidence of vascular invasion; and (c) a pancreatic mass less than 2 cm in diameter surrounded by normal parenchyma.

Ultrasonography of the pancreas is faster, is less expensive, and requires no intravenous or oral contrast. However, the examination may be limited by the presence of bowel gas, especially in the region of the body and tail of the pancreas. It is still a good screening examination for pancreatic carcinoma if an adequate view of the pancreas can be obtained. The findings on sonography are similar to those on CT. Focal pancreatic masses of decreased echogenicity suggest the diagnosis of carcinoma.

Endoscopic retrograde cholangiopancreatography (Fig. 24.18B) can be used as an ancillary diagnostic test in patients in whom the diagnosis of pancreatic carci-

noma is suspected but the CT scan is equivocal. Encasement or obstruction of the pancreatic duct may be seen. At times a brush biopsy of the pancreatic duct is obtained to document the diagnosis; and if there is obstruction of the common bile duct, a stent can be placed endoscopically.

Islet Cell Tumors of the Pancreas

The preoperative localization of islet cell tumors of the pancreas is difficult. Fewer than half of these lesions can currently be imaged by CT. The scans must be performed after oral ingestion of contrast material and then repeated with multiple bolus injections of intravenous contrast material. Islet cell tumors, when detected, are small, enhancing masses that may distort the margins of the pancreas or may be completely within the contours of the gland.

Sonography can demonstrate focal hypoechoic masses with well defined margins. A hyperechoic capsule may be present. In the proper clinical setting, a lesion with this appearance is compatible with an islet cell tumor.

If CT and US are negative and there is a strong clinical suspicion of an islet cell tumor, angiography and transhepatic venous sampling should be considered to confirm the diagnosis and demonstrate the location of the tumor(s) preoperatively.

Cystic Neoplasms of the Pancreas

Microcystic adenomas and mucinous cystic neoplasms of the pancreas are uncommon. Each may contain calcifications that can be detected on plain films of the abdomen.

Microcystic adenomas have a variable US appearance, but two basic patterns have been described. The first is an echogenic mass with well defined margins (usually a mass composed of multiple tiny cysts), and the second is a larger hypoechoic mass with thin walls. CT of these lesions is also variable, with heterogeneous (multiple tiny cysts) or homogeneous (larger cysts) patterns of enhancement.

Mucinous cystic neoplasms are usually larger than the microcystic adenomas. Sonographically, they are uni- or multilocular anechoic masses with posterior wall acoustic enhancement, which confirms the cystic nature of the mass. Internal septations may also be detected. CT demonstrates a well encapsulated mass with attenuation numbers close to those of water. Internal septations are often not detected even when seen sonographically.

QUESTIONS

1. The most common benign neoplasm of the liver is:
   a. Hepatic cyst.
   b. Hepatic adenoma.
   c. Hepatic hemangioma.
   d. Hepatocellular carcinoma.
2. Which of the following is diagnostic of hepatocellular carcinoma?
   a. Tumor in the hepatic veins.
   b. Tumor in the portal vein.
   c. Tumor in the hepatic artery.
   d. All of the above.

3. The best way to differentiate presinusoidal cirrhosis from postsinusoidal cirrhosis is:
   a. Hepatic arteriography.
   b. CT arterial portography.
   c. Hepatic venography (free and wedge).
   d. Ultrasonography.
4. The best imaging procedure for diagnosing acute cholecystitis is:
   a. Ultrasonography.
   b. Computed tomography.
   c. Oral cholecystography.
   d. ^{99m}Tc-IDA scintigraphy.
5. The modality of choice for the diagnosis of obstructive jaundice is:
   a. ^{99m}Tc-IDA scintigraphy.
   b. Ultrasonography.
   c. Computed tomography.
   d. ERCP.
6. Computed tomographic findings in acute pancreatitis include all of the following *except:*
   a. Enlargement of the pancreas.
   b. Indistinct margins of the pancreas.
   c. Pancreatic and peripancreatic fluid collections.
   d. Air in the pancreas.

SELECTED REFERENCES

Liver

Birnbaum BA, Weinreb JC, Sanger JJ, et al. Definitive diagnosis of hepatic hemangiomas: MR imaging versus Tc-99m-labeled red blood cell SPECT. *Radiology* 1990;176;95–101.

Brodsky RI, Friedman AC, Maurer AH, et al. Hepatic cavernous hemangioma: diagnosis with ^{99m}Tc-labeled red cells and single photon emission CT. *AJR* 1987;148:125–129.

Ferrucci JT, Freeny PC, Stark DD, et al. Advances in hepatobiliary radiology. *Radiology* 1988;168;319–338.

Foley WD, Jochem RJ. Computed tomography focal and diffuse liver disease. *Radiol Clin North Am* 1991;29:1213–1233.

Freeny PC, Marks, WM. Hepatic hemangioma: dynamic bolus CT. *AJR* 1986;147:711–719.

Heiken JP, Weyman PJ, Lee KT, et al. Detection of focal hepatic masses: prospective evaluation with CT, delayed CT, CT during arterial portography, and MR imaging. *Radiology* 1989;171:47–51.

Kudo M, Ikekubo K, Yamamoto K, et al. Distinction between hemangioma of the liver and hepatocellular carcinoma: value of labeled RBC-SPECT scanning. *AJR* 1989;152:977–983.

Marn CS, Bree RL, Silver TM. Ultrasonography of the liver, technique and focal diffuse disease. *Radiol Clin North Am* 1991;29:1151–1170.

Nelson RC, Chezmar JL. Diagnostic approach to hepatic he-mangiomas. *Radiology* 1990,176:11–13.

Nelson RC, Chezmar JL, Sugarbaker PH, et al. Preoperative localization of focal liver lesions to specific liver segments: utility of CT during arterial portography. *Radiology* 1990; 176:89–94.

Pagani JJ. Intrahepatic vascular territories shown by computed tomography (CT). *Radiology* 1983;147:173–178.

Stark DD, Felder RC, Wittenberg J, et al. Magnetic resonance imaging of cavernous hemangioma of the liver: tissue-specific characterization. *AJR* 1985;145:213–222.

nenberg E. Fine needle transhepatic cholangiography: re-flections after 450 cases. *AJR* 1981;136:85–90.

Pedrosa CS, Casanova R, Lezana AH, Fernandez C. Computed tomography in obstructive jaundice. Part II. The cause of obstruction. *Radiology* 1981;139:635–645.

Pedrosa CS, Casanova R, Rodriguez R. Computed tomography in obstructive jaundice. Part I. The level of obstruction. *Radiology* 1981;139:627–634.

Weissmann HS, Frank MS, Sugarman LA, et al. Role of ^{99m}Tc-IDA cholescintigraphy in evaluating biliary tract disorders. *Gastrointest Radiol* 1980;5:215–223.

Biliary Tract

Baron RL. Computed tomography of the biliary tree. *Radiol Clin North Am* 1991;29:1235–1250.

Berk RN (moderator), Ferrucci JT Jr, Fordtran JS, Cooperberg PL, Weissmann HS. The radiological diagnosis of gallblad-der disease. *Radiology* 1981;141:49–56.

Choy, D, Shi EC, MacLean RG, et al. Cholescintigraphy in acute cholecystitis: use of intravenous morphine. *Radiology* 1984;151:203–307.

Cohen SM, Kurtz AB. Biliary sonography. *Radiol Clin North Am* 1991;29:1171–1198.

Drane E. Nuclear medicine techniques for the liver and biliary system update for the 1990s. *Radiol Clin North Am* 1991; 29:1129–1150.

Ferrucci JT Jr, Adson MA, Mueller PR, Stanley RJ, Stewart ET. Advances in the radiology of jaundice: a symposium and review. *AJR* 1983;141:1–20.

Fig LM, Wahl RL, Stewart RE, et al. Morphine-augmented he-patobiliary scintigraphy in the severely ill: caution is in or-der. *Radiology* 1990;175:467–473.

Grund FM, Reinke DB, Larson BW, et al. Hepatobiliary imag-ing: the diagnostic use of intravenous morphine in fasting patients. *Am J Physiol Imag* 1986;1:26–32.

Kim EE, Pjura G, Lowry P, et al. Morphine-augmented cho-lescintigraphy in the diagnosis of acute cholecystitis. *AJR* 1986;147:1177–1179.

Laing, FC, Jeffrey RB Jr, Wing VW, et al. Biliary dilatation: defining the level and cause by real-time US. *Radiology* 1986;160:39–42.

Mueller PR, Harbin WP, Ferrucci JT Jr, Wittenberg J, VanSon-

Pancreas

Baker ME, Cohan RH, Nadel SN, et al. Obliteration of the fat surrounding the celiac axis and superior mesenteric artery is not a specific CT finding of carcinoma of the pancreas. *AJR* 1990;155:991–994.

Balthazar EJ, Robinson DL, Megibow AJ, et al. Acute pancre-atitis: value of CT in establishing prognosis. *Radiology* 1990;174:331–336.

Dunnick NR, Doppman JL, Mills SR, McCarthy D. Computed tomographic detection of nonbeta pancreatic islet cell tu-mors. *Radiology* 1980;135:117–120.

Gunther RW, Klose KJ, Rückert K, et al. Islet cell tumors: de-tection of small lesions with computed tomography and ul-trasound. *Radiology* 1983;148:485–488.

Jeffrey RB Jr. Sonography in acute pancreatitis. *Radiol Clin North Am* 1989;27:5–17.

Johnson CD, Stephens DH, Charboneau JW, et al. Cystic pan-creatic tumors: CT and sonographic assessment. *AJR* 1988; 151:1133–1138.

Leutmer PH, Stephens DH, Ward EM. Chronic pancreatitis: re-assessment with current CT. *Radiology* 1989;171:353–357.

Mathieu D, Guigui B, Valette PJ, et al. Pancreatic cystic neo-plasms. *Radiol Clin North Am* 1989;27:163–176.

Rossi P, Allsion DJ, Bezzi MS, et al. Endocrine tumors of the pancreas. *Radiol Clin North Am* 1989;27:129–161.

Schulte SJ, Baron RL, Freeny PC, et al. Root of the superior mesenteric artery in pancreatitis and pancreatic carcinoma: evaluation with CT. *Radiology* 1991;180:659–662.

Steiner E, Stark DD, Hahn PF, et al. Imaging of pancreatic neo-plasms: comparison of MR and CT. *AJR* 1989;152:487–491.

25

Melanoma, Sarcoma, Lymphoma

Ronald N. Kaleya

MELANOMA

Melanoma is now the seventh most common cancer in the United States, accounting for 2% to 3% of all malignancies and 1.5% of cancer deaths. Melanoma usually arises in the skin, but it also occurs in the anus, vulva, vagina, upper aerodigestive tract, and uveal tract. The incidence of cutaneous malignant melanoma (CMM) has increased more than that of any other cancer, doubling every 5 to 10 years over the past three decades. Approximately 41,000 new cases and 7,500 deaths are anticipated in 1998 in the United States. Coincident with the higher incidence, the virulence of the disease has decreased dramatically, with most of the patients presenting with thinner, more localized, and thus more curable lesions. The 5-year cancer specific survival for patients with CMM has increased from 35% in 1930 to more than 85% in 1990. Putting this increased risk into perspective, the lifetime risk for CMM was 1 : 1500 for a person born in 1935 compared to 1 : 75 for a child born in 2000.

Pathogenesis

Several factors have been associated with increased risk for CMM. These risk factors, genetic and environmental, have not been causally related to the develop-

ment of melanoma. They are simply markers of propensity.

Environmental Risk Factors

The relation between solar radiation and CMM has been popularized. However, distinct from basal and squamous skin cancers, which occur at chronically sun-exposed sites (head, neck, hands), no such clear association exists for CMM. Additionally, CMM occurs more frequently in city dwellers and in office workers rather than outside laborers. For these reasons, cumulative sun exposure is not clearly related causally to melanoma. Furthermore, if cumulative sun exposure were etiologically significant, the melanoma risk would increase linearly with age, which is true only for lentigo maligna melanomas.

Evidence supporting an actinic etiology of melanoma comes primarily from epidemiologic studies that have shown an increased rate of melanoma in people living closer to the equator within a single country. Migration studies have also revealed increased rates of melanoma for patients who moved to a more sunny environment than their native country. In fact, the rate of melanoma increases with the length of time the person remains in the new environment. Others have associated the risk of melanoma with the severity and number of sunburns especially while a child and adolescent. Therefore it is probable that severe intermittent sun exposure rather than total actinic exposure places the patient at increased risk for development of melanoma.

Genetic Risk Factors

Several phenotypic characteristics are markers of increased melanoma risk (Table 25.1). Among them are fair complexion, red or blonde hair color, and a tendency to burn or freckle rather than tan. Eye color, once thought to be associated with increased risk, is not an independent risk factor.

Personal or family history of melanoma places the patient at increased risk of developing CMM. Approximately 3% to 5% of patients with a past melanoma develop a second primary during their lifetime. First degree relatives of a patient with melanoma have twice the risk of melanoma as the general population. Familial melanoma accounts for 8% to 12% of CMM. Patients with familial melanoma tend to have a higher incidence of atypical moles, earlier development of melanoma, and multiple primaries. Owing to an increased awareness, however, they also tend to present at an earlier stage and therefore have a better overall survival. Other genetic risk factors include abnormalities on chromosomes 1p, 6q, 7, and 9. Some of these chromosomal changes are found in familial atypical multiple mole melanoma syndrome (FAMMM) or atypical mole syndrome, which has previously been called the dysplastic nevi syndrome or the B-K mole syndrome. Additionally, rare chromosomal defects such as xeroderma pigmentosum, an autosomal recessive defect in DNA repair, is associated with increased melanoma incidence.

Atypical Mole Syndrome
(FAMMM, Dysplastic Nevi Syndrome)

Atypical mole syndrome (AMS) appears in both familial and sporadic settings. It is characterized by the presence of atypical (dysplastic) moles, which when multiple are considered potential precursors to melanoma as well as a marker for increased risk of developing melanoma. Although several clinical and pathologic characteristics of the atypical moles set them apart from junctional and compound nevi, no clear definition has been formulated for their diagnosis. Therefore they are seen in a spectrum of clinical and pathologic entities.

The "typical mole" tends to be symmetric, is less than 5 mm, has uniform contour and color, and is sharply circumscribed. It is most commonly located in sun-exposed areas. In contrast, atypical moles are more likely to have indistinct borders, irregular contours, variegated colors (fried egg- or target-shaped), are larger (more than 5 mm), and can be located in sun-protected areas. Histologically, they tend to have a nested pattern of growth, nuclear atypia, indeterminate circumscription, and asymmetry. The National Institutes of Health (NIH) has suggested that the term "atypical mole" be used with the clinical entity and the term "nevi with architectural disorder" for those that show histologic changes of atypia.

The classic triad of the AMS includes the presence of more than 100 moles, one mole larger than 6 mm, and at least one with "atypical features." The syndrome has an autosomal dominant inheritance pattern with varying penetrance. The nevi are frequently larger than 8 mm in diameter, develop after age 35, and occur in areas that are not exposed to the sun. The latency period for the development of CMM is unknown. The lifetime risk has been stratified by the number of relatives with the syndrome and melanoma (Table 25.2). The lifetime risk of melanoma approaches 100% for patients who have two family members with AMS and melanoma. These patients should be examined thoroughly every 3 to 12 months, and the examination should include epiluminescence (surface) microscopy. Photographs of specific moles should be obtained to document that they are static lesions. The patient should perform self-examination with a full-length mirror and a hand-held mirror every 1 to 2 months. All moles should be charted and measured carefully. Any change in a mole on a patient with AMS should undergo biopsy to confirm its benign status.

TABLE 25.1. *Phenotypic characteristics predisposing to melanoma*

Hair color: blonde or red >> brown or black (2–3 times
    lifetime risk)
Skin color: fair >> olive or black (10 times lifetime risk)
Presence of >20 nevi on body
Tendency to burn or freckle with sun exposure
Prior melanoma: 3–6% develop a second melanoma
    (900-fold risk)
Family history of melanoma
Increased: blood type O, HLA DR4, GM2 expression
Decreased risk: HLA DR3

TABLE 25.2. *Lifetime risk of melanoma in patients with atypical mole syndrome*

Kindred type	Descriptive name	Characteristics	Risk
A	Sporadic	One relative has DN	27 ×
B	Familial	>Two relatives have DN	30–40 ×
C	Sporadic and melanoma	One relative has DN and melanoma	?
D1	Familial and melanoma	>Two relatives have DN and one has melanoma	?
D2	Familial and melanoma	>Two relatives have DN and melanoma	150 ×
D3	Familial and melanoma	Personal history of melanoma as well	500 ×

Source: Adapted from Kraemer KH, et al. Dysplastic nevi and cutaneous melanoma. *Lancet* 1983:1076.
DN, dysplastic nevi syndrome (FAMMM syndrome)

Giant Congenital Nevi

Congenital nevi are present in 1% of neonates. Some of these nevi involve large portions of the body or portions of the face. By convention small congenital nevi are those with a diameter less than 1.5 cm, intermediate moles are those between 1.5 and 2.0 cm, and giant congenital nevi are those that are larger than 20 cm in diameter or that encompass an orbit or a major portion of the face. The natural history of the giant nevi is unclear. Only 5% progress to melanoma. Excision eliminates the risk but may leave the child irreparably scarred. The small nevi do not pose an increased lifetime risk of melanoma.

Therapy for the intermediate and giant nevi should be individualized, considering the relatively small increase in risk and the potential disfigurement. Options for treatment include excision and grafting, excision after tissue expansion of the adjacent normal skin, curettage, dermabrasion and ruby laser therapy. In most cases, treatment is withheld until the child is 6 months old for the giant nevi and until adolescence for the other nevi.

Pathology

Melanoma is divided into several distinct forms by its histologic characteristics, gross appearance, prognosis, and the duration of the respective radial and vertical growth phases. Nodular melanoma is considered monophasic because there is either a short or absent radial growth phase. The superficial spreading, acral lentiginous and lentigo maligna melanomas are considered to be biphasic with a variable radial growth phase preceding the vertical growth phase.

Superficial Spreading Melanoma

Superficial spreading melanoma (SSM) is the most common type of melanoma, comprising approximately 70% of cases seen in the United States. It usually arises near or from a pre-existing nevus. Although this type of melanoma can arise at any time after puberty, the peak incidence is during the fourth to fifth decade of life. SSMs are usually brought to medical attention when the lesion begins to bleed, becomes pruritic, or enlarges, a slow change in the precursor lesion can often be elicited retrospectively.

The SSM has been reported to be more common in women in some reviews, but this is not universally accepted. It is, however, more prevalent on the legs of women and the backs of men.

The SSMs are typically flat and have irregular or notched borders with an average diameter of 2 cm at diagnosis. The invasive lesions tend to be larger than 2 cm, with loss of Langer's lines of the adjacent skin. Although most are blue or black, the color is often variegated. White or gray areas are frequently seen within the lesions. Ulceration is uncommon, occurring in about 10% to 15% of cases at diagnosis. SSM has an intermediate prognosis.

Nodular Melanoma

Nodular melanoma (NM) accounts for 15% to 30% of cases. This type has a male predilection (2 : 1), has a peak incidence during the fifth to sixth decades, and does not arise from a preexisting nevus. These lesions tend to develop and progress more rapidly than the SSM. NM may be more aggressive than SSM because it has an earlier vertical (invasive) growth phase.

The NM commonly affects the trunks of men and the lower extremity of women. The lesions are raised, symmetric, and generally darker than their SSM counterparts. Although only 5% of NMs are amelanotic, most primary amelanotic melanomas are of the nodular type. Approximately half of the NMs are ulcerated at the time of diagnosis. The prognosis of NM is significantly worse than that of SSM.

Lentigo Maligna Melanoma

Also known as the Hutchinson's freckle, lentigo maligna melanoma (LMM) accounts for only 4% to 10% of melanomas. It occurs in areas of severe actinic skin damage and exhibits a prolonged radial growth phase and a growth phase. It is common during the seventh to eighth decades of life and rarely if ever occurs before age 50. There is a slight female predominance that may be partly attributed to the longer life expectancy of women.

The LMM commonly occurs on the temporal and malar regions of the face and the dorsal surface of the hands. It is typically larger than 3 cm and appears as a light brown stain on the skin. The margins of the lesions tend to be convoluted. LMM rarely recurs locally after excision and does not metastasize. LMM has a good overall prognosis.

Acral Lentiginous Melanoma

Acral lentiginous melanoma (ALM) comprises 2% to 8% of melanomas in Caucasians and 35% to 60% of those found in the black population. The incidence of ALM peaks during the seventh decade of life. Most of these lesions are located on the soles of the feet and the palms of the hands. They exhibit an early vertical growth phase and therefore have a relative poor prognosis. ALMs are frequently larger than 3 cm at diagnosis. Though characteristically flat, nodularity may develop later in the course. The borders are irregular, and the lesions are tan or brown. Most mucosal melanomas are of this subtype.

Subungual Melanoma

Subungual melanomas (SMs) are rare, accounting for only 2% to 3% of melanomas in the white population but a much higher percentage in the black population. Almost 75% are located on the great toe or thumb. They are often noted when the nail becomes detached from the underlying nail bed. Regional nodes are involved in more than 35% of cases at the time of diagnosis. SM occurs late in life and has a poor prognosis. Unlike the other types of melanoma, the prognosis is not related to tumor thickness but rather to (a) destruction of the nail bed; (b) location in the toe compared to other digits; (c) bony invasion; (d) lack of pigmentation; and (e) nodal involvement.

Differential Diagnosis

Several benign lesions can be mistakenly diagnosed as melanoma. In general, acquired benign melanocytic nevi tend to be smaller than 7 mm in greatest diameter, symmetric, and uniformly pigmented (Table 25.3). In contrast, melanomas tend to be larger than 8 mm and have variegated color and asymmetric borders. More reliable indicators of melanoma are a change in size or color, the development of nodularity, ulceration, pruritus, and the discovery of a new pigmented lesion after age 40.

The British have devised an ABCDE and seven-point checklist for diagnosing melanoma by nondermatologists (Table 25.4). The sensitivity and specificity of this system are 79% and 96%, respectively.

TABLE 25.3. *Differential diagnosis*

Seborrheic keratosis: Waxy; unchanging; verrucous raised and sharply delineated.
Junctional nevus: Usually <5 mm and rarely >10 mm; uniform pigmentation; preservation of Langer's line. Melanocytes at dermoepidermal junction. Rarely occurs after age 40.
Compound nevus: Palpable but similar to junctional nevus. May have excessive hair.
Dysplastic nevus: Nevus with architectural distortion and cytologic atypia; preserved epidermal rete architecture. Difficult to distinguish from melanoma *in situ.*
Halo nevus: Can undergo spontaneous regression. Differentiated from melanoma by symmetry and cytologic maturation.
Hemangioma: Bleeds more profusely than melanoma. Blanches with pressure.
Blue nevus: Less than 5 mm. Pigmented basal cell/squamous cell carcinoma; long history; pearly nodules surrounding lesion.
Subungual hematoma: Can be drained by nail puncture. Moves with nail growth.

TABLE 25.4. *Historical and clinical features of a suspicious skin lesion and a seven-point checklist for diagnosis of melanoma*

Historical features
  Change in color
  Change in size
  Bleeding
  Tenderness or pain
  Pruritus
  Family or personal history of melanoma
  Tendency to sunburn
  Prior sunburn frequency

Clinical features
  A: Asymmetry: Lesion is bisected visually, and the two halves are not identical.
  B: Border irregularity: Border is not smooth or straight and is irregular or ragged.
  C: Color variegation: More than one shade of pigment is present.
  D: Diameter: It is >6 mm.
  E: Elevation: Lesion is elevated above the skin surface.
  Inflammation
  Crusting or bleeding
  Sensory change

Checklist
  Major criteria (2 points for each one present): change in shape, size, or color
  Minor criteria (1 point for each one present): inflammation, crusting or bleeding, sensory change, or diameter >6 mm
  If score is more than 3, biopsy is indicated.

Source: Adapted from Whited JD, et al. *JAMA* 1998;279:696.

Prognostic Factors

Factors that help predict survival include the depth of invasion or the tumor thickness, the presence or absence of ulceration, lymph node involvement, and dissemination of disease.

1. *Sex.* The incidence of melanoma is equal in men and women. The latter have thinner lesions that are more likely to be located on the extremity and less commonly ulcerated. Even when stratified by all pathologic risk factors, there is a survival advantage for women, site for site and stage for stage.

2. *Age.* Age at onset may be prognostically significant. Older patients present with thicker lesions. The median thickness of melanoma during the third decade is 1.1 mm compared to 2.8 mm for patients in the seventh decade of life. However, when stratified by thickness, survival is equivalent. The Intergroup Melanoma Trial showed a significant improvement in survival for patients less than 60 years of age who underwent an elective node dissection compared to those who were simply observed.

3. *Anatomic setting.* The anatomic site of the primary lesion is an important prognostic variable, with extremity lesions, excluding the hands and feet, indicating better survival than the head, neck, and trunk primaries, respectively. The purported poorer prognosis for lesions of the posterior back, arms, neck, and scalp (BANS area) has not been confirmed for clinical stage I melanoma. Only the scalp lesions have a poorer prognosis. The BANS area lesions tend to behave more aggressively when the regional nodes are involved (clinical stage II).

4. *Pregnancy.* Approximately one-third of women who develop CMMs are in the childbearing age group. Women who develop melanoma during pregnancy tend to have thicker lesions, but there is no survival decrement. Furthermore, pregnancy does not influence survival or recurrence rates in women previously treated for melanoma.

Staging

Several staging systems have been developed for CMM. The clinical staging system (Table 25.5) helps define the initial workup, whereas the pathologic staging systems are better for determining definitive therapy and prognosis. Because tumor depth or thickness is not included in the evaluation, the clinical staging system is inadequate. In addition most (87%) patients fall into clinical stage I disease, thus not allowing adequate comparisons of therapy in view of the prognostic importance of tumor thickness.

TABLE 25.5. *Clinical staging system for melanoma*

Stage	Criteria
I	Localized primary melanoma
IA	Localized recurrent melanoma
II	Metastases to regional nodes or in-transit metastases
III	Disseminated disease

Clark's microstaging system determines the level of the tumor by the depth of invasion into the layers of the skin (Table 25.6). This system tends to be subjective and requires multiple sections and a committed pathologist. The Breslow microstaging system is less subjective and has become the present standard (Table 25.7). The thickness of the tumor (reported in millimeters) is determined using an ocular micrometer.

The American Joint Commission on Cancer (AJCC) has created a pathologic TMN staging system using all of the prognostic variables (Table 25.8). Because all prognostic variables are included, this staging system stratifies the patients better and allows improved comparisons of results.

Surgical Treatment of Cutaneous Melanoma

Indications for Biopsy

Any pigmented lesion that enlarges, has variegated colors or irregular borders, changes color, develops nodularity or becomes ulcerated should undergo biopsy. Pigmented lesions that develop after age 40 should be closely evaluated. In addition, any time there is doubt about the nature of a pigmented lesion, the lesion should be biopsied.

Options for Biopsy

Excisional biopsy is recommended for lesions less than 2 cm in diameter. The excision should include both underlying fat and 1 to 3 mm of adjacent normal skin to permit orientation by the pathologist. The resultant defect may be closed primarily without the use of a skin flap or skin graft. In cases of a benign lesion, excision is definitive therapy.

TABLE 25.6. *Clark's microstaging system for melanoma*

Level	Criteria
I	Confined to the epidermis; no invasion of the basement membrane
II	Into papillary dermis
III	Through papillary dermis, abutting reticular dermis
IV	Into reticular dermis
V	Into subcutaneous fat

TABLE 25.7. *Breslow microstaging system for melanoma*

Diameter (mm)	Clark		Melanoma designation
0–0.75 IA	II	T_1	Thin
0.76–1.50 IB	III	T_2	
1.51–4.00 IIA	IV	T_3	Intermediate
>4.00 IIB	V	T_4	Thick

(handwritten annotations: "Depth" over "Diameter"; "Clark" heading; IA, IB, IIA, IIB in column)

An incisional biopsy is reserved for larger lesions. The surgeon should choose the clinically thickest part of the lesion and perform the biopsy at that site. It is preferable to include normal skin and subcutaneous tissue to allow pathologic orientation of the specimen. Punch biopsies are acceptable but should be at least 5 mm in diameter.

Shave biopsies and electrodesiccation of pigmented lesions are mentioned only to condemn them. These techniques invalidate all subsequent attempts to stage the disease accurately and have an enormous impact when planning definitive therapy.

The prognosis for a subungual melanoma is not determined by thickness or depth of invasion; therefore the biopsy needs only to confirm the presence of melanoma pathologically. After removing a piece of the nail, a portion of the lesion can be excised. Lesions involving the nail matrix should be excised horizontally and those of the nail bed longitudinally. Because all or some of the lesion can be attached to the nail plate, the nail itself should be submitted for pathologic evaluation. In cases where the tumor has fungated through the nail, the exophytic component can be excised to obtain the specimen.

Orientation of the Biopsy

The biopsy on the extremities should be oriented along the axis of the extremity, whereas those on the trunk should be performed transversely. Primary closure of the definitive wide excision can be performed more easily if the initial biopsy is oriented properly.

Preoperative Assessment

The natural history of melanoma is unpredictable. The most common sites of metastasis are, in order of frequency: nodes and adjacent skin, lung, liver, brain,

TABLE 25.8. *TMN staging of cutaneous malignant melanoma (AJCC 1992 staging system for cutaneous melanoma)*

Stage	Criteria	Patients (%)	Survival (%)
IA	Localized disease, <0.75 mm, or level II (T1N0M0)	47	>85 at 10 years
IB	Localized disease, 0.76–1.5 mm, or level III (T2M0N0)		
IIA	Localized disease, 1.51–4 mm, or level IV (T3N0M0)	38	60 at 10 years
IIB	Localized disease, >4.00 mm, or level V (T4N0M0), satellites within 2 cm of primary tumor		
IIIA	Limited nodal metastases (TxN1M0), nodal metastases <3 cm in diameter	13	Median 3 years
IIIB	Advanced regional disease (TxN2M0), nodal metastases >3 cm, in-transit metastases		
IV	Metastatic disease (TxNxM1-2)	2	Median 10 months

and bones. Most other visceral sites, such as the bowel, heart, eye, and bladder, are rare except in autopsy series. Therefore once melanoma is diagnosed and prior to embarking on definitive therapy, the patient should undergo an extent-of-disease workup determined by the clinical stage of the disease.

In patients with clinical stage I disease a complete blood count, chest radiography, and liver function tests are performed. If these tests are normal, definitive therapy can be undertaken without further evaluation. Patients with laboratory abnormalities or palpable nodal disease (clinical stage II) may require a computed tomography (CT) scan of the primary nodal drainage basin, the liver, and perhaps the brain. All patients should be examined for a second primary.

Margins of Resection

The controversy concerning optimal lateral margins of resection has been resolved with the Intergroup Melanoma Trial. In this trial intermediate thickness melanomas (1 to 4 mm) were randomized to 2- versus 4-cm margins. The overall local recurrence rate was 3.8%; and the individual local recurrence rates were 2.3%, 4.2%, and 11.7% for lesions 1 to 2 mm, 2 to 3 mm, and 3 to 4 mm, respectively. The wider margins did not provide a statistically significant decrement in local recurrence. Only 11% of the wounds required a skin graft, which reduced the cost and morbidity of the local treatment. Presently, the recommendations for margins vary with the Breslow thickness of the primary lesion. *In situ* melanoma is treated with 0.5 to 1.0-cm margins. Invasive lesions less than 1 mm in depth (thin

melanoma) can be treated with 1 cm margins without an appreciable increase in local recurrences; 2-cm margins are adequate for 1- to 4-mm melanomas. Melanomas thicker than 4 mm are treated with 2- to 3-cm margins. (These recommendations have not been supported by randomized trials.) Most of these excisions can be done on an ambulatory basis and usually can be closed primarily. Skin grafts are generally reserved for patients with large primaries or those with local satellitosis.

Melanomas located on the head, neck, and face pose a difficult oncologic and cosmetic problem. Although there are no good rules governing these resection margins, margins twice the largest diameter of the lesion are employed by many surgeons.

Mucosal melanomas are generally advanced at the time of initial therapy and tend to fail locally irrespective of the margins of resection. Similarly, anorectal melanoma and vaginal melanoma are associated with a dismal survival. With rectal melanoma, abdominoperineal resection seems to improve local control but not overall survival. Patients with localized and small rectal melanomas can be adequately treated with local excision.

Subungual melanoma in a digit other than the thumb is best treated with distal interphalangeal amputation. Melanoma involving the thumb can be treated with interphalangeal amputation. These recommendations are a reasonable compromise between the potential functional deficits and the possibility for cure.

Lesions involving the pinna can be treated with a wedge resection of the pinna, including the cartilage, with rotation of the remaining ear to achieve a reasonable cosmetic result. Melanoma on the sole must be treated in a fashion that maintains as much of the innervated weight bearing surface as possible. Melanoma overlying the female breast should be treated similar to any other truncal lesion. Mastectomy is not indicated.

Depth of Resection

The controversy of whether to include the deep fascia during primary resection of a melanoma has largely been resolved. There does not seem to be a difference in local recurrence rates, time to local recurrence, or survival for stage I melanoma regardless of whether the fascia is resected.

Closure of the Defect

Local random flaps can be used to close the defect created during the initial treatment of CMM. Skin grafts can be used for large defects when needed. The use of skin grafts does not affect the outcome of the local therapy.

Treatment of Regional Nodes in Clinical Stage I Melanoma

The role of elective lymph node dissection (ELND) continues to be a controversial area in the treatment of stage I melanoma. Underlying this debate is the fact that a large percentage of patients with clinically uninvolved regional nodes have occult nodal micrometastases when the nodes are examined pathologically (Table 25.9). The patients with thin melanomas (less than 1 mm) rarely have microscopic involvement of the regional nodes and are therefore not candidates for ELND. The patients with thick lesions (more than 4 mm) frequently have microscopic nodal disease but have a high incidence of distant failure, again making them poor candidates for ELND.

TABLE 25.9. *Nodal metastases by thickness for clinical stage I melanoma*

Thickness (mm)	Stage I patients (%)	% With micrometastases (%)
<0.75	39	0
0.76–1.50	27	14–25
1.51–4.00	22	37–51
>4.00	12	54–62

The patients with intermediate thickness melanomas are those who could potentially benefit from prophylactic regional lymph node dissection. Considering that 85% of patients present with clinical stage I disease, and about half of these patients have intermediate-thickness lesions, more than 40% of patients with melanoma are possible candidates for ELND. Of these, only one-third harbor micrometastases at the time of ELND. Therefore about 15% of all patients with melanoma could achieve potential benefit from ELND.

Argument for ELND

Based on the assumption that micrometastases in regional lymph nodes, at least in part, give rise to disseminated disease, ELND could theoretically delay or eliminate this progression. Several retrospective studies have shown statistically significant improvements in disease-free and overall survival of patients who underwent ELND for intermediate thickness melanoma. Furthermore, survival in retrospective studies is as much as 40% higher for patients with micrometastases in the regional nodes (clinical stage I, pathologic stage II) as for patients with palpable nodal disease (clinical stage II).

The two prospective randomized studies not showing a survival advantage for ELND were seriously flawed. The World Health Organization (WHO) trial included an excess of women, who are known to have a low rate of nodal metastases. Additionally, critics of this study suggest that there may have been inconsistent clinical staging at some of the participating institutions, thereby introducing an element of bias into the study. Furthermore, complete pathologic and clinical data were available for fewer than half of the patients.

Stratification with respect to two important prognostic variables, tumor thickness and the presence of ulceration, was not done in this study. When the data were reanalyzed using these two criteria, it was found that there were more ulcerated lesions in the group that did not undergo node dissection. When analyzed with respect to ulceration and thickness, patients in the intermediate-thickness group treated with ELND had a statistically better survival at 10 years.

The Mayo Clinic trial evaluating the use of ELND, delayed ELND, and therapeutic node dissection did not show a survival advantage for node dissection. Again, the study was seriously flawed. Most of the lesions were distal to the knee, most of the patients were women, and relatively few patients fell into the intermediate-thickness group. At 10 years the ELND and delayed node dissection groups are now showing statistically insignificant survival advantage. A recent analysis of the WHO trunk melanoma trial also suggests a survival advantage for male patients with melanomas more than 1.5 mm in thickness.

The Intergroup Melanoma Trial randomized patients with 1- to 4-mm melanomas to ELND versus observation. This study included stratification by thickness, primary site, and ulceration. The results supported elective node dissection in male patients less than 60 years of age with 1- to 2-mm melanomas. The survival benefit was statistically significant. In addition, pathologic staging is necessary because there is a clinically proved adjuvant therapy for patients with nodal metastases.

Argument Against ELND

The opponents of ELND suggest that the progression from micrometastases to systemic disease has never been adequately proved and that systemic disease may in fact be present at the time of primary treatment. In a prospective evaluation of patients treated with wide local excision alone carried out by the WHO, about half of the melanomas recurred. Distant metastases, with or without local and regional recurrence, were the first site of recurrent disease in half of the patients. This finding undermines the suggestion that there is an orderly progression from primary site to regional nodes to systemic spread.

Furthermore, opponents of ELND have suggested that the retrospective studies supporting the efficacy of ELND may have resulted from a selection bias with respect to their patient populations. Therefore the retrospective data, though encouraging, should be disregarded. The results of the prospective trials should be the only basis for determining the efficacy of ELND. Only the Intergroup Trial showed a survival benefit for ELND and only in a small subset of patients. The opponents of ELND suggest that subset analysis may introduce type II error into the interpretation of this trial.

Furthermore, the opponents of ELND point out that almost 70% of patients undergoing ELND have pathologically negative nodes and do not benefit from the procedure. These patients do, however, have the full spectrum of morbidity associated with regional lymphadenectomy.

Alternative Treatment of Regional Nodes: Lymphatic Mapping and Sentinel Node Biopsy

Donald Morton described a reasonable approach to the management of the regional nodes in stage I melanoma. His group performs lymphoscintigraphy and identifies the primary nodal drainage area. A marker dye is injected subdermally around the primary, and the nodes draining this area are exposed surgically. The marker dye highlights the "sentinel node," which is resected and examined in frozen sections. If the node contains metastatic disease, a lymphadenectomy is performed. When no metastatic melanoma is found, the incision is closed without further treatment. This method uses the available information to the maximal benefit of the patient. It has been adopted by most centers treating large numbers of melanoma patients.

Summary of Recommendations for Treatment of Regional Nodes in Stage I Melanoma

The available data do not confirm the need for ELND. Currently, the decision to (or not to) perform an ELND must be made by the surgeon treating the disease. In Europe, ELND is not routinely performed. The patients are examined every 3 months for regional and distant recurrence. The American College of Surgeons Patient Care Evaluation Study showed that most general surgeons have abandoned the practice of ELND. In the major cancer centers in the United States, lymphatic mapping and sentinel node biopsy procedure is practiced almost universally. It is becoming the standard of care for the treatment of regional nodes.

ELND: Which Node Group?

The extremities have fairly constant lymphatic drainage, but drainage from the trunk and head and neck regions can be ambiguous in as many as half of the cases. Multiple-node groups and unexpected drainage patterns can be found in these areas. The failure to demonstrate a survival advantage for ELND in the past may have resulted from resection of the wrong nodal groups. ELND should therefore be directed by preoperative lymphoscintigraphy in these cases. Technetium-labeled filtered sulfur colloid and human serum albumin have been used for lymphoscintigraphy. The ongoing ELND study for head and neck melanoma requires preoperative lymphoscintigraphy prior to node dissection.

Morbidity of Node Dissection

The morbidity rate associated ELND is considerable, ranging from 25% to 81%. About 8% of patients develop lymphedema associated with functional deficits. Approximately one-fourth of patients develop lymphedema that does not impair function. Wound infection rates range from 4% to 45%. The mortality may be 3% following the procedure. The average hospitalization is 8 days.

ELND for Head and Neck Melanoma

The ELND for intermediate-thickness melanoma of the head and neck is another area of controversy. The results from retrospective studies have and have not supported a survival advantage for ELND. There appears to be a decrease in regional recurrence rates with neck dissection. Based on these findings, elective neck dissections should be considered for the treatment of head and neck primary lesions. Most surgeons now use one of many modified neck dissection techniques that preserve the internal jugular vein, sternocleidomastoid muscle, and accessory nerve rather than using the classic radical neck dissection. As for other anatomic sites, sentinel node biopsy may be the best alternative to elective node dissection.

Extent of Node Dissection

The axillary dissection performed for upper extremity melanoma requires full dissection of levels I, II, and III. The pectoralis minor should be sacrificed. The groin dissections should initially include the inguinal (superficial) nodes. These nodes are examined by frozen section; and if involved, the iliac and obturator nodes are dissected. About 25% to 50% of patients with inguinal node involvement also have iliac node disease. Approximately 10% to 20% of patients with iliac node disease survive 5 years.

Treatment

Clinical Stage II Disease

Patients with clinically palpable lymphadenopathy should undergo therapeutic lymph node dissection (TLND) simultaneously with the treatment of their primary lesion if there is no evidence of systemic disease. Some surgeons also perform isolated hyperthermic perfusion (IHP) at the time of TLND. The efficacy of IHP is based on retrospective studies and has been challenged. The 5-year survival is about 20% in these cases.

Stage II Disease with an Unknown Primary

Treatment of stage II disease without a known primary should be TLND. The survival is the same as for other patients with stage II disease. The mucous membranes, vagina, and anus are examined to uncover the occult primary.

In-Transit Disease

In-transit disease is defined as subcutaneous or cutaneous metastases more than 2 cm from the primary lesion. There are several options for therapy, including isolated perfusion, tourniquet occlusion infusion, irradiation, intralesional therapy, cryotherapy, or systemic immunotherapy. There are no good prospective randomized trials to support the use of IHP. Retrospective and anecdotal evidence shows IHP to be effective in some cases.

Locally Recurrent Melanoma

Several series have reported 20% five-year survival following resection of localized metastatic melanoma. Favorable prognostic factors for survival following resection of recurrent melanoma include regional versus distant recurrence; recurrence of an extremity versus a head, neck, or trunk primary; nodal versus nonnodal recurrence; and a disease-free interval of more than 1 year.

Adjuvant Therapy for High-Risk Melanoma

Patients with thick primary melanomas (more than 4 mm), in-transit disease, and regional nodal metastases relapse in more than 50% of cases. A recent trial using interferon alpha-2b versus observation revealed a significant increase in both disease-free and overall survival in the treatment arm. Disease-free survival increased from 26% to 37%, and the overall 5-year survival increased from 36% to 47%. Presently, routine adjuvant therapy is recommended consisting of 20 million U/m^2 per day i.v. × 5 for 4 weeks followed by 10 million Units/m^2 3 times a week for 11 months.

Advanced Disease

About one-third of patients with a single metastatic site can be rendered disease-free by surgery. Isolated brain metastases should be resected to improve quality of life. There is no good chemotherapy for this disease. Immunotherapy, including interleukin-2 (IL-2)-LAK cell therapy and tumor necrosis factor, has only marginal, short-lived effects. Tumor vaccines, monoclonal antibodies, and other biologic response modifiers are still investigational treatments for advanced disease. Paclitaxel has produced some encouraging results in small clinical trials.

SOFT TISSUE SARCOMA

The soft tissue sarcomas (STSs) are a heterogeneous group of malignancies. There are at least 50 types of STS, each with different histologic and biologic characteristics. The peripheral nerve sheath tumors are included in the discussion of STS, though they are not considered sarcomas. Although different STSs have clearly different biologic behavior, they are treated as a homogeneous group because they have a similar natural history and management.

The STSs can occur at any age. STS in pediatric patients is not discussed in this section. The median age for STS in adults is 49 years, and 90% occur in Caucasians. The annual incidence of adult STS is 6,600. The lesions generally present as a painless mass that gradually enlarges. Symptoms are associated with encroachment of other organs (e.g., iliofemoral thrombosis with pelvic sarcomas). Because there are no distinguishing historical features of STS, the diagnosis is frequently delayed even under medical observation.

These tumors tend to invade locally. A pseudocapsule, comprised of compressed tumor cells and normal tissue, is frequently present. The STSs disseminate almost exclusively by the hematogenous, rather than the lymphatic, route. Lymph node metastases are uncommon except in the synoviosarcomas, high-grade malignant fibrous histiocytomas, and epithelioid sarcomas. The lung is the most common site of metastasis for all STSs. Liver metastases are seen more frequently with the visceral and retroperitoneal sarcomas.

Common Soft Tissue Sarcomas

The most common soft tissue sarcomas are listed in (Table 25.10).

Liposarcoma

There are several subtypes of the liposarcomas, including the well differentiated, myxoid, and pleomorphic varieties. These tumors commonly arise in the thigh, groin, shoulder, and popliteal spaces. The well-differentiated liposarcoma is rare, has a prominent pseudocapsule, and is associated with a 70% five-year survival. The other, more common, poorly differentiated liposarcomas are associated with a 20% five-year survival.

Malignant Fibrous Histiocytomas

The diagnosis of malignant fibrous histiocytoma (MFH) has increased over the past two decades with the use of immunohistochemical and cytokeratin staining techniques. There are several subclassifications of the MFH, the most common being the malignant histiocytic fibrous histiocytoma. These tumors tend to occur in the deep soft tissues of the buttocks, thighs, arms, and neck; and they infiltrate widely. They are more likely to have high-grade histology.

Leiomyosarcoma

Leiomyosarcomas can occur anywhere in the body but have a high incidence in the retroperitoneum and visceral sites. They have been reported to arise from blood vessel smooth muscle. Although survival is associated with the grade, a small collected series looking only at this subtype showed that leiomyosarcomas in the extremities behave aggressively.

TABLE 25.10. *Common soft tissue sarcomas*

Lesion	%
Liposarcoma	22
Leiomyosarcoma	19
Malignant fibrous histiocytoma	17
Fibrosarcoma	10
Synovial sarcoma	7
All others	25

Fibrosarcoma

Many fibrosarcomas have been reclassified as MFH; therefore some of the common wisdom concerning fibrosarcomas is no longer applicable. There are several subtypes, ranging from locally aggressive to frankly malignant.

Dermatofibrosarcoma protuberans (malignant fibroblastic fibrous histiocytoma) is a low-grade fibrosarcoma of the trunk with a propensity for local recurrence. Metastases are rare, and wide excision is the most appropriate therapy for this tumor.

Desmoid tumors are classified as abdominal and extraabdominal subtypes. The abdominal desmoids occur in women of childbearing age and may be associated with hormonal influences and the trauma of cesarean section. They usually arise from the aponeurosis of the rectus abdominis muscle. Treatment is wide local excision. Estrogen receptors have been identified in some of these tumors, but the significance of this finding remains unclear. There is an association with scarring and some of the polyposis syndromes. In the latter cases the tumors may become extensive and locally aggressive. These tumors may regress with the addition of some of the nonsteroidal antiinflammatory drugs. This response is not predictable or well documented.

The extraabdominal desmoids tend to occur in men in their thirties and forties. Though metastases are rare, they do occur. The locally aggressive nature of these lesions can cause significant morbidity and disability.

Diagnosis

Etiology

' Most sarcomas arise without an identifiable cause. Trauma has been associated with the abdominal desmoid tumors (Table 25.11). Approximately 10% of patients with Von Recklinghausen's disease develop neurofibrosarcoma. Radiation therapy has been implicated in the development of sarcomas. Generally these radiation-induced sarcomas occur more than 10 years after therapy in poorly accessible areas of the head and neck; they respond poorly to therapy and have a rapidly progressive course. Chronic lymphedema following surgical lymphadenectomy or radiation therapy for breast cancer or melanoma is related to the development of lymphangiosarcoma of the affected extremity (Stewart-Treves syndrome).

TABLE 25.11. *Etiology and predisposing factors for soft tissue sarcomas*

Trauma
  Fracture site: fibrosarcoma
  Burn: dermatotofibrosarcoma protuberans
  Foreign body: fibrosarcoma
Chemical
  Alkylating agents
  Vinyl chloride, Thorotrast, arsenic: hepatic angiosarcoma
Radiation
  Both orthovoltage and megavoltage
  Latency 2–25 years
  MFH, extraskeletal osteosarcoma, fibrosarcoma
Lymphedema
  Stewart-Treves syndrome (60% had radiation therapy)
  Latency 8.6 years
  Lymphangiosarcoma
Genetic
  Von Recklinghausen's disease: neurofibrosarcoma
  Gardner syndrome: desmoid fibrosarcoma of the mesentery
  Li-Fraumeni cancer family syndrome
  p53 Gene mutations: rhabdomyosarcoma
  Synovial sarcoma: t(x:16)(p11.2; q11.2)

MFH, malignant fibrous histiocytoma.

Several organic and inorganic chemicals are associated with hepatic angiosarcoma (Table 25.11). The androgenic anabolic steroids are notably included in this group.

Distribution of Soft Tissue Sarcomas in Adults

Sarcomas arise from mesodermally derived tissue and therefore occur where there is the greatest amount of muscle bulk. Half of the sarcomas occur on the extremities, one-fourth in the retroperitoneum, and one-fourth on the trunk and head and neck region (Table 25.12).

Prognostic Factors

Survival

Several factors predict outcome, not all of which are independent of one another. Because some of the variables are dependent, there seems to be confusion in the literature as to which factors are the most important prognostic variables.

TABLE 25.12. *Sites of soft tissue sarcomas*

Site	%
Extremities	54 (two-thirds in lower limb)
Retroperitoneum	24 (60% retroperitoneum, 20% genitourinary, 20% visceral)
Trunk	17 (66% abdominal, 17% thoracic, 17% buttock)
Head and neck	4

Histologic grade has the most prominent effect on survival, followed by the tumor size, depth, and site. All of these factors are independent. Patients with peripheral extremity sites tend to do better than those with proximal extremity locations. Retroperitoneal lesions have a worse prognosis than the proximal extremity lesions.

Some studies show better survival for young patients than older patients, but this finding has not been reproduced in all of the large studies. Histology and necrosis are not independent variables for survival but, rather, a function of the tumor grade. Certain lesions always have high-grade histology and therefore have a poor prognosis. Included among them are the tenosynoviosarcomas, epithelioid sarcomas, and adult rhabdomyosarcomas.

Local Recurrence

Grade, size, and depth of the primary do not affect the incidence of local recurrence. An inadequate margin of resection, however, does predict a higher frequency of local recurrence. Local recurrence is not a predictor of systemic failure.

Staging

There are several staging systems for sarcomas. Because grade is such an important prognostic variable, it is the basis of the American Joint Commission on Cancer staging system (Table 25.13). This staging system is currently undergoing reevaluation because assignment to high, intermediate, and low grades is difficult. Furthermore, size has become an important prognostic factor irrespective of the grade of the lesion.

Treatment

Surgical Management

Indications for Biopsy

Any soft tissue mass that is enlarging or more than 5 cm in diameter and persists for more than 1 month should undergo biopsy. In addition, any new and enlarging mass in the adult should be considered for biopsy.

Options for Biopsy

The surgical management of a sarcoma is determined by the location, size, and grade of the tumor. Therefore biopsy must be performed as the initial procedure. The pathologist requires a relatively large, fresh specimen to classify a sarcoma accurately. Fine-needle aspiration biopsies are inadequate for initial evaluation of a suspected STS because the pathologist cannot classify the tumor, immunohistochemical staining cannot be done, grade cannot be determined, and frequently the pathologist cannot determine if the lesion is benign or malig-

TABLE 25.13. *TMNG staging of soft tissue sarcomas and survival*

Stage	Criteria	5-Year survival (%)
IA (G1T1N0M0)	Grade 1, <5 cm	82
IB (G1T2N0M0)	Grade 1, >5 cm	
IIA (G2T1N0M0)	Grade 2, <5 cm	67
IIB (G2T2N0M0)	Grade 2, >5 cm	
IIIA (G3T1N0M0)	Grade 3, <5 cm	46
IIIB (G3T2N0M0)	Grade 3, >5 cm	
IIIC (GxT1–3N1M0)	Any grade or size, +nodes, no mets	
IVA (GxT3N0–1M0)	Bone or blood vessel invasion, no mets	10
IVB (GxTxNxM1)	Metastatic disease	

mets, metastases.

nant. Core needle biopsies are acceptable if several cores of tissue are retrieved. An excisional biopsy is recommended for small tumors, whereas larger tumors should undergo an incisional biopsy. The biopsy incision is oriented along the axis of the extremity or in a manner that does not compromise a subsequent definitive operation. Improperly oriented biopsy incisions can limit the reresection option or necessitate more extensive, debilitating surgery.

Preoperative Evaluation

Low-Grade Lesions. Most extremity and trunk melanomas metastasize to the lungs, whereas the visceral and retroperitoneal sarcomas metastasize to the lungs and liver. Low-grade lesions metastasize in only 15% of cases. Therefore, a chest radiograph is the only required preoperative test for extremity and trunk sarcomas. A CT scan or magnetic resonance imaging (MRI) of the lesion allows better definition of the anatomic setting of the tumor and may help when planning the resection. MRI is considered the best test because bony artifacts are eliminated, multiple planes can be reconstructed, and the patient is not exposed to radiation. If an MRI scan is obtained, both T1- and T2-weighted images must be done for best definition of the tumor.

High-Grade Sarcomas. Chest tomograms or chest CT is suggested because these lesions have a propensity to metastasize to the lungs.

Retroperitoneal or Visceral Sarcomas. Abdominal CT scans are mandatory. These tumors tend to be avascular, so angiography or vena cavagraphy should be used judiciously.

Options for Resection

Despite the radiosensitivity of these tumors, irradiation alone does not cure sarcomas. Therefore the surgeon must be included in the treatment of this disease. Sarcomas should be treated by a team of physicians that includes a radiotherapist, medical oncologist, and surgeon. The surgeon must ultimately decide the scope of the resection as determined by the anatomic setting of the tumor, its proximity to vital structures, its grade, the potential for cure, and the potential functional impairment that may result from ablative surgery. In addition, the patient must be willing to undergo the planned resection.

Margins of Resection

The resection should be planned to have as wide a margin as possible to prevent local recurrence. At a minimum, the margins of resection must be pathologically free of tumor.

Limited margin resections (**LMRs**) are those where the margins are not pathologically involved, but the tumor is only one to two high-power microscope fields from the edge of the specimen. The LMR is not recommended because local recurrences occur in up to 90% of patients. LMS is considered adequate local therapy when combined with radiotherapy.

Wide margin resections (**WMRs**) require a margin of 2 to 3 cm and is the minimal procedure if used as the sole modality. Usually the recommended 2- to 3-cm margins cannot be achieved owing to anatomic constraints (i.e., bones, arteries, nerves).

Muscle group resection is the prototype function-sparing but oncologically sound procedure. It is applicable to the lower extremity exclusively. Because the proximal and distal portions of a muscle divided during a wide local resection perform no function, these procedures are no more disabling than the WMR. A problem arises when one of the margins of resection is close and radiotherapy (RT) is required. The RT must encompass the entire resection bed, necessitating larger radiation portals and higher overall doses with increased risk of radiation-induced complications. Muscle group resections and compartment resections provide no oncologic benefit over routine WMR.

Amputation causes significant functional impairment and has not been shown to provide a survival benefit. Amputations should be avoided if a conservative limb-sparing option exists.

General Guidelines for Specific Sites

Sarcomas near or abutting neurovascular structures, bone, or joints or in the distal extremity are difficult to resect with adequate margins. For these lesions, amputation must be among the curative options. If the mass is in close proximity to the pelvis, a hemipelvectomy should be considered. The internal hemipelvectomy preserves the leg for cosmetic, not functional purposes. Reconstruction of the pelvis has been done with autoclaved autologous pelvic bone or preserved bone. Similarly, sarcomas near the shoulder or scapula may require intrascapulothoracic amputation (forequarter amputation) when no curative conservative option is available.

Although buttectomy alone has a 25% to 35% local recurrence rate for lesions of the gluteal region, more extensive resections have not been shown to improve local control and function. The sciatic nerve should be preserved if it is not involved.

Amputation is recommended for tumors involving the popliteal or antecubital fossae. Margins are limited by the nerves, arteries, and veins traversing these spaces and by the joint itself. A limited margin resection with radiotherapy may be considered for the patient who refuses amputation. Locally recurrent disease following limited margin resection and irradiation requires amputation.

Half of the sarcomas on the hands or feet treated by local resection recur locally. All patients with local recurrence in this site have died of their disease. Therefore some form of local amputation is recommended.

Sarcomas of the trunk are difficult to treat because the margins of the abdominal and thoracic walls are thin, precluding adequate deep margins. The surgeon and the patient must be prepared to resect ribs and close the large defects with flaps and prosthetic materials.

The mean diameter of a retroperitoneal sarcoma is about 20 cm at presentation. Leiomyosarcomas (25%), liposarcomas (21%), and fibrosarcomas (12%) are the most common types. These tumors should be resected through a transabdominal approach because 79% require resection of an adjacent structure or organ to achieve complete resection. Half of theses tumor recur and require reresection. The recurrences can appear more than 5 years after the initial therapy. These patients should be followed by serial CT scans of the abdomen every 3 to 6 months. Recurrences are treated with repeated resection when possible.

Visceral (gastric and intestinal) sarcomas usually present with vague pain, bleeding, and a palpable abdominal mass. Several approaches have been proposed including some radical procedures, but no survival advantage has be shown for the more radical procedures. Therefore the therapy currently in vogue is wide local resection.

Trends in Sarcoma Treatment

There is no universal treatment for soft tissue sarcomas. The anatomy, site, and potential for long-term sur-

vival must be considered before embarking on function-impairing surgery. Presently the trend is toward more conservative resections with the use of adjuvant radiation therapy (brachyradiotherapy or external irradiation).

Adequate local treatment of the primary tumor does not improve long-term survival. Patients undergoing less than optimal local therapy for a primary sarcoma in the extremity have the same long-term survival as the patient undergoing "adequate" local therapy. This finding suggests that tumor dissemination may precede primary therapy, or it may reflect inherent biologic characteristics of the sarcomas.

Adjuvant Therapy

Adjuvant radiation therapy reduces local recurrences but does not change the overall mortality associated with sarcoma of the extremity. Adjuvant irradiation is not beneficial in patients with retroperitoneal or visceral sarcomas. In general, for sarcomas of the extremity, adjuvant radiation therapy is used in situations where the margins are free but close to the tumor and for all high-grade sarcomas irrespective of the adequacy of the resection margins. The radiation therapy can be administered externally or with the use of interstitial catheters (brachyradiotherapy).

Forty percent of sarcoma patients die as a result of systemic, hematogenous metastases. Systemic adjuvant chemotherapy makes empiric sense in this situation. Several prospective and randomized trials have shown a small increase in the disease-free interval but no survival benefit. Routine adjuvant chemotherapy is not advocated.

Alternative Therapy

Herman Suit advocated preoperative (neoadjuvant) radiation therapy in patients with extremity sarcomas. Despite a high incidence of local wound complications, survival and local control rates are comparable to that found with other methods of treatment.

Treatment of Recurrent Disease

Eighty percent of recurrences are noted within 2 years of initial therapy. The routine follow-up for a patient with sarcoma includes chest radiography every 3 months, chest CT every 6 months, and a physical examination of the site of the primary every 3 months. Imaging studies of the areas of the primary can be considered.

About 15% of sarcomas fail locally. If no distant metastases are present, local reresection or amputation is undertaken. Approximately 60% of patients undergoing complete resection of a locally recurrent sarcoma survive 5 years. This excellent survival may reflect the biologic behavior of the tumor rather than the efficacy of the reoperative surgery. The recurrence rate for retroperitoneal sarcomas is higher, and the long-term survival is lower.

The lung is the most common site of metastatic disease from soft tissue sarcomas. In situations where pulmonary metastases are noted prior to treatment of the primary lesion, the patient must be carefully evaluated. If the primary lesion and the metastases appear resectable on preoperative studies, the patient is a candidate for staged surgery. The primary is resected first. In cases where lung metastases are noted on follow-up examination, they are resected if possible.

Lung metastases are generally located peripherally, and resection does not sacrifice much lung parenchyma. If the lesions are bilateral, a median sternotomy approach is used. Pulmonary functions (including FEV-1) should be obtained preoperatively to determine whether the patient can tolerate thoracotomy. Median survival for metastasectomy is 20 months, with 30% of patients surviving 5 years. The survival is not affected by the histology, number of metastases, or the site of recurrence.

Advanced Disease

In general, treatment of advanced sarcomas is poor. The active agents include doxorubicin, DTIC, ifosphamide, cyclophosphamide, actinomycin D, and cisplatin. At best, 20% of patients respond to chemotherapy. In the current trials, median survival increased from 4 months to 8 months.

LYMPHOMA

The surgeon's role in the treatment of nonintestinal lymphomas is limited to diagnosis, assessment of the extent of disease, evaluation of residual disease, and support during chemotherapy and radiation therapy.

Lymph Node Biopsies

Nodes are excised (not incised) if possible because the stromal architecture is important to the diagnosis. All nodes should be presented to the pathologist fresh without formalin fixation, allowing immunohistochemical analysis and immunophenotyping. In the future, the treatment of certain types of lymphomas will be based on the immunophenotype rather than the histologic class of the tumor.

Hodgkin's Disease

Hodgkin's disease can be treated with irradiation, chemotherapy, or both. Patients with localized disease, stages 1A or IIA, are candidates for RT alone. If RT is considered, it is imperative that the extent of disease be determined surgically at the time of a staging laparotomy, as radiation fields depend on the extent of the disease: 25% are down-staged (worse disease), and 15% are up-staged (less disease than suspected). In 30% of patients the therapy is altered by the results of the staging laparotomy.

Staging Laparotomy

The purpose of the staging laparotomy is to assess accurately the extent of disease; therefore it is essential that all suspicious lymph nodes be biopsied. The abdomen is explored thoroughly. All nodes that were seen to be abnormal on the preoperative lymphangiogram must be removed, and their removal must be confirmed with intraoperative radiographs. The splenic hilar, celiac, porta hepatis, mesenteric peripancreatic, paraaortic, paracaval, and iliac nodes are examined. The spleen is removed as well. Several liver biopsies, both core and wedge biopsies, of both lobes are performed. Large areas of residual disease are marked with surgical clips.

The staging laparotomy is not performed if radiation therapy is not considered a reasonable treatment option for Hodgkin's disease at the treating institution. In addition, patients with B-type symptoms (weight loss, fevers, sweats, pruritus) all subjected to chemotherapy and therefore should not undergo a laparotomy. Other contraindications for staging laparotomy include bone marrow involvement, extranodal lymphoma, mediastinal involvement, and co-morbid conditions, which make general anesthesia a significant risk to the patient. Although splenectomy can attenuate the pancytopenias associated with aggressive chemotherapy, it is not an adequate indication for splenectomy in lymphoma patients.

Non-Hodgkin's Lymphoma

The most common type of non-Hodgkin's lymphoma is diffuse histiocytic lymphoma. These patients present late with stage III or IV disease. Staging laparotomy is not useful because all patients receive chemotherapy as their primary treatment. Occasionally, posttreatment laparotomy is needed to define residual disease.

Gastrointestinal Lymphomas

Gastrointestinal (GI) lymphomas represent 1% to 4% of all GI neoplasms. The GI tract is the most common extranodal site of lymphoma. Most are B cell lymphomas. About 55% occur in the stomach, 25% in the small intestine, and 20% in the colon. The incidence of gastric lymphoma peaks at age 62, whereas the other GI lymphomas occur at around age 50. These patients present with GI bleeding, obstruction, perforation (9% to 47%), abdominal pain, nausea, weight loss, and fatigue.

There is no controversy with regard to the role of surgery in the small intestinal and colonic lymphomas. Most can be resected, and survival is fairly good with surgery alone. These tumors are discovered almost always at exploratory surgery for a bowel obstruction or bleeding.

In contradistinction, gastric lymphomas are frequently diagnosed preoperatively. Controversy still exists as to the primary role of surgery for gastric lymphoma. For stage I gastric lymphoma, radiotherapists report up to a 70% cure rate without perforations. Surgeons report a 40% incidence of perforation following RT and a 60% incidence of bleeding. Chemotherapy alone is attended by at least a 13% incidence of perforation.

In general, GI lymphomas that can be completely resected are associated with an 83% five-year survival. The addition of RT seems to be beneficial, whereas the addition of chemotherapy does not. Early-stage lymphomas can be treated with either surgery or RT alone or with a combination of the two. The treatment of advanced GI lymphoma must be individualized.

QUESTIONS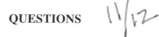

Select one answer.

1. Risk factors for the development of melanoma include all of the following *except:*
   a. Fair hair.
   b. Light complexion.
   c. Green eyes.
   d. Multiple nevi.
2. The classic triad of the dysplastic nevi syndrome includes all of the following *except:*
   a. Patient with more than 100 moles.
   b. One mole larger than 8 mm.
   c. Superficial spreading melanoma of one of the moles.
   d. One mole with atypical histologic features.
3. True statements with respect to melanoma include all of the following *except:*
   a. Melanoma is increasing at a rapid rate.
   b. Most melanomas are more common in outdoor laborers than office workers.
   c. Melanoma has become less virulent.
   d. Melanoma is associated with xeroderma pigmentosum.
4. True statements with respect to superficial spreading melanoma include all of the following *except:*
   a. SSM is the most common form of melanoma.
   b. Approximately half of the lesions are ulcerated at presentation.
   c. SSMs arise from or near a preexisting nevus.
   d. SSM has an immediate prognosis.
5. True statements with respect to nodular melanoma include all of the following *except:*
   a. NM is more common in females.
   b. Ulceration is common.
   c. Most amelanotic melanomas are of the nodular type.
   d. The lesions are raised and generally darker than the SSM counterparts.
6. True statements with respect to the prognosis of subungual melanomas include all of the following *except:*
   a. Prognosis is related to destruction of the nail bed.

b. Prognosis is related to the thickness of the tumor.
c. Prognosis is related to bony invasion.
d. Prognosis is related to the location of the lack of pigmentation.

7. Acceptable biopsy methods for a pigmented lesion include all of the following except:
   a. Excisional biopsy.
   b. Punch biopsy.
   c. Shave biopsy.
   d. Incisional biopsy.

8. Optimal resection for melanomas of various sites include all of the following *except:*
   a. Subungual melanoma of the thumb: interphalangeal amputation.
   b. Subungual melanoma of the third digit: distal interphalangeal amputation.
   c. Melanoma on the female breast: mastectomy.
   d. Melanoma of the thigh, 3 mm deep: wide local excision with 3-cm margins.

9. The following are true statements with respect to clinical stage II melanoma *except:*
   a. If no primary is found the patient should receive chemotherapy.
   b. Therapeutic node dissection is not indicated.
   c. Common sites of metastases include regional nodes, lung, liver, brain, and bones.
   d. About 20% of patients with positive regional nodes survive 5 years.

10. Adequate local therapy for a soft tissue sarcoma includes all of the following *except:*
    a. Neoadjuvant radiation therapy followed by excision.
    b. Wide margin resection.
    c. Limited margin resection.
    d. Amputation.

11. True statements with respect to soft tissue sarcomas include all of the following *except:*
    a. Lymphatic metastases are common and require lymphadenectomy when present.
    b. Hematogenous spread is most common.
    c. The pseudocapsule is made up of fibrous tissue and no tumor.
    d. Lung metastases are the most common sites of initial failure.

12. Prognostic factors influencing survival include all of the following *except:*
    a. Size.
    b. Grade.
    c. Location.
    d. Histology.

SELECTED REFERENCES

Balch CM, Milton GW, eds. *Cutaneous melanoma.* Philadelphia: JB Lippincott, 1985.

Devita VT, Hellman S, Rosenberg SA, eds. *Principles and practice of oncology.* Philadelphia: JB Lippincott, 1990.

Economou SG, ed. *Adjuncts to cancer surgery.* Philadelphia: Lea & Febiger, 1991.

McKenna RJ, Murphy GP, eds. *Fundamentals of surgical oncology.* New York: Macmillan, 1986.

Sabiston DC, ed. *Textbook of surgery: the biological basis of modern surgical practice.* Philadelphia: WB Saunders, 1991.

Shiu MH, Brennan MF, eds. *Surgical management of soft tissue sarcoma.* Philadelphia: Lea & Febiger, 1989.

26

Neurosurgery

James T. Goodrich and David F. Jimenez

HEAD INJURY

Epidemiologic Aspects

Head injuries represent the leading cause of death in the 2- to 42-year-old age group and account for significant morbidity in the United States. Each year 10 million Americans sustain a head injury for which medical attention is obtained. There are some 40,000 fatalities per year in the United States (i.e., 20/100,000) from head injury. Among them, 70% result from motor vehicle accidents, and 50% to 60% occur within the first 24 hours after injury. Among patients with multiple injuries, the head is the most commonly involved area. A review of the records of fatal road accident victims showed that 75% were found to have significant injury to the central nervous system (CNS) (i.e., brain and spinal cord) at autopsy.

Types of Head Injury

Head injuries are classified according to the tissue affected (skull, blood vessels, brain parenchyma), the type of external force applied, and the resulting pathologic changes. The following sections outline the types of external trauma, specify the major types of injury they cause, and summarize their management.

Blunt Head Injury

Contact

Contact injury results when an object strikes the head with sufficient force to cause tissue damage. The surface area of the object that comes into contact with the head is relatively small (e.g., a lead pipe or baseball bat). Often the object is accelerating as it meets the skull, and there may be shearing effects. Most tissue damage is local: skull fracture, epidural hematoma, brain contusion adjacent to the area of impact.

Deceleration

The area of impact is larger with a deceleration injury than with a contact injury—as when the head's motion is stopped by a windshield or sidewalk. Tissue damage for the most part is due to sudden dissipation of momentum or shearing forces, resulting in intracranial injuries such as subdural hematoma, contrecoup contusion, or diffuse damage to axons.

Penetrating Head Injury. Typically, penetrating head injuries are more devastating than blunt injuries. The pathologic injuries to the brain tend to vary with the type of penetrating object: icepick, screwdriver, bullet, and so on. The depth of penetration and the structures injured determine the outcome and prognosis.

Gunshot Wounds. As our urban population has expanded and the younger generation has come to rely increasingly on high-power side arms, gunshot wounds (GSWs) have come to account for a major proportion of injuries seen in emergency rooms. The switch from the low-power, low-velocity bullets of the "Saturday night special" to the high-power, high-speed bullets of the 9-mm rapid repeating weapon has also increased the severity of gunshot injuries. The injury caused by a bullet depends more on its *velocity* than on its mass. The shock wave spreading out from the bullet may transiently elevate intracranial pressure. The damage due to the gunshot includes not only direct traumatic effects as the bullet passes through brain but also the *ricochet* potential inside the skull. Hematomas often form as a result of torn blood vessels, adding to morbidity and mortality. The bullet or missile can also cause penetration by bone fragments.

Effects of External Forces on the Skull and Its Contents

Skull Fractures

Skull fractures are classified according to their morphology (e.g., linear, stellate, comminuted, depressed), their location (e.g., calvarial, basilar), and whether the overlying soft tissue is also involved (compound).

Linear Fractures

A linear fracture occurs whenever a hard object strikes the cranial vault with enough force to cause a temporary deformational change in the skull but without depression of the bone elements. The diameter of the object is usually larger than 5 cm, thereby reducing the risk of skull penetration in the typical instance. The presence of a simple linear skull fracture demonstrates that a considerable amount of energy has been transmitted to the head. Unless associated with an altered level of consciousness or a focal neurologic deficit, this type of fracture has little surgical significance. However, if a linear skull fracture crosses the midline or a suture of the calvarium, the patient requires further workup, and an underlying hematoma must be ruled out. Linear fractures of the calvarium are radiolucent and have well defined margins. They do not have sclerotic borders, nor do they bifurcate as vascular structures do.

Depressed Fractures

Depressed skull fractures are similar to linear fractures except that greater forces of impact are involved, and the object's surface area at the point of contact is typically smaller, thereby concentrating the amount of kinetic energy transmitted to the skull. The mortality associated with depressed fractures is 11%; 15% of patients have permanent neurologic deficits. Between 5% and 7% of skull fractures are associated with intracranial hematomas. Other major problems associated with this type of fracture include lacerations of the dura and concomitant injuries of the parenchyma (Fig. 26.1).

The decision as to when to intervene surgically varies from center to center. It is generally agreed, however, that when a fracture lowers the outer table of bone below the inner table, débridement and elevation

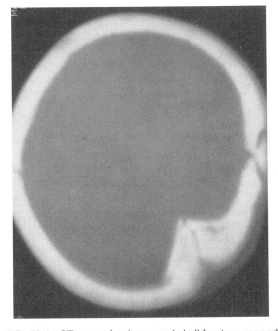

FIG. 26.1. CT scan of a depressed skull fracture caused by a sharp-edge object (tomahawk). There is an in-driven piece of calvarial bone with the outer table below the inner table with compression of the underlying brain. There is an additional fracture just anterior that is not depressed and a linear fracture on the opposite side of the skull.

should be performed. Other situations requiring surgical intervention include depressed fractures over the sagittal sinus, motor strip, or dominant angular gyrus (i.e., speech area) as well as those in which bone fragments appear sharp on radiographs. A computed tomography (CT) scan with bone windows is often the best basis on which to determine the need for surgical intervention. In the case of a sagittal sinus fracture, magnetic resonance angiography (MRA) can be done to rule sagittal sinus occlusion, a potentially devastating situation.

Basilar Fractures

Any of the bones that constitute the base of the skull—ethmoid (cribriform plate), frontal (orbital roof), sphenoid, temporal (squamous and petrous portions), and occipital bones—can be fractured. Such fractures are caused by direct impact (occiput, mastoid, or supraorbital areas) or by energy transmitted from trauma to the mandibular or facial region. The incidence of basilar skull fractures after head injury ranges between 3.5% and 24.0%.

Clinically, basilar skull fractures are manifested by cerebrospinal fluid (CSF) rhinorrhea (11%), otorrhea (5%), meningitis (4%), pneumocephalus, hemotympanum, facial nerve palsy, Battle's sign (ecchymosis over the mastoid prominence), or racoon's eyes (periorbital ecchymosis). Basilar skull fractures can be difficult to resolve on CT scan. To assist in locating a CSF fistula, a CT scan is performed after intrathecal injection of contrast material (e.g., iohexol).

Basilar skull fractures rarely require surgical intervention. If a CSF fistula is present, an indwelling lumbar spinal drain is placed as the first line of treatment (typically for 7 to 10 days) to divert CSF away from the leak site. If spinal drainage fails, surgical intervention to repair the site of leakage is required. For basilar skull fractures involving the temporal bone and petrous ridge, the facial nerve can become entrapped and swollen. If signs of improvement do not appear after initiation of steroid treatment, surgical decompression is required to save the nerve.

Intracranial Hemorrhage

Intracranial hemorrhage types are listed in Table 26.1. The associated mortality is shown as well.

TABLE 26.1. *Mortality from intracranial hemorrhage*

Type of hemorrhage	Mortality (%)
Acute subdural	50
Acute intraparenchymal	30–60
Acute epidural	10–20

Subarachnoid Hemorrhage

Subarachnoid hemorrhage (SAH) is the most common form of intracranial hemorrhage following head injury, and it may occur as a result of trivial or severe trauma. SAH has little if any significance from a surgical standpoint with one exception. Blood in the subarachnoid space can interfere with the reabsorption of CSF, leading to a communicating type of hydrocephalus that may require treatment, such as ventriculoperitoneal shunting (see below). SAH occurs because of shearing or tearing of the plial vessels, allowing blood to diffuse throughout the subarachnoid space. Clinically, SAH may produce meningismus (i.e., stiff neck), photophobia, and headaches. In some patients SAH is associated with bizarre and maniacal behavior.

Subdural Hematoma

After subarachnoid hemorrhage, subdural hematomas (SDHs) are the most common type of posttraumatic intracerebral hemorrhage. SDHs result from a laceration or tearing of the "bridging" veins between the cortex and the venous sinuses, direct laceration of the cortical vessels, or contusion of the cortex with bleeding into the subdural space from torn pia–arachnoid membranes. They develop in the anatomic space between the inner layer of the dura and the arachnoid membrane.

The SDHs are found in 9% to 13% of all severe head injuries. They may be classified as a simple SDH (i.e., hematomas not associated with brain injury) or a complicated SDH (those associated with laceration of the parenchyma and intracerebral hematomas). The mortality associated with simple SDH is about 22%, whereas for complicated SDH it is 50% to 90%. Seventy percent of the intracerebral hematomas, lacerations, and contusions associated with SDH arise from contrecoup injuries; therefore most are located in the temporal and frontal lobes, the areas most susceptible to this type of injury.

Subdural hematomas are also categorized according to the time period between injury and the appearance of the clinical symptoms.

Acute Subdural Hematoma

Acute subdural hematomas (ASDHs) are defined as those that produce symptoms within 48 hours after the injury. They are most commonly associated with a severe head injury. Frequently, the impact that produces the ASDH also causes severe injury to the underlying brain parenchyma. ASDH is associated with high morbidity and mortality rates (60% in young patients and 90% in elderly patients).

The clinical presentation and course are determined by two factors: the severity of the injury at the time of impact and how rapidly the hematoma develops. The quality of consciousness varies from sustained loss of consciousness (17%), to fluctuations from lucidity to unconsciousness (17%), impaired consciousness with lucid intervals (13%), and unimpaired consciousness (29%). Clinical findings can include anisocoria (dilation of the pupil), contralateral hemiparesis, abducens palsy, hemiparesis, decerebration, aphasia, and seizures. Anisocoria and contralateral hemiparesis are referred to as Kernohan's sign, and in 85% of patients they indicate the site of the hematoma (i.e., the side on which anisocoria appears).

The radiographic appearance of an ASDH on CT scan is that of a hyperdense crescentic mass adjacent to the inner table of the skull and overlying the affected hemisphere (Fig. 26.2). A significant midline shift and a mass effect are commonly observed. For smaller hematomas with little mass effect, the gyral pattern of the brain can be seen to be outlined, helping to differentiate the subdural hematoma from the epidural hematoma. Although most commonly found over the convexity, ASDHs may also be found in the interhemispheric space, along the tentorium, and in the posterior fossa, the last being an ominous finding.

Early definitive treatment (i.e., surgical evacuation within the first 4 hours) has been shown to reduce mortality significantly: Patients who undergo operation within 4 hours have a mortality rate of 30% compared with 90% for patients in whom operation is delayed beyond 4 hours. If a CT scan is not available and the patient is deteriorating, the order of trephination placement on the side of the dilated pupil is (a) temporal, (b) frontal, and (c) parietal. If necessary, these burr holes

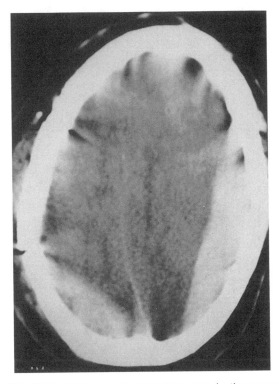

FIG. 26.2. A 72-year-old man was seen in the emergency room after falling down a flight of stairs. There are two acute subdural hematomas: in the left parietooccipital and right occipital regions. The increased density of fresh hemorrhage is evident here in both of the subdural hematomas.

can be connected to develop the "question mark" craniotomy flap used in patients with trauma.

Subacute Subdural Hematoma

The subacute subdural hematoma (SSDH) produces neurologic deficits after more than 48 hours but less than 2 weeks after the injury. Typically, the patient has a history of trauma with or without loss of consciousness followed by gradual improvement but then neurologic deterioration, with findings that may include hemiparesis, cranial nerve deficits, and depressed mental status.

Evacuation of the hematoma is warranted if there is an impending risk of herniation or if midline shift is significant and cerebral compression is seen on the CT scan. Treatment consists in (a) formal craniotomy if the clot is solid or (b) trephination with external drainage if the clot has significantly liquefied. The gradual decrease in density of a SSDH on CT scan (Fig. 26.3) evolves over 10 to 12 days, with the hematoma becoming isodense with the brain parenchyma; this change can make the diagnosis of SSDH difficult. In these cases the only clues to the presence of a SSDH may be obliteration of the sulci and a lateralizing shift of the ventricles.

Chronic Subdural Hematoma

The chronic subdural hematoma (CSDH) presents more than 2 weeks after the injury. Its incidence is estimated to be 1/100,000 to 2/100,000 per year. Most patients are elderly or of late middle age. Typically, 20% to 50% of the patients have no history of trauma. Predisposing factors for CSDH include alcoholism, epilepsy, shunting procedures for hydrocephalus, and anticoagulation therapy.

Approximately 7 to 10 days after bleeding into the subdural space, a semipermeable membrane forms around the clot. Fibroblasts migrate in from the surrounding meninges and establish a thin inner and a thick outer membrane around the hematoma. How the hematoma expands is unclear. One hypothesis states that as red blood cells and hemoglobin molecules break down the osmotic pressure increases, leading to inflow of CSF through the semipermeable membrane. In some studies in which the albumin/γ-globulin and albumin/total protein ratios in subdural fluid, serum, and the hematoma have been examined, the results indicate that the osmolality of the hematoma does not change with time. It is likely that albumin diffuses across the membrane, and that recurrent bleeding into the clot accounts for the enlargement of the CSDH.

The clinical presentation of a CSDH may be variable. The more typical picture is of slowly progressive symptoms, such as hemiparesis (45%), hemianopsia (7%), oculomotor palsy (11%), and impaired consciousness (53%), which develop 3 to 4 weeks after the injury.

The CT scan appearance of a CSDH is that of an isodense lesion, often lenticular in shape. Commonly, there can be a mixture of hypodense and hyperdense areas, indicating recent hemorrhage into CSDH (Fig. 26.4).

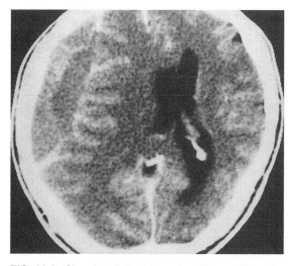

FIG. 26.3. Chronic subdural hematoma in a patient who had fallen out of bed. A large frontotemporal, nearly isodense hematoma can be seen with pronounced shift and mass effect with obliteration of the frontal horn plus falcine and cingulate herniation of the brain.

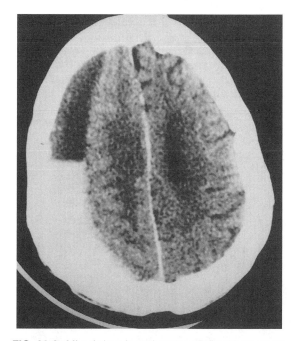

FIG. 26.4. Mixed chronic and acute subdural hematoma with blood layering out, seen here as the bright white contrast to the isodense superior chronic component. The mass effect of this hemorrhage has obliterated the lateral ventricle.

If a CSDH becomes symptomatic, the treatment of choice is surgical evacuation. Craniotomy, burr holes, and twist drill craniostomies have been used successfully. The most commonly used surgical treatment is twist drill trephination over the site of maximal clot thickness. After drainage, external catheters are left in place for 24 to 48 hours to assist in the removal of any residual fluid. The patient is kept supine to decrease the likelihood of hematoma reaccumulation. Because of the natural atrophy of the brain with aging, recurrence has been reported in up to 45% of patients; however, about 75% of these patients are able to return to normal functioning even when small residual hematoma remains.

Subdural Hygroma

Subdural hygromas represent about 10% of all traumatic intracranial mass lesions. Hygromas are collections of a clear, xanthochromic, or slightly bloody fluid in the subdural space. They are thought to arise from tears in the arachnoid membrane that allow escape of CSF into the subdural space. Most patients are asymptomatic. Those who become symptomatic present with symptoms similar to those of an ASDH or CSDH. The CT scan, the diagnostic approach of choice, shows crescentic areas of hypodensity with a density signal similar to that of CSF. In contrast to a CSDH, there are no membranes and no enhancement after contrast infusion. Patients who are symptomatic undergo trephination or twist drill craniotomy. Because recurrence is common, the patient requires frequent follow-up.

Epidural Hematoma

The epidural hematoma (EDH) is defined anatomically as a collection of blood between the skull's inner table and the dura mater. The incidence of EDH is low (0.4% to 4.6%) compared to that of an ASDH (50%). The source of bleeding is arterial in 85% of the cases and venous in 15%. The middle meningeal artery is the most common source of bleeding in middle fossa EDHs. About 70% occur laterally over the hemispheres with the pterion as the epicenter. The remaining 30% have a frontal, occipital, or posterior fossa location.

In the "textbook" presentation of an EDH (which occurs in only 10% to 30% of cases) there is (a) brief loss of consciousness following the injury, (b) restoration of consciousness (the so-called *lucid interval*), and then (c) progressive obtundation, hemiparesis, anisocoria, and coma. It must be remembered that a lucid interval can also occur in such conditions as SDH. The appearance of the lucid interval depends on the rate at which the expanding clot enlarges. Other clinical presentations include headaches, emesis, seizures, and hyperreflexia. Approximately two-thirds of the patients have anisocoria (85% ipsilateral to the EDH) and contralateral hemiparesis secondary to midbrain compression from a herniated uncus (temporal lobe). *Kernohan's phenomenon* (a dilated pupil contralateral to the EDH and ipsilateral hemiparesis) occurs in about 15% of patients. These clinical findings result from compression of the opposite cerebral peduncle against the tentorial notch by the expanding hematoma. CT scans show a high-density lenticular (biconvex) area adjacent to the skull that does not cross suture lines (Fig. 26.5).

Only patients who become symptomatic are treated. A large craniotomy is performed to expose and control the bleeding site and then evacuate the hematoma. The mortality rate, even with surgical treatment, varies between 15% and 43%. Mortality rates are low in children

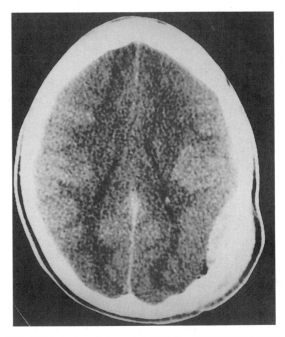

FIG. 26.5. Left parietooccipital acute epidural hematoma. The characteristic "lens shape" hemorrhage is present.

(5%) and much higher in the elderly (35% to 45%). Patients who have had periods of wakefulness before surgery have a better prognosis; those who are decerebrating or in a coma have a mortality higher than 50%.

Cerebral Contusion

Like contusions elsewhere in the body, those affecting the cerebrum are composed of areas of hemorrhage, necrosis, and infarction. Contusions occur in brain areas underlying the site of an external impact (coup lesion) but also commonly on the side of the skull opposite from the site of impact (countrecoup lesion). The temporal poles and undersurfaces of the frontal lobes are the most frequent sites of contusion. The CT scan shows areas of increased density mixed with areas of hypodensity, indicating hemorrhage and edema, confirming the diagnosis (Fig. 26.6). Small or deep lesions are managed conservatively. Large lesions with mass effect are often removed surgically. The mortality rate

varies from less than 5% to 60%, depending on the size of the contusion, its location, and the associated injuries. Contusions of the brain stem are seen after a shear-type injury and carry a poor prognosis in terms of functional recovery.

Shaken Baby Syndrome/ Nonaccidental Injury Syndrome

One of the most difficult situations in an emergency room is that of reaching a diagnosis for the child presenting with a head injury whose history is inconsistent with the findings. Most states now require the reporting of any suspected cases of child abuse. Recently pediatric neurosurgeons have described clinical findings that might help identify the child who has been subjected to a nonaccidental injury (NAI), the terminology currently preferred for the entity formerly referred to as "shaken baby syndrome" (Table 26.2).

Depressed Skull Fracture in the Young Child

When is a skull fracture likely to result from abuse? When a fracture occurs on the front or side of the head, the examiner must carefully obtain a history, as these locations are suggestive of an abuse injury. Children have a primitive protective reflex, the Moro reflex, so when they fall forward, their outstretched hands break the fall. A fracture on the back of the head is usually not due to abuse. When the young child falls backward (e.g., out of a crib), no protective reflex comes into play.

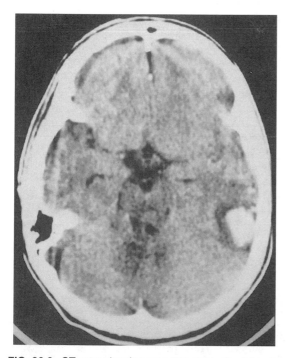

FIG. 26.6. CT scan showing an acute contusion injury to the left temporal region with fresh intraparenchymal blood with surrounding reactive edema.

TABLE 26.2. *Identifying the infant with a nonaccidental injury*

1. Uncertain history or one that seems to be at odds with the physical findings.
2. New onset of seizures associated with (a) *retinal hemorrhages* (due to a sudden elevation of intracranial pressure, subhyloid bleed); (b) *intradural surface hemorrhages* on CT or MRI.
3. Additional findings of new or *healing fractures* of long bones, in particular *rib fractures* (usually pathognomonic for NAI). Bruise marks and/or fingernail marks on the upper arm are potential signs of abuse.
4. *Long-term findings:* enlarging head, slowed development, failure to thrive, hyperirritability, and increased muscle tone.

It is vitally important that the history matches the mechanism of injury.

Radiographic Findings of NAI

A finding that once was commonly categorized as benign external hydrocephalus has recently become recognized as a sequela to NAI. In a brain that has been "shaken" (i.e., subjected to repeated rapid acceleration–deceleration cycles), the plial and dural bridging vessels are torn and so bleed. As the blood is resorbed, the CSF circulating pathways can be partially occluded, and with time the brain atrophies and pulls away from the skull. As a result of the lack of CSF resorption the skull continues to enlarge, and these children typically have a head circumference in the greater than 95% category. These findings are best detected by CT or magnetic resonance imaging (MRI). For lack of a better term, it has been called the shriveled walnut sign (Fig. 26.7). The developmental outcome in these children is

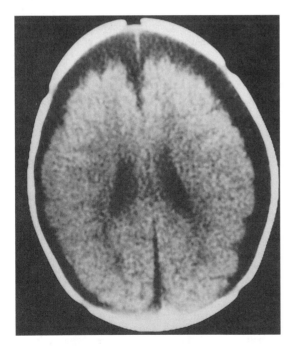

FIG. 26.7. CT scan of a 8-month-old child suspected of sustaining a nonaccidental injury. The shriveled walnut sign is present here with the brain pulled away from the skull secondary to the original hemorrhage and then atrophy.

poor. Their development is often moderately to severely delayed, and they often require long-term care.

Posttraumatic Syndrome

Often forgotten during management of a head injury is the posttraumatic syndrome, a common sequela in a patient who has lost consciousness as the result of a head injury. Table 26.3 lists the conditions commonly seen with posttraumatic syndrome. These findings may be immediate or may not develop for several days. With aggressive pain management and physical therapy the syndrome can be adequately treated.

Management of Head Injury

A detailed discussion of the cerebral dynamics and physiologic responses after a head injury is beyond the scope of this chapter, but certain basic principles must be kept in mind when managing the head-injured patient. A critical parameter for adequate brain function and survival after an injury is blood flow to the neurons and supporting glial structures. Cerebral blood flow (CBF) is difficult to quantitate without recourse to invasive monitoring, but the cerebral perfusion pressure (CPP), which is directly proportional to the CBF, can be calculated:

$$CPP = MAP - ICP$$

where MAP is the mean arterial pressure, and ICP is the intracranial pressure. This is a simple but fundamental concept in the management of head injury. The CPP in a normal adult is higher than 50 mm Hg. The therapeutic endpoint is simply that of maintaining an adequate perfusion pressure of the brain. With head injuries, the variable that compromises CPP is an increase in ICP. The treatment of elevated ICP is logically aimed at ma-

TABLE 26.3. *Posttraumatic syndrome: clinical findings*

Headache (mild to excruciating)
Neck stiffness and muscle spasm
Irritability
Forgetfulness
Postural vertigo (dizziness)
Enuresis
Disturbance in sleep patterns
Episodic aggressive behavior
Decline in school performance (impaired concentration)

nipulating the three major tissues that make up the cerebral compartment: brain parenchyma, CSF volume, and blood volume.

In the case of elevated ICP, the brain parenchyma can be manipulated therapeutically by means of osmotic diuretic agents, which dehydrate cells (by removing free water) and thus reduce cerebral volume. Typically, mannitol is used in the range of 0.25 to 1.0 g/kg; the dose is repeated every 6 hours until a serum osmolality of 300 to 310 mOsm (exceeding 320 mOsm is counterproductive) is reached (Table 26.4). Mannitol should be used only in cases where there is impending brain herniation or progressive neurologic deterioration. Diuresis is not recommended in patients without signs of significantly increased ICP. Furosemide can also be used with mannitol. Blood electrolytes must be closely monitored during diuresis to avoid rapid or extreme alterations. When diuresis is used, the blood volume and pressure must be kept up (i.e., euvolumia) to maintain adequate brain perfusion, which is always the end goal. A Foley catheter must be in place.

The CSF volume can be manipulated by placing an external ventricular drain via a ventriculostomy and removing CSF. It can also be adjusted by giving furosemide, which is thought to decrease CSF production by interfering with chloride transport at the choroid plexus level.

Hyperventilation (via endotracheal intubation) can be used to decrease the size of the intracranial blood volume compartment, thereby reducing ICP (Tale 26.4). Respiratory alkalosis produces a reflex vasoconstriction of the cerebral vasculature, reducing the total blood volume. A distinct disadvantage, and one that must be kept in mind, is that the blood volume can be so lowered that adequate perfusion of the brain is compromised, a condition called iatrogenic cerebral ischemia. The recommendations now for hyperventilation are to maintain a tidal volume and respiratory rate that maintain the Pco_2 within 30 to 35 mm Hg. The response of the brain to hyperventilation is rapid, but the effect

TABLE 26.4. *General principles for managing the head-injured*

Mannitol (0.25–1.00 g/kg): serum osmolality of 300–310 mOsm)
Hyperventilation (Pco_2 30–35 mm Hg)
Barbiturates (only in refractory patients that fail other modalities)
Steroids (no longer used)

TABLE 26.5. *ICP levels*

Level	mm Hg
Normal	1–10
Slightly increased	11–20
Moderately increased	21–40
Severely increased	>40

Patients who present with ICP >40 mm Hg have an extremely poor prognosis even with aggressive management.

ceases after 48 to 72 hours, when the kidneys adjust the blood pH to normal levels.

Steroids (glucocorticoids) were once commonly administered to head-injured patients (and unfortunately are still used by some physicians). Several large randomized trials have provided evidence that steroids exert no beneficial effect on morbidity and mortality in head-injured patients, and today steroids are no longer used by major academic centers for their treatment.

Other measures used for management of head injury patients are sedation, muscle paralysis, head elevation, control of systemic hypertension, and hyperglycemia. The use of barbiturates (Table 26.4) is reserved for patients with severe head injury who have become refractory to all other medical and surgical management; its

TABLE 26.6. *Summary of initial evaluation of head injury*

1. Provision for *adequate airway* and ventilation
2. Observations of *vital signs:* evaluate for associated injuries
3. State of *consciousness*
4. *Neurologic* examination
5. GCS evaluation
6. *History* of trauma
   a. Mechanism of injury
   b. Loss of consciousness (immediate? and how long)
   c. Progression of symptoms (lucid interval)
   d. Drug use or other medical history (which might contribute to neurologic findings)
7. Associated *injuries:* cervical spine radiographs (rule out fractures or injury to at least C7)
8. *Prognostic* factors: better outcomes seen with the following:
   a. High GCS score (>13)
   b. Younger age
   c. Good pupillary response to light
   d. Normal intracranial pressure
   e. Brainstem reflexes present
   f. Epidural >> subdural > intraparenchymal injury

aim is to provide cerebral protection by decreasing the cerebral metabolic rate ($CMRO_2$). Once commonly used for head injury, barbiturates are now reserved for patients with severe injury, low Glasgow Coma Scale (GCS) scores, and high ICPs (Table 26.5).

In summary, the initial evaluation of a head injury includes a careful history, physical examination, and a neurologic evaluation. The protocol and prognostic factors are outlined in Table 26.6.

SPINAL CORD INJURY

Epidemiology

Spinal cord injury most commonly affects the young, with the victims mostly male and in their second or third decades. The most common etiology remains vehicular accidents, followed by falls, sporting injuries, and more recently penetrating gunshot injuries. The most common injury site is the mid to low cervical spine. The outcomes of such injuries are evenly divided between quadriplegia and paraplegia. The mortality rate is as high as 40% in quadriplegics.

Definitions

Incomplete Spinal Injury

With an incomplete spinal cord lesion some residual motor or sensory function remains below the level of the lesion. Possible residual findings include sensation or movement of the extremities, voluntary rectal sphincter contraction, or voluntary toe movement. The three types of incomplete lesion include the Brown-Sequard syndrome (cord hemisection), central cord syndrome, and anterior cord syndrome.

Complete Spinal Cord Lesions

A complete spinal cord lesion is one in which no motor or sensory functions are preserved below the lesion. As many as 5% of these patients progress to incomplete lesions, but most recover no function.

Spinal Shock

Often there is confusion between spinal and neurogenic shock. Spinal shock refers to the loss of motor, sensory, and reflex functions below the level of the lesion that occurs immediately following the injury and spontaneously resolves 6 to 16 weeks later. Resolution does not mean improvement of neurologic function, but, rather, a change from a lower motor neuron lesion to an upper motor neuron lesion with concomitant hyperreflexia, hypertonia, and spasticity. By definition, spinal shock is associated with a complete lesion. Neurogenic shock refers to the condition of the patient who presents in a sympathectomized state with bradycardia, hypotension, and hypothermia.

Stability of the Cervical Spine

Cervical spine stability can be understood by dividing the spine into three functional columns or components: an anterior column made up of the anterior longitudinal ligament and anterior half of the vertebral body and disk; a middle column made up of the posterior longitudinal ligament and the posterior half of the vertebral body and disk; and a posterior column composed of the bony arch along with all associated ligaments: ligamentum flavum, supraspinous and interspinous ligaments, facet joints, and capsular ligaments. It is generally considered that a spine is stable if only one column is disrupted and unstable if two or three columns are damaged.

Types of Cervical Spine Injury

Atlantooccipital Dislocation

Atlantooccipital dislocations make up 1% of spinal injuries; they are also known as craniocervical injuries. These injuries can be immediately fatal or present with minimal neurologic deficits. Most fatalities result from anoxia secondary to a low bulbar/high cervical injury that affects the respiratory center.

Atlas (C1) Fractures

Also known as Jefferson fractures (Fig. 26.8), atlas (C1) injuries comprise about 15% of cervical fractures. The ring of C1 is broken in at least two places, with the mechanism of injury most commonly axial loading. Because of the large size of the spinal canal at this level, these patients rarely present with neurologic deficits. The anteroposterior (AP) "open-mouth" view shows lateral displacement of the lateral masses of C1.

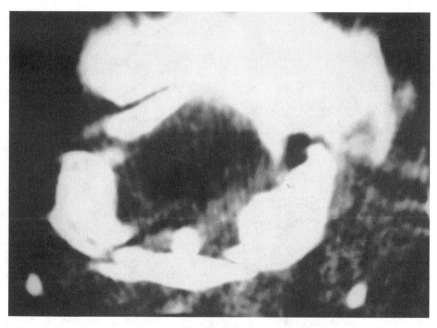

FIG. 26.8. Axial CT scan of the C1 showing a burst fracture (Jefferson fracture) that occurred during a motor vehicle accident where the patient was thrown into the windowshield. There are multiple fractures in the ring of C1 (i.e., a burst fracture).

Axis (C2) Fractures

Hangman's Fracture

The hangman's fracture is through the pedicles of C2 (Fig. 26.9) at the pars interarticularis. The usual mechanism of injury is hyperextension. As with C1 fractures, neurologic deficits are rare. It is diagnosed with plain films or CT scans.

Odontoid Fractures

Fractures through the body or the dens of C2 (Fig. 26.10) are classified as type I, II, or III odontoid fractures (Table 26.7). These injuries are usually caused by hyperflexion with resultant displacement of C1 on C2. Most patients have no neurologic deficit but complain of neck pain.

Subaxial Fractures

Several fracture patterns affect the cervical spine. The most commonly affected area is the C5–6 level, as it has the greatest mobility in the cervical spine. Injuries include burst fractures, teardrop fractures, subluxations, locked (or jumped) facets, and fractures of spinal processes (spinous or transverse). Cervical spine stability can be assessed by the use of dynamic spinal films (flexion-extension) and by looking for movement between the vertebral bodies (Fig. 26.11). Lower cervical injuries are associated with a higher rate of neurologic damage because the spinal cord/spinal canal ratio is less than that at higher cervical levels.

Management

Field Management

1. Immobilization of any patient suspected of having a spinal cord injury is imperative. It may be accomplished with the use of a hard collar (Philadelphia) or sandbags.
2. Systemic blood pressure must be maintained to prevent further injury secondary to ischemia. Pressors and intravenous fluids are used as necessary.

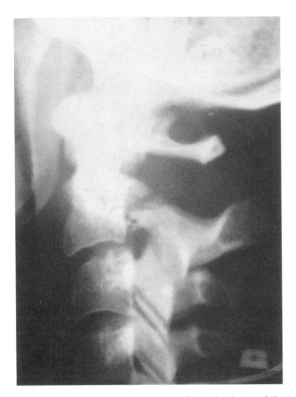

FIG. 26.9. Lateral spine radiograph from the base of the skull to C4. A hangman's fracture of C2 can be seen. The clues here are the widened interspinous distance between C1 and C2, and a fracture that can be seen in the lamina of C2 with downward disarticulation of the C2 lamina.

3. Adequate oxygenation must be maintained. (If intubation is necessary, caution is taken not to hyperextend the neck.)

Hospital Management

1. Immobilization is continued.
2. A thorough neurologic examination is performed.
3. A nasogastric tube is inserted to decompress the stomach and prevent functional ileus.
4. A Foley catheter is placed.
5. Steroids are given.

A recent prospective trial with assessment at 6 weeks and 6 months found methylprednisolone to be beneficial for both complete and incomplete cord injuries. The medication must be administered within 8 hours of injury to be effective. The drug is given at 30 mg/kg i.v. bolus followed by a continuous infusion of 5.4 mg/kg/hr for 23 hours.

Atlantooccipital dislocation is treated by means of stabilization and surgical fusion. Monitoring for apnea during the first 48 hours is also considered. Treatment of Jefferson fractures and C2 fractures requires halo immobilization for 8 to 16 weeks. The outcome is excellent in most cases. Depending on the level and type of fracture, unstable fractures may be treated with skeletal traction (e.g., Gardner-Well tongs) or weights, halo immobilization, or surgical fusion (e.g., plates, screws, or wiring).

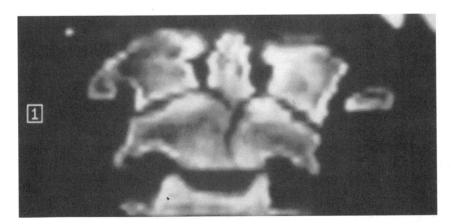

FIG. 26.10. CT reconstruction of a type III odontoid fracture. There is a fracture through the base of the dens extending into the body of C2.

TABLE 26.7. *Odontoid fractures*

Type	Location	Stability	Treatment
I	Tip of the dens	Stable	Rarely required
II	Through base of the dens	Unstable	Surgical fusion
III	Extending through body of C2	Stable	Halo immobilization

Decompressive surgery is reserved for patients with incomplete injuries who demonstrate external compression and those who, after reduction and alignment, still show (a) progression of neurologic deficits, (b) complete block by myelogram, (c) presence of bony fragments or soft tissue/hematomas in the canal, causing cord compression, or (d) compound fractures or penetrating trauma.

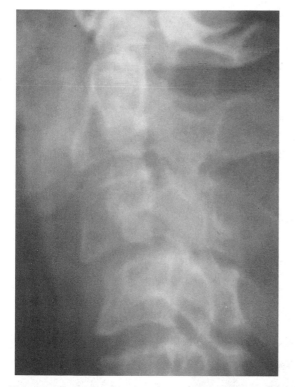

FIG. 26.11. Subtle but obvious subluxation fracture of C3 on C4. The diagnostic clue here is the lack of alignment of the edges of C3 on C4. Flexion/extension views would most likely show this malalignment even more dramatically.

Contraindications to surgical treatment include presentation with complete spinal cord injury after 24 hours, medical instability, and central cord syndrome. Patients should be studied with plain films, CT scans, and MRI.

BRAIN TUMORS

Epidemiology

In almost 25% of all patients with cancer the brain and its coverings are affected at some time in the clinical course. The average mortality ranges between 6/100,000 and 8/100,000 per year in the United States. Analysis of mortality rates for primary brain neoplasms indicates that the age-specific curve rises to a maximum during the seventh and eighth decades. The overall age-adjusted mortality rate is higher for men and for Whites.

Classification

Historically, classification of brain tumors has been based on their histologic features. A classification based on the embryonic origins of neural tissues is presented in Table 26.8. Table 26.9 shows the approximate incidence of each type of tumor.

Clinical Presentation

The clinical findings associated with brain tumors reflect their anatomic location and effect on function. A progressive neurologic deficit is the most common presentation (68%) of brain tumors. Such a deficit may be caused by any of several mechanisms: (a) direct compression of neural tissue; (b) direct destruction or invasion by tumor cells; or (c) alteration of normal regional blood supply by the tumor. Other common clinical findings include headaches (54%), seizures (26%), and mo-

TABLE 26.8. *Classification of brain tumors*

Origin	Tumor
Neural tube derivatives	
Glial cells	
Astrocytes	Astrocytoma
	Glioblastoma multiforme
Oligodendrocytes	Oligodendroglioma
Ependymocytes	Ependymomas
	Choroid plexus
	papilloma/carcinoma
Neurons	Medulloblastoma (PNET)
	Ganglioma
	Ganglioglioma
Neural crest derivatives	
Schwan cells	Schwanoma (acoustic
	neuroma)
	Neurofibroma
Arachnoid cell	Meningioma
Melanocyte	Primary CNS melanoma
Other cells	
Adenohypophyseal cells	Pituitary adenoma
Vascular cells	Hemangioblastomas
Notochord	Chordoma
Adipose cell	Lipoma
Germ cell	Germinoma
Other	Craniopharyngioma
	Teratoma

tor weakness (45%). Typically, signs and symptoms of progressive and generalized increased ICP are detected: decreased or cloudy mentation and consciousness, papilledema, vomiting, and Cushing's triad or phenomenon (bradycardia, systemic hypertension, and irregular

TABLE 26.9. *Frequency distribution of brain tumors in adults and children*

Tumor	%
Adults	
Glioblastoma	52.0
Meningioma	18.0
Astrocytoma	10.0
Pituitary adenoma	7.0
Neurolemoma	1.5
Medulloblastoma	1.3
Ependymoma	1.3
Children	
Medulloblastoma/astrocytoma	24.0
Brain stem	9.0
Glioblastoma	20.0
Ependymoma	8.0
Craniopharyngioma	5.6
Meningioma	1.5
Pinealoma	2.0

respirations). Increased ICP may result from an increase in tumor size or from hydrocephalus secondary to blockage of CSF circulation pathways. Cerebral edema (of the vasogenic type), associated with many brain tumors, is also a common cause of increased ICP (Fig. 26.12).

Whereas the clinical presentation of supratentorial tumors holds to the pattern described above, the presentation of infratentorial tumors varies in that seizures are rare. Most posterior fossa tumors present with signs and symptoms of increased ICP, headache, nausea, vomiting, ataxia, vertigo, diplopia, and lower cranial nerve (VII, VIII, IX, X, XII) deficits. These findings are caused by compression of the pons and medulla and their respective cranial nerves (Fig. 26.13).

Diagnosis

The state of the art method for brain tumor diagnosis is MRI, usually with contrast (gadolinium) enhance-

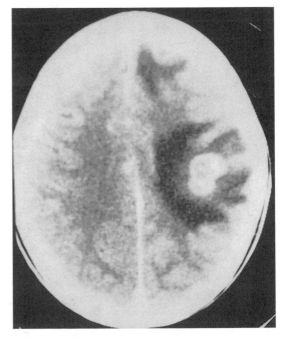

FIG. 26.12. Axial CT scan of an intraaxial brain tumor with contrast enhancement and surrounding edema. There is a hint of edema in the anterior pole of the frontal lobe, suggesting a second lesion, most likely metastatic tumors.

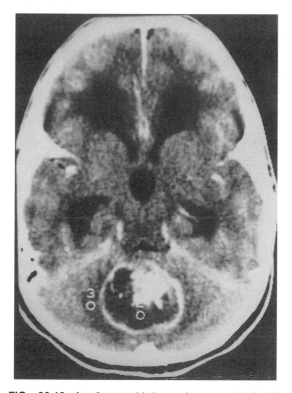

FIG. 26.13. An 8-year-old boy who presented with ataxia, severe headaches, and VI nerve palsy. This CT scan shows a ring enhancing mass in the posterior fossa with a cystic component and a tumor nodule that brightly enhances. The ventricles are dilated, causing hydrocephalus secondary to the fourth ventricle being occluded. At surgery it was found to be a medulloblastoma.

ment. CT scanning is also valuable, especially for assessing bony involvement and planning the surgical approach. Cerebral angiography has become less important, but it continues to provide information that is critically important in relation to surgical decision making. Ventriculography, brain scanning, and pneumoencephalography no longer play a role in diagnosis. Depending on tumor location and histologic makeup, serum endocrine levels [prolactin, growth hormone, cortisol, luteinizing hormone (LH), follicle-stimulating hormone (FSH), triiodothyronine (T_3), and thyroxine (T_4)] and tumor markers [human β-chorionic gonadotropin (βhCG), carcinoembryonic antigen (CEA), and α-fetoprotein (AFP)] may be measured to aid in diagnosis.

Management: Clinical Classification and Treatment

Astrocytoma

Astrocytomas are the most common primary intraaxial brain tumor, presenting in about 12,000 cases per year in the United States. Various classifications have been proposed for grading astrocytomas. The Kernohan system divides astrocytomas into grades I to IV, based on histologic findings, with grade I being the most benign and grade IV the most malignant. At present a three-category system is most frequently used: low-grade astrocytoma (Kernohan grades I and II), anaplastic astrocytoma (Kernohan grade III), and glioblastoma multiforme (Kernohan grade IV). This classification is based on the degree of anaplasia, cellular pleomorphism, number of mitoses, neovascularity, and necrosis (Fig. 26.14).

For certain types of astrocytoma (childhood cystic cerebellar astrocytoma and pilocystic astrocytoma), surgery is the principal mode of treatment, with gross

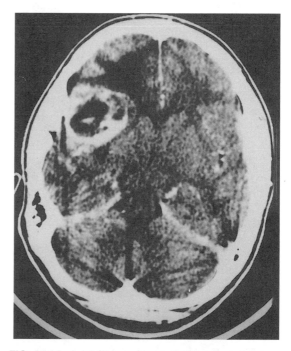

FIG. 26.14. Axial CT scan demonstrating a contrast-enhancing lesion in the right temporal lobe with surrounding edema, shift, and obliteration of the ventricle. At surgery it proved to be an anaplastic astrocytoma.

total surgical resection ideal. For most other astrocytomas surgery is only part of the treatment: Radiation therapy and chemotherapy are also administered. Glioblastomas have the worse prognosis, with a 1-year survival of 30% compared to 60% for anaplastic astrocytomas. The 5-year survival rate of patients with malignant astrocytomas remains at less than 5%.

Meningioma

Meningiomas account for 15% to 20% of primary intracranial tumors, with a peak incidence at 45 years and a female/male ratio of 2:1. Approximately 25% of adolescent patients with neurofibromatosis also develop meningiomas. These tumors are slow-growing and arise from arachnoid cells. They are parasagittal in 20%, in the convexity in 15%, in the sphenoid bone in 30%, and in the falx in 10% (Fig. 26.15). Commonly associated with meningiomas is an overlying hyperostosis of the

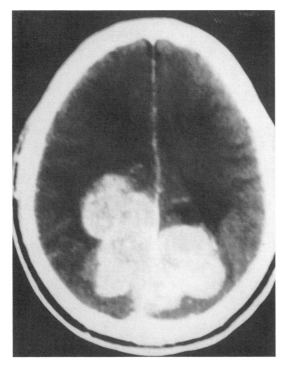

FIG. 26.15. A 55-year-old man presented with visual loss and severe headaches. A large parafalcine meningioma is evident on this contrast-enhanced CT scan.

bone. These tumors are extraaxial and with rare exception (i.e., those with sarcomatous changes) are histologically benign.

The extent of surgical removal is the most important factor in determining long-term outcome; complete excision implies cure, but it is not always possible. Incompletely resected tumors are reported to recur at rates of 37% to 85%. However, the 5-year survival rate for patients with meningioma is high, with 90% to 92% typically reported, indicating an excellent prognosis. Irradiation may be used as an adjunctive treatment for incompletely resected meningioma.

PITUITARY TUMORS

As with other CNS tumors, a number of classifications have been used to systematize pituitary tumors. Light-microscopic classification divides them into acidolphils [prolactin, growth hormone, or thyroid-stimulating hormone (TSH) producers], basophils (ACTH, LH, FSH producers), and chromophobes (typically nonsecreters). Pituitary tumors can be separated into functional (secreting) and nonfunctional tumors. More specifically, they can be categorized according to the hormone they produce (e.g., prolactinomas). Their clinical presentation is either as an endocrinologic disturbance (e.g., Cushing's disease) or a mass effect (e.g., visual field deficits).

Clinical Presentation

Cushing Syndrome

Cushing syndrome is caused by hypercortisolism due to excessive ACTH production. Patients typically have centripetal obesity, moon facies, hirsutism, buffalo hump, striae, hypertension, and diabetes mellitus. The diagnosis is normally based on a positive dexamethasone suppression test and appropriately elevated hormones.

Acromegaly

Acromegaly results from hyperproduction of growth hormone. The patient presents with increased hand or foot size, frontal bossing, prognathism, macroglossia, hypertension, carpal tunnel syndrome, and soft tissue swelling.

Pituitary Apoplexy

Pituitary apoplexy refers to the abrupt onset of neurologic deterioration, usually associated with headaches, visual deterioration or loss, ophthalmoplegia, and decreased mental status. It is caused by an abrupt hemorrhage within the tumor or by necrosis of the tumor with swelling.

Progressive Visual Loss

With a pituitary tumor, progressive visual loss is caused by a mass effect of a tumor that extends above the sella to encroach on the optic chiasm. The most common visual loss is progressive bitemporal hemianopsia resulting from compression of the medial retinal fibers in the chiasm. This finding is easily demonstrated with a gross (finger-based) visual fields examination.

Treatment

Secreting pituitary tumors can be treated pharmacologically using dopamine agonists (bromocriptine), somatostatin analogs (octreotide), serotonin antagonists, and antiinflammatory drugs (dexamethasone). Surgical treatment is indicated for Cushing's disease, prolactinomas (prolactin level over 500 ng/mL), acromegaly, large tumors causing mass effect, and pituitary apoplexy. Radiation therapy is not routinely recommended postoperatively. Patients should be followed yearly; and if after reoperation a recurrence cannot be resected and the tumor continues to grow, radiation therapy is indicated.

CONGENITAL MALFORMATIONS

Hydrocephalus

Cerebrospinal fluid is normally produced in the adult at a rate of 500 mL per day. If resorption or flow is blocked, hydrocephalus results. Its estimated prevalence is 1.5% with an incidence of 2/1000 live births. Hydrocephalus is classified as communicating (malabsorption of CSF at the arachnoid villi) or noncommunicating (blockage of CSF circulation proximal to the arachnoid granulations). The etiologies of hydrocephalus include congenital conditions such as stenosis of the aqueduct (38%), Chiari II malformation/myelomeningocele (29%), and Dandy-Walker malformation. Acquired conditions such as meningitis, intraventricular hemorrhage (e.g., bleeding from an aneurysm), intraventricular hemorrhage (IVH) due to prematurity, or tumors blocking normal CSF pathways can also cause hydrocephalus.

For the most part, hydrocephalus is a surgical condition, although in certain situations patients with hydrocephalus can be managed medically until normal CSF resorption resumes. For this purpose the carbonic anhydrase inhibitor acetazolamide is used. Multiple spinal taps are performed routinely in infants with posthemorrhagic hydrocephalus with significant success in that the patients do not go on to require shunting. Nevertheless, for most types of hydrocephalus, a ventricular shunt to the peritoneum, cardiac atrium, or pleural cavity is regularly constructed. Ventriculoperitoneal shunting is the preferred mode of shunting. If hydrocephalus is caused by tumor blocking CSF pathways, tumor removal to allow normal circulation usually results in resolution of the symptoms.

Spina Bifida

Spina bifida occulta is defined as congenital absence of the spinal vertebral elements (spinous process and lamina). The defect is covered with normal skin and often presents as an incidental finding on radiographs. Spina bifida occulta occurs in approximately 20% to 30% of the U.S. population. Spina bifida aperta refers to the condition in which, in addition to maldevelopment of the vertebral element, the overlying skin and subcutaneous tissue fail to close, exposing the underlying neural elements.

Meningocele

Meningocele refers to a skin- or membrane-covered cystic midline mass that is typically found in the lumbodorsal region in 10% of patients with spina bifida. The dorsal halves of the vertebrae are missing at one or several levels. The contents of the sac comprise CSF and meninges; no neural elements are present. The prognosis and results are excellent after surgical treatment.

Myelomeningocele

Myelomeningocele represents the most common form of neural tube defect, with an incidence of 2/1,000 to 3/1,000 live births (Figs. 26.16, 26.17). Recent recommendations regarding the nutritional importance of folic acid during pregnancy may help reduce the incidence substantially. This condition represents failure of the posterior neuropore to close. The clinical findings vary with the level of the lesion. The most severe and debilitating forms are myelomeningoceles at the thoracic level; the least severe are located at the low lumbar and sacral levels.

The neurologic examination discloses sensory and motor changes below the level of the lesion. Varying degrees of anesthesia, weakness, or paralysis of the

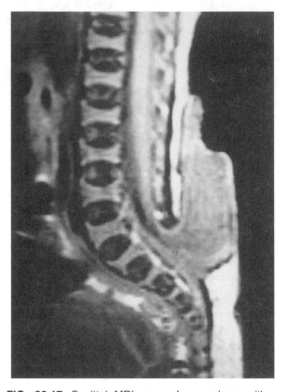

FIG. 26.17. Sagittal MRI scan of a newborn with a myelomeningocele. The cord can be seen coming down to and out of the myelomeningocele defect. A large, patent fluid-filled sac can be seen at the lumbosacral junction.

lower extremities are common, as are urinary and fecal incontinence and orthopedic abnormalities (clubfoot, scoliosis, hip dislocation). The coincidence of hydrocephalus with spina bifida is high, ranging from 75% to 90%. Treatment involves surgical closure of the defect with a lifetime of follow-up care to deal with multiple problems regarding ambulation, bladder care, orthopedic problems, and so on.

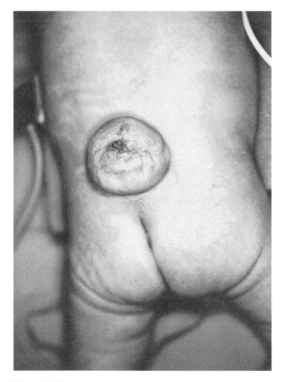

FIG. 26.16. Newborn with a large lumbosacral myelomeningocele. The skin is stretched and dilated, with the neuroplacode seen in the center under a thin, diaphragm-like skin covering.

Encephalocele

Encephaloceles make up a group of congenital anomalies that produce varying degrees of protrusion of neural tissue through a cranial bone defect. The pathogenesis reflects failure of the anterior neuropore to close and fuse on about the 25th day of gestation. In the United States the most common location is the occipital area, but other locations include the frontal, parietal, and frontal bones. Frontoethmoidal and basal encephaloceles are found less often.

The clinical presentation of an encephalocele is a bulging lesion in any of the aforementioned locations that may be apparent at birth. Lesions at the anterior cranial base rarely offer evidence of their presence at birth but, rather, do so later in life by obstructing airway passages or by the development of hypertelorism.

Treatment consists in surgical removal and closure. The prognosis depends on the size of the lesion (i.e., amount of brain involved) and its location. Posterior encephaloceles, those that occur in the posterior fossa and occipital region, have a high incidence of associated hydrocephalus, ranging from 30% to 60%.

Dermal Sinus Tract

The dermal sinus tract typically begins at the skin surface and communicates internally with the subarach-noid space. It is lined with epithelium or sometimes with sebaceous and hair material. The lesion is most commonly found at either end of the neural tube, along the midline. The two most frequent locations are the nasion and the lumbosacral region. Although innocent in appearance, its potential for producing meningitis is high; indeed, such tracts should never be probed or injected with contrast, as it may precipitate the infection. The lesion can be confused with the pylonidal sinus tract; but because the latter lesion does not communicate with the subarachnoid space, it does not cause meningitis.

Treatment requires complete removal. The lesion must be followed intrathecally and the associated dermoid lesion removed.

VASCULAR DISORDERS

Cerebral Aneurysms

As in any other part of the body, an aneurysm of a cerebral vessel represents a weakening of the vessel

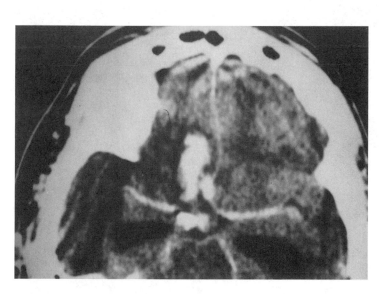

FIG. 26.18. Axial CT scan of a 37-year-old woman who suddenly developed the "worst headache of my life" and rapidly became obtunded. This CT scan shows an acute hemorrhage in the region of the circle of Willis with fresh blood layering out over the middle cerebral arteries and the parasellar area. An angiogram demonstrated a large anterior communicating artery aneurysm (see Fig. 26.19).

wall leading to dilatation and possible rupture. The most common site is at an arterial bifurcation. In the United States approximately 28,000 cerebral aneurysms rupture per year and are associated with high morbidity and mortality rates. About 90% to 95% of cerebral aneurysms are located in the carotid system and 5% to 15% in the vertebrobasilar system. The etiology may be congenital (berry aneurysms), atherosclerotic, embolic, infectious, or associated with other medical conditions such as polycystic kidney disease, fibromuscular dysplasia, connective tissue disease, coarctation of the aorta, and the like. Aneurysms most commonly present with a subarachnoid hemorrhage and a severe, explosive headache (commonly described as the "worst headache of my life") along with photophobia and meningismus. It is diagnosed by lumbar puncture (presence of fresh blood), CT scan (subarachnoid bleeding), MRI, and angiography (Figs. 26.18, 26.19). Surgical treatment includes isolating the neck of the aneurysm and applying a surgical spring clip. Some cases may be treated with balloon occlusion via an endovascular approach.

Arteriovenous Malformations

Arteriovenous malformations form as a result of failed development of a capillary bed between the arterial and venous circulations. Their presentation is most commonly due to hemorrhage (e.g., subarachnoid hemorrhage) or a intracerebral clot and associated neurologic deficit. Seizures are not uncommon and are thought to be due to chronic ischemia caused by blood flow "steal."

Treatment involves evacuation of the clot (if present) and surgical excision, if possible. Endovascular obliteration of small lesions is sometimes possible, but most require surgical treatment.

INFECTIONS

Brain Abscess

Brain abscesses are loculated infections found intraparenchymally. They are approximately twice as common in men. At present, acquired immunodefi-

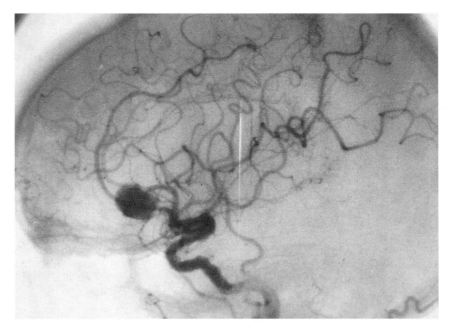

FIG. 26.19. Angiogram obtained from the patient in Fig. 26.18 shows a large bulbous contrast-containing aneurysmal structure at the point of the anterior communicating artery.

ciency syndrome (AIDS) has become the most significant factor in the development of a brain abscess. The clinical presentation is nonspecific and mostly related to the increase ICP (headaches, nausea, vomiting, lethargy). *Streptococcus* is the most frequent pathogen (30% to 50%). Multiple organisms can be cultured up to 80% of the time and typically include anaerobes. In AIDS patients *Toxoplasma* is the most common cause of brain abscess. Pathophysiologic mechanisms include (a) hematogenous spread [lung abscess, cyanotic and congenital heart disease (left-to-right shunt)], pulmonary arteriovenous fistulas, endocarditis, empyema, and bronchiectasis; (b) contiguous spread from nearby infected sinuses; (c) dental extractions; and (d) introduction of organisms as a sequela to penetrating cranial trauma or neurosurgical procedures.

Treatment depends on the age of the abscess. Early in the infection (less than 2 weeks) and in the cerebritis stage, antibiotics alone may be used. If there are signs of elevated ICP, neurologic findings, or the abscess is close to the ventricles (an ominous sign because of the possibility of rupture), surgical evacuation is the treatment of choice in conjunction with intravenous antibiotics for 6 to 8 weeks.

Subdural Empyema

The subdural empyema is an extremely serious infection of the CNS. The infection forms in a preexisting space whose lack of barriers allows easy spread. Such a space permits only poor penetration of antibiotics. The subdural empyema is seen in the subdural space, not within the brain substance, as seen with an abscess. The subdural empyema commonly starts within the paranasal sinuses (60% to 75%) or from a site of otitis (15%). Patients present with fever (more than 90%), focal neurologic deficits (80% to 90%), meningismus (80%), headaches, and seizures. The severe inflammatory reaction with resulting thrombophlebitis of cerebral veins causes high morbidity and mortality.

Subdural empyema is a neurosurgical emergency, and surgical evacuation with irrigation is the treatment of choice, along with antibiotics. Once neurologic deficits occur, their reversal is rare, and a mortality rate of 20% is found even today.

Spinal Epidural Abscess

The spinal epidural abscess is an infection localized to the spinal canal, found in the epidural space; it occurs with an incidence of 1/10,000 hospital admissions. The thoracic level is the most common location, followed by lumbar and cervical levels. Hematogenous spread accounts for up to 50% of cases. Foci of infections include the skin, abdominal contents, endocardium, urinary tract, lower respiratory tract, and pharynx or oral cavity. Another mechanism is local extension of infections such as decubitus ulcers, psoas abscesses, abdominal wounds, mediastinitis, and pharyngitis.

Patients with a history of diabetes, intravenous drug use, or AIDS are at high risk. *Staphylococcus aureus* is cultured in more than 50% of cases. The patients typically present with severe back pain over the involved segments, bowel and bladder dysfunction, motor weakness, sensory changes, and abdominal distension.

Treatment consists in surgical evacuation with intravenous antibiotics. Patients with marked neurologic deficits rarely improve.

QUESTIONS

Select one answer.

1. The lesion most likely to cause neurologic injury and permanent sequelae is:
   a. Basilar skull fracture.
   b. Subdural hematoma.
   c. Epidural hematoma.
   d. Subarachnoid hemorrhage.
2. Subdural hygromas:
   a. Are common following head injury.
   b. Are made up of a blood collection.
   c. Show as hyperdense lesions in a CT scan.
   d. Are treated with burr holes and twist drills.
3. A complete spinal cord lesion is seen in which of the following?
   a. Anterior spinal syndrome.
   b. Central cord syndrome.
   c. Brown-Sequard syndrome.
   d. Spinal shock.
4. Jefferson fracture is a fracture of the:
   a. Odontoid process.
   b. Ring of C1.

c. Pedicle of C2.

d. Pars interarticularis of C3.

5. Which of the following is the most common brain tumor in an adult?

   a. Ependymoma.

   b. Low-grade astrocytoma.

   c. Glioblastoma multiforme.

   d. Pituitary adenomas.

6. Cushing's disease is associated with an increase of which of the following hormones?

   a. Somatostatin.

   b. ACTH.

   c. TSH.

   d. GnRH.

7. Hangman's fracture refers to a fracture of which of the following?

   a. Odontoid process.

   b. Ring of C1.

   c. Pedicle of C2.

   d. Pars interarticularis of C3.

8. Which of the following is the most common type of myelodysplasia?

   a. Encephalocele.

   b. Dermal sinus tracts.

   c. Myelomeningocele.

   d. Meningocele.

Indicate whether each statement is true or false.

9. Neurogenic shock and spinal shock are the same clinical entity.

10. Tachycardia is associated with Cushing's phenomenon.

11. Meningiomas are usually benign tumors.

12. Subdural empyemas can be treated expectantly.

13. Type III odontoid fractures should be treated with surgical fusion.

14. Chronic subdural hematomas are usually treated with craniotomy and evacuation.

15. Subarachnoid hemorrhage is the most common form of hemorrhage following head injury.

SELECTED REFERENCES

Bracken MB, Shepard MJ, Collins WF. A randomized, controlled trial of methylprednisolone or naloxone in the treatment of acute spinal cord injury. *N Engl J Med* 1990;322: 1405–1411.

Burger PC. Classification and biology of brain tumors. In: Youmans JR, ed. *Neurological surgery.* Philadelphia: WB Saunders, 1990;2967–2999.

Dwan PS, Becker DP. Closed head injury: management dilemmas. In: Long DM, ed. *Current therapy in neurological surgery-2.* Toronto: BC Decker, 1989;173–175.

French BN. Abnormal development of the central nervous system. In: McLauren RL, Venes JL, eds. *Pediatric neurosurgery.* Philadelphia: WB Saunders, 1989;9–34.

Marmarou A, Tabaddor K. Intracranial pressure: physiology and pathophysiology. In: Cooper RR, ed. *Head injury.* Baltimore: Williams & Wilkins, 1982;115–128.

Okazaki H. *Fundamentals of neuropathology,* 2nd ed. New York: Igaku-Shoin, 1989;95–114.

Plum F, Posner JB. *The diagnosis of stupor and coma,* 3rd ed. Philadelphia: FA Davis, 1986;153–176.

Ramsey RG. *Neuroradiology,* 2nd ed. Philadelphia: WB Saunders, 1987;103–129.

Schoenberg BS. *Neurobiology of brain tumors.* Baltimore: Williams and Wilkins, 1991;3–18.

Young W, Ransohoff J. Injuries to the cervical cord. In: The Cervical Spine Society Editorial Committee, ed. *The cervical spine.* Philadelphia, JB Lippincott, 1989;464–525.

27

Anesthesia

Elizabeth A.M. Frost and Mosses Bairamian

Advances in anesthetic techniques and monitoring, the development of new drugs, and better perioperative preparation have ensured that many more and complicated procedures may be safely performed on very ill patients. In contrast to 100 years ago, when approximately 25% of patients who received chloroform anesthesia suffered severe, often fatal cardiac dysrhythmias, mortality due to anesthesia may now be as low as 1/500,000 procedures. Analysis of anesthesia administered at the Harvard group of hospitals to more than 300,000 relatively healthy individuals after the introduction of safety monitoring standards (see below) in 1985 showed no major intraoperative injury from anesthesia. Also, The American Society of Anesthesiologists (ASA) closed-claims database, which analyzes insurance companies' malpractice suits against anesthesiologists, points out that the severity of anesthesia-related injuries is decreasing, substantiating the safety of anesthetic practice in the United States. Nearly all mishaps (technical or due to errors in judgment) can be identified through monitoring early enough to prevent most major patient injuries.

Complications do arise, however, from interactions among anesthetic drugs, underlying disease, and surgical intervention. The most common problems include misplaced endotracheal tubes, pulmonary aspiration, hypotension, cardiac dysrhythmias, drug interaction, adverse drug effects, and machine failure. Improved pre-

anesthetic preparation, discussion with the patient and family, and close communication with the surgical team can reduce mortality and morbidity to close to zero.

PREANESTHETIC CARE

The most important aspects of preanesthetic evaluation are listed in Table 27.1.

Previous Anesthetic Experiences and Family History

Any previous complications associated with anesthesia must be determined. Such problems and possible solutions might include the following.

1. Difficult intubation, previous tracheostomy. Regional anesthesia might be preferable. In 1993 the ASA developed guidelines for practical management of the difficult airway. Awareness of these guidelines further increases safety (Table 27.2, Fig. 27.1).
2. Prolonged nausea or vomiting postoperatively (PONV). Factors that increase the incidence of PONV include young age, absence of preexisting medical conditions, female gender, site of surgery (laparoscopic gynecologic procedures, ear and eye procedures), and history of motion sickness. Nitrous oxide

TABLE 27.1. *Areas to explore during preparation of a patient for anesthesia and surgery*

Previous anesthetic experiences
Medical assessment
Medications
Personal habits
Physical examination
Laboratory data
Family history

and narcotics should be avoided and propofol used. A nasogastric tube should be passed at the conclusion of surgery to empty the stomach. Antiemetic drugs, such as ondansetron (Zofran), droperidol, and promethazine are useful prophylactically.

3. Allergic drug reaction. The causative agent should be identified and alternative drugs or techniques sought.
4. Delayed return to consciousness. Long-acting drugs such as diazepam and lorazepam are avoided, especially in older patients; and drug dosages are reduced.
5. Organotoxicity (e.g., hepatitis associated with halothane, renal dysfunction after methoxyflurane, hallucinations or delirium after ketamine). Anesthetic technique should be modified or other agents used.

A family history of anesthetic difficulties is sought. A history of unexplained, unexpected anesthetic death in family members, particularly if fever was noted, raises the suspicion of malignant hyperthermia (MH) susceptibility. MH is a genetically determined muscle disease.

TABLE 27.2. *Difficult airway algorithm*

1. Assess the likelihood and clinical impact of basic management problems
   a. Difficult intubation
   b. Difficult ventilation
   c. Difficulty with patient cooperation or consent
2. Consider the relative merits and feasibility of basic management choices
   a. Nonsurgical technique for initial approach to intubation vs. surgical technique for initial approach to intubation
   b. Awake intubation vs. intubation attempts after induction of general anesthesia
   c. Preservation of spontaneous ventilation vs. ablation of spontaneous ventilation
3. Develop primary and alternative strategies

In humans the mode of transmission appears to be an autosomal dominant trait. A specific pair basechange in the gene that encodes the ryanodine receptor of hormone-sensitive lipase has been identified. This receptor represents the calcium channel of the sarcoplasmic reticulum of muscle that controls calcium release, initiating muscle contraction. The gene raised the hope for a simple DNA-based diagnostic test. Subsequent studies, however, have shown that the other encoding proteins may also be responsible for MH, conferring heterogeneous genetic character.

The syndrome is often undiagnosed until the susceptible patient is exposed to a "triggering" agent such as volatile anesthetic agents, succinylcholine, or stress. The incidence of MH is 1:3,000 to 1:15,000 in pediatric patients and 1:50,000 to 1:100,000 in the general population. The clinical picture is one of poor relaxation, tachypnea, tachycardia, ventricular ectopy, cyanosis, hyperthermia, acidosis, hyperkalemia, myoglobinuria, and cardiovascular collapse. Late complications include disseminated intravascular coagulation, renal failure, muscle swelling with entrapment syndromes, and coma. The etiology is associated with abnormal elevation of intracellular calcium. Patients with MH frequently have other evidence of muscle disease, such as ptosis, hernia, scoliosis, and muscle cramps. They avoid coffee and caffeinated beverages (Coca Cola), which cause muscle weakness. Plasma creatine phosphokinase (CPK) is elevated in about 70% of MH patients. If the syndrome is suspected, a neurologic consult should be sought or referral to an MH center made. Muscle biopsy may be indicated.

The best diagnostic test to date is the halothane–caffeine contracture test. The test involves removal of 1 to 2 g of muscle and testing for contracture response to halothane and caffeine. In MH-positive cases, contracture in response to halothane and a left-shifted dose response to caffeine are demonstrated. The test is available in only a few centers in the United States and is time-consuming and expensive. Rather than delay surgery for diagnostic testing, patients should be treated as MH-susceptible and nontriggering agents used.

Other diagnostic tests that are less specific include calcium uptake, calcium ATPase test, platelet ATP depletion, calcium release from lymphocytes, and the myophosphenylase test. Elevated CPK levels are more diagnostic if familial increases are also demonstrated.

If elective surgery is planned, regional anesthesia is recommended, although no technique is considered

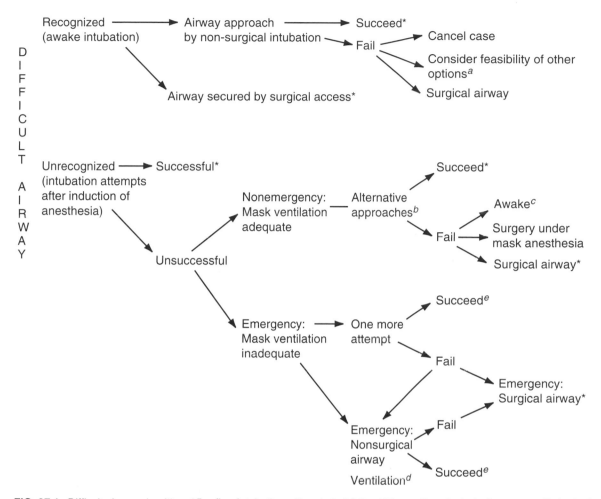

FIG. 27.1. Difficult airway algorithm. *Confirm intubation with exhaled CO_2. [a]Other options include (but are not limited to) surgery under mask anesthesia, surgery under local anesthesia infiltration or regional nerve blockade, or intubation attempts after induction of general anesthesia. [b]Alternative approaches to difficult intubation include (but are not limited to) use of different laryngoscope blades, awake intubation, blind oral or nasal intubation, fiberoptic intubation, intubating stylet or tube changer, light wand, retrograde intubation, and surgical airway access. [c]See awake intubation. [d]Options for emergency nonsurgical airway ventilation include (but are not limited to) transtracheal jet ventilation, laryngeal mask ventilation, or esophageal-tracheal combination tube ventilation. [e]Options for establishing a definitive airway include (but are not limited to returning to the awake state with spontaneous ventilation, tracheotomy, or endotracheal intubation.

completely safe. Prophylactic dantrolene is rarely used. The intravenous preparation 2.5 mg/kg is given over 30 minutes preoperatively. Outpatient care with oral dantrolene is not recommended because of the side effects of muscle relaxation, nausea, and dizziness.

"Safe" drugs for the MH patient include barbiturates, benzodiazepines, narcotics, rocuronium, vecuronium, pancuronium, mivacurim, atracurium, *cis*-atracurium, propofol, ketamine, and probably nitrous oxide. Calcium salts, digitalis, and catecholamines are also safe. Drugs to be avoided include succinylcholine, isoflurane, halothane, enflurane, desflurane, and sevoflurane.

Intraoperative therapy for an MH response includes discontinuing all triggering agents, hyperventilation, correction of acidosis, cooling the patient, and administration of dantrolene 2.5 mg/kg i.v. The patient should be monitored in the intensive care unit (ICU) for several days and dantrolene kept available, as recrudescence is likely.

The neurolept malignant syndrome may be related to MH. It is characterized by fever, muscle destruction, acidosis, and death. It is precipitated by haloperidol and phenothiazines. The syndrome responds to dantrolene and bromocriptine (a dopamine agonist). Autonomic disorders such as occur in Riley-Day or Shy-Drager syndromes should be identified because severe hypotension may be induced by anesthetic agents in these patients.

Sodium pentobarbital given intravenously may cause sudden, severe demyelination in patients with the porphyrias. The presence of atypical pseudocholinesterase is a rare inherited condition. Succinylcholine and mivacurium (nondepolarizing, short-acting muscle relaxants) are broken down slowly, and prolonged neuromuscular paralysis occurs.

Patients may express specific concerns about losing control of consciousness or awakening intraoperatively. Reassurance and, if appropriate, use of local or regional anesthetic techniques are indicated. Intraoperative awareness is less likely with inhalation techniques, combined with a short-acting benzodiazepine (midazolam) or propofol (Diprivan) due to the amnestic properties of the latter. An awareness monitor is available (Aspect, Boston, MA). Patients may be advised that cerebral activity can be noninvasively monitored continually and anesthetic dosages adjusted to ensure adequate depth of unconsciousness without recall.

Medical Assessment

Frequently, patients with multisystem disease undergo surgical procedures. If time permits, patients should be brought under the best possible medical control prior to elective surgical intervention. Several organ systems require special attention (Fig. 27.2).

Cardiovascular System

Blood pressure should be stable. However, a diastolic pressure up to 110 mm Hg or less should not prove deleterious provided the patient is stable intraopera-

tively and throughout the recovery period. A baseline electrocardiogram (ECG) should be available. Recent changes in pattern or rhythm must be investigated for possible myocardial infarction. If the patient has suffered a heart attack during the preceding 3 to 6 months, surgery should be postponed if possible. The risk of reinfarction is less than 6% if surgery is undertaken within 3 months of infarction, 2.5% at 3 to 6 months, and 2% after 6 months.

Congestive cardiac failure must be treated preoperatively with digitalis, diuretics, antidysrhythmic agents, and positive-pressure ventilation if necessary.

Mitral valve prolapse (MVP), reported to occur in up to 17% of healthy individuals, is considered to be the most common cardiac valvular abnormality. Although the anesthetic course may be uneventful, complications may arise for the first time during the perioperative period, including life-threatening dysrhythmias, mitral regurgitation, and infective endocarditis. Prophylactic antibiotic administration to prevent bacterial endocarditis is recommended for patients undergoing oral or urologic surgery. Adequate premedication is essential. Drugs causing tachycardia or having an α-adrenergic blocking effect should be avoided. Hyoscine, because of its negative chronotropic effect, is preferable to atropine. Prevention of hypovolemia, acidosis, hypercarbia, hypokalemia, and overdose is essential.

Potentially dysrhythmic agents such as epinephrine are best avoided to prevent diagnostic confusion. Inhalation anesthesia is recommended. However, most patients with MVP usually have an uneventful anesthetic episode, and care is taken to prevent their unnecessary identification as cardiac cripples.

Respiration

Respiratory status must be assessed in patients with clinical pulmonary disease, including a history of exercise tolerance, severity of cough, quality and quantity of sputum production, and history of recent upper respiratory infection. Routine pulmonary function tests (PFTs) and arterial blood gas analyses during the preoperative evaluation of most surgical patients are no longer recommended (normal values are shown in Table 27.3). PFTs are indicated prior to lung resection. There is no evidence that a mild upper respiratory infection will progress to pneumonia if anesthesia is ad-

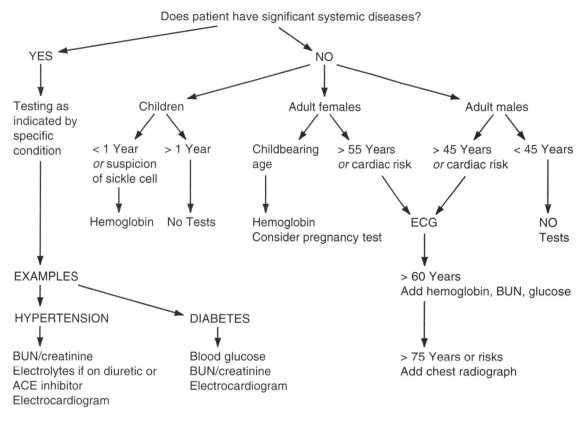

FIG. 27.2. Preoperative testing algorithm.

ministered. In the case of elective surgery, for better patient comfort and well-being, anesthesia should probably be postponed until optimal conditions prevail. Most patients with acute respiratory failure tolerate general anesthesia well and do not develop hypoxemia or severe deterioration in pulmonary status intraoperatively.

Renal System

Many anesthetic drugs (e.g., nondepolarizing muscle relaxants such as vecuronium and pancuronium) are excreted through the kidneys. Thus assessment of renal function, such as volume, specific gravity, urinary electrolytes, blood urea nitrogen (normal 20 mg/dL), serum creatinine (normal 1 mg/dL), and creatinine clearance

(normal 120 mL/min), is indicated in patients in whom kidney failure is suspected.

Central Nervous System

Patients with central nervous system (CNS) disease are often highly sensitive to narcotic and depressant drugs. For medicolegal reasons, for diseases such as multiple sclerosis, Parkinson's disease, and amyotrophic lateral sclerosis, regional anesthesia has often been avoided because of the possibility of developing new neurologic lesions coincidental with the procedure, although no scientific evidence has substantiated the risk. Preexisting neurologic lesions, such as deficit following a cerebrovascular accident (CVA), and peripheral neuropathy associated with diabetes mellitus, when properly evalu-

TABLE 27.3. *Normal values for assessment of respiratory function*

Parameter	Normal
Respiratory values	
Rate	12–35/min
Rhythm	Regular
Tidal volume	4–8 cm³/kg (250–500 cm³)
Vital capacity	20–55 cm³/kg (1.51–41.00)
Negative inspiratory pressure	−40 to −80 cm H_2O
Dead space/tidal volume (Vd/Vt)	0.3
Arterial blood gases	
pH	7.35–7.45
Pa_{CO_2}	34–45 mm Hg
Pa_{O_2}	95–100 mm Hg
CO_2 content	26–28 mEq/L
Bicarbonate (HCO_3^-)	22–28 mEq/L
O_2 saturation	
Arterial	94–100%
Venous	60–85%
O_2 content	
Arterial	15–23 vol/dL
Venous	10–16 vol/dL
Pulmonary function tests[a]	
FVC (forced vital capacity)	4.74 L
FEV$_1$ (forced expiratory volume in 1 s)[b]	3.87 L
FEV$_3$ (forced expiratory volume in 3 s)[b]	4.41 L
PEFR (peak expiratory flow rate)	8.97 L/sec
MMF (midmaximal flow rate)	3.08 L/sec
ERV (expiratory reserve volume)	0.96 L
RV (residual volume)	1.77 L
TLC (total lung capacity)	6.56 L
RV/TLC ×100%	27%
FRC (functional residual capacity)	2.73 L
IC (inspiratory capacity)	3.78 L

[a]Normal arterial blood gas and pulmonary function test values (70-kg man age 50).
[b]Expressed as a percentage of the FVC, FEV[1] = 83% (i.e., 3.87 L is 83% of 4.74 L), and FEV[2] is 97% (i.e., 4.41 L is 97% of 4.74 L).

ated and documented are not contraindications for neural blockade. Patients with hemiplegia or those severely burned may be hyperkalemic. Succinylcholine, which increases serum potassium levels, should be avoided.

Patients with myasthenia gravis on anticholinesterase therapy should have their medication continued throughout the operative period. Premedication is best avoided. Use of small doses of succinylcholine is not contraindicated, but prolonged neuromuscular blockade may result. The use of nondepolarizing relaxants is probably not warranted. Increased duration of narcotic effects also occurs.

Gastrointestinal System

Fluid and electrolyte imbalance is often associated with gastrointestinal disease. Hypovolemia, compensated in the awake state, may cause severe, prolonged hypotension during anesthesia. Hypokalemia and metabolic alkalosis may contribute to cardiac instability intraoperatively. Intestinal obstruction may result in a "full stomach" and pose the risk of aspiration during intubation. This complication may be avoided by using the Sellick maneuver: Cricoid pressure compresses the esophagus and prevents regurgitation of gastric contents. (The technique is also used in emergency situations when the patient has just eaten and in the pregnant patient in labor.)

Closed gas spaces are often caused by intestinal obstruction. Nitrous oxide, which is 34 times more soluble than nitrogen, expands the gas volume by replacing nitrogen. It should be avoided, as surgical closure may be hampered by dilated intestinal loops.

Metabolic and Endocrine Considerations

Endocrinopathies should be identified and treated preoperatively. Uncontrolled thyrotoxicosis can cause cardiovascular collapse intraoperatively. Manipulation of pheochromocytomas results in severe hypertension. Treatment requires phenoxybenzamine and (acutely) phentholamine or sodium nitroprusside infusion.

Allergies

Any allergic history should be identified. Asthmatic attacks may be provoked by sodium thiopental, intubation, or β-adrenergic drugs (e.g., propranolol). Treatment requires a β-agonist inhaler, epinephrine, and deep inhalation anesthesia. Premedication with diphenhydramine may be useful in susceptible individuals. In circumstances such as latex allergies, protocols for the perioperative period exist to ensure use of latex-free materials to avoid disastrous events (Table 27.4). Latex (natural rubber) sensitivity has become a major concern among health care workers. Between 1988 and 1992 a total of 1,118 cases and 15 deaths were reported to the Food and Drug Administration (FDA). Patients with rubber-induced anaphylaxis make up 10% of the total number of those with anaphylactic reactions to anesthetic drugs. Health care workers, especially operating room personnel, are prone to develop latex hypersensitivity due to continuous occupational exposure.

Documentation of Medications

There is an exponential incidence of adverse drug interactions in relation to the number given. Drug surveys show that an average of 8 to 11 drugs are prescribed for a hospitalized patient. During normal anesthesia and surgery an additional 5 to 10 drugs or more may be given. Many of the drugs are multicomponent preparations. Complications approximate 45% when more than 20 drugs have been ingested.

Commonly used drugs that interact with anesthetic agents to cause increased sedation are listed in Table 27.5. To avoid complications, simple drugs are given only when necessary, and anesthetic dosages should be modified. It behooves the entire surgical team to consider carefully the indications before adding drugs to the patient's therapeutic armamentarium. Drugs that should be continued up to and including the day of surgery are antihypertensive medications, propranolol,

TABLE 27.4. *Latex and health are personnel*

High risk patients
  Group 1: patients, especially children, with myelodysplasia, congenital orthopedic defects, and genitourinary anomalies
  Group 2: patients undergoing barium enema procedures with latex balloon tip
  Group 3: patients with occupational exposure to latex product manufacturing
  Group 4: health care providers and other employees, including household workers, who frequently wear latex gloves (6% workers affected)
Symptoms and treatment
  Contact dermatitis (type IV hypersensitivity reaction)
    Symptoms: itching, burning, and erythema shortly after contact; eczema
    Treatment: avoid contact with allergen, topical treatment, rarely systemic
  Latex-induced anaphylaxis (type I hypersensitivity reaction)
    Symptoms: cardiovascular (hypotension, tachycardia, dysrhythmias), respiratory (bronchoconstriction), cutaneous (erythema, rash), hemostasis (coagulation abnormalities)
    Treatment: supportive
Operative care
  Awareness: history of individuals at risk; high index of suspicion
  Prophylactic regimen: steroids, diphenhydramine, and H_2 blockers
  Latex allergy-identifying band; sign on the operating room
  Latex-free operating room; identify latex-free products and latex-containing products
  Prepare latex-free cart

TABLE 27.5. *Commonly used medications that may interact with anesthetic agents to cause increased sedation[a]*

Maintenance medications
  Cardiovascular
    Antihypertensive drugs
    Antidysrhythmic agents
    Digitalis glycosides
    Diuretics
  Antibiotics
  Psychotropic drugs
    Lithium
    Monoamine oxide inhibitors
    Phenothiazine derivatives
    "Street drugs"
  H_2 receptor antagonists
    Cimetidine
    Ranitidine
  Chemotherapeutic agents
  Immunosuppressant drugs
Intravenous agents
  Narcotics
  Barbiturates
  Benzodiazepines
  Ketamine
  Trimethaphan
Inhalation agent
  Nitrous oxide
  Halothane
  Enflurane
  Isoflurane
  Desflurane
  Sevoflurane
Muscle relaxants

[a]Patients subjected to anesthesia frequently have other medical problems. Pharmacologic interaction with anesthetic agents can increase sedation or neuromuscular paralysis.

L-dopa, insulin, steroids, phenytoin, and narcotics (especially if the patient is dependent). Drugs that should be discontinued are the monoamine oxidase inhibitors (MAOIs), which can cause cardiovascular reactions and profound sedation in combination with anesthetic agents. If a patient on an MAOI presents emergently for anesthesia, recommended narcotics include fentanyl or morphine rather than meperidine. Hypertension should be treated with direct-acting vasodilators.

Hypotension responds to fluids or direct-acting pressors (or both). Special attention is paid to patients receiving steroids (they may require increased dosages), hypoglycemics (half-life is 2 days; hypoglycemia, unrecognized under anesthesia, may occur if the patient is fasted preoperatively), digitalis (an adequate dose under anesthesia may be toxic in the awake state), diuretics (low and severe hypotension may be induced during anesthesia), and Phospholine Iodide eyedrops (typical cholinesterase prolongs the action of succinylcholine).

Intravenous vancomycin has been recommended as prophylaxis for methicillin-resistant staphylococcal infection in patients allergic to penicillin, although there have been no clinical efficacy studies. Concomitant administration of vancomycin and anesthetic agents has been associated with increased frequency of hypotension, flushing, erythema, and urticaria. Infusions of vancomycin should be given slowly and completed prior to anesthesia.

Personal Habits

Smokers may have acute and chronic respiratory changes. Oxygen-carrying capacity is decreased through the production of carbon monoxide, as is functional residual capacity. Postoperative desaturation, atelectasis, and pneumonic infiltrates may occur. Baseline respiratory therapy instruction is valuable.

The patient who is chronically addicted to alcohol usually requires more anesthesia because enzyme induction systems have been mobilized, and thus anesthetic agents are metabolized faster. Liver function should be known because many agents depend on hepatic breakdown. During acute intoxication, less anesthesia is needed.

Drug abusers present special problems to the surgical team. Drug interaction, withdrawal, venous access, pulmonary problems, hepatitis, infection, cardiac involvement, and altered sensorium affect anesthetic manage-ment. Drug withdrawal should not be attempted perioperatively.

Physical Examination

Preanesthetic evaluation includes recording the vital signs. Of particular importance is the ability to open the mouth and documentation of the state of dentition. The presence of a tracheostomy scar should alert the clinician to the possibility of granulomatous tissue within the trachea, which may hamper free passage of an endotracheal tube. Neck movement should be checked and the ability to intubate assessed. Particularly in patients with advanced diabetes or carotid artery or cervical spine disease, neck extension should be possible without neurologic changes.

Chest auscultation is also necessary, with special attention paid to the quality of breath and cardiac sounds. Pathologic murmurs should be sought. Documentation of ASA physical status classification in the preanesthetic assessment provides a "tool" for subsequent examination of anesthetic morbidity and mortality, rather than an estimate of anesthetic risk (Table 27.6). An Allen test, which assesses the adequacy of the radial and ulnar blood supply to the hand, should be recorded in all patients in whom invasive arterial monitoring is planned. Most importantly, a plan for anesthesia including postoperative pain management must be presented to and accepted by the patient. Whenever feasible, doc-

TABLE 27.6. *ASA physical status classification*

Physical status	Criteria
1	Healthy patient
2	Mild systemic disease, no functional limitations (asthma, chronic bronchitis, diabetes mellitus, hypertension, obesity)
3	Severe systemic disease, functional limitation (angina, history of myo cardial infarction, uncontrolled hypertension, or diabetes mellitus)
4	Systemic disease, constant threat to life (advanced pulmonary, renal, or hepatic dysfunction; congestive heart failure; unstable angina)
5	Moribund, patient is not expected to live if not operated
6	Organ harvest

Add (E) for emergency operation.

umentation should note a discussion of alternate anesthetic techniques.

Evaluation of Laboratory Data

Studies have questioned the application of standardized routine testing in all patients, especially in young, healthy, ambulatory individuals. Considerable interinstitutional variability exists. Generally, testing should be performed within a few days of surgery. Guidelines recently introduced by the ASA are shown in Table 27.7.

Several tests are commonly performed. A complete blood count includes a hematocrit close to 30% and hemoglobin above 9 g. In chronically uremic patients much lower values are tolerated. The serum potassium level should be more then 3 mEq, although lower values may be accepted in emergency situations. Blood urea nitrogen and creatinine levels give some indication of renal function. Baseline glucose levels indicate appropriate fluid management. Liver function tests, if appropriate, are done. Elevated CPK levels may indicate

MH but are also commonly found in athletes. A baseline EGG is usually requested for all patients over 45 years of age, as is chest radiography. A pregnancy test should be performed on all women in whom pregnancy cannot be ruled out.

AVAILABLE ANESTHETIC TECHNIQUES

Surgical anesthesia may be achieved by general, regional, or local techniques; the latter tow may be combined with conscious sedation. Selection of method depends on the location, duration, and complexity of the operative procedure, the patient's age and physical status, and the personal preference of the physician and patient.

General Anesthesia

General anesthesia is accomplished by intravenous injection of an hypnotic, such as an ultrashort-acting

TABLE 27.7. *Indications for laboratory testing[a]*

Test	Indications
Hemoglobin	Menstruating females; children <1 year old or with suspected sickle cell disease; history of anemia, blood dyscrasia or malignancy, congenital heart disease, chronic disease states; age >60 years
WBC count	Suspected infection or immunosuppression
Platelet count	History of abnormal bleeding or bruising, liver disease, blood dyscrasias, chemotherapy, hypersplenism
Coagulation studies	History of abnormal bleeding, anticoagulant drug therapy, liver disease, malabsorption, poor nutritional status
Electrolytes, blood glucose, BUN/creatinine	Patients with hypertension, diabetes, heart disease, or disease states with the potential for fluid-electrolyte abnormalities. Patients taking digoxin, diuretics, steroids, or angioleusin-converting enzyme (ACE) inhibitors
Liver function tests	Patients with liver disease, history of or exposure to hepatitis, history of alcohol or drug abuse, drug therapy with agents that may affect liver function
Pregnancy test	Patients in whom pregnancy cannot be reliably ruled out by history (some suggest all females of childbearing years)
Urinalysis	No indication during preanesthetic evaluation; surgeon may request that infection be ruled out before certain surgical procedures, particularly those involving prosthetic implants
Electrocardiogram	Men >45 years old, women >55 years old; history of symptoms of cardiac disease; history of hypertension, diabetes, morbid obesity, significant pulmonary disease, cocaine abuse
Chest radiograph	Patients with symptoms of pulmonary disease, airway obstruction, cardiac disease, malignancy, history of heavy smoking, age >75 years
Cervical spine flexion/ extension	Patients with rheumatoid arthritis or Down syndrome

[a]No laboratory test is indicated merely because the patient is undergoing anesthesia or surgery. Laboratory tests should be chosen according to specific indications, based on a comprehensive history and physical examination.

barbiturate (sodium thiopental), propofol, or etomidate. Intubation of the trachea may be facilitated by succinylcholine (a depolarizing muscle relaxant with a duration of action of 5 minutes) or more commonly by one of the intermediate-acting nondepolarizing relaxants, such as mivacurium, rocuronium, atracurium, or vecuronium. Administration of succinylcholine has been associated with K^+ release, especially in comatose, plegic, paretic, and burn patients. Fasciculation may increase abdominal pressure and cause regurgitation in nonfasting patients. The anesthetic state is continued by administration of inhalation or intravenous drugs, often combined with nitrous oxide.

Inhalation agents include halogenated compounds such as desflurane, sevoflurane, isoflurane, halothane, and enflurane, which are all nonexplosive. The two new inhalation anesthetics, desflurane and sevoflurane, have rapid onset/offset characteristics, allowing easy titration, with rapid emergence and recovery. Like isoflurane, they cause minimal cardiovascular depression. Sevoflurane does not irritate the patient's upper airway, making it an ideal induction agent in patients with difficult vascular access (e.g., children). Excretion of inhalation agents is through the lungs, and only small portions (0.02% for desflurane and 0.2% for isoflurane) are metabolized. None is hepatotoxic or nephrotoxic. (The by-product of sevoflurane after exposure to soda lime, compound A, might be nephrotoxic in rates, but clinical experience supports the drug's safety in humans.) Nitrous oxide is usually used as a carrier gas in equal concentration with oxygen. Use of this gas in not recommended for neurologic procedures (detrimental cerebral effects), intestinal obstruction (increases the volume of entrapped gas), or eye surgery when air or sulfur hexafluoride ($SF6$) has been used (intraocular hypertension may result). Moreover, if repeat surgery is necessary within 7 to 10 days of craniotomy or eye surgery, nitrous oxide should be avoided because intermarginal or intraocular air is absorbed slowly. Muscle relaxants may be used as dictated by surgical requirements.

Intravenous anesthesia involves bolus or continuous infusion of narcotics (meperidine, morphine, fentanyl, sufentanil, alfentanil, remifentanil), tranquilizers (midazolam, diazepam, lorazepam), hypnotics (barbiturates, propofol, etomidate), and muscle relaxants (mivacurium, rocuronium, cis-atracurium, vecuronium, atracurium, pipecronium, doxacurium, pancuronium, and curare). Nitrous oxide is used for its analgesic properties. Ketamine causes a dissociative anesthesia accompanied by salivation, hallucinations, and delayed return to consciousness. Its main use is for burn dressing changes. It is not recommended for outpatient use.

Propofol (Diprivan) provides rapid onset of anesthesia and equally prompt recovery because of fast metabolism and extensive distribution. The overall incidence of nausea and vomiting is low. Transient local pain on intravenous injection may be prevented by prior infusion of lidocaine. The drug may be used as an induction agent or, if given by infusion, as a maintenance anesthetic. Remifentanil (Ultiva), the latest addition to the narcotic family, is also rapidly metabolized by nonspecific cholinesterases. Rapid clearance of this drug, which has a clinical effect that measures in minutes, confers on it maximum flexibility in titration and dissipation of effect as soon as the administration is discontinued. Such drugs prove particularly valuable for ambulatory cases and for procedures of short duration.

Regional Anesthesia

Regional anesthesia is achieved by spinal, epidural, or caudal block, specific nerve blocks (e.g., brachial plexus, femoral, sciatic, celiac), or Bier block (arm or leg intravenous injection of local anesthetic after exsanguination of the extremity). Indications for spinal anesthesia include patient preference, difficult airway, and possibly respiratory infection. Contraindications include patient refusal, shock, skin sepsis, elevated intracranial pressure, spinal cord disease, peripheral nerve deficit, coagulopathies, prostatism, the headache-prone patient, and respiratory inadequacy. Complications are listed in Table 27.8. Therapy includes volume replacement, vasopressor administration, and (rarely) respiratory support. Regional anesthesia is seldom a safer technique than well monitored general anesthesia.

TABLE 27.8. *Complications associated with spinal anesthesia*

Sympathetic paralysis → hypotension, bradycardia
Respiratory difficulties ;→ hypoxia, hypercarbia
Nausea, vomiting → aspiration
Restlessness → confusion
Wears off too soon; does not "take"
Urinary retention
Headache
Neurologic sequelae

Documented benefits of epidural anesthesia are reduced intraoperative blood loss and decreased incidence of deep venous thrombosis, especially with hip and limb surgeries. Advantages of epidural anesthesia if a catheter has been placed for repeated injection of local anesthetic solutions include longer duration of postoperative pain relief and sympathectomy, which may be beneficial after vascular surgery or limb reattachment. Easy administration of intrathecal narcotics may be continued for hours or days. Complications include intravascular injection and accidental dural puncture, causing total spinal blockade with cardiorespiratory complications.

Local anesthetic agents may be divided into esters (metabolized in the plasma by pseudocholinesterase) and amides (metabolized in the liver) (Table 27.9). The most common drugs used are lidocaine 1%, tetracaine 1%, and bupivacaine 0.5%. Ropivacaine 1% (Naropin), introduced recently, is an amide local anesthetic with a kinetic and potency profile similar to that of bupivacaine but with a greater margin of safety regarding cardiac toxicity. Local anesthesia or field block is usually performed by the surgeon using 0.5% to 1% lidocaine. The safe limit for injection is 30 to 40 mL of a 1% solution. Complications that are drug-related are caused by allergy (usually esters), overdose, and intravascular injection (Table 27.10).

Monitoring

The ASA has outlined standards for basic intraoperative monitoring that have been adopted by all states. These standards, which apply to all anesthesia care, are as follows.

TABLE 27.9. *Commonly used local anesthetics listed in order of potency*

Esters
  Procaine (600 mg)
  Chloroprocaine (800 mg)
  Tetracaine (20 mg)
Amides
  Mepivacaine (300 mg)
  Lidocaine (300 mg) = 30 cc of 1%
  Etidocaine (300 mg)
  Bupivacaine (75 mg) = 30 cc of 0.25%
  Ropivacine (75 mg)

Maximum dosage is in parentheses.

TABLE 27.10. *Complications that may be caused by overdose or intravascular injection of local anesthetics*

Drug	Complication
Lidocaine	Sedation; thick speech
Procaine	hypotension; perioral numbness
All drugs	CNS changes: tinnitus, strange taste, dizziness, visual disturbances, disorientation, shivering, twitching, tremor, coma, convulsions
	Cardiovascular signs: hypotension, bradycardia, PR prolongation, widening QRS
	Respiratory distress

1. Qualified anesthesia personnel shall be present in the room throughout the conduct of all general anesthetics and monitored anesthesia care.
2. During all anesthetics, the patient's oxygenation, ventilation, circulation, and temperature shall be continually evaluated.

To ensure adequate oxygenation, an oxygen analyzer with a low oxygen concentration limit alarm must be functional in all anesthetic machines. Also, during all anesthetics, a quantitative method of assessing oxygenation, such as pulse oximetry, must be employed.

Appropriate ventilation is ensured by monitoring the end-tidal CO_2 concentration. An audible disconnect alarm must be incorporated in all anesthetic machines.

Circulation is monitored by continuous ECG display, and blood pressure and heart rate are evaluated at least every 5 minutes. Continuous measurement of temperature is another requirement. All information is usually charted every 5 minutes. Many monitors are now able to store information and provide a hard copy of trends.

Additional monitoring used with increasing frequency includes mass spectrometry, portable units utilizing infrared absorption, and Raman scattering technologies for respiratory gas and anesthetic agent measurements, fluid balance, pulmonary artery pressure, cardiac output, neuromuscular transmission, and (in neurosurgical patients) Doppler ultrasonography, intracranial pressure measurements, electroencephalography, power spectral analysis, bispectral index, and evoked potentials recording. Transesophageal echocardiography is useful for cardiac surgery and neuro surgery and during hepatic transplantation.

CAUSES OF DELAYED RETURN TO CONSCIOUSNESS

Following anesthesia, most patients are returned to the postanesthetic care unit (PACU) in varying degrees of consciousness. Occasionally, if an anesthetic technique has combined regional block with sedation and the patient is considered "recovered and discharged from anesthetic care," he or she may be transferred directly to the ward or ambulatory unit. The most common causes of unresponsiveness postoperatively include the following.

Prolonged anesthetic effect or overdose
Respiratory insufficiency
Drug interaction
Intraoperative catastrophe
Hypothermia
Fluid and electrolyte imbalance
Allergic or atypical drug response
Preoperative condition

Prolonged Anesthetic Effect or Overdose

By far the most frequently observed cause of delayed return of consciousness postoperatively is a prolonged effect of anesthetic agents or overdose of these drugs. The diagnosis is made by checking premedication, examining the anesthetic record, or assessing neuromuscular transmission. Treatment is both supportive and specific in the use of narcotic antagonists or reversal of muscle relaxants.

Any patient still unresponsive after administration of an anesthetic must be monitored meticulously. Oxygen-enriched, humidified air is given routinely, and the ECG is monitored continuously. If respiration is inadequate, ventilation must be supported. Blood pressure and pulse are charted at least every 15 minutes and the temperature recorded hourly. Whenever possible, comatose patients who have been extubated are maintained in a lateral position to minimize the possibility of aspiration. Pulse oximetry is used routinely in the PACU. Although high-dose narcotics are no longer in use, if overdose occurs patients who have received large amounts may require ventilatory support for many hours despite administration of narcotic antagonists.

Low-dose inhalation anesthesia (1% halothane or isoflurane or 1.5% enflurane) is usually associated with prompt return to consciousness postoperatively. Newer generations of anesthetic agents (inhalation, intravenous and muscle relaxants) with significantly shorter half-lives and rapid redistribution phase may eliminate the concern about overdose, making them ideal agents for use during outpatient and same-day surgery.

Respiratory Insufficiency

All degrees of ventilatory inadequacy, from mild depression to overt failure, may occur and can readily predispose to prolonged unconsciousness. Common causes of postoperative respiratory insufficiency include the following.

1. Intraoperative hyperventilation, which reduced CO_2 stores; hypoventilation occurs as CO_2 reaccumulates
2. Anesthetic agents
3. Fluid overload
4. Operative site (e.g., upper abdomen) causing pain and diaphragmatic splinting
5. Intraoperative complications
6. Aspiration
7. Preexisting disease

Accurate diagnosis depends on close observation, clear communication between the surgeon and anesthesiologist, blood gas reports, appropriate radiographs, and preoperative history. Therapy depends on the cause and includes supplemental oxygen, assisted ventilation, narcotics, bronchodilators, and fluid replacement as necessary.

Drug Interaction

As already noted, the incidence of complications rises sharply after ten drugs have been given. Combinations of drugs that commonly delay responsiveness postoperatively include muscle relaxants, antibiotics, tranquilizers, diuretics, digitalis, and narcotics. For example, combinations of small doses of midazolam (Versed) and fentanyl cause apnea in about 50% of otherwise healthy individuals.

Intraoperative Catastrophe

An intraoperative catastrophe, although uncommon, may occur, and the patient is admitted to the PACU comatose. The most important factor is early and continued communication between all medical personnel. Some possible causes include shock, myocardial infarction, rupture of an intracranial aneurysm, or severe hypoxia.

Hypothermia

Regulation of body temperature is impaired (poikilothermic state) during anesthesia. If the procedure is prolonged or if the operative site has been continuously irrigated with cold solution, the core temperature may decrease as much as 6°C, especially in children. At this low level, the depressant effects of all anesthetic agents are exaggerated.

Certain physiologic and metabolic effects are seen with hypothermia. Almost all organ functions are affected; or note are the increase in blood viscosity by 2% to 3% per degree centigrade decrease in temperature. Hypothermia promotes platelet aggregation, contributing to further increase in resistance in blood flow especially in the capillaries. Coagulation is impaired, owing to the decrease in coagulation factor activity. The cardiovascular system initially responds with cutaneous constriction manifested by shivering and increased oxygen consumption. If the temperature is allowed to drop below 30°C, cardiac dysrhythmias herald ventricular fibrillation and cardiac standstill. (In some circumstances, however, controlled hypothermia is desirable and beneficial for organ protection, especially during cardiac and neurosurgical procedures.) Uncontrolled hypothermia can be detrimental. In one study body temperature less than 35°C was associated with a threefold increase in the incidence of surgical wound infections, compared to normothermia.

During warming, which must be performed gradually to prevent skin burns in areas of low perfusion, the ECG must be monitored for ventricular dysrhythmias. Care must be taken to avoid sudden elevation of the limbs, which might push large quantities of relatively cold peripheral blood toward the heart. The respiratory status must also be closely watched, particularly if the patient has received nondepolarizing muscle relaxants, because recurarization may occur as the body is warmed.

Malignant hyperthermia may be triggered by stress in the recovery room. Therapy requires changing all breathing circuits, hyperventilation with 100% oxygen, cooling blankets, infusion of cold fluids, correction of metabolic acidosis, dantrolene (1 mg/kg i.v., repeated up to 10 mg/kg), glucose and insulin (to treat hyperkalemia), and furosemide and fluids (to prevent acute renal failure from myoglobin deposition). Procainamide has also been used. Calcium-containing drugs and β-adrenergic stimulants should be avoided. The patient may be severely hypokalemic for the next several days, requiring potassium replacement.

Fluid and Electrolyte Imbalance

Fluid and electrolyte imbalance occurs most frequently in elderly, debilitated, hypertensive patients who are maintained on diuretic therapy. During bowel manipulation particularly, large volumes of fluid may be lost from the circulation and not adequately replaced intraoperatively because of the risk of precipitating congestive heart failure. Serum electrolytes should be measured postoperatively in all patients after extensive intestinal surgery.

Diabetic patients who are usually fasted preoperatively but may have received insulin are also prone to hyper or hypoglycemic states. Infection, stress, and especially steroid administration may increase blood glucose values to high levels. Therefore in all patients with a diabetic history, urinalysis should be performed as soon as the patient is admitted to the PACU. At least a small quantity of glucose should be detected to ensure that the patient is not in hypoglycemic coma. Bedside estimations of blood glucose are accurate only to about 100 mg/dL; and although this test may be suitable for a rough estimate, it is no substitute for the standard laboratory glucose test. Patients in hyperglycemic coma require an immediate rapid injection of approximately 40 U of regular insulin. Replacement of large volumes of fluid is usually necessary, and supplemental potassium should be added to each bottle because insulin decreases serum potassium levels. Patients in hypoglycemic coma usually respond within 5 minutes to a rapid injection of 50 mL of 50% dextrose in water.

Allergic or Atypical Drug Response

Minor variations in response to any drug are common. Occasionally, the response is such as to interfere with return to consciousness postoperatively. Some of the drugs that can cause problems during the perioperative period include the following.

1. Penicillin (rash, respiratory distress, laryngeal edema)
2. Droperidol (neurologic changes, coma)
3. Diazepam (prolonged coma)
4. Muscle relaxants (muscle paralysis)
5. Narcotics (respiratory depression)
6. Ketamine (hallucinations)
7. Barbiturates (prolonged coma)

It is important to remember that the response to narcotics is variable, and 25 mg meperidine (demerol) postoperatively depresses respiration in most patients.

Preoperative Condition

A patient's postoperative condition can be correctly evaluated only with knowledge of the preoperative status. A patient who is comatose before surgery in all likelihood will remain so for some time afterward. The verbal recovery room report must include a description of the preoperative pathology.

CONCLUSIONS

Adequate anesthesia is essential to the good outcome of surgical procedures. Inducing such a state carries the potential of causing severe, life-threatening complications. An understanding of the requirements and problems on both sides of the "ether screen" minimizes perioperative morbidity and mortality and improves operating conditions.

QUESTIONS

Select one answer.

1. If a patient taking MAO inhibitors presents for surgery, which of the following should be avoided:
   a. Desflurane.
   b. Remifentanil.
   c. Meperidine.
   d. Morphine sulfate.
2. Uncontrolled hypothermia can cause all of the following *except:*
   a. An increase in blood viscosity.
   b. Normal ECG findings.
   c. A decrease in coagulation factors.
   d. Shivering with increased oxygen consumption.
3. The following apply to latex allergy:
   a. No true allergens can be documented.
   b. Anaphylactic reaction is rare.
   c. Difficult to identify a group at risk.
   d. Awareness is a key factor in avoiding untoward events.
4. Sevoflurane, a halogenated agent:
   a. Should be avoided in patients with cardiac disease.
   b. Is associated with hepatoxicity.
   c. Has limited use due to slow onset/offset characteristics.
   d. Is considered an ideal induction agent because it does not irritate the airway.
5. Which of the following is least commonly associated with nausea and vomiting?
   a. Fentanyl.
   b. Etomidate.
   c. Propofol.
   d. Midazolam.
6. With regional anesthesia:
   a. Patient refusal is an absolute contradiction.
   b. Documented benefits of epidural anesthesia include reduced blood loss and fewer instances of deep venous thrombosis.
   c. Postoperative pain relief is improved.
   d. All of the above.
7. Malignant hyperthermia-susceptible patients:
   a. Should have the "halothane–caffeine contracture test" before planned surgery.
   b. May be given succinylcholine.
   c. Should be pretreated with oral dantrolene.
   d. Usually avoid coffee and caffeinated beverages.
8. A patient with an incarcerated hernia presents for surgery. He suffered a myocardial infarction 6 weeks ago. The risk for perioperative reinfarction is:
   a. Dependent on the type of anesthesia.
   b. About 6%.
   c. Negligible, as he is now asymptomatic.
   d. Over 30%.
9. Patients with mitral valve prolapse:
   a. Should not receive any premedication, as atropine causes tachycardia.
   b. Represent about 10% of all patients with cardiac valvular disease.
   c. Must be monitored carefully, as ventricular fibrillation is easily provoked by isoflurane.
   d. Usually have an uneventful anesthetic.

10. Administration of succinylcholine:
    a. Is safe in the burn patient 2 weeks after injury.
    b. Causes fasciculations.
    c. Results in diaphragmatic paralysis of about 20 minutes.
    d. Is the drug of choice for myasthenia gravis patients.
11. Lidocaine:
    a. Is an amide local anesthetic.
    b. May cause slurred speech if more than 250 to 300 mg is administered.
    c. Results in sedation.
    d. All of the above.

SELECTED REFERENCES

American Society of Anesthesiologists. New clarification of physical status. *Anesthesiology* 1963;24:11.

American Society of Anesthesiologists: Statement on routine preoperative laboratory and diagnostic testing. Approved by House of Delegates on October 14, 1987. Amended on October 13, 1993;775.

ASA. Practice guidelines for management of the difficult airway: a report by the American Society of Anesthesiologists task force on management of the difficult airway. *Anesthesiology* 1993;78:597.

ASA. Standards for basic anesthetic monitoring. Approved by House of Delegates in October, 1986. Amended on October 13, 1993.

Barash PG, Cullen BF, Stoeltinng RK. *Clinical anesthesiology,* 3rd ed. Philadelphia: Lippincott-Raven, 1997.

Eichorn JH, et al. Prevention of intraoperative anesthesia accidents and related severe injury through safety monitoring. *Anesthesiology* 1989;70:572.

Frost E. *Post anesthesia care unit,* 2nd ed. St. Louis: Mosby, 1990.

Frost E. *Preanesthetic assessment 1, 2, 3.* Boston: Birkhauser, 1988, 1989, 1991.

Frost E. *Preanesthetic assessment 4, 5.* New York: McMahon Publishing Group, 1994, 1996.

Frost E, Goldiner P. *Post anesthetic care unit.* Norwalk, CT: Appleton & Lange, 1990.

Katz J, Benumof J, Kadis LB. *Anesthesia and uncommon diseases,* 4th ed. Philadelphia: WB Saunders, 1997.

Roizen MF, Fleisher LA. *Essence of anesthesia practice.* Philadelphia: WB Saunders, 1997.

Stoelting RK, Diedoref SF. *Anesthesia and coexisting disease,* 3rd ed. New York: Churchill Livingstone, 1993.

Tinker JH, Dull DL, Caplan RA, Ward RJ, Cheney FW. et al. Role of motoring devices in prevention of anesthetic mishaps: a closed claims analysis. *Anesthesiology* 1989; 71:541.

Twersky RS. *The ambulatory anesthesia handbook.* St. Louis: Mosby, 1995.

28

Orthopedic Surgery

Neil J. Cobelli and Andrew Stein

The objective of this chapter is to provide a simplified overview of the major areas of orthopedic surgery including trauma, adult orthopedics, and brief elements of pediatric orthopedics. By its nature, any overview greatly simplifies areas of controversy, and in those instances the effort is made to present the most widely held opinions. Areas where the orthopedic surgeon and general surgeon overlap, especially within the management of polytraumatized patients are stressed. The remainder is intended to provide a method of quick and easy review of specific entities within orthopedics.

TRAUMA

Polytrauma

Management of the polytraumatized patient represents an area in medicine in which a coordinated team approach by multiple subspecialties has a significant impact on the outcome. The older concepts of stabilizing a patient for several days prior to dealing with less life-threatening injuries such as long bone fractures and pelvic fractures have just about been put to rest. In 1990 the number one cause of death for patients between the ages of 1 and 39 was multiple trauma. Most deaths during the first hour af-

ter injury are due to head injury and shock. It is estimated that at least one-third of these deaths are potentially preventable.

Early orthopedic intervention in the management of polytraumatized patients has the greatest impact on that group of patients who survive the first few hours but are nonetheless seriously injured.

The two greatest causes of death late in the management of polytraumatized patients are adult respiratory distress syndrome (ARDS) and infection. The management of the patient's orthopedic injuries can have a significant impact on these entities. Beginning in the early 1980s it became clear that stabilization of pelvic fractures and long bone fractures led to distinctly improved outcome for polytraumatized patients.

In 1982 Goris et al. demonstrated that individuals managed by early surgical stabilization of long bone and pelvic fractures spent an average of 6 days on a respirator for ARDS and had a late death rate of 10%. Those managed by conservative means spent an average of 26 days on a respirator and had a late mortality rate of 55%. Studies by Riska and Myllynen (1982) supported the concept that early stabilization of fractures improved long-term outcome. Of 629 patients treated between 1967 and 1974, a total of 384 treated conservatively had an ARDS rate of 22%, whereas 245 treated surgically had an ARDS rate of 4.5%. Another study by the same authors of 211 patients between 1975 and 1978 showed that patients managed by early stabilization of long bone fractures had an ARDS rate of only 1.4%.

Not only does early operative intervention lead to a decrease in ARDS, it makes mobilization of the patient substantially easier. It is easier to transport the patient for tests and makes achievement of an upright posture possible. This, of course, leads to benefits such as lower incidences of pneumonia, urinary tract infection, and decubitus ulcer. Finally, the ability to mobilize a patient makes it substantially easier to meet his or her nutritional needs, leading to further reduction in the late death rate. Provided the patient can be managed adequately in terms of hematocrit and oxygenation, at the current time there is no doubt that polytraumatized patients, especially those with femoral shaft and pelvic fractures, benefit greatly from early stabilization of fractures.

Open Fractures

Commonly, patients with serious trauma also have open fractures. Early management of the open fracture involves three basic concepts: irrigation and débridement of the open wound, stabilization of the soft tissue envelope, which may involve closure by secondary intention, by skin graft, or by muscle flap. Recreation of the soft tissue envelope leads to an environment more conducive to bone healing and protects against infection.

The classification of open fractures by the Gustilo method has prognostic significance. Open fractures that are of a low-energy type with a small wound of compounding in general do well. These fractures have much the same prognosis as closed fractures. A grade I fracture is a fracture with a low-energy fracture pattern (i.e., little in the way of comminution, little or no soft tissue loss, and a wound of compounding 1 cm or less). A grade II open fracture is a fracture that may have mild comminution of the fracture site; there may be a small amount of soft tissue loss, and the wound of compounding shows an opening 1 to 5 cm in the skin. There is little or no crush injury component to the soft tissue injury. Grade III fractures, which are subdivided into subtypes A, B, and C, show a high-energy fracture pattern, usually with marked comminution on the radiograph. There may be moderate to severe tissue loss and a significant element of crush. The wound of compounding is, in general, 5 cm or more. A type III-A fracture has no exposed bone at the end of the irrigation and débridement procedure. Type III-B has exposed bone remaining, and type III-C has an associated vascular injury.

The likelihood of complications such as infection and nonunion increases with each grade, although most complications are seen with type III-B and III-C fractures. Early management of these fractures via the methods stated above leads to improved outcome of the specific fracture, positively benefiting management of the patient as a whole.

REGIONAL TRAUMA

A variety of fractures in locations throughout the body are discussed briefly. Emphasis is on general forms of management and specific complications that can be expected in any particular area. The concept of acceptability of fracture position is involved in the management of most diaphyseal fractures. Although the position may not be anatomic, it should be close enough that there is no functional or cosmetic disability. Fractures into joints frequently lead to severe functional disability with only small displacement of the fracture fragments. This disability can be compounded by prolonged immobilization. Intraarticular fractures are therefore frequently dealt with operatively to diminish the degree of functional disability, whereas many diaphyseal and metaphyseal fractures can be treated conservatively.

Fractures of the Clavicle

Clavicle fractures, especially through the medial and middle thirds, are treated conservatively. This treatment involves a sling in the adult and possibly a figure-of-eight bandage in the child. Fractures along the outer third at the acromioclavicular junction can lead to marked displacement because of disruption of the ligamentous complexes, and it may require fixation. Fractures of the central portion of the clavicle are occasionally associated with injuries to the subclavian vessels.

Fractures of the Proximal Humerus

Fractures of the proximal humerus involving the surgical neck can be grouped into two general categories: impacted or displaced. Fractures in which the fragments have been driven together have an innate stability. This type of fracture can be treated conservatively with early immobilization in a sling and then various exercise programs within a week or two. The fractures that have displacement of the fragments tend to require operative treatment.

Fractures that involve the surgical neck and tuberosities of the proximal humerus have been subclassified by Neer. Those that involve displacement of the neck fracture and displacement of both tuberosities are treated by prosthetic replacement. Fractures with displacement of the shaft and single tuberosity may be dealt with by open reduction and internal fixation. These same fractures, when associated with a dislocation, are often treated by a prosthetic replacement. The rationale has to do with the remaining blood supply to the humeral head fragment and the likelihood of survival of the humeral head. With displaced surgical neck fractures with both tuberosities off or one tuberosity and the head dislocated, the likelihood that the nutrient blood supply has been disrupted is high.

In cases where the tuberosities are intact but the surgical neck fracture is displaced, the fracture can frequently be close-reduced but may redisplace. Stabilization with some form of intermedullary rod or percutaneous wire fixation may be necessary.

Fracture of the Greater Tuberosity

Nondisplaced fractures of the greater tuberosity are treated similarly to stable or impacted fractures of the surgical neck. The arm is immobilized for a short time (2 to 3 weeks), and then rapid mobilization occurs. Displaced fractures of the greater tuberosity involve disruption of the rotator cuff in addition to the mechanical difficulties caused by displacement of the tuberosity. These injuries are generally dealt with operatively.

Fractures of the Humeral Shaft

Fractures of the humeral shaft can be successfully treated conservatively. They are managed with 3 to 4 weeks of immobilization followed by a period of another 3 weeks of limited motion. Full motion is initiated around the sixth week.

The structure most likely to be injured is the radial nerve. This is especially true of fractures at the junction of the middle and distal thirds.

Controversy exists over the indications for surgical treatment of humeral shaft fractures. Patients who present for initial evaluation with an intact radial nerve but who then lose function of the radial nerve during fracture reduction are clearly in need of an open reduction and internal fixation with simultaneous exploration of the radial nerve. A relative indication may exist in patients who present with a radial nerve injury initially. These injuries most often prove to be a neuropraxia rather than nerve entrapment. Further indications include polytraumatized individuals and patients with pathologic fractures.

Fractures of the Supracondylar Region of the Humerus

Fractures of the supracondylar region of the humerus tend to occur most commonly in children and the elderly. In both situations, they can be managed successfully conservatively. For fractures that are either not acceptably reducible or present in a young adult population, surgical management with open reduction and internal fixation with wires or plate and screws is often the treatment of choice. Structures at risk for injury, especially during the childhood years, include primarily the brachial vessels.

Fractures of the Radial Head

Nondisplaced fractures of the radial head are treated with minimal immobilization for 7 to 10 days, followed by active range of motion exercises of the extremity. Fractures of the radial head with displaced fragments are treated by open reduction and internal fixation or excision of the fragment. Fractures of the radial neck are treated in a similar manner if only minimally displaced. Displaced fractures of the radial neck are treated with radial head excision to permit recovery of full supination and pronation.

Fractures of the Olecranon

Displaced fractures of the olecranon represent an avulsion fracture of the triceps mechanism. As such, they require open reduction and internal fixation to reconstruct the muscular attachment. The most common technique involves tension band wiring of the displaced fracture, which permits immediate mobilization of the extremity. Fractures that are nondisplaced can be treated by conservative means, as the triceps mechanism is intact. Care must be taken to mobilize these individuals early to prevent loss of function.

Fractures of the Radial Shaft

Displaced fractures of the radial shaft in adults are treated by open reduction and internal fixation. Generally only severe open fractures lead to associated injury of the radial artery and median nerve. Nondisplaced fractures can be treated by casting.

Fractures of the Ulnar Shaft

Proximal ulnar fractures with associated radial head dislocation are referred to as Monteggia fractures. This fracture is dealt with by plate-and-screw fixation of the ulna. It rarely requires operative intervention at the radial head–capitellar joint, as the fracture generally reduces with ulnar reduction. Fractures of the ulnar shaft that are the result of a direct blow are commonly referred to as nightstick fractures. These fractures can be treated with minimal immobilization and early range of motion exercises of the extremity if it is only minimally displaced.

Fractures of the Radius and Ulna

Two-bone fractures of the forearm are treated operatively in adult patients if there is any displacement whatsoever. Failure to do so leads to pronounced loss of supination and pronation.

Fractures of the Distal Radius

Many eponyms are attached to fractures of the distal radius. The most common is the Colles fracture, which involves fracture of the distal radius with dorsal displacement and angulation of the distal fragment. Classically, it is described as a small fracture of the ulnar styloid as well. A fracture that has displacement in the opposite direction is frequently referred to as a Smith's fracture. Treatment of this type of fracture depends on the age of the patient. The single major factor in determining treatment is the degree of intraarticular involve-

ment. In an elderly population with a wholly or primarily extraarticular fracture, most of these fractures can be treated conservatively with closed reduction and application of a cast for 4 to 6 weeks.

In a younger population, this fracture represents a high-energy injury and has a high degree of associated intraarticular involvement. It has a poor prognosis unless restoration can be anatomic or near-anatomic in nature. The primary mode of operative treatment at this time is application of an external fixator with concomitant K-wire fixation of intraarticular fragments, either percutaneously or through a limited open incision, frequently including a bone graft. Extensive fractures may require plate fixation.

Fractures of the Scaphoid

Fracture of the scaphoid is one of the most commonly missed injuries about the wrist. The injured individual may report having sprained the wrist some time ago, and initial radiographs may be completely unremarkable. Careful attention must be given to physical examination of these individuals, looking for pain on palpation of the anatomic snuff box of the wrist. When in doubt, they must either be treated for several weeks or have a fracture ruled out with a bone scan.

Nondisplaced fractures of the scaphoid recognized early and treated conservatively have an excellent prognosis and heal uneventfully. Those that are missed, with treatment initiated late, have a much higher incidence of nonunion and frequently require surgical intervention. Displaced fractures of the scaphoid are probably best treated with either wire or screw fixation (Herbert screw). Fractures diagnosed late may require the above form of fixation, an additional bone graft, or both.

Fractures of the Pelvis

Fractures of the pelvis occur in two situations. They can involve relatively low-energy trauma, such as a slip and fall against the edge of a bathtub, or be the result of a high-speed trauma, such as a fall from a height or an automobile accident. Fractures that represent relatively low-energy household accidents occur frequently in the elderly. They present as fractures of the pubic symphysis, pubic rami, or ischium. These injuries are managed with observation, analgesia, and rapid mobilization of the patient.

High-energy pelvic fractures are grouped by the proposed mechanism of injury. Although no injury happens according to a rigid set of rules, where a force is exerted from a single direction, the concept of the mechanism of injury is helpful prognostically and therapeutically in managing pelvic fractures. The first of the three major mechanisms of injury is external rotation, commonly referred to as open-book injuries (Fig. 28.1A). Here the two wings of the pelvis rotate apart with the pelvic opening anteriorly. The second major mechanism of injury is lateral compression (Fig. 28.1B), where a force is applied to the lateral aspect of one side of the pelvis, driving the two sides of the pelvis together, as in a fall onto the lateral portion of the pelvis. The final mechanism of injury is a sheer fracture (Fig. 28.1C). This represents a vertical shearing force delivered to one side of the pelvis, translocating one side superiorly and posteriorly relative to the contralateral side.

For each mechanism of injury, there is a range, from relatively stable to unstable injuries. Several broad generalizations can be made. External rotation injuries tend to be at the more stable end of the spectrum relative to vertical shear injuries, which tend to be at the more unstable end of the spectrum. Disruption of the posterior elements, through the bone or ligamentous structures, is the key to bony stability and is an indicator of severity. Fractures that completely disrupt and posteriorly dislocate the structures about the sacrum lead to a much higher mortality rate than those that leave these structures intact.

Acetabular Fractures

Fractures through the hip socket can occur with or without dislocation. Fractures that are essentially nondisplaced can be dealt with conservatively through traction and movement of the joint. Fractures that have displaced to any significant degree must be dealt with operatively through relatively complex surgical approaches. The associated structure most likely injured is the sciatic nerve as it exits the sciatic notch. Fractures of the acetabulum that involve the posterior column of the acetabulum have a higher incidence of injury to the sciatic nerve.

Hip Fractures

Fractures of the proximal femur are commonly referred to as hip fractures. There are several major types of hip fracture; the most common classifications differentiate the fracture types anatomically. The first major classification is the subcapital hip fracture, which occurs through the junction of the neck and head of the femur (Fig. 28.2). The second major type is the intertrochanteric fracture, which occurs in the area between the greater and lesser trochanters. These fractures are frequently subgrouped into fractures of the base of the neck, intertrochanteric, and pertrochanteric (which extend beyond the lesser trochanter) (Fig. 28.3). For all intents and purposes, the management and prognosis are identical throughout the intertrochanteric region.

Fractures about the hip occur primarily in an elderly population. When they occur in a younger population, they represent a high-energy injury.

Subcapital Fractures

The blood supply to the femoral head travels along the capsule of the hip through the region of the femoral neck and enters the head of the femur at the neck–head junction (Fig. 28.2). As a result, fractures that occur through the femoral neck–head junction tend to disrupt the blood supply to the femoral head if displaced. The most widely accepted classification system is referred to as the Garden classification of subcapital hip fractures. A Garden 1 fracture is of the subcapital region and is impacted with mild valgus displacement, or it is an incomplete fracture. A Garden 2 fracture is complete but nondisplaced. A Garden 3 fracture is in varus, and a Garden 4 fracture is a fracture that is completely displaced from the femoral neck. Treatment depends on the degree of displacement and the physiologic age of the patient. In patients who have a nondisplaced or impacted valgus fracture or who have displaced fractures but are physiologically under the age of 65 (the cutoff is individual), the fracture is likely to be treated by pin or screw fixation of the femoral head.

In individuals who are elderly with displaced fractures, the fracture is treated by prosthetic replacement.

FIG. 28.1. Fractures through the pelvis occur by three major mechanisms of injury: external rotation injury (**A**); lateral compression injury (**B**); and vertical shear injury (**C**).

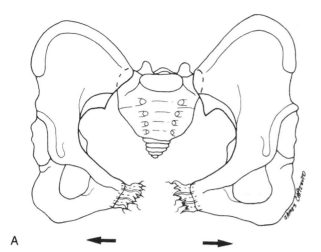
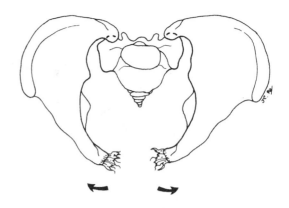

A

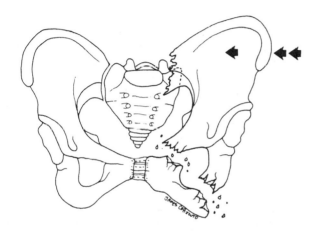
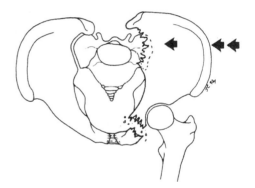

B

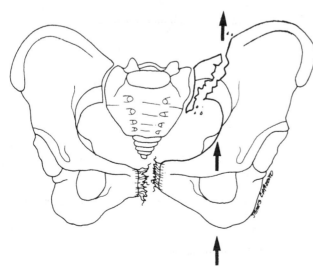
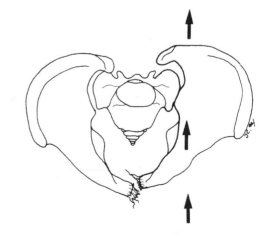

C

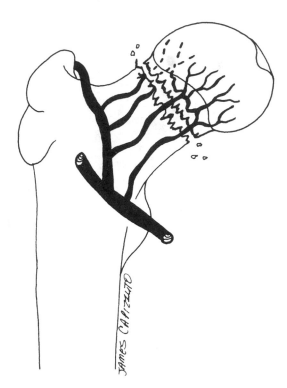

FIG. 28.2. Vessels nourishing the femoral head enter at the neck–head junction. Displaced fractures in this region lead to disruption of the vasculature to the femoral head.

This practice decreases the incidence of a second operation to deal with a fracture that has not healed, has displaced, or has had the femoral head undergo avascular necrosis. It also allows rapid mobilization of the patient with full weight-bearing and requires little cooperation on the part of the patient, which is especially useful in an elderly population with diminished mental capacity.

Intertrochanteric Fractures

Intertrochanteric fractures require operative intervention. The major classifications of intertrochanteric fracture have to do with fracture stability. The more stable the fracture pattern, the more likely the patient is to be able to bear weight on the fracture without difficulty after surgery (Fig. 28.3). Most intertrochanteric frac-

tures are currently treated by some variation of a sliding screw-and-plate device (Fig. 28.4). The term "nailing a hip" stems from earlier days when large nail-like appliances were utilized. For today's treatment, a large screw is placed up into the proximal fragment and head of the femur, and a plate is placed over it, which allows sliding at the junction of the plate and screw. Newer devices involve intermedullary rods with transfixation screws that go up into the head and neck, but in most cases they have no distinct advantage over the more traditional treatment.

Fractures of the Femoral Shaft

Fractures of the femoral shaft occur in the region between the lesser trochanter and the supracondylar region of the femur. These fractures, unless contraindicated, are treated operatively. Such repair allow rapid mobilization and prevents the difficulties encountered with prolonged traction. Skeletal traction can be used successfully to treat these fractures when absolutely necessary, but the time and disability involved for the patient are much greater than if it is treated surgically.

Surgical treatment today involves placement of an intermedullary rod. Image intensifiers allow placement of these rods through "closed" techniques; that is, the surgical incision is made at a site distant to the fracture, usually in the region of the greater trochanter. The rods are then placed over a guidewire after reaming the femoral canal.

Highly comminuted fractures or fractures that have a good deal of shortening are treated with interlocking intermedullary rods, which have transfixion screws placed through the intermedullary rod proximally and distally to augment fixation (Fig. 28.4B).

Supracondylar Fractures of the Femur

Supracondylar fractures of the femur occur most commonly in elderly patients; in younger patients they are the result of high-energy trauma. Although they also can be dealt with by skeletal traction, the common treatment involves plates and screws. This allows rapid mobilization of the joint and rapid return to normal activities for the patient. Fractures in this region can also involve individual condyles of the femur. This intraarticular fracture is treated by open reduction and internal fixation if there is any displacement.

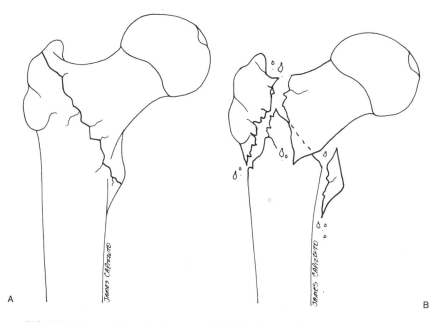

FIG. 28.3. Intertrochanteric features. **A:** Stable fracture. **B:** Unstable fracture.

Fractures of the Tibial Plateau

Fractures of the weight-bearing surface of the proximal tibia are common in all adult age groups. The more common plateau to be fractured is the lateral one, but isolated medial plateau fractures and bicondylar plateau fractures are seen. These fractures occur when the condyle of the femur drives down through the tibial plateau, splitting or depressing the weight-bearing surface. These fractures are treated by elevating the weight-bearing surface, maintaining its position with a bone graft, and fixing the fracture fragments with plates and screws or screws alone. Fractures that are less extensive are amenable to treatment through a combination of arthroscopic visualization of the fracture surface and percutaneous screw fixation of the fracture fragments.

Fractures of the Patella

Displaced fractures of the patella represent disruption of the quadriceps mechanism of the leg. Nondisplaced fractures can be treated with immobilization for a period of 6 to 12 weeks, but displaced fractures must be treated by open reduction and internal fixation. The preferred treatment involves some form of tension-band wiring, which allows early range of motion of the knee.

Fractures of the Tibial Shaft

Nondisplaced fractures of the tibial shaft or fractures that can be reduced into acceptable alignment can be treated conservatively with a long leg cast. It is widely agreed that early weight-bearing on this type of fracture leads to an improved union rate. Fractures that cannot be maintained in acceptable alignment and fractures that cause shortening of the tibial shaft are dealt with operatively. Treatment is most commonly an intermedullary rod placed through an incision distant from the fracture site. This "closed" intermedullary nail allows rapid return to normal activities. Fractures that are highly comminuted or demonstrate excessive shortening of the extremity require interlocking screws placed proximally and distally through the intermedullary nail to preserve position and length.

Fractures of the tibial shaft are the most common form of open fracture. Management of open tibial frac-

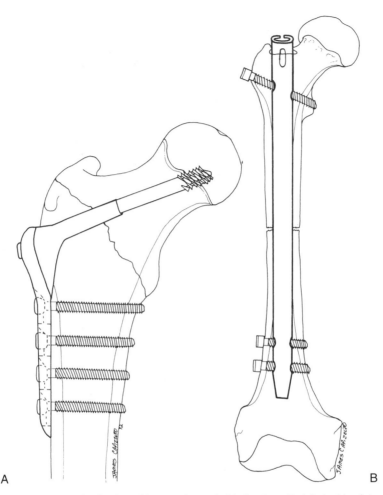

A   B

FIG. 28.4. A: Typical device for fixation of intertrochanteric hip fracture. **B:** Interlocking intermedullary nail.

tures is one of the most time-consuming and difficult elements of orthopedic surgery. These fractures must be attended to at the time of injury with irrigation, débridement, and stabilization of the fracture. The modalities of stabilization are external fixation of the fracture and, more commonly in recent years, intermedullary fixation. External fixation represents construction of an exoskeleton with pins placed above and below the fracture site and rods of metallic or composite material placed between the pins to hold the position and length.

The injured tibia with a high-grade open injury to the soft tissues has a high potential for infection. The common method for placing intermedullary rods involves reaming the medullary canal. The further damage done by reaming has been demonstrated to increase the potential for infection in high-grade open fractures. Therefore intermedullary nails that can be interlocked proximally and distally, and that can be placed without reaming, have been developed. For open grade I and II fractures, these devices are proving to be beneficial, as they eliminate many of the difficulties encountered with external pin fixation. Controversy still exists about grade III open fractures, but both external fixators and unreamed intermedullary nails are being utilized effectively.

Ankle Fractures

Ankle fractures involve one malleolus (lateral or medial), two malleoli (bimalleolar fracture involving both lateral and medial), or three malleoli (a trimalleolar fracture involving the lateral, medial, and posterior malleoli). Displaced ankle fractures may also involve dislocation of the talus from underneath the tibia.

Unimalleolar fractures are lateral or medial malleolar fractures. The more common is the lateral malleolus involving an eversion injury of the ankle. These fractures, if not associated with secondary ligamentous damage to the opposite side of the ankle, can be treated conservatively in a short leg cast.

If a bimalleolar fracture is essentially nondisplaced or it can be reduced to an acceptable position, it or bimalleolar equivalents (fractures of one malleolus with disruption of the ligaments on the opposite side) can be treated in a long leg cast. Displaced bimalleolar fractures are treated with open reduction and internal fixation involving plates and screws in the lateral malleoli and screws in the medial malleoli. Trimalleolar ankle fractures are uncommonly nondisplaced. These fractures are generally treated by open reduction and internal fixation, which allows early mobilization of the joint. The posterior malleolus can be difficult to get to, and small fractures of the posterior malleoli involving less than 25% of the articular surface are not generally fixed. Those involving 25% or more of the joint surface can undergo open reduction and internal fixation.

Fractures of the Foot

Fractures of the midfoot and hind foot occur with impact loading, such as a fall from a height, or violent twisting injuries. Fractures of the talar neck can be nondisplaced or displaced. Nondisplaced fractures that are truly anatomic have a reasonably good prognosis and can be treated conservatively. They are uncommon. Displaced fractures require open reduction and internal fixation. The higher the degree of initial displacement, the worse the prognosis.

In the past fractures of the calcaneus were universally treated conservatively, with a uniformly mediocre to poor result for severe fractures. In recent years, more and more attempts are proving successful with open reduction and internal fixation of calcaneal fractures.

Still, displaced calcaneal fractures, even with open reduction and internal fixation, can lead to a high degree of long-term disability for the patient.

Fractures of the Metatarsals

Fractures of the metatarsals can generally be treated conservatively. Multiple fractures or fractures grossly displaced can be treated with percutaneous pinning or open reduction and pin or screw fixation.

Fractures of Toes

Fractures of the toes with minimal displacement or those capable of being reduced are treated by taping the injured toe to an unaffected toe. Multiple phalangeal fractures or those grossly displaced may require pin fixation.

SPINAL FRACTURES

Evaluation of the polytraumatized patient for serious spinal injury represents one of the highest priorities when caring for these individuals. During early resuscitation and transportation efforts care must be taken to immobilize the cervical spine, utilizing backboards and in general treating the individual as if he or she has an unstable spinal injury until a thorough evaluation can take place.

History taking should focus on the mechanism of injury, presence of transient motor or sensory loss, loss of consciousness, impairment secondary to drugs and alcohol, and severe facial and head trauma. The treating physician must be aware of spinal cord injury as a potential cause of hypotension secondary to loss of sympathetic tone. In contrast to hypovolemic shock, neurogenic shock is characterized by warm extremities but generally not tachycardia or diaphoresis.

Orthopedic management, although obviously concerned with the general condition of the patient and the neurologic state, also encompasses the concept of spinal stability with regard to fractures. Fractures that include gross dislocations are clearly unstable, which presents management difficulties in the neurologically compromised individual and potential for further injury in the neurologically noncompromised individual. The three-column theory of spinal stability has gained popularity in an effort to categorize the potential for instability of nondislocated fractures of the vertebrae, especially those referred to as burst fractures. These fractures tend to occur with axial loading and may well explode the vertebral body and posterior elements.

The bony spine is divided into three columns: anterior, middle, and posterior (Fig. 28.5). The anterior column includes the anterior longitudinal ligament and the anterior half of the vertebral body. The middle column includes the posterior half of the vertebral body and the posterior longitudinal ligament. The posterior column is made up of the remaining structures in the posterior elements including pedicles, lamina, facet joints, and spinous processes. Fractures that completely disrupt two of the three columns are considered to be orthopedically unstable. Management is discussed under specific regions of the spine.

Fractures of the Cervical Spine

Adequate radiographs of the cervical spine are essential for evaluation of injuries in this region. These include, at least, anteroposterior (AP), lateral, and open-mouth odontoid views. Care must be taken that all vertebrae from C1 through the top of T1 are visualized. During initial evaluation, management consists at least of a collar or sandbag (or both) until the evaluation is completed.

Fractures of C1: Jefferson Fracture

Fracture of the C1 posterior arch secondary to an axial load is referred to as a Jefferson fracture. Relatively nondisplaced fractures are treated with halo immobilization for a 3-month period. For displaced fractures with involvement of the lateral masses and more than 6.9 mm of widening on the open-mouth view, treatment consists in 6 weeks of cervical traction followed by a halo vest for the remainder of the 3 months. Fortunately, because of the wide canal diameter in this region, cord injuries are uncommon.

Injuries to the transverse ligament can occur with C1 arch fractures. The normal atlantoaxial distance as visualized on a lateral view is less than 5 mm. If this distance is increased to more than 5 mm, it is indicative of atlantoaxial instability; and C1–2 wiring and fusion are required to prevent cord compression. Atlantooccipital

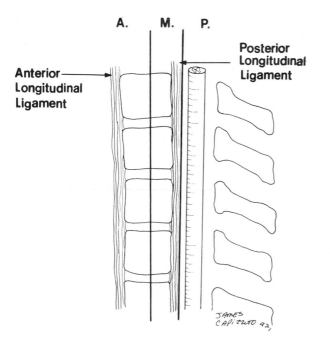

FIG. 28.5. The spine is divided into three columns. The anterior column is the anterior longitudinal ligament and the anterior one-half of the disk and vertebral body. The middle column is the posterior one-half of the disk and vertebral body and the posterior longitudinal ligament. The posterior column is made up of the pedicles, lamina, facet joints, spinous processes, and interspinous ligaments.

ligamentous disruption can also occur; and if the patient survives it, occiput–C2 fusion is indicated.

Odontoid Fractures

Fractures of the odontoid are best visualized through the open-mouth view. Nondisplaced fractures are, in general, managed by 3 months of halo immobilization. Fractures are generally divided into three types. Those involving the odontoid itself are classified as type 1; those involving the junction of the odontoid and the body of the axis are type 2; and those fracturing down through the body of the axis are type 3. If displacement of more than 5 mm occurs in these higher-type fractures, C1–2 posterior wiring and fusion are performed.

Fractures of C2: Hangman's Fracture

A fracture occurring through the posterior elements of C2 is referred to as a hangman's fracture. These injuries are usually treated successfully with halo immobilization for several months. When associated with dislocation, the injuries may be irreducible and require open reduction, wiring, and fusion.

Fractures of Cervical Vertebrae C3 through C7

Because of the small diameter of the canal in the C3 to C7 region, neurologic injuries are often associated with fractures of these vertebrae. Fractures considered to be stable in this region can be treated successfully with immobilization. Unstable fractures in this area require reduction, stabilization, and fusion. This regimen often requires combined anterior decompression, anterior bone graft with a block of bone, and posterior wiring and fusion.

Facet Injuries

Facet injuries can be purely ligamentous disruptions with dislocation or can involve fractures. Dislocations with displacement of less than 25% of the vertebral body may well represent only single-facet dislocation, whereas larger displacements represent bilateral facet dislocations. Initial management is traction through skull tongs to attempt to achieve reduction. Significant facet injuries generally necessitate posterior wiring and single-level fusions.

Fractures of the Thoracic and Lumbar Spine

Anterior compression fracture occurs with hyperflexion caused by abrupt deceleration. If less than the anterior 40% of the body is involved and other studies indicate no significant disruption of the posterior structures of the posterior longitudinal ligament, these injuries are treated with a brace. Injuries that involve more than 40% and those to the middle column or the posterior elements are thus considered unstable, and operative treatment is indicated. Operative management involves posterior instrumentation (e.g., Harrington, Cotrel/Dubousset, Luque) and local fusion.

Burst Fractures

Burst fractures occur with sudden deceleration injuries. The concept of stability has been discussed previously. Unstable fractures must be managed operatively. The method for dealing with retropulsed fragments is controversial. Many fragments reduce with distraction. The need for immediate decompression of retropulsed fragments remains controversial.

Pathologic Fractures

Pathologic fractures of the spine can occur at any level. The most common causes are metastatic tumor, multiple myeloma, and osteoporosis. A pathologic fracture occurs when relatively minor trauma causes a significant structural abnormality within a bone. Fractures secondary to metastatic lesions, if stable, may be managed conservatively in conjunction with treatment directed at the tumor in that locale. If unstable, they may require fixation as described above.

Compression fractures in the elderly secondary to osteoporosis are managed with rest initially, followed by rapid mobilization as tolerated, analgesics, and at times braces.

DISLOCATIONS

Acromioclavicular Joint Dislocation

Dislocation of the acromioclavicular (AC) joints are also known as shoulder separations. The degree of displacement of the joint is a reflection of the severity of ligamentous disruption. A grade 1 AC joint separation represents only a partial disruption of the ligamentous structures; there is still joint integrity, and the joint does not dislocate even under load. A grade 2 AC joint separation involves complete disruption of the AC ligaments with some integrity through he coracoclavicular ligaments. This joint is displaceable under load. Finally, a grade 3 AC separation involves complete disruption of both the AC ligaments and the coracoclavicular ligament complex, and the joint is dislocated even at rest.

Treatment for these injuries varies widely through the more severe grades. Grade 1 injuries are universally treated with a sling; grade 2 and grade 3 injuries may simply be treated with a sling or may be aggressively repaired surgically.

Shoulder Dislocations

Dislocations of the glenohumeral joint can be anterior or posterior. Some individuals are classified as having multidirectional instability after numerous dislocations. The most common is an anterior glenohumeral dislocation. In a younger age group, this is almost always accompanied by disruption of the fibrocartilaginous structure known as the labrum from the glenoid or bony socket of the shoulder joint. This relatively avascular structure may well not heal back to the bony glenoid, which leads to a potential for redislocation with an appropriately applied force through the joint.

Elderly individuals may dislocate with low-energy trauma and in a higher percentage of cases may leave the labrum intact and simply tear through other soft tissue structures. This leads to a lower likelihood of redislocation.

First dislocations in all age groups are treated by immobilization. The shoulder is immobilized for a minimum of 3 weeks, and then an exercise regimen is begun that only slowly introduces the motions of abduction and external rotation. Individuals who have undergone multiple dislocations require surgical reconstruction. A variety of procedures exist, many of which limit external rotation and abduction. Several of the more commonly performed procedures involve reconstruction or reattachment of the labral structures and capsule of the shoulder (Bankaart procedure).

The structure most likely to be injured is the axillary nerve, which can lead to denervation of the deltoid and loss of sensation over the lateral aspect of the upper arm. Chronic dislocations in the elderly are sometimes recognized late, and attempts at closed reduction can have disastrous effects on the vascular structures of the axilla. These structures may be scarred and adhere to the shoulder capsule; and on attempts at reduction there are reports of rupture of the brachial artery.

Elbow Dislocations

Elbow dislocations can be anterior, posterior, medial, or lateral. The most common dislocation is posterior. It represents a rather severe injury, and there can be injury to associated vascular structures anteriorly and to the median and ulnar nerves. These can be managed with closed reduction and splint for several weeks and then mobilization of the elbow joint. Occasionally, residual instability requires reconstruction of ligaments.

Wrist Dislocations

Dislocations about the wrist can occur through the carpals and distal radius or through the carpal bones themselves. The most common dislocations involve the scapholunate joint. This can involve a fracture of the scaphoid and is then known as a transscaphoid perilunate dislocation. Dislocations of the lunate itself can occur. Regardless of the particular type of dislocation, they frequently require surgical reconstruction, as the ligamentous disruption leads to long-term instability at the wrist if it is not reconstructed.

Hip Dislocations

Dislocations of the hip can be anterior or posterior. Posterior dislocations are far more common and are generally brought on by a blow to the knee in a flexed position. The classic position on dislocation is that of a shortened extremity held in a flexed, adducted, and internally rotated position. With anterior dislocations there is a shortened extremity in an externally rotated position. Posterior dislocations are associated with a significant incidence of injury to the sciatic nerve. They may be accompanied by fractures of the acetabulum or fractures of the femoral head (Pipkin fractures).

Treatment involves rapid closed reduction of the joint. If plain films and a computed tomography (CT) scan reveal no evidence of any debris within the joint and no associated fractures, conservative management may be all that is necessary. If there are associated fractures, they may require open reduction and internal fixation. There is a significant incidence of debris within the joint with a fracture, which should be removed via irrigation and débridement of the joint.

Knee Dislocations

Knee dislocations can be anterior or posterior. They are equally devastating and have a high incidence of associated injury to the popliteal vessels. After relocation of the knee, even in the face of normal pulses, an angiogram is required to rule out an intimal tear of the artery. These dislocations are associated with devastating consequences on the function of the joint. A number of ligaments are disrupted depending on the direction of the dislocation. The patient may have disrupted the anterior cruciate, posterior cruciate, and medial and lateral collateral ligaments. Extensive reconstructive surgery is necessary to obtain adequate knee function.

Ankle Dislocations

Ankle dislocations occur most often in conjunction with fractures and have been discussed under ankle fractures.

Subtalar Dislocations

Dislocations of the hind foot and mid foot around the talus occur with violent twisting injury. They may be reduced closed or may require open reduction and pin fixation. One fracture of this region that frequently requires open reduction and pin fixation is the Lisfranc fracture dislocation, which is a fracture dislocation of the metatarsals from the tarsals. A variety of patterns exist based on the direction of the four lateral digits and involvement of the base of the first metatarsal. This fracture dislocation must be reduced anatomically and held with pins percutaneously, at least; frequently it requires open reduction and pin fixation.

SPORTS INJURIES

As the field of sports medicine expands, more and more injuries are being considered sporting injuries.

Each sport or activity has an area of the musculoskeletal system that can be overtaxed or injured by that particular activity. The more common entities dealt with by sports medicine orthopedic surgeons are discussed here.

Shoulder Injuries

Recurrent shoulder dislocation (see Shoulder Dislocations, above) require reconstruction in the active adult. As sophistication within the area of arthroscopic surgery of the shoulder has increased, a broader spectrum of abnormalities has been recognized. At the core of most of these entities is the glenoid labrum. Shoulder arthroscopy has allowed recognition and remedy of loose bodes within the shoulder joint, excision of labral tears that cause locking of the shoulder, diagnosis of shoulder subluxation in contrast to frank dislocation, and diagnosis of multidirectional instability. Although many of these entities can be dealt with directly through the arthroscope, some controversy still exists over reconstruction of shoulder dislocations.

A number of arthroscopic procedures exist for stabilization of the shoulder. The standard of comparison, however, remains an open reconstruction of the labrum and anterior capsule.

Knee Ligament Disruption

Advances in the field of sports medicine have led to an increased awareness of ligamentous injuries about the knee. Increased diagnostic acumen has led to a greater number of diagnoses of serious knee ligament abnormalities at an early stage. The ability to deal with them surgically has helped decrease the likelihood of crippling arthritic degeneration later in life. Disruption of anterior and posterior cruciate ligaments with associated medial collateral or lateral collateral ligament instabilities leads to an increase in abnormal motion within the knee. These abnormal motions result in torn menisci and early degenerative changes.

The most common entity causing substantial instability within the knee is rupture of the anterior cruciate ligament. This injury frequently has associated lateral side instability, which in the long term leads to degenerative changes within the knee. In the short term it frequently prevents individuals from participating in sporting activities as they did in the past. The patient experiences a sense of the knee giving way during attempts to plant the extremity and pivot. Tests such as the Lachman test (a test for the ability to translocate the tibia anteriorly on the femur) and a "pivot shift" test, which recreates the giving-way episode, help diagnose the entity.

A number of procedures have been utilized to reconstruct an anterior cruciate ligament. Currently, the most promising procedures involve arthroscopic replacement of the deficient ligament with a substitute tendon graft. The most common grafts are autologous patellar tendon bone grafts. These procedures, whether performed for substitution of an anterior cruciate or posterior cruciate ligament, although technically demanding, can lead to substantially improved performance.

Meniscal Injuries

Injuries to the menisci are due to acute trauma or the accumulation of trauma over time; commonly referred to as degenerative menisci. Clinical presentation of pain with flexion or extension beyond a certain point, inability to fully flex or fully extend the knee, pain over the joint line, swelling within the joint, and a history of trauma are indicative of a possible meniscal injury. Magnetic resonance imaging (MRI) has helped confirm the diagnosis of injuries to the meniscus but is no substitute for a careful history and physical examination. Arthroscopic meniscal surgery with resection of the damaged portion of the meniscus and recontouring of the remaining menisci is the treatment of choice. Peripheral tears in select individuals can be effectively repaired.

ADULT ORTHOPEDIC SURGERY: ARTHRITIS

Arthritis simply means inflammation of a joint. Two major categories of arthritis are recognized: those that are a result of a local phenomenon, such as posttraumatic arthritis or osteoarthritis, and those that are, in general, thought to be a manifestation of a more generalized or autoimmune phenomenon, such as rheumatoid arthritis or psoriatic arthritis. These major categories of arthritides can be distinguished by the patient's presentation. Rheumatoid-type arthritides tend to be polyarthritides. They present with multiple joint involvement; and generally all joints of the body are at risk. Osteoarthritis occurs commonly in a few joints and is uncommon in others. The weight-bearing joints of the

hips and knees, small joints of the spine, and base of the thumb are common sites, whereas shoulders, ankles, and wrists are less common. In the major weight-bearing joints such as the hips or knees, rheumatoid arthritis presents radiographically as diffuse narrowing of the joint space with a reactive osteopenia. Osteoarthritic degeneration tends to be more pronounced through the weight-bearing surfaces and frequently has hypertropic (osteophyte formation) bony reaction.

When conservative management has failed in either type, surgical management is appropriate. The most commonly replaced joints for arthritic degeneration are the hips and knees. Shoulder replacements and elbow replacements are less commonly performed but function reasonably well, especially in patients with rheumatoid arthritis. Replacement of finger joints in rheumatoid arthritis also is successful. Replacement of wrist and ankle joints has been tried, but at present there are few well recognized functioning prostheses. Treatment in these areas is fusion of the joint.

Both hip and knee prostheses have undergone substantial improvement in design over the last decade. Current prosthetic implants can be expected to function at a reasonably high performance level for many years depending on the age and general condition of the patient. The use of cement fixation of the prosthesis remains an area of controversy. Relatively sedentary patients in their late seventies and eighties who require total hip or total knee replacement can predictably undergo cemented joint replacement and feel confident that the joint will perform adequately for the remainder of their lives, barring uncommon complications such as infection. The cemented total joint replacement in this age group remains the standard by which all other methods must be judged.

Individuals in their fifties who require total joint replacement, especially active individuals who have only single-joint involvement, cannot expect a cemented total joint replacement to perform for the remainder of their lives. These implants fail at the bone–cement interface in a substantial percentage of cases. The advent of porous coated prostheses that allow, at least theoretically, a biologic interlock via bony ingrowth into the interstices of the prosthesis, in theory, offer longer performance. Early performance reports appear promising.

In today's orthopedic practice, patients in their fifties or younger in most cases, if otherwise suitable, have uncemented prostheses placed. In many practices, those in their late seventies and above routinely have cemented prostheses, although this is not universally so. In between, the decisions are individualized, based on the patient's overall condition and the surgeon's general experience, whether to receive a cemented prosthesis, an uncemented prosthesis, or a hybrid (one component cemented, other components not cemented).

In general, the performance level of hip and knee replacements, given today's technology, is good. The longevity, although affected by age and activity level, is acceptable.

SOFT TISSUE INFLAMMATION AND ABNORMALITIES

Almost any soft tissue structure in the body, be it ligament, tendon, or muscle, can be inflamed or irritated. This can lead to acute or chronic pain syndromes, loss of function, and rupture of a tendon or musculotendinous junction. Several problems mentioned here occur commonly, and their presentation and treatment are discussed.

Shoulder Impingement Syndrome

Shoulder impingement syndrome is a descriptive term for a broad spectrum of painful problems about the shoulder. Into this category fall a variety of shoulder problems including bursitis, tendinitis, rotator cuff inflammation, and painful arc syndrome. The patient usually presents complaining of weeks to months of pain in and about the shoulder. The pain is most commonly anterior, although it can present as lateral, posterior, or even anterior deltoid insertion. The patient frequently denies any specific trauma that could have caused the pain. In many cases the patient relates an activity or a trauma that seemed to start the problem, but this is not universal. Patients often complain that the pain is worse at night, awakens them from sleep, and forces them to rise early in the morning. They report that the pain is brought on within a reproducible arc of motion, which can be anywhere from just a few degrees of abduction to the extreme limits of abduction, external rotation, or forward flexion. The problem can be acute in nature, being present only a few days, or chronic, lasting many months.

The term impingement syndrome arises from the fact that the space between the humerus and the acromion is a relatively fixed distance and that a number of structures including the rotator cuff, subacromial bursa, and biceps tendon all must glide within this space without difficulty. When inflammation begins within this region, the swelling within the soft tissue structures causes impingement on the bony undersurface of the acromion. Many structures have been implicated as the initiating cause, from a tight coracoacromial ligament in young muscular individuals to osteophyte formation underneath the acromion in the elderly. The problem may be simple inflammation of the biceps tendon or subacromial bursa or a mechanical defect into the rotator cuff.

Initial management of all of these entities is conservative, with antiinflammatory drugs, either oral or locally injected, and maintenance of motion of the shoulder to prevent adhesive capsulitis. For the cases that fail on conservative management, resection of the underside of the acromion, by open means or arthroscopic technique, may be indicated or excision and repair of the damaged area of the rotator cuff (or both).

Lateral Epicondylitis

Inflammation of the origin of the extensor tendons of the forearm is commonly referred to as tennis elbow. This inflammation, also called lateral epicondylitis, is an abnormality of the extensor origin. It may be brought on by repetitive activities, such as tennis or working on an assembly line, but in many cases it is idiopathic in origin.

Most of the patients are handled conservatively. Initial treatment may involve oral antiinflammatory drugs or, more commonly, steroids by injection. Splints and a simple exercise regimen may also be used. Most of the individuals settle down on this type of regimen, but some do not. In those individuals, especially those in whom the etiology is the performance of a repetitive task, release of the extensor origin may be required. Several procedures exist for this, most with an excellent outcome.

deQuervain Syndrome

Stenosing tenosynovitis of the first extensor compartment of the wrist is commonly referred to as deQuervain syndrome. Patients present with pain over the distal radial aspect of the radius. They report pain with activities that require them to deviate the wrist ulnarly or that require twisting the wrist, such as opening a door or a jar. The presentation is frequently accompanied by a small nodule in this area. Initial treatment is conservative, with local injection, antiinflammatory drugs, or splint. Surgery is reserved for recalcitrant cases.

Trochanteric Bursitis

Similar to individuals presenting with pain about the shoulder secondary to bursitis, inflammation of the abductor musculature about the hip is common. It is sometimes confused with sciatica, but these individuals are usually distinctly tender over the greater trochanter. Treatment, again, involves either nonsteroidal agents or local injection, with a high likelihood of improvement.

Pes Anserine Bursitis

Inflammation of the medial side of the knee is one of the more common soft tissue complaints seen in an orthopedist's office. A variety of soft tissue inflammations are grouped under this term. Whether the inflammation is of a pes anserine tendon at its insertion, a small bursa underneath the medial collateral ligament, or the ligament itself is difficult to ascertain. Frequently, there is an underlying cause for the inflammation. Many individuals who suffer from it have early degenerative changes within the medial compartment of the knee. Treatment is conservative with rest, antiinflammatory drugs, and possibly local injection.

Achilles Tendon

Inflammation or rupture of the Achilles tendon occurs during the third through fifth decades most commonly. Complete ruptures are often associated with unusual physical activity. The "weekend warrior" syndrome, in which a rather sedentary individual plays a high-demand sport on a weekend and suddenly feels a tearing sensation in the calf, is a common presentation. The patient presents with an inability to actively plantar-flex the foot; although dorsiflexion is present, pain may limit the excursion. Positioning the patient supine on a table with the knee flexed and the foot held in a neutral position while the calf is squeezed (Thompson test) leads to plantar flexion of the foot with an intact Achilles tendon. With a ruptured tendon, no movement

of the foot occurs. This test is reliable for diagnosing complete rupture of the Achilles tendon.

Chronic inflammation of the Achilles tendon can present as soreness at the musculotendinous junction with a nodule forming in this area. It can lead to rupture with ordinary activities, such as stepping off a curb.

Treatment of a ruptured Achilles tendon, if diagnosed early in the active adult, remains controversial. Excellent results are reported with management in a plantar flexion cast if the diagnosis is made in a 24- to 48-hour period. Because performance athletes have shown slightly better results with operative treatment, it is unclear if there are any benefits from this type of treatment in the average individual. The choice for conservative versus operative management, however, remains one for the individual surgeon based on his or her expertise and experience.

Plantar Fasciitis

A painful heel is commonly referred to as a "heel spur." The tough plantar fascia of the foot can become inflamed at its origin. If calcification has occurred at this site, radiographs may show a spur at the anteroinferior aspect of the tuber of the calcaneus. The presence of the spur, however, is not necessary for the diagnosis, and many individuals are asymptomatic even when the spur can be seen.

Treatment overwhelmingly is conservative, with nonsteroidal drugs, heel pad appliances, or local injection. It is uncommon to treat this entity surgically.

Low Back Pain

Abnormalities of the lower back account for more time lost from work, more compensation payouts, and more time in the orthopedic surgeon's office than any other orthopedic problem. The spine is made up of a series of small joints, each of which is constrained by numerous ligaments. In addition, the disk exists between the vertebral bodies in close association with numerous neurologic structures. Most adults at some time in their lives experience an episode of low back pain. It may be a problem only a few days, or it may last as long as several months. Fortunately for doctors and patients alike, the most episodes of low back pain are self-limited. With rest, support, and education, the preponderance of patients are returned to normal activities in a relatively brief time. The individual who suffers from recurrent bouts, low back pain that does not respond within a relatively short time, and of course those who have low back pain associated with neurologic findings may have structural abnormalities that require surgical intervention.

The individual who presents with a history of only several days of back pain related to some traumatic incident (it may have been a mild incident) and who has improved and had no neurologic findings, no neurologic complaints, no radiation of pain to the leg indicative of a possible radiculopathy, and normal plain radiographs can be confidently managed conservatively. Those patients who do not fall into this type of presentation—those who complain of radicular symptoms, frequent recurrence, or specific reproduction of their symptoms with a particular activity—all warrant further workup. This workup may include a CT scan, MRI, and myelogram.

A *herniated nucleus pulposus,* or "slipped disk," classically represents a disruption of the hard outer ring of the disk (annulus fibrosis) with extrusion of the gelatinous nucleus pulposus of the disk and possibly fragments of the hard annulus. Classically, patients present with back pain and pain radiating down the leg below the knee into the leg and foot. They may present with weakness of motor function in the distal extremity and decreased sensation in a dermatomal distribution. Straight-leg raising produces pain radiating down the leg, and the patients in general are quite incapacitated. In the absence of hard neurologic findings, most individuals with a documented herniated disk on MRI, CT scan, or myelogram may well settle down conservatively. Those who present with a neurologic deficit and those who fail to improve on several weeks of bed rest warrant surgical intervention for decompression of the nerve root. Today's workers' compensation system creates significant numbers of people who have the potential for large secondary gain and make sorting out the problem much more difficult.

Another common entity, seen primarily in elderly patients, is *spinal stenosis.* The classic presentation is that of pain in the buttocks radiating into the leg with exercise. The complaints may sound much like vascular claudication and, in fact, probably represent vascular claudication of the spine. Typically, the pain is reproducible with the same activity or distance walked each episode. Pain may also be brought on by standing erect for any period of time. One feature differentiating it from vascular claudication is that patients frequently report that to feel better they must sit down or bend forward and put their hands on their thighs. This flexed position increases room within the spinal canal for the neural elements, diminishing the symptoms. Treatment is surgical decompression.

TUMORS

Whether a lesion is a primary bone tumor or a metastatic lesion, accurate description of the presentation usually yields a narrow differential diagnosis. Age and past medical history are particularly relevant to the differential diagnosis of bone tumors. The most frequent metastatic tumors of bone generally affecting patients over 50 years of age arise from primary breast, prostate, lung, renal, and thyroid carcinomas. Multiple myeloma is the most frequent primary bone tumor and occurs with a peak incidence during the seventh decade. Osteosarcoma is the most frequent primary bone sarcoma and usually occurs during the second decade.

Benign Bone Tumors

Bone Cysts

Simple bone cysts usually presenting in the first and second decade are recognized most often after fracture. Primarily metaphyseal lesions in active individuals, they are recognized when a fracture occurs. After allowing the fracture to heal, current treatment recommendations include intraoperative irrigation of the cyst and installation of steroids. Occasionally, multiple injections or curettage and bone grafting are required.

Aneurysmal Bone Cyst

Aneurysmal bone cysts present during the second and third decades as rapidly expansile, locally aggressive lesions. They appear much as simple bone cysts. Treatment is curettage and bone grafting.

Nonossifying Fibroma

Seen during the first to third decades of life, nonossifying fibromas, which are cortical lesions, have a characteristic radiographic presentation. They are well circumscribed eccentric cortical lesions in the metaphyseal region of long bones. No treatment is required.

Osteoid Osteoma

Osteoid osteoma occurs during the second decade primarily. The patient usually complains of night pain frequently relieved by aspirin. Osteoid osteoma commonly occurs about the spine and may present as scoliosis. The classic radiograph shows a sclerotic lesion with a small radiolucent nidus centrally. Treatment is block resection and bone grafting.

Osteochondroma

Osteochondromas are also referred to as exostoses. These are primarily benign bony excrescences with cartilaginous caps that occur during the second and third decades of life. They may be either isolated lesions or part of a hereditary syndrome (multiple hereditary exostoses). Malignant degeneration of the cartilaginous cap has been reported. Isolated exostoses are rare but are slightly more common in the hereditary multiple form of the disease. Individuals presenting with pain or other indications of rapid growth are best treated by excision of the lesion.

Malignant Tumors of Bone

Multiple Myeloma

Plasma cell myeloma of bone usually presents after the fifth decade. The classic radiographic appearance is that of a lytic lesion (without a sclerotic border) that causes endosteal erosion, cortical expansion, or both. Bone scans are considered less sensitive than the skeletal survey in this entity, as the scan may well be negative even with large lesions present on radiographs. Treatment involves internal fixation for stability as necessary and local radiotherapy.

Giant Cell Tumor of Bone

Giant cell tumor of bone is an epiphyseal lesion of the bone. It presents during the third through fifth decades with a spectrum from low-grade to high-grade

malignancy. Although uncommon, these tumors can metastasize to the lung. Treatment of low-grade tumors involves curettage and bone graft. Recurrences and more highly malignant tumors require wide excision.

Ewing Sarcoma

Radiographically, Ewing sarcoma (presenting during the second decade) has an elongated permeative appearance on radiographs and frequently has abundant periosteal new bone formation. The differential diagnosis includes metastatic neuroblastoma, infection, osteosarcoma, and lymphoma. Current treatment includes irradiation and chemotherapy, although some centers recommend wide excision, especially in expendable bones such as the fibula or after recurrences.

Osteosarcoma

Osteosarcoma presents as a rapidly growing metaphyseal sarcoma during the second and third decades of life. It penetrates the cortical barrier early, causing periosteal new bone formation and frequently a soft tissue mass. The periosteal reaction may have the classic radial or sunburst pattern. Because metastases occur early, surgical treatment is combined with chemotherapy. Surgical treatment includes aggressive limb salvage techniques, amputation, and occasionally resection of isolated pulmonary metastases.

PEDIATRICS

Fractures

Children are subject to most of the same fractures as adults. They, however, have a more complex situation in their bony anatomy due to the presence of growth plates. The cartilaginous growth plates sandwiched between the metaphysis and epiphysis creates a composite structure with different properties than those of adult bone. Although the higher metabolic activity of children's bone allows a greater percentage of bony remodeling after fracture, damage to the growth plate from fracture leads to deformities that are progressive rather than static, as in the adult. The Salter Harris classification has been developed as a prognostic aid for dealing with fractures through the growth plate (Fig. 28.6).

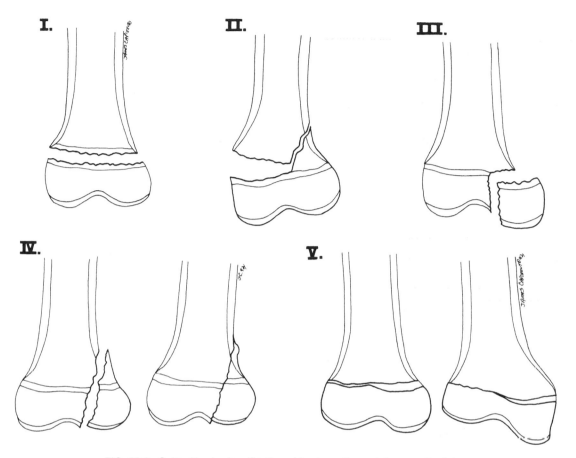

FIG. 28.6. Salter Harris classification of fractures through the growth plate.

Salter I Fractures

A Salter I fracture is a transverse fracture through the growth plate that in general is nondisplaced and frequently not visible on radiographs. It is therefore commonly diagnosed clinically. The prognosis for normal growth is excellent.

Salter II Fractures

Salter II fracture occur transversely through the growth plate at the same level as a Salter I, but they exit through the metaphysis before completely transversing the growth plate. These fractures may or may not be displaced and, although of a slightly higher severity than a Salter I fracture, with acceptable reduction carry a good prognosis, as the resting or germinal layer of the growth plate has remained unaffected.

Salter III Fracture

Salter III fractures involve a transverse fracture of the growth plate with exit across the germinal layer of the growth plate out through the epiphysis of the bone. Not only do these fractures involve the articular surface, leading to a potential for functional abnormality, they also disturb the germinal layer. If sufficient area has been damaged, it can lead to cessation of growth of all or a portion of the growth plate, with increasing anatomic and functional deformity resulting.

Salter IV Fracture

Salter IV fractures occur in line with the longitudinal axis of the bone. They cross the growth plate in a perpendicular manner and, as with Salter III fractures, affect the articular surface of the joint and germinal layer of the epiphyseal plate.

Salter V Fracture

Salter V fractures cause crush of the growth plate, greatly affecting the germinal layer. As such, they have high potential for growth abnormality and increasing deformity.

Treatment

Salter I and II fractures, if they can be adequately reduced, can be maintained in a cast and treated conservatively. Salter III and IV fractures have the potential to be treated conservatively if completely nondisplaced. However, because of the potential for late displacement and the rapidity with which this type of fracture solidifies even when nondisplaced, many surgeons opt for pin fixation. Displaced fractures of this category require surgical intervention.

All of these fractures, and Salter V fractures as well, require close monitoring for growth abnormality. These growth abnormalities can be dealt with if there is local tethering of the growth plate through resection of the area of tethering. If an entire growth plate or the major portion of a growth plate has been affected, epiphysiodesis or obliteration of the growth plate in that extremity or the contralateral one (or both) may be necessary.

Long-standing limb length abnormalities may require surgery for limb elongation. A variety of external fixation devices are available that can lead to excellent results in skilled, competent hands.

Child Abuse

Child abuse is a problem of extraordinary proportion. Although potential for abuse, whether physical, psychological, or sexual, is always difficult to assess, the suspicion of child abuse carries a moral, ethical, and in many states legal obligation to report. There are no specific fractures or fracture patterns that are pathognomonic of child abuse, but there are situations that may be indicative. Fractures of long bones in nonambulatory children, especially those with spiral patterns, are uncommon in situations other than child abuse. Although clearly some situations can cause this type of injury that are not child abuse, all too often the ultimate etiology is either some sort of physiologic abnormality or child abuse. The wrenching or twisting of an extremity is the source of this type of fracture.

A second presentation that is highly suspicious is multiple fractures of differing ages within a single individual. This, again, is either indicative of a physiologic abnormality or more commonly child abuse.

Slipped Capital Femoral Epiphysis

The slipped capital femoral epiphysis usually occurs early in the adolescent years. It is more common in boys. A short, stocky stature or tall, thin stature seems to predominate. Patients are usually in a growth spurt and complain of pain about the hip or knee. When a patient in this age group complains of achiness about the knee, a thorough examination and radiographs of the hip are a must. Treatment involves maintaining the position of the femoral head with pins or screws until the femoral epiphyseal plate stops growing. A significant incidence of bilaterality exists, and caution must be taken to observe the contralateral side.

QUESTIONS

Select one answer.

1. Early operative fixation of long bone and pelvic fractures in polytrauma patients reduces the risk of all of the following except:
   a. Sepsis.
   b. Negative nitrogen balance.
   c. ARDS.
   d. Fat embolism
   e. Malunion or nonunion.
2. Principles for managing high-grade complex open fractures include all of the following *except:*
   a. Intravenous antibiotics.
   b. Thorough irrigation and débridement.
   c. Cast immobilization.
   d. Meticulous soft tissue care.
   e. Careful assessment of compartment pressures.
3. The nerve most commonly injured in anterior shoulder dislocations is the:

a. Suprascapular nerve.
b. Ulnar nerve.
c. Median nerve.
d. Axillary nerve.
e. Long thoracic nerve.

4. Posterior dislocations of the hip most commonly injure which nerve?
   a. Femoral nerve.
   b. Obturator nerve.
   c. Sciatic nerve.
   d. Peroneal nerve.
   e. Interosseous nerve.

5. Vascular compromise has been associated with all of the following injuries *except:*
   a. Clavicle fracture.
   b. Knee dislocation.
   c. Patella fracture.
   d. Sternoclavicular joint dislocation.
   e. Supracondylar fracture of the humerus.

6. Which of the following scenarios warrants operative exploration of the radial nerve after closed manipulation of a fracture of the shaft of the humerus?
   a. No radial nerve function at the time of the initial physical examination.
   b. No radial nerve function on presentation and without improvement after closed manipulation.
   c. Intact radial nerve function at presentation and after closed reduction, but no function at the initial office visit 1 week after the fracture.
   d. Intact radial nerve function on presentation but no function after closed reduction.
   e. Intact radial nerve function on presentation, after manipulation, and at subsequent office visits.

7. A 23-year-old male motorcyclist presents to the emergency department with bilateral closed femoral fractures. He is placed in bilateral traction and admitted. Twenty-four hours later, he is confused and tachypneic. The most likely diagnosis is:
   a. Pulmonary embolism.
   b. Myocardial infarction.
   c. Fat embolism.
   d. Urinary tract infection.
   e. Stroke.

8. The most common primary bone malignancy is:
   a. Osteosarcoma.
   b. Synovial sarcoma.
   c. Multiple myeloma.
   d. Malignant fibrous histiocytoma.
   e. Chondrosarcoma.

9. The position in which a patient with a posterior dislocation of the hip holds the affected extremity is:
   a. Abducted, flexed, and externally rotated.
   b. Abducted, flexed, and internally rotated.
   c. Adducted, flexed, and internally rotated.
   d. Adducted, flexed, and externally rotated.
   e. Abducted, extended, and internally rotated.

10. Which of the following types of childhood Salter fractures of long bones is associated with the highest likelihood of subsequent growth arrest?
    a. Type I.
    b. Type II.
    c. Type III.
    d. Type IV.
    e. Type V.

11. The most important diagnostic test in an adolescent with knee pain and normal knee radiographs is:
    a. Ipsilateral hip radiographs.
    b. Ipsilateral femur radiographs.
    c. AP pelvis.
    d. Bilateral hip radiographs.
    e. Ipsilateral tibia radiographs.

12. A young female patient presents with pain with an L5 radiculopathy and weakness of the extensor hallucis longus on the right. The level of the herniated disc most likely is:
    a. L2–3.
    b. L3–4.
    c. L4–5.
    d. L5–S1.

SELECTED REFERENCES

Crenshaw AH. *Campbell's operative orthopedics,* 8th ed, vol 4. St. Louis: CV Mosby, 1991.

Denis F. The three column spine and its significance in the classification of acute thoracolumbar spinal injuries. *Spine* 1983;8:817.

Evarts CMcC. *Surgery of the musculoskeletal system.* New York: Churchill-Livingstone, 1990.

Goris RJ, Gimbrere JS, Van-Niekerk JL, Shoots FJ, Booy LH. Early osteosynthesis prophylactic mechanical ventilation in the multitrauma patient. *J Trauma* 1982;22:895.

Gustilo RB, Anderson JT. The prevention of infection in the treatment of one thousand and twenty-five open fractures of long bone. *J Bone Joint Surg Am* 1976;58:453.

Hoppenfeld S. *Physical examination of the spine and extremities.* Norwalk, CT: Appleton-Century-Crofts, 1976.

Riska EB, Myllyen P. Fat embolism in patients with multiple injuries. *J Trauma* 1982;11:891.

29

Selected Principles of Plastic Surgery

Robert D. Goldstein, Bruce Greenstein, and Robert Bibi

This chapter deals with the various aspects of hand surgery and principles of soft tissue coverage.

HAND ANATOMY

Surface Anatomy

The surface anatomy of the hand is separated into a volar surface and a dorsal surface. The thenar musculature relates to the thumb and the hypothenar musculature to the little finger. Starting proximally, the joints are called the metacarpophalangeal (MCP) joint, proximal interphalangeal (PIP) joint, and distal interphalangeal (DIP) joint. The thumb does not have a joint. Full motion at the MCP joint is approximately 85 degrees, at the PIP joint 110 degrees, and at the DIP joint 65 degrees.

Nerve Supply to the Hand

The median nerve innervates the pronator muscles (teres and quadratus), two of the three wrist flexors (flexor carpi radialis, palmaris longus), all of the superficialis tendons, the two radial flexor profundus tendons (index and long), the flexor pollicis longus, the thenar intrinsic muscles (abductor pollicis brevis, opponens pollicis, and one-half of the flexor pollicis brevis), and the radial two lumbrical muscles. Its sensory distribution is to the radial three and one-half digits (thumb, index, long, and radial half of the ring finger).

The ulnar nerve supplies innervation to one wrist flexor (flexor carpi ulnaris), the two ulnar flexor profundi (ring and little), and all the remaining intrinsic muscles of the hand, including the hypothenar musculature (abductor, opponens, flexor digiti V), the interossei, the little and ring lumbricals (the adductor pollicis and one-half of the flexor brevis), and the palmaris brevis. Its sensory branches supply the dorsum of the ring and little fingers as well as the palmar aspect of the little and ulnar border of the ring finger.

The radial nerve supplies all of the extensor muscles of the hand and wrist, including the abductor pollicis longus and the supernator of the hand, the triceps, and the branchioradialis muscles. It has a dorsal sensory branch to the dorsum of the thumb, index, and long fingers.

Sensibility in the hand is best tested by moving two-point discrimination. Median intrinsic function is best demonstrated by thumb opposition (bringing the thumb out of the plane of the rest of the hand). Ulnar intrinsic muscles are tested by crossing the index and long fingers over each other or abducting and adducting the little finger.

Tendons of the Hand

Muscles that power the hand are divided into extrinsic muscles (having their muscle bellies in the forearm and tendon insertion in the hand) and intrinsic muscles (having their origin and insertion within the hand). The extrinsic muscles include the long extensor tendons, which are arranged in six compartments on the dorsum of the wrist. They are essentially MCP joint extenders.

The superficial flexor tendons function as PIP joint flexors, and the profundus tendons function as DIP joint flexors.

The intrinsic muscles include the thenar muscles (the abductor pollicis brevis, which is the most superficial and important for opposition; the opponens pollicis, which rotates the thumb; the flexor pollicis brevis; and the adductor pollicis), the lumbrical muscles, the interosseous muscles, and the hypothenar muscles. The MCP joints are flexed by the intrinsics. The lumbrical muscles have their origin from the profundus tendon and insertion into the dorsal expansion. They function to flex the MCP joint and extend the interphalangeal joint.

Sublimis function is tested by stopping the motion of the distal joints of the fingers on each side of the finger being tested as the finger is flexed. The common profundus tendons are then blocked in extension. Profundus function is tested by blocking superficialis function by holding the middle phalanx extended.

Vascular Anatomy

The hand and fingers are supplied by a deep and a superficial vascular arch. The deep arch is the dominant arch. The ulnar artery is the dominant arterial supply to the hand in 80% of cases. Adequacy of hand circulation is checked by capillary refill in each fingertip and the Allen test. For the Allen test both arteries are occluded at the wrist. After flexion and extension of the fingers several times, each artery is released separately, and circulation is monitored by the appearance of capillary refill to all of the five digits.

FLEXOR TENDON INJURIES

We have witnessed a revolution in the management of flexor tendon pathology, especially treatment of injuries in the region of the digital fibrous sheath, popularly classified as "no man's land." Flexor tendon injuries may be defined by various zones of injury that are used to describe and manage tendon injuries at different anatomic locations.

Zone V Injuries

Zone V injuries are those in the forearm. Repairs at this level often yield favorable results because the intramuscular location of the tendons and the generous supply of adventitial tissues allow good motility.

Zone IV Injuries

Zone IV injuries are in the carpal tunnel. Injuries at this level are problematic because the tendons are in a tightly closed space, and often there are associated neurovascular injuries, especially to the median nerve.

In general, when all the superficial and deep flexors are cut at the same level, only the index superficial and deep tendons are repaired. The purpose is to avoid adherence of the superficialis to the profundus tendons, resulting in tendon excursion limited to that of the shorter superficial flexors.

Zone III Injuries

Zone III injuries are those in the palm between the carpal tunnel and the first annular pulley (the start of the digital fibrous sheath). The results of repairs at this level are reasonably good (although not as good as in the forearm), and all tendons can be repaired at this level, especially if the deep and superficial flexors have been cut at different locations.

Zone II Injuries

Zone II injuries are in "no man's land." This is the region of the tight digital fibrous sheath extending from the first annular pulley at the MCP joint to the insertion of the sublimis tendon after its decussation onto the middle phalanx. Experienced surgical management of injuries at this location and patient compliance with a carefully prescribed postoperative therapeutic regimen are critical if optimal results are to be obtained. In the past, injuries at this level were reconstructed exclusively with the secondary use of tendon grafts, often involving multiple, staged procedures including sheath reconstruction with a Silastic rod.

Studies of tendon healing and nutrition at this level have demonstrated the importance of atraumatic handling of tissues and careful preservation of both the vascular and synovial tendon nutritional sources. Thus handling of tendons is via their cut ends, and repairs with minimal compression are performed. Proper suture placement, preservation of vincula, repair of both superficialis and deep tendons, and sheath closure must all be considered if primary repairs are to be done at this level.

Postoperatively, the patient is splinted and subjected to a vigorous hand therapy regimen. Most commonly, dynamic traction is utilized following repairs. Limited active extension results in reflex flexor muscle relaxation, allowing the range of motion of the repaired flexor tendon through the sheath. This circumscribed range of motion limits the formation of adhesions. The finger is passively returned to a flexed position via a rubber band sutured to the nail and attached to the volar dressing. A passive range of motion technique performed daily by experienced therapists has also been utilized recently, with reported results similar to those ascribed to dynamic traction techniques. The use of dynamic traction or controlled passive notion by experienced hand surgeons (or both) has resulted in significant improvement in the results of primary repairs in zone II injuries.

Ruptured repairs, joint contractures, and adhesions remain significant complications. Secondary surgery requiring tenolysis or staged tendon grafts (or both) may be required to salvage satisfactory results in this region.

The best results for primary repairs of tendon grafts are in the 12- to 50-year age group. Tendon grafts are almost always performed in multiple stages, with excision of the scarred tendon and sheath and preservation of as many pulleys as possible, especially the critical arcuate (A2) pulley at the proximal portion of the proximal phalanx and the middle phalangeal arcuate (A4) pulley, and placement of a Silastic rod. At any time after 6 weeks, when satisfactory passive range of motion has returned, the rod may be replaced with a tendon graft, usually either a palmaris or plantaris tendon.

Zone I Injuries

Zone I injuries are distal to the insertion of the superficialis tendons and are therefore limited to the profundus tendon. If adequate distal length of tendon is present, end-to-end repairs are performed. Otherwise, tendon advancement of up to 1 cm is accomplished. In the latter case, a trough is made in the distal phalanx, and the proximal cut end of the profundus tendon is advanced into it. Reasonable results can be anticipated with carefully performed repairs at this level.

Flexor tendon repairs should be undertaken only when wound conditions are satisfactory. Ideally, repairs are performed within 1 week through a closed, healing, noninfected wound.

EXTENSOR TENDON INJURIES

Mallet Finger

The mallet finger may be a result of either an open or closed injury. Either a laceration of the dorsum of the DIP joint or forced flexion of an actively extended finger may result in loss of full extension of the distal joint. A closed injury with a large associated fracture (30% of the joint surface) may require reduction and fixation of the fracture. Open lacerations are sutured, including repair of the severed tendon. Following repairs, the fingers are splinted. Closed injuries without major fractures and late open injuries may be treated successfully by splinting in extension for a period of 6 weeks to 3 months. This regimen yields relatively uniformly good results, only rarely requiring secondary operative repairs. Untreated late mallet fingers may result in swan-neck deformities, where the PIP joint is hyperextended and the DIP joint is held in flexion. Repairs of this deformity are complex.

Boutonnière or Buttonhole Deformity

The boutonnière deformity is a result of an open or closed injury to the extensor tendon over the middle phalanx or PIP joint. This injury allows the lateral bands to slip volar to the PIP joint axis. The extensor mechanism shifts proximally, resulting in DIP joint hyperextension and PIP joint flexion. Early injuries may be treated with prolonged periods of splinting in extension because the extensor tendons are capable of healing via the formation of functional scar. Several techniques for secondary surgical repairs have been described, the simplest involving shortening of the functional scar and repair of the tendon.

Extensor Tendon Injuries of the Hand, Wrist, and Forearm

Injuries at the level of the hand, wrist, and forearm are repaired end to end. Because of intertendinous attachments, such tendons are held in place and do not tend to retract. Late repairs of finger extensor tendons are possible several weeks after injury. An exception is the extensor pollicis longus tendon. Here, early repair is critical because permanent early retraction of the tendons can occur. The prognosis following repair of isolated extensor injuries is good. When they are associated with other injuries such as fractures of the metacarpals and digits, adhesions that are difficult to treat may result.

INFECTIONS

All infections of the hand are considered serious because severe functional and aesthetic deformities may result. Infections in the hand tend to be "closed-space" infections with little room for collections of large quantities of pus. Delayed recognition and treatment may result in osteomyelitis, skin necrosis, and amputation. In general, antibiotics play a supportive role to adequate surgical drainage and débridement. Splinting of infected hands and digits has been shown to increase the speed of resolution of infectious problems. Prolonged rehabilitation therapy following an infection may be necessary to avoid unfortunate sequelae.

Paronychia

Paronychia, an infection of the soft tissues around the fingernail, is usually caused by *Staphylococcus aureus*. Long-standing chronic paronychia is often fungal in origin. The tissue around the nail is usually red, swollen, and painful. Direct incision into the abscess just above the nail is often adequate to treat these infections. Rarely, it is necessary to raise a flap of skin overlying the proximal nail fold, where damage to the ger-

minal matrix of the nail may result in severe ungual deformity. Improperly treated paronychia may result in felons and osteomyelitis. In diabetics, paronychia and felons are serious infections. Careful follow-up observation is necessary. Hospital admission and intravenous antibiotics should be considered in these cases.

Felon

Felons are pulp space infections of the digits, often caused by *Staphylococcus aureus*. Tight septa attach the volar tip skin of the digits to the terminal phalanges, dividing the fat pad into multiple compartments. Adequate drainage requires division of these septa to open all of the involved spaces. A popular incision is a subungual "hockey stick" type, extending from the anterodistal border of one side of the fingertip around to the proximal portion of the nail on the opposite side, with the incision carried down to the bone. Proper placement of the incision is critical to divide all of the septa and to avoid necrosis of the fat pad. Improperly treated felons can result in osteomyelitis of the terminal phalanx.

GRAVE INFECTIONS OF THE HAND

Acute Suppurative Tenosynovitis

The digital fibrous sheath is a tight, closed compartment. Small quantities of pus present in the tendon sheath manifest dramatically. Kanavel's classic signs for the recognition of tenosynovitis are (a) swelling of the involved digit, (b) exquisite pain with passive extension, (c) tenderness elicited by palpation over the sheath, and (d) the patient maintaining the finger in slight flexion (to avoid extension). Because of the relation of the little finger and thumb to the ulnar and radial bursae, respectively, infections of these digits may spread to the wrist. The classic horseshoe abscess involves the spread of infection from the ulnar to the radial bursa. *Staphylococcus aureus* is the most common causative organism, although mixed infections have become more common.

Treatment involves the employment of intravenous antibiotics and surgical drainage. Drainage with continuous irrigation has been used successfully. A multiply perforated catheter is placed into the sheath via a palmar incision. A counterincision is made over the lateral aspect of the distal phalanx. The catheter is irrigated for 48 hours with a continuous drip of plain or antibiotic saline solution, after which the catheter is withdrawn. Most patients have done well with this therapy. For late neglected infections, wide drainage and excision of necrotic tissues occasionally are necessary.

Midpalmar and Thenar Space Infections

A fascial septum extending from the third metacarpal to the palmar fascia at the level of the long finger separates the midpalmar and thenar spaces. The posterior border of the thenar space is the adductor pollicis muscle. The midpalmar space posterior border is the interosseous muscles, and the flexor tendons of the ulnar three digits are the anterior boundary. Infections in this area manifest as dorsal swelling, pain, tenderness, and occasionally palmar erythema or fluctuance.

Thenar space infections are drained via a dorsal incision of the first web space. A transverse palmar incision is made at the points of fluctuance, parallel to the distal palmar crease, to drain a palmar abscess. Drains are placed, and intravenous antibiotics are used as an adjunct. Again, the most common causative organism is *Staphylococcus aureus*. The infection may be a sequela of acute tenosynovitis of the long and ring fingers.

Superficial Lymphangitis

Following an abrasion or superficial puncture wound of the hand, a rapidly spreading superficial lymphangitis may develop in 24 to 48 hours. The hallmark of this entity is red streaking, extending from the point of injury linearly up the forearm and arm. Constitutional symptoms and general signs of infection may be present, such as fever, tachycardia, and leukocytosis. Most infections are due to *Staphylococcus aureus* or streptococci. Dog bites may become infected with *Pasteurella multocida,* which requires penicillin for treatment. When treating human bites, one must be aware of the possibility of *Eikenella* infections, which usually require treatment with a cephalosporin. Infections secondary to herpes simplex (herpetic whitlow) show signs of vesicle formation. No surgical treatment is indicated, and generally the goal of therapy is to prevent secondary infection. Without secondary infection, there is usually a self-limiting process.

VOLKMANN ISCHEMIC CONTRACTURE

Volkmann ischemic contracture is the result of a cascade of pathology in which arterial or venous insufficiency to the musculature in the relatively tight fascial compartments of the arm and forearm result in muscle swelling and necrosis, in turn causing secondary fibrosis and contracture. Three are sensory disturbances and motor weakness. Normal compartment pressures are 0 to 8 mm Hg; with a compartment syndrome, these pressures rise to 30 to 50 mm Hg. The etiology of Volkmann-type injuries includes massive crush, supercondylar fractures of the elbow, elbow dislocations, high-pressure injection injury, crush injury, emboli, snake bite, and radial and ulnar fractures. The classic deformity in this syndrome is flexion contracture of the wrist and all five digits. Claw hand deformity secondary to intrinsic paralysis is present, as are median and ulnar nerve sensory changes.

Prevention of the secondary deformities of Volkmann ischemic contracture requires adequate and expeditious fasciotomy. This often means decompression of the carpal tunnel, the volar forearm (both the superficial and deep compartments), the dorsal musculature, and the intrinsic muscles of the hand.

FINGERTIP INJURIES

When treating fingertip injuries, one goal is to obtain the earliest possible healing in the simplest fashion. The best functional and aesthetic results are also goals of treatment of these injuries. At first, one should always consider the simplest method of closure. This frequently involves débridement of the amputated tip skin and suturing this portion on as a full-thickness skin graft harvested from the hypothenar area, lateral border of the foot, or thigh may be used. Grafts are applicable only in those settings where significant amounts of exposed bone are not present or when débridement of exposed bone may result in only minimal shortening of the involved digit. In the case of the thumb, length is critical for function, and every effort should be made to preserve functional length.

When wound conditions do not allow simple coverage techniques, local flaps must be considered. In the case of tangential injuries with exposed bone and shortage of volar skin, bilateral laterally based V–Y advancement flaps (Kutler) should be considered to cover the fingertip. In cases where there is sufficient volar skin and the flap does not cross the flexion crease, volar V–Y advancement flaps (Kleinert–Atasoy) are performed for closure of amputations. These flaps are based on subcutaneous pedicles and can be considered neurovascular island flaps. They must be performed properly to ensure appropriate flap viability and maintenance of sensibility.

If local flaps do not suffice, regional flaps are considered. These are cross-finger flaps, thenar flaps, and, of special utility in the thumb, volar advancement flaps, as described by Moberg and Snow. The volar flaps involve elevation of the entire volar skin via bilateral midaxial incisions and advancement with the thumb held in mild to moderate flexion. After healing, the thumb can be stretched out to full extension. These flaps are safest in the thumb, where a sufficient blood supply limits the risk of dorsal skin necrosis and the flexed position is least likely to result in capsular joint contracture.

If regional flaps are not available, distant flaps should be considered, transferred either as pedicled flaps (such as the groin flap) or as free vascularized flaps. The temporal fascial flap has gained popularity for coverage of large hand defects. It causes minimum donor-site deformity and can provide thin, broad coverage for the hand; it requires microsurgical techniques.

In the case of fingertip amputations in children, allowing secondary healing should be considered in cases where skin is not available for amputated specimens, because the final healed result may equal that of grafted digits. Donor-site deformity is eliminated in these cases, even if prolonged healing time is needed.

Crush injuries to the fingertip that result in subungual hematomas and distal fingertip fractures require removal of the nail plate for exploration of the nail bed. The disrupted nail bed must be repaired to ensure normal nail growth.

TRAUMATIC AMPUTATIONS

Digital amputations are a common work-related injury and are frequent emergency treatment dilemmas. With the advent of successful digital neurovascular repairs performed under microscopic magnification, functional recovery of replanted parts has significantly altered the outlook for patients with mutilating devascularizing injuries. General indications for replantation

are multiple digital amputations, thumb amputations, and single-digit amputations in young patients or those with special occupational requirements.

In general, amputations of border digits (index and little finger at the level of zone II, or "no man's land"), severe crush or contamination, and patients with medical illnesses that contraindicate the long surgical intervention and anesthesia necessary are not replantation candidates. Proper handling of the amputated parts prior to transfer to replantation centers is critical if microvascular repairs are to be attempted. The amputated specimens should be transported with the patient, even if deemed unreplantable, because they can often be utilized for "spare parts" such as vein, skin, and nerve grafts.

Because of the severe functional disability associated with major amputations, attempts should be made to replant these parts when feasible if they have not been subjected to prolonged warm ischemic periods.

HAND DISORDERS

Carpal Tunnel Syndrome

The median nerve, along with the nine flexor tendons to the digits, passes through the carpal tunnel underneath the transverse carpal ligament at the wrist. Carpal tunnel syndrome is a compression neuropathy and may be associated with pregnancy, rheumatoid arthritis, wrist fractures, diabetes, thyroid disease, and chronic renal failure. Most cases are idiopathic.

Patients complain of numbness and tingling in the radial three and one-half digits (i.e., thumb, index, long, and radial border of the ring finger). Often the pain occurs at night and is relieved by dependency. In cases of long duration, there can be thenar wasting secondary to muscular atrophy. Tapping over the wrist may produce an "electric shock" type of response over the median nerve with paresthesias (positive Tinel sign). For Phalen's test, the wrist is held in flexion for 1 minute, eliciting symptoms. Nerve conduction studies and electromyography, when performed, demonstrate slowing of nerve conduction and denervation activity in involved muscles (fasciculations, fibrillations).

In early cases with sensory involvement, only splinting and local injection of steroids may be needed. Long-standing cases and those with motor involvement are treated surgically. An incision is made ulnar to the thenar crease in the palm. It may be continued onto the distal forearm for a short distance by an incision that crosses the wrist crease at a 60-degree angle. The nerve is identified in the proximal portion of the incision and protected as the transverse carpal ligament is opened from the wrist to the superficial palmar arch. The anterior epineurium is split until a normal fascicular pattern is noted pouting out of the nerve (external neurolysis). Internal dissection (internal neurolysis) is reserved by most surgeons for treatment failures. A tenosynovectomy of the neighboring flexor tendons is performed.

Stenosing Tenosynovitis (Trigger Finger)

Any of the five digits may be involved in stenosing tenosynovitis. Snapping of the flexor tendon as it passes under the first annular pulley located at the level of the MCP joint is the early sign of the syndrome. Often the involved digit starts locking in flexion, as the thickened tendon catches under the pulley. The tendon may be painful to palpation at the MCP joint.

Treatment initially consists in steroid injection underneath the involved pulley and splinting. If this fails, surgery is performed through a small transverse incision, usually located in the distal palmar crease. The first annular pulley is identified and then divided.

DeQuervain Syndrome

DeQuervain syndrome is most often a nonspecific tenosynovitis, as are carpal tunnel syndrome and trigger finger. The first dorsal wrist compartment tendons, the abductor pollicis longus and extensor pollicis brevis, are involved. Pain over the area of the radial styloid that may radiate up the arm and down to the thumb is present. The pain is elicited by active use of the thumb when grasping and may be demonstrated by the Finklestein test. With a positive Finklestein test, pain is produced when the thumb is grasped by the other digits and the wrist is ulnar-deviated.

Splinting and a steroid injection are tried as the first therapeutic modality. If these fail, the first dorsal compartment is decompressed surgically. A transverse incision is made over the radial styloid, with care taken to avoid injury to the radial nerve sensory branches. A linear incision is made through the dorsal carpal ligament, and the tendons are removed from the compartment.

Ganglions

Ganglions are the most common tumors of the hand. They are cystic lesions that arise from joints and tendon sheaths. The most common ganglions are dorsoradial, volar wrist ganglions, and retinacular cysts of the flexor tendon sheaths. Ganglions may cause pain and cosmetic deformities. They can be distinguished from solid masses by transillumination. Dorsal wrist ganglions almost always arise from the scapholunate ligament.

Operative treatment involves complete excision, including the attachment to the ligament, which is removed by cutting a window of tissue surrounding it in the scapholunate ligament, thus leaving an opening into the joint. Care must be taken to avoid injuries to the radial sensory nerve branches coursing over near these ganglions. Volar radial ganglions should be distinguished from arterial lesions, such as radial artery aneurysms. When there are strong suspicions of vascular pathology, investigative studies such as technetium-99m flow studies or ultrasonography may be able to distinguish the ganglion from the vascular lesion.

Glomus Tumors

Glomus tumors are characteristically found subungually in the hand; and although there are nonpainful lesions of this kind, they are rare. Most glomus tumors are associated with paroxysmal, severe, radiating pain. Subungual lesions may be exceptionally small and difficult to locate. Occasionally, they are visible only as a small area of salmon or bluish discoloration underneath the nail. They are derivatives of the glomus body, a normal arteriovenous anastomosis, and are benign lesions.

These tumors require surgical excision. Attempts should be made to preserve the overlying nail bed during operative removal to minimize postoperative nail deformity.

Dupuytren Contracture

Dupuytren contracture is a proliferation and contracture of bands of the palmar aponeurosis between the skin and the flexor tendons. It occurs most frequently in the ring and little fingers. It begins as a nodule and progresses to include fibrous bands extending to the digits, pulling them down into a flexed position. It is a slow process and is generally painless and nonulcerating. The condition affects only extension, not flexion. The fibrous process closely involves the digital nerves. Dupuytren contracture is generally thought to be hereditary and not work-related. The disease occurs in a male/female ratio of approximately 8:1.

Patients with Dupuytren diathesis are diagnosed by (a) a strong family history, (b) early age of onset, (c) ectopic areas of involvement such as Peyronie disease of the penis and contractures of the foot, and (d) associated diseases such as epilepsy, alcoholism, cirrhosis, pulmonary tuberculosis, and diabetes. The disease is often bilateral and associated with knuckle pads on the dorsum of the hand.

Management is conservative early on, with stretching exercises and therapy. The tabletop test is useful for determining the timing of surgical intervention: Operation is indicated when the patient is unable to flatten his or her hand on a tabletop. In the patient without the diathesis, conservative surgery often suffices. It consists of a subtotal fasciectomy. A longitudinal incision is made over the band of contracture, and the involved tissue is excised after careful identification and preservation of the digital neurovascular bundles, the incision is then closed with multiple Z-plasties.

Total fasciectomy is performed in patients with a diathesis, by removing the entire palmar aponeurosis, including resection into the involved fingers. Skin grafts may be necessary. An open technique was designed by McCash to avoid palmar hematomas after extensive dissection. The incisions are left open following fasciectomy, and during the 4 to 6 weeks, of secondary healing the patient is involved in an exercise regimen and dressing changes. In the usual case the patient is splinted for a week postoperatively, and active range of motion is started upon removal of the splint.

PRINCIPLES OF SOFT TISSUE COVERAGE

The decisions that concern appropriate wound closure include such factors as the site of tissue loss, the presence of contamination or infection, the exposure of underlying vital structures, the need to perform pre- or postoperative radiation therapy, or the need to perform secondary procedures in the same operative field.

Free Skin Grafts

A skin graft is a segment of dermis and epidermis that has been completely separated from its blood supply and donor-site attachment before being transferred to another area of the body. Skin grafts are generally classified according to their thickness. Split-thickness skin grafts include the epidermis and part of the dermis. This graft is versatile and popular, and it is likely to survive on its recipient site. The donor site heals rapidly by reepithelialization, and large amounts of donor material can be obtained with little morbidity. Its main disadvantage is that it undergoes a greater degree of soft tissue contracture; and, depending on its thickness, hair follicles and sebaceous glands may not be included in the graft.

Full-thickness skin grafts comprise the entire thickness of the skin, both the dermis and the epidermis. Because of its thickness, this type of graft is less likely to take and is slower to vascularize. It requires optimal conditions for complete take. In its favor, it has less tendency to undergo contracture and generally gives a superior cosmetic result.

Initial graft take is by diffusion of nutrients from the bed to the skin graft. Vascular inoculation can be completed within 48 to 72 hours, with capillary blood flow and neovascularization. Factors leading to graft loss include fluid collections, hematomas or seromas between the graft and the graft bed, shearing forces between the graft and the graft bed, an improper recipient bed, or bacterial contamination of more than 10^5 bacteria per gram of tissue.

Flaps

When conditions dictate that direct closure or skin graft is not appropriate, a flap is needed. A flap is a unit of tissue transferred from a donor site to a recipient site while maintaining a continuous blood supply through a vascular pedicle. Flaps can be defined by their blood supply or their donor tissue. Those defined by their blood supply include random-pattern flaps, axial-pattern flaps, myocutaneous flaps, and fasciocutaneous flaps. Those defined by their donor tissue include cutaneous flaps, myocutaneous flaps, or osseocutaneous flaps.

Flaps are preferred in the following situations: (a) for covering densely scarred areas or areas of functional stress; (b) for covering bone with poor padding; (c) for covering tendons (tendons must be placed in tissue that allows gliding); (d) for covering nerves; and (e) for areas where secondary surgical procedures may be necessary.

Random pattern flaps obtain their blood supply through the subdermal plexus of vessels and are generally limited to a length/width ratio of 1:1. Axial pattern flaps have a direct cutaneous axial vessel that supplies a segment of skin and can be raised to much longer length/width ratios (3:1). Myocutaneous flaps have their skin supplied via myocutaneous perforators from the deep axial vessels supplying the muscle. The underlying muscle provides bulk and a filler for soft tissue deadspace and ensures an adequate blood supply to the overlying skin.

Soft Tissue Expansion

It is well known that skin, both dermis and epidermis, has the ability to contract and stretch. Advantage can be taken of this phenomenon in a controlled fashion through the technique of soft tissue expansion. With this technique a deflated Silastic balloon is placed underneath normal skin adjacent to an area that must be removed. Over a period of time, the balloon is inflated with saline injections, thereby stretching the skin over the balloon. Enough skin can be generated to allow movement of the skin, to remove the adjacent tissue, and to cover the defect.

During the course of soft tissue expansion, a number of changes can be expected. There is thickening and hyperplasia of the epidermis, with increased melanocytic activity. There is thinning and increased collagen synthesis in the dermis. The adipose tissue is the most sensitive and shows compression, with either necrosis or some contour deformities that may be permanent. Muscle function is retained during soft tissue expansion, but there may be thinning and compression of the muscles. There is an enhancement of the vascularity to the overlying skin, which has been demonstrated by the increase in capillaries, arterioles, and venules. Finally, with respect to the dermal appendages, there seem to be no changes in hair follicles, sebaceous glands, sweat glands, sensory nerves, and end receptors.

QUESTIONS

Select one answer.

1. Injuries to the profundus tendon can be missed if:
   a. The median nerve has been cut along with the tendon.
   b. The wrist is not held in neutral position while testing the flexor tendons.
   c. The superficialis tendons are not blocked by holding the middle phalanx extended.
   d. All of the above.
2. The adequacy of the circulation of the hand is determined by:
   a. Finkelstein maneuver.
   b. Addison maneuver.
   c. Allen test.
   d. Phalen's test.
3. Primary repair of flexor tendons in "no man's land" is successful when:
   a. Both superficialis and deep tendons are repaired.
   b. The patient is allowed active extension and passive flexion during the postoperative period.
   c. When passive traction is utilized.
   d. All of the above.
4. When performing tendon surgery in "no man's land," the following pulleys are critical to preserve:
   a. A-2 and A-4 pulley.
   b. A-1 and A-3 pulley.
   c. Cruciate pulleys.
   d. All of the above.
5. Rupture of the extensor tendon at its insertion at the distal phalanx may result in:
   a. Mallet finger deformity.
   b. Recurvatum deformity.
   c. Swan-neck deformity.
   d. None of the above.
   e. All of the above.
6. Acute separative tenosynovitis:
   a. Is a closed-space infection in the distal pulp.
   b. Most commonly caused by *Streptococcus*.
   c. May present as a tender, swollen finger.
   d. Can usually be managed with intravenous antibiotics.
7. Contraindications to replantation of amputated digits include:
   a. A thumb in a young patient.
   b. A thumb in a 20-year-old manual laborer.
   c. A complete amputation of the hand at the level of the wrist.
   d. A complete amputation of the index finger at the level of the proximal phalanx.
   e. A gunshot wound to the hand.
8. Dupuytren contracture:
   a. Occurs most frequently in the ring and little finger.
   b. Is frequently thought to be a work-related condition.

c. Is frequently quite painful.

d. Prevents the patient from making a full fist.

9. A full-thickness skin graft:

   a. Shows a greater degree of contracture than a split-thickness skin graft.

   b. Shows a lesser degree of contracture than a split-thickness skin graft.

   c. Is used to cover exposed extensor tendon devoid of paratenon.

   d. Is more likely to take when the bacterial contamination is greater than 10^5 per gram.

10. The blood supply to the skin of a myocutaneous flap is derived from:

   a. The subdermal plexus of vessels.

   b. A named axial vessel.

   c. An unnamed axial vessel.

   d. Myocutaneous perforators.

11. In the course of soft tissue expansion, which of the following is most sensitive to the pressure forces of the expander?

   a. Muscle.

   b. Dermis.

c. Epidermis.

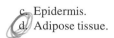

d. Adipose tissue.

SELECTED REFERENCES

Beasley RW. *Hand injuries.* Philadelphia: WB Saunders, 1981.

Burton RI, McFarland GB, et al. American Society for Surgery of the Hand: *The hand: examination and diagnosis,* 3rd ed. New York: Churchill Livingstone.

Flatt AE. *The care of minor hand injuries.* St. Louis: CV Mosby, 1972.

Flynn JE. *Hand surgery,* 3rd ed. Baltimore: Williams & Wilkins, 1982.

Georgiade N, Georgiade G. *Essentials of plastic, maxillofacial and reconstructive surgery,* 2nd ed. Baltimore: Williams & Wilkins, 1900.

Green DP. *Operative hand surgery.* New York: Churchill Livingstone, 1982.

Kaplan EB. *Functional and surgical anatomy of the hand,* 2nd ed. Philadelphia: JB Lippincott, 1965.

Lister G. *The hand: diagnosis and indications.* Edinburgh: Churchill Livingstone, 1977.

Smith JW, Sherrell JA, eds. *Grabb and Smith's plastic surgery,* 4th ed. Boston: Little, Brown and Company, 1991.

30

Urologic Surgery

Peter L. Stone

The general surgeon is often confronted with signs and symptoms that suggest pathologic processes involving the genitourinary system. During elective or emergency surgical procedures, unanticipated urologic conditions or problems may be encountered. Multiple trauma victims frequently present with gross or microscopic hematuria as the only manifestation of possibly severe urinary tract injury. Accurate diagnosis and appropriate management in such situations requires a fundamental knowledge of urologic conditions, surgical techniques, and available diagnostic tools. Such knowledge also helps minimize iatrogenic injury to genitourinary structures during unrelated general surgical procedures. This chapter reviews the more common urologic neoplasms and conditions, genitourinary injuries, and urologic emergencies. Clinical presentation, diagnosis, and treatment are emphasized.

RENAL MASSES

Cysts and Benign Tumors

Renal cysts are the most common mass lesions in the kidney, both clinically and at autopsy. Renal cysts are found in approximately 50% of individuals over the age of 50 and are of no clinical significance except to be distinguished from malignancy. Ultrasonography, computed tomography (CT), and magnetic resonance imaging (MRI) are highly accurate in diagnosing benign renal cysts. Occasionally, however, the benign nature of complex cysts (i.e., cysts with thickened or irregular walls, inhomogeneous fluid, calcifications, loculations) can be determined only by surgical excision. Although most renal cysts are asymptomatic, they may cause hematuria, pain, abscess formation, or calyceal or renal pelvic obstruction.

Adult polycystic kidney disease (APKD) is an autosomal dominant condition with a high degree of penetrance. Usually symptoms arise between the ages of 30 and 40. The most common initial symptom is pain in the lumbar region followed by hematuria. Liver cysts are found in approximately 30% of patients with APKD. APKD is also associated with a 10% to 20% incidence of cerebral aneurysm. Treatment, for the most part, is medical with regard to the associated progressive renal failure.

Angiomyolipoma is a benign renal hamartoma that can manifest clinically as pain, retroperitoneal hemorrhage, gross hematuria, or an abdominal mass. Bilateral or multiple angiomyolipomas are commonly associated with tuberous sclerosis, a clinical syndrome classically characterized by mental retardation, epilepsy, and sebaceous adenomas of the face. Solitary renal hamartomas are most often found in women between the ages of 40 and 60. These tumors are most accurately diagnosed by CT scan or MRI, both of which clearly demonstrate the characteristic fat content. An isolated symptomatic angiomyolipoma can be treated initially by angiographic embolization. If embolization fails, surgical removal is necessary.

Renal cortical adenoma, usually an incidental radiographic or autopsy finding, is the most common benign parenchymal neoplasm. By definition, benign renal adenomas are less than 3 cm in diameter. These neoplasms have a propensity to grow and eventually metastasize once they are more than 3 cm; they should be extirpated in patients with a life expectancy of more than 10 years.

Other benign renal tumors, such as fibroma, lipoma, cholesteatoma, leiomyoma, and hemangioma, are exceedingly uncommon. Because radiologic techniques are often inconclusive for defining such tumors, surgical removal is generally necessary and results in partial or total nephrectomy.

A functional renin-secreting juxtaglomerular tumor is rare. They are typically no larger than 2 to 3 cm in diameter and are often undetectable radiographically. Juxtaglomerular tumor should be suspected in a young patient with hypertension, hyperaldosteronism, and high serum renin levels. A high differential renal vein renin ratio confirms the diagnosis.

Malignant Tumors

Renal cell carcinoma (clear cell adenocarcinoma) accounts for approximately 3% of adult malignancies, with a 2 : 1 male/female ratio. A higher incidence occurs in chronic hemodialysis patients, those with adult polycystic kidney disease, and those with von Hippel-Lindau disease, in which multiple and bilateral renal carcinomas are characteristic.

The classic clinical triad of pain, hematuria, and flank mass occurs in no more than 10% of cases. Associated clinical disturbances include erythrocytosis caused by excessive erythropoietin production, hypercalcemia, hypertension, fever, and weight loss. Hepatic dysfunction in the absence of hepatic metastases occurs in up to 20% of cases.

A suspicion of renal tumor is usually based on the excretory urogram, (intravenous pyelogram, IVP) or nephrosonogram; CT scanning without and with intravenous contrast is a highly sensitive diagnostic tool for renal carcinoma. With the advent of CT scanning, the indications for angiography have become limited to cases where parenchyma-sparing procedures are considered or where the CT findings are equivocal.

Renal cell carcinomas spread by direct extension and by invasion into adjacent structures and regional lymphatics. The most common sites of distant spread are the lungs, liver, and bone. Approximately one-third of patients initially present with metastatic disease. Renal carcinoma has a characteristic propensity for extension and occasionally invasion into the renal vein or inferior vena cava in the form of a tumor thrombus. This thrombus may extend as far cephalad as the right atrium without invading the vessel wall(s). It is now widely accepted that patients with caval extension and tumor otherwise confined to the kidney are amenable to surgical cure. MRI has the capacity to demonstrate exquisitely the extent of tumor thrombus in the venous system. Inferior venacavography is also useful except in cases where thrombus has occluded the inferior vena cava. Involvement of regional lymph nodes, extension through Gerota's fascia, invasion into adjacent organs, and distant metastases portend a poor prognosis.

Radical nephrectomy, which includes *en bloc* removal of the kidney, the surrounding perirenal fat, and the ipsilateral adrenal gland, continues to serve as the only effective treatment for renal cell carcinoma. Renal parenchyma-sparing procedures such as partial nephrectomy or tumor enucleation with an adequate margin are indicated in patients with a solitary kidney, synchronous bilateral renal cell carcinomas, or a poorly functioning contralateral kidney. Every attempt is made to remove tumor thrombus from the inferior vena cava, particularly if there is no evidence of tumor invasion elsewhere. Cardiopulmonary bypass may be required in cases with supradiaphragmatic or right atrial tumor thrombus extension.

The treatment of metastatic renal cell carcinoma in the form of chemotherapy or radiotherapy has been generally unsuccessful. Unusual with renal carcinomas, patients with a solitary metastatic lesion (e.g., bone, lung, brain) and tumor otherwise confined to the kidney have a 20% to 30% five-year survival after surgical removal of all tumor. Occasional partial regressions or significant stabilization of disease has resulted from treatment with vinblastine, CCNU, percutaneous angioinfarction, progesterone, and interferons. Investigations with monoclonal antibodies and interleukin-2/LAK therapies are hopeful.

Transitional cell carcinoma of the renal pelvis accounts for approximately 7% to 8% of renal tumors. An increased risk for the development of upper tract urothelial tumors is associated with Balkan nephropathy, analgesic abuse, and cigarette smoking. Squamous cell carcinoma of the upper tracts, though rare, is usually associated with chronic inflammation secondary to calculi, infection, or both. The treatment of choice for a localized transitional cell tumor of the renal pelvis is total nephroureterectomy with contiguous excision of a cuff of bladder mucosa.

Other primary renal tumors include sarcomas of all types, hemangiopericytoma, and oncocytoma. Of interest, oncocytomas are often histologically indistinguishable from the eosinophilic or granular cell types of renal adenocarcinomas. The electron microscopic finding of cells packed with mitochondria is pathognomonic for oncocytoma. Metastatic tumors in the profusely vascular renal parenchyma are not uncommon, particularly at autopsy. *lymphoma most common*

Discovery at Surgery

The general surgeon occasionally discovers an unsuspected renal mass or congenital renal anomaly at operation. All renal masses should be palpated thoroughly without opening Gerota's fascia. Further exploration is not warranted; a well planned workup can be performed postoperatively. Intraoperative puncture and aspiration of a renal mass should be confined to situations where a solid mass is highly suspected and is located in a region difficult to puncture via a percutaneous route. The importance of recognizing renal anomalies cannot be overstated. Ectopic, horseshoe, and pancake kidneys have been mistaken for pathologic processes and have been partially or completely excised.

PROSTATE

Prostatic Carcinoma

Prostatic carcinoma is the most common malignancy now clinically diagnosed in men. Second only to cancer of the lung, it accounts for 14% of cancer deaths in men in the United States. Afro-American men are affected almost twice as often as Caucasian men in the United States. About 75% to 80% of prostatic tumors are located in the periphery of the posterior region of the prostate and are often palpable by digital rectal examination (DRE). Any suspicious prostatic area should be biopsied via the transrectal or transperineal route. With the now common use of office-based transrectal ultrasonography (TRUS), US-guided biopsies are routine. The differential diagnosis of a prostatic nodule includes tuberculosis, granulomatous prostatitis, infarct, calculi, metastatic focus from another primary tumor, and postsurgical scarring. Management of prostatic carcinoma depends on the clinical stage of disease (Table 30.1). A staging workup consists of an excretory urogram with or without renal US, chest radiography, prostate-specific antigen (PSA) assay, bone scan, and routine blood work. Although the specificity and sensitivity are relatively low, gross pelvic lymph node involvement can be initially evaluated by pelvic CT or MRI.

The DRE in conjunction with a PSA assay (a protease produced by the prostatic epithelium) is the accepted method for initially detecting prostate cancer. The likelihood of prostatic malignancy generally increases as the PSA titer rises. It should be noted that benign prostatic hypertrophy (BPH) can also cause elevated PSA levels, on the order of up to 0.33 ng/mL for every gram of BPH. PSA can also be elevated in the presence of inflammation, urinary retention, infarction, and prostatic manipulation (cystoscopy, catheterization, biopsy). In two studies, a 4% to 9% positive biopsy rate was noted in men with normal PSA and DRE. The PSA assay is of most value when used as a comparative parameter over time (i.e., PSA velocity) in patients being treated for prostate cancer to assess treatment success and rate of progression.

Transrectal US is the definitive modality for measuring the size of the prostate or suspicious nodules and to detect extracapsular or seminal vesicle extension of cancer. TRUS is useful for detecting centrally or anteriorly situated foci of prostate cancer or suspicious areas. TRUS also allows accurately guided biopsies of suspicious or site-specific areas of the prostate.

Laparoscopic pelvic lymph node dissection offers a low-morbidity pathologic staging procedure for patients at high risk for stage D1 disease. Candidates with high risk factors for nodal spread such as poorly differentiated histology, PSA over 50 ng/mL, and evidence of capsular penetration are candidates for laparoscopic pelvic node dissection. Additionally, patients opting for

TABLE 30.1. *Staging prostatic carcinoma*

Description	Stage UICC, AJCC (1992)	Jewett
Disease localized to prostate, clinically unsuspected, incidental histologic finding	T1	A
Histology		
Well-differentiated tumor involving < 5% of resected tissue	T1a	A1
Moderately to poorly differentiated tumor or well-differentiated tumor involving > 5% of resected tissue	T1b	A2
Tumor identified by elevated PSA-prompted biopsy	T1c	A3
Nodule involvement		
Palpable prostatic nodule(s) confined to gland	T2	B
Half a lobe or less	T2a	B1
More than half a lobe but not both	T2b	
Tumor in both lobes	T2c	B2
Extension		
Tumor locally extending beyond capsule	T3	C
Metastases		
Distant metastases		D
Pelvic lymph nodes only	N1–3	D1
Bones, lung, etc.	M	D2

radical perineal prostatectomy, radioactive seed implantation, and external beam radiation with high suspicion of nodal disease may be staged laparoscopically.

More than 95% of prostate cancers are adenocarcinomas. The remaining 4% to 5% are considered ductal carcinomas arising from the central portion of the gland. Histologically, they are transitional cell, mixed, or endometrioid carcinomas.

Prostate cancer often causes few if any specific symptoms. Prior to the advent of PSA, up to 75% of men with prostate cancer were initially diagnosed with metastatic disease-related symptoms: bone pain, weight loss, sciatica, lower extremity edema, anemia, and azotemia. Hematuria, occurring in fewer than 15% of prostate cancer patients, is more commonly associated with infection and obstruction. Many patients present with bladder outlet obstructive symptoms that are commonly caused by coexisting BPH.

Prostate cancer spreads by local extension and by lymphatic and hematogenous routes. Extension into the urethra, seminal vesicles, and trigone is common with advanced disease. One or both ureteral orifices may become obstructed by invasion. In decreasing order of frequency, the obturator, hypogastric, external iliac, presacral, and paraaortic nodes may become involved. Blood-borne metastases are most common to bone and invariably are osteoblastic. The pelvis, lumbar spine,

femur, thoracic spine, and ribs are the most frequent sites of bone involvement. The most common visceral sites of metastasis are the lung and liver.

The appropriate therapy for patients with prostate cancer depends on the clinical stage of disease, the patient's life expectancy, and the patient's general medical condition. Curative surgical procedures are indicated in patients with tumor clinically confined to the prostate gland, who have a life expectancy of more than 10 to 15 years, and who are medically stable. Pelvic lymphadenectomy is performed in conjunction with (requiring frozen sections) or prior to definitive surgery employing the laparoscopic technique.

The retropubic or perineal approaches are the accepted forms of radical prostatectomy (prostatoseminal vesiculectomy). The most common complications are rectal injury, incontinence, impotence, and stricture at the vesicourethral anastomosis. A potency-sparing radical retropubic prostatectomy has gained wide acceptance. If the disease is organ-confined, the nerve-sparing procedure is associated with an approximately 90% fifteen-year survival rate. The overall return-of-potency rate is approximately 65%. Definitive external beam radiotherapy is reserved for similarly staged patients who are greater surgical risks or refuse surgery. The 1990s have seen a resurgence of interest in interstitial radioactive seed implantation therapy for prostate cancer. Irid-

*Surgery c̄ better survival ā radiation (p̄ breaks)
— but ∅ good studies   Rx*

ium-192 or palladium-103 seeds can be implanted via a transperineal approach utilizing US guidance as an ambulatory procedure. Long-term follow-up is not yet available to assess its treatment efficacy compared to the more traditional external beam therapy. The 15-year survival rate of men with comparably staged disease who receive radiotherapy is on the order of 65% to 75%. Many patients with a shorter life expectancy (less than 10 years) and low-stage, low-grade disease do well without any therapy ("wait and watch").

Normal prostatic cells and many populations of prostatic cancer cells are dependent on androgen to function. The goal of hormonal therapy for prostate cancer is to eradicate or inhibit androgenic stimulation of the tumor. Bilateral orchiectomy (surgical castration), equally effective injectable luteinizing hormone-releasing hormone (LHRH) agonists (medical castration), and less effective oral estrogens (diethylstilbestrol) act to decrease the level of circulating testosterone. Complete androgen ablation can be accomplished by adding oral flutamide or nilutamide, each of which inhibits the production of adrenal androgenic metabolites in surgically or medically castrated men. Hormonal manipulation is indicated in patients with evidence of metastatic disease or progression of the primary disease, or in patients unsuitable for surgery or irradiation.

Benign Prostatic Hypertrophy

Benign prostatic hypertrophy is probably the most common neoplasm in men; it is an almost universal phenomenon of aging. BPH originates exclusively from the periurethral prostatic tissue. As this benign adenomatous neoplasm enlarges, the surrounding normal prostatic tissue becomes compressed, eventually forming a "surgical" capsule. With enlargement comes prostatic urethral obstruction and its associated constellation of symptoms, often referred to as "prostatism." Obstructive symptoms include hesitancy, decreased force and caliber of the urinary stream, terminal or postvoid dribbling, a sense of incomplete emptying, and urinary retention. These problems must be considered separate from irritative voiding symptoms, such as dysuria, frequency, and urgency, which suggest infection or some other inflammatory process. Hematuria occurs much more commonly with BPH than with prostatic cancer.

The workup of a patient with suspected BPH includes urinalysis, urine culture, blood urea nitrogen and creatinine levels, PSA assay, acid phosphatase assay, and uroflometry. Excretory urography or renal and pelvic sonography can document upper tract changes, the presence of bladder calculi, the degree of bladder emptying, and the presence of intravesical prostatic enlargement. Cystourethroscopy is essential for accurately assessing the entire lower urinary tract prior to considering surgical intervention.

Patients with mild symptoms and no significant abnormalities on routine investigation require reassurance and yearly follow-up. Patients with more severe symptoms or evidence of bladder or upper tract deterioration require pharmacologic or surgical intervention. Indications for surgical intervention include renal failure due to obstructive uropathy, persistent hematuria, recurrent urinary tract infections, significant urinary retention, bladder calculi, and bothersome symptoms unresponsive to medical therapy.

The objective of the various surgical approaches is to enucleate the adenomatous neoplasm from the surrounding compressed prostatic tissue, which is to remain. Generally, open prostatectomy is reserved for patients with glands weighing more than 60 to 100 g, depending on the individual surgeon. Suprapubic prostatectomy through a bladder incision is most appropriate when a large intravesical median lobe, bladder calculi, or diverticula require removal or excision. Retropubic prostatectomy through a prostatic capsular incision is usually associated with less blood loss. Smaller glands can be resected via the transurethral route.

Transurethral resection of the prostate remains the gold standard of endoscopic prostatectomy. Newer endoscopic surgical approaches under investigation and use and at times the object of controversy include transurethral incision of the prostate, transurethral laser incision of the prostate, laser ablation, vaporization, transurethral microwave hyperthermia, and endoscopic insertion of a metal alloy prostatic stent.

Noninvasive pharmacologic regimens to alleviate symptoms and signs related to BPH objectively and subjectively must be discussed and offered to appropriate patients. Terazocin (1 to 10 mg qhs) or doxazocin (1 to 8 mg qhs) are α-adrenergic antagonists, traditionally used as antihypertensives, that have a significant, measurable effect on relaxing the urethral internal sphincter mechanism, which includes the smooth muscle within the prostate and bladder neck. Numerous studies have consistently shown dose-dependent improved symptomatic relief, improved urodynamic parameters, and limited side effects in men treated for symptomatic BPH. Finasteride, an α-reductase inhibitor, inhibits the transformation of testosterone to the more peripherally active form, dihydrotestosterone (DHT), thereby effecting DHT-sensitive organs such as the prostate. Finasteride 5 mg daily for a 4- to 6-month period decreases prostatic volume by an average 20% and objectively alleviates symptoms in about 50% of patients with acceptable minimal side effects.

BLADDER

Urothelial (transitional cell) carcinoma is the most common histologic type of bladder tumor (about 95%) and occurs three times more frequently in men than women. Proved and proposed etiologic agents include industrial chemicals such as benzidine and 2-naphthylamine, cigarettes, artificial sweeteners, coffee, phenacetin, cyclophosphamide, and pelvic irradiation. Most patients with transitional cell carcinoma initially present with superficial disease and usually do not progress to more invasive disease if followed and treated appropriately. The likelihood of recurrence increases in patients with multiple tumors, high-grade lesions, and urothelial cell changes, such as severe atypia or carcinoma *in situ* (CIS) in other areas of the bladder. Most of the patients with more aggressive, muscle-infiltrating tumors present *de novo* without a history of superficial disease.

Painless hematuria, microscopic or gross, is the most common presenting sign or symptom. Irritable bladder symptoms frequently occur in patients with invasive tumors. A routine workup consists in urine cytologic examination, an IVP to determine the presence of upper tract abnormalities, bimanual examination, and cytoscopy. After biopsies are done, the tumor may be resected, fulgurated, or ablated by Nd:YAG laser. Random bladder biopsy specimens are obtained to evaluate normal-appearing mucosa for urothelial atypia or CIS. Recurrent superficial tumors may be repeatedly resected, fulgurated, or ablated by laser. Intravesical instillation of bacille Calmette Guérin (BCG) has become a standard form of treating recurrent superficial tumors and CIS in properly selected patients. BCG and instillation of mitomycin C, doxorubicin, or thiotepa can markedly reduce the frequency of recurrences or eradicate the disease. Muscle-invading tumors require extirpative surgery. Segmental cystectomy is reserved for the solitary lesion in which a 2-cm tumor-free margin can be achieved. More diffuse, invasive disease with no evidence of metastatic spread requires radical cystectomy with pelvic lymph node dissection. Laparoscopic pelvic node dissection is indicated in patients at high risk for metastatic lymph node involvement. Those with positive nodes are spared cystectomy and can proceed with appropriate chemotherapeutic regimens.

Preoperative, neoadjuvant, cisplatin-based chemotherapeutic regimens (e.g., methotrexate, vinblastine, doxorubicin, cisplatin = MVAC) with or without preoperative radiotherapy has been shown to down-stage selected patients. Definitive radiotherapy is indicated in patients considered at high surgical risk or with a shortened life expectancy. Some patients refuse surgery in favor of radiotherapy despite its decreased effectiveness because voiding and sexual function are preserved. Conversely, potency/nerve-sparing procedures in conjunction with continent urinary diversion or ileal neobladder reconstruction have evolved to minimize postoperative quality of life changes in selected patients. Urethrectomy should be included in patients with involvement of the trigone or prostatic urethra, or with CIS; otherwise a 10% to 20% urethral recurrence rate can be expected.

Metastatic disease most commonly occurs in bone, lung, and liver. After radical cystectomy, 25% to 50% of patients with muscle-invading tumors develop metastatic disease within 3 to 5 years. Partial regression and control of the progression of metastatic disease has been achieved with various chemotherapeutic agents, most notably cisplatin-based regimens.

Approximately 5% of bladder carcinomas are of the squamous cell variety. Chronic infection or inflammation, chronic foreign body irritation, and schistosomiasis are associated with the development of squamous cell carcinoma of the bladder. Radical cystectomy is the most effective form of treatment, with the 5-year survival 15% to 50%. Adenocarcinoma represents fewer than 1% of bladder tumors. It typically arises from the trigone or from a urachal remnant at the bladder dome. A higher incidence occurs in patients with a history of bladder extrophy.

TESTICULAR NEOPLASMS

Testicular tumors are the most common solid tumors in men between the ages of 20 and 34 in the United

[handwritten at top: Ileal conduit – Hyperchloremic acidosis]

States. Seminoma, the most common histologic type, rarely occurs below the age of 10. Yolk sac tumors predominate during infancy and childhood. More than 90% of primary testicular malignancies are germinal tumors (seminoma, embryonal carcinoma, teratocarcinoma, teratoma, and choriocarcinoma). Simultaneous or metachronous bilateral testicular tumors occur in 2% to 3% of cases. Epidemiologic studies have calculated the risk of testicular cancer in cryptorchid patients to be 3 to 14 times the normal incidence. Among the patients with a history of cryptorchidism and subsequent development of testis tumor, approximately 20% develop a malignancy in the contralateral descended testis.

Most patients present with a painless nodule, swelling, or altered consistency of the testis. Approximately 10% of patients initially present with symptoms attributable to metastatic disease. Another 10% complain of a painful scrotal swelling that is frequently misdiagnosed and treated as epididymitis. Such patients should undergo exploration if no improvement occurs after 2 weeks of conservative management.

The most important diagnostic step is prompt radical orchiectomy through an inguinal incision. Specific serum tumor markers are measured prior to surgery: α-fetoprotein (AFP) produced by yolk sac cells, β-subunit of human chorionic gonadotropin (β-hCG) produced by syncytiotrophoblasts, and lactic acid dehydrogenase (LDH). Approximately 10% of patients with seminoma have an elevated β-hCG level; 90% of patients with nonseminomatous germ cell tumors have either or both AFP and β-hCG elevations. Following orchiectomy, persistent elevation of tumor marker levels strongly suggests residual tumor. Unfortunately, up to 20% of patients with postorchiectomy normalization of tumor marker levels develop metastatic disease.

The histology of the tumor and results of a metastatic workup determine subsequent management. Postorchiectomy evaluation consists of excretory urography, chest tomography or CT, abdominal CT scan, and tumor marker assays. Testicular tumors initially spread via the lymphatics. The primary lymphatic drainage of the right testis is to the interaortocaval nodes and right renal hilar region; the left testis drains into the paraaortic and left renal hilar areas.

Seminoma is exquisitely sensitive to radiation therapy. Postorchiectomy irradiation to the retroperitoneum and ipsilateral inguinopelvic regions (2500 to 3000 rad) in patients with seminoma produces a cure in up to 90% of cases with a negative metastatic workup (stage A).

TABLE 30.2. *Staging testicular tumors*

Stage	Description
A or II	Tumor limited to testis alone
B1 or IIA	Tumor involving retroperitoneal lymph node < 2 cm
B2 or IIB	Retroperitoneal lymph nodes 2–6 cm on CT
B3 or IIC	Retroperitoneal lymph nodes > 6 cm on CT
C or III	Tumor above the diaphragm or involving abdominal solid organs

[handwritten: lymphoma most common Testicular met in men >5t]

Stage B seminoma responds well to retroperitoneal irradiation and platinum-based combination chemotherapy. Stage C seminoma is treated with primary chemotherapy similar to that for nonseminomatous tumors. The staging of testicular tumors is outlined in Table 30.2.

Retroperitoneal lymph node dissection is indicated in patients with nonseminomatous germ cell tumors (NSGCTs) with a negative metastatic workup (stage A) or after adjuvant chemotherapy for stage B disease. Extremely compliant patients with organ-confined, stage A NSGCTs can be observed knowing that there is a 20% recurrence rate. These patients require an abdominal CT scan, chest radiography, and tumor markers every 3 months for the first 2 years followed by follow-up evaluations every 6 months for the next 3 years.

Combination chemotherapy with cisplatin, etoposide, and bleomycin (BEP) has remarkably improved overall and disease-free survival in patients with more advanced metastatic testicular cancer. A cure rate of approximately 50% can be achieved in patients with NSGCT involving multiple organs (stage C). Choriocarcinoma, which accounts for 3% of testicular tumors, has the worst prognosis, as it usually presents as a metastatic process.

GENITOURINARY TRAUMA

Renal Trauma

A high index of suspicion and accurate assessment of traumatic renal injuries allow maximal renal salvage and avoidance of complications from missed or delayed diagnosis. Approximately 5% to 10% of cases of penetrating abdominal trauma sustain renal injury. Conversely, 80% of patients with penetrating renal injuries have injuries to other intraabdominal organs such as liver, colon, spleen, and stomach (in decreasing order of frequency). Renal injury should be considered in any patient who sustains blunt trauma to the abdomen, lower chest, or spine. Such injury is most commonly secondary to motor vehicle accidents, falls, and contact sports. Renal injury following minor blunt trauma is not uncommon in patients with preexisting hydronephrosis, renal tumor, renal cystic disease, or vascular malformation. Rapid deceleration can cause disruption of the ureteropelvic junction and renal arterial intimal tear, resulting in thrombosis.

Several investigations with large numbers of patients have allowed more refined, organized criteria to emerge in the diagnosis and management of renal trauma. Radiographic evaluation, if feasible, is required for all patients with penetrating injuries to the abdomen with or without microscopic or gross hematuria. Radiographic imaging of the kidney has been found to be unnecessary in the adult patient with blunt trauma, stable blood pressure (over 90 mm Hg systolic), microscopic hematuria (fewer than 5 RBC/HPF), and no clinical indication of flank trauma (e.g., lower rib or lumbar transverse process fractures, flank bruises, seat-belt marks). All injured pediatric patients with any degree of hematuria must be assessed radiographically.

High-dose infusion excretory urography (IVP) remains the mainstay of diagnostic modalities for evaluating the upper urinary tract in trauma cases (Fig. 30.1). IVP often identifies the extent of injury and, equally important, documents the presence and function of the contralateral kidney. Major trauma, such as deep renal laceration, avulsion/fracture, or vascular occlusion is suggested by incomplete, poor, or nonvisualization of

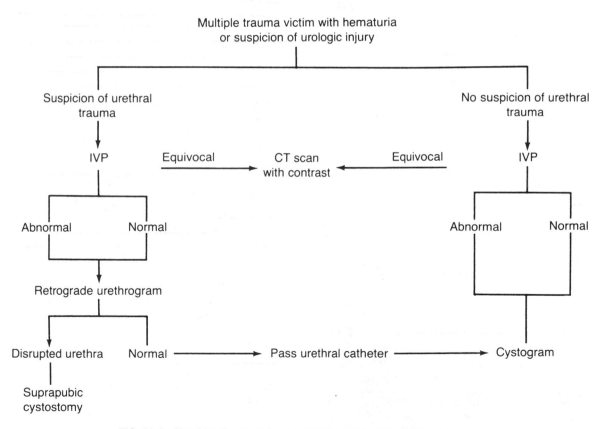

FIG. 30.1. Algorithm for urologic assessment of the multiple trauma victim.

the kidney. Relatively stable patients with an equivocal IVP require radiographic staging by CT scan, which is noninvasive, reliable, and extremely sensitive; other visceral injuries are better delineated as well. In trauma patients, where abdominal CT is indicated for other reasons, an IVP is unnecessary. Complete nonvisualization of the kidney on IVP, although often because of benign contusion with subcapsular hematoma, requires further evaluation. Contrast CT scan can exquisitely document perfused renal parenchyma. Invasive, time-consuming angiography is indicated only when CT scanning is unavailable or is necessary to evaluate some other injury.

Almost all patients with penetrating renal injuries require surgical exploration because of the need to assess and repair associated visceral injuries. The occasional patient with a solitary stab wound to the flank with rapidly clearing hematuria, a negative IVP, normal abdominal examination, and negative peritoneocentesis may be treated with bed rest and parenteral antibiotics. Minor lacerations documented preoperatively with or without urinary extravasation can be left unexplored unless active bleeding is suspected. All other penetrating renal injuries require débridement of devascularized tissue to prevent delayed hemorrhage and abscess formation, primary approximation of renal parenchymal margins, closure of the collecting systems when possible, and extraperitoneal drainage of the renal fossa. Exploration of renal injuries should be performed only after control of the renal pedicle is achieved in an attempt to reduce the rate of nephrectomy.

For nonpenetrating renal injuries, a widely employed classification is helpful for determining appropriate treatment.

Class I: renal contusion

Class II: minor cortical laceration, with or without renal capsular disruption, without urinary extravasation

Class III: major cortical laceration with urinary extravasation, a large perinephric hematoma, or both

Class IV: multiple lacerations; shattered kidney

Conservative, nonoperative management is appropriate for class I and II injuries, which comprise approximately 85% of patients with blunt renal trauma. Although somewhat controversial, most authors advocate early surgical intervention for class III injuries to minimize the risk of developing perinephric abscess, secondary hemorrhage, hypertension, or ischemic atrophy. Class IV injuries require surgical exploration and frequently nephrectomy.

A renal pedicle injury demonstrated by contrast abdominal CT scan or angiography requires immediate surgical intervention. When associated with renal lacerations and urinary extravasation, nephrectomy is warranted, particularly when other intraabdominal injuries are present. Restoration of renal function may be achieved in up to 80% of pedicle injuries if surgery is performed within 12 hours after the injury; success rates decline rapidly thereafter. Most commonly bypass grafting with autologous vein is employed. Use of synthetic grafts is to be avoided because of possible contamination from other abdominal injuries.

Occasionally, the general surgeon or urologist is confronted intraoperatively with an unexpected retroperitoneal hematoma. In the absence of life-threatening hemorrhage, intraoperative IVP should be done. The presence of bilateral kidney function rules out major pedicle injury. Further exploration would be required only if gross urinary extravasation was demonstrated or parenchymal injury causing an expanding hematoma was present. When one or both kidneys are not functioning, immediate aortography is indicated. If the renal arteries are shown to be patent, nonfunction is due to contusion or acute tubular necrosis. When a renal pedicle injury is identified, immediate repair may be attempted.

Ureteral Trauma

The proper management of ureteral injury depends on early recognition, awareness of the presence of associated injuries, and the mechanism of injury. A missed ureteral injury frequently results in infection, fistula, or stricture formation. The ureter is fixed only at its junctions with the renal pelvis and bladder. Above the pelvic brim, the ureter is attached to the undersurface of the posterior peritoneum. The blood supply to the ureter is segmental and unpredictable; dissection must therefore be performed outside the adventitial sheath. In a further attempt to avoid undue injury to the ureteral blood supply, the surgical approach to the ureter should be lateral above and anterior below the pelvic brim.

More than 95% of ureteral injuries due to violence are caused by gunshot wounds. At least 10% of such patients have a normal urinalysis. Excretory urography delineates the injury in approximately 90% of cases. High-velocity injury to the ureter requires wide débridement because of the blast effect. One must assume a high-velocity injury if the bullet is not visible on radiographs and knowledge of the weapon is unavailable. When injury to an unsevered ureter is suspected, stenting the ureter and adequate Penrose drainage minimize delayed extravasation and allow healing to take place. More serious concern about healing necessitates excision and repair of the injured area. Although rare, severe blunt trauma of the deceleration type may cause avulsion of the ureter from the renal pelvis.

The presence and proper management of associated injuries in patients with external traumatic ureteral injuries is crucial to ureteral integrity. Pancreatic or duodenal injury must be drained away from the site of ureteral repair in conjunction with ureteral stenting or nephrostomy diversion (or both). Stenting and nephrostomy drainage are also useful in patients with ureteral and large bowel injuries.

The gravity of iatrogenic injury to the ureter lies not so much in the injury itself but in the failure to recognize it. Such injury most commonly occurs during abdominal hysterectomy, colon resection with surrounding inflammation, abdominoperineal resection, and aortic or iliac aneurysm resection. Preoperative IVP is most useful in any patient undergoing surgery in the retroperitoneal space. More secure visualization or palpation of the ureter can be achieved by initiating a diuresis with furosemide to produce a bolus of urine. Preoperative catheterization may assist in ureteral identification when a distorted course is anticipated. Suspected ureteral injury may be more easily confirmed or ruled out by intravenous methylene blue or indigo carmine.

Iatrogenic ureteral injury may result from ligation, crushing, avulsion, devascularization, or transection. When a ureter is clamped or ligated, damage is minimal if the injury is recognized and resolved immediately. The ureter should be stented for 5 to 7 days. A partial transection of less than half the circumference of the ureter without vascular compromise can be repaired with simple sutures and drainage. With more severe transection or suspected vascular compromise, completion of the transection, débridement to healthy tissue, and ureteroureterostomy should be performed. Unfortunately, many iatrogenic injuries are not recognized until the postoperative period.

Early during the postoperative period, fever, ileus, flank pain, uriniferous drainage, hematuria, or an abdominal mass may suggest ureteral injury. IVP can accurately diagnose the injury in almost all cases. Blood urea nitrogen and creatinine assays in urinary drainage fluid show levels 20 to 30 times the normal serum values.

The following general principles are important to proper ureteral repair.

1. Successful repair requires a tension-free anastomosis.
2. Only absorbable suture material is used. Nonabsorbable sutures act as a nidus for calculus formation if in contact with urine.
3. Attempt at watertight closure is unnecessary and may cause vascular compromise.
4. Proximal urinary diversion (nephrostomy tube, intraureteral stent) in all but the most uncomplicated cases acts as a safety valve and is worth the minimal risk and time needed to achieve it.
5. Adequate wound drainage is essential because extravasated urine can delay epithelialization and cause periureteral fibrosis and infection.

The choice of surgical repair depends on the location and extent of ureteral injury. Pyeloplasty techniques are employed for ureteropelvic junction injuries. Ureteroureterostomy with opposing spatulated ends is adequate for upper and middle one-third injuries. A defect of up to 5 to 6 cm can sometimes be bridged without undue tension because of the inherent mobility of the ureter. A ureteral injury close to the bladder is usually amenable to ureteroneocystotomy (i.e., reimplantation). With more extensive injuries of the distal one-third, a psoas hitch or a Boari flap may be necessary to attain a tension-free anastomosis.

A variety of Silastic or polyurethane nonmigrating (pigtail configurations on each end) internal ureteral stents are now available. These stents can be placed intraoperatively through the open wound/ureterotomy, with the proximal end coiled in the renal collecting system and the distal end in the bladder. Cystoscopic stent removal can be performed in 6 to 8 weeks in an office or outpatient setting.

Long ureteral defects are usually associated with high-velocity missile injuries with multiple organ damage. In this setting, it is prudent to ligate the proximal ureter and insert a nephrostomy tube via a small renal pyelotomy incision through the dependent lower pole exiting from a separate skin stab wound. If the kidney is also injured, nephrectomy is indicated. If the patient survives, ileal interposition or autotransplantation can be considered 3 to 6 months later.

Bladder Trauma

The empty bladder is well protected by the bony pelvis, whereas the full bladder is much more vulnerable. The weakest part of the bladder and thus the most likely point of rupture is the superior portion, or dome, which is covered by peritoneum. In children the bladder is a more intraabdominal organ and is more likely to sustain intraperitoneal rupture. Most bladder injuries (more than 90%) are secondary to blunt trauma and are usually associated with pelvic fracture(s). Approximately 85% of patients with bladder injuries have gross hematuria.

Once a bladder injury is suspected, cystography with a postdrainage film is done. An IVP is not an adequate study to assess the nature and extent of possible bladder injury. If a urethral injury is also suspected, a urethrogram must be obtained prior to inserting a catheter. Retrograde urethrography should be performed first in any male patient with blood at the urethral meatus, scrotal or perineal hematoma, or abnormal position of the prostate on rectal examination. With only simple contusions the bladder is intact. Extraperitoneal rupture is radiographically characterized by flame-like configurations of contrast. Intraperitoneal rupture results in extravasation of contrast into the peritoneal cavity, often outlining portions of bowel. When associated with pelvic fracture, the bladder often assumes a teardrop shape on cystography because of surrounding hematoma.

Proper management of a bladder injury or rupture includes delineation of the extent of injury if possible, repair of the wall, adequate diversion of urine, and perivesical drainage. Intraperitoneal injuries should be explored routinely. Lacerations are closed in one to two layers using absorbable suture material. In male patients a 24F to 28F suprapubic cystotomy tube (e.g., Malecot catheter) is used to drain the bladder. In female patients a 24F to 26F urethral catheter is usually adequate for urinary drainage. Suprapubic or urethral catheters are removed at 7 to 10 days after cystography demonstrates the absence of extravasation. Extraperitoneal bladder injuries may be treated conservatively with a urethral catheter, particularly when there is no other reason for surgical intervention.

Urethral Trauma

Urethral injuries are much more common in male patients because of the length and the fixation of the urethra to the pubic bone by the puboprostatic and suspensory ligaments. Injury to the anterior urethra, which extends from the urogenital diaphragm to the external meatus, usually results from straddle, penetrating, or crush injuries. Extravasation limited by Buck's fascia is confined to the penis. Extravasation limited by Colles' fascia, which is continuous with Scarpa's fascia, may extend into the abdominal and chest walls because of its peripheral attachments to the coracoclavicular fascia, the fascia lata of the thigh, and the triangular ligament posteriorly.

Suspicion of an anterior urethral injury, often presenting with blood at the urethral meatus and difficulty or inability to void, requires retrograde urethrography. Contrast material that is suitable for intravenous use should be used exclusively. Patients are encouraged not to void to prevent possible urinary extravasation. Penetrating injuries must be débrided. If conditions permit, primary repair may be performed; otherwise a suprapubic cystostomy tube may be placed and the repair delayed. Perineal extravasation of urine and blood secondary to blunt urethral trauma requires adequate local drainage. If the injury is minor, primary repair may be performed and an indwelling urethral catheter left in place for 10 days. Suprapubic diversion is employed with more extensive urethral ruptures, which are more easily and effectively repaired once inflammation has subsided.

Most posterior urethral injuries are associated with pelvic fractures. Such injuries occur in 5% to 10% of patients with a pelvic fracture. Although not universal, blood at the urethral meatus occurs frequently. Careful rectal examination may reveal a superiorly displaced urethral disruption at the level of the urogenital diaphragm. Although somewhat controversial at present, initial urologic management is confined to suprapubic cystostomy placement, rather than an attempt at emergent primary repair of posterior urethral injuries. Restoration of urethral continuity by a variety of reconstructive techniques can be performed 3 to 4 months later. The morbidity associated with either emergent or delayed repair includes impotence, stricture formation, incontinence, and additional urologic procedures.

RENAL CALCULUS DISEASE

Renal calculus disease is a common urologic condition occasionally deceptive in its clinical presentation.

The patient often complains of severe flank or abdominal pain that may be associated with nausea, vomiting, and fever. Acute renal or ureteral colic may simulate acute cholecystitis, appendicitis, intestinal obstruction, or pancreatitis. Findings highly suggestive of nephrolithiasis include costovertebral punch tenderness, absence of peritoneal signs, microscopic hematuria, or pyuria. A plain abdominal radiograph often confirms the diagnosis, because 85% to 90% of renal calculi are radiopaque. Uric acid calculi are radiolucent; cystine and struvite (infection) stones are relatively nonopaque but are usually faintly visible. Excretory urography is a more definitive radiographic means of determining the nature and position of renal calculi.

Approximately 70% to 75% of renal calculi are predominantly composed of calcium oxalate. The most common cause of calcium oxalate stone formation is intestinal hyperabsorption of calcium, often in conjunction with inadequate fluid intake. Less common causes include regional enteritis, short bowel syndrome, and bypass surgery for obesity. Primary hyperoxaluria is a rare congenital enzymatic defect in the metabolism of glyoxylic acid characterized by diffuse calcium oxalate deposition in the kidney, causing renal failure.

Numerous metabolic diseases are associated with calcium stone formation. Primary hyperparathyroidism accounts for 2% to 4% of renal calculi and most calcium phosphate (brushite) stones. Another cause of brushite stones is renal tubular acidosis (RTA), particularly the more common type II, proximal RTA. Cystinuria, a congenital defect in proximal tubule reabsorption of cystine, ornithine, lysine, and arginine (COLA), is manifested clinically only by cystine stone formation. Vitamin D intoxication, sarcoidosis, prolonged immobilization, medullary sponge kidney, metastatic or parathyroid hormone-producing neoplasms, milk alkali syndrome, and hyperthyroidism are all associated with calcium stone formation.

Uric acid calculus disease is related to a combination of hyperuricosuria, abnormally low urine pH, and inadequate fluid intake. Approximately 25% of patients suffering from gout form renal calculi composed of or containing uric acid. Patients with gastrointestinal disorders such as ulcerative colitis and those requiring colostomy or ileostomy lose substantial amounts of bicarbonate and water through the intestinal tract. The kidneys respond by excreting a more concentrated, acidic urine, an ideal environment for uric acid precipitation. A high incidence of uric acid stones occurs in patients with gout

or the rare Lesch–Nyhan syndrome, in those undergoing chemotherapy, and in patients with an unusually high-purine diet. The prevention of uric acid stone formation requires alkalinization of the urine with sodium bicarbonate (by mouth) when appropriate, allopurinol in patients with uric acid overproduction, and adequate hydration.

Persistent urinary tract infection with urease-producing (i.e., urea-splitting) organisms accounts for 5% to 10% of renal caculi. *Proteus mirabilis* is the most common bacterium associated with infection or struvite stones. These calculi are composed of magnesium ammonium phosphate admixed with smaller amounts of calcium phosphate and carbonate crystals. They are soft, relatively radiolucent calculi that often form casts of the renal collecting system and hence are termed "staghorn calculi." Antibiotic therapy is useful in the acutely septic patient or perioperatively to prevent resistant organisms from forming.

The various surgical approaches to renal calculi are beyond the scope of this brief review. New techniques have been developed that markedly restrict the need for open surgery. Extracorporeal shock wave lithotripsy (ESWL) allows completely noninvasive stone disintegration by focusing shock waves at the stone through a water–skin interface under fluoroscopic or sonographic control. ESWL has an approximately 95% success rate in treating renal calculi less than 2 cm in diameter. Larger renal calculi (over 3 cm) or staghorn calculi are routinely removed by initial percutaneous endoscopic debulking using an ultrasonic lithotrode followed, if necessary, by ESWL of the remaining fragment(s). These techniques are associated with few major complications, shortened hospital stays, and more rapid return to normal daily activities compared with open surgical procedures.

UROLOGIC EMERGENCIES

Renovascular Emergencies

Renal artery aneurysms represent approximately 1% of all arterial aneurysms; 75% are noncalcified and prone to rupture. Hypertension, gross or microscopic hematuria, and upper quadrant abdominal bruit are commonly associated with fibromuscular dysplasia, a disease process more common in young adults. Once selective arteriography delineates the lesion, urgent autologous saphenous vein aortorenal bypass with or without excision of the aneurysm is indicated if (a) the aneurysm is 2 cm or more in size, (b) intramural clot is present, or (c) renal artery occlusive disease is present.

Embolic phenomena affecting the kidney occur with 2% to 3% of all arterial emboli. Severe flank and lower back pain and hematuria are manifestations of renal infarction. Nonvisualization of the kidney on IVP should prompt arteriography to establish the diagnosis and the location of the embolus. If more than 2 to 3 hours has elapsed from the time of embolization to diagnosis, embolectomy cannot salvage the kidney unless collaterals or incomplete occlusion is evident. Heparinization must be started immediately to prevent further propagation of thrombus.

Testicular Torsion

Torsion of the spermatic cord obstructs the venous blood supply, causing edema, hemorrhage, and eventual obstruction of arterial blood supply. Torsion most commonly occurs during the second decade of life at or near puberty. Approximately 20% to 30% of cases, however, are seen in men over 20 years of age. Failure to intervene promptly results in irreversible testicular infarction. An acute scrotal condition in an adolescent or young man should be considered torsion unless proved otherwise. The differential diagnosis includes acute epididymitis, which is the most common cause of scrotal swelling and pain, acute orchitis, strangulated hernia, traumatic hematocele or hydrocele, and torsion of the appendix testis.

The clinical history and physical findings in patients with testicular torsion are, unfortunately, of limited value. A horizontal testicular lie, upward testicular retraction because of a shortened spermatic cord, and acute onset in the face of normal urinalysis strongly suggest torsion minimalor. No relief of pain on raising the testis (a negative Prehn's sign) is unreliable. When available, a ^{99m}Tc pertechnetate testicular scan is highly sensitive for demonstrating the characteristic reduced blood flow in patients suffering from torsion. Color Doppler sonographic scanning has been shown to be as sensitive and specific as the radionuclide scan. The color Doppler technique, however, is not yet readily available.

Torsion occurs within the tunica vaginalis (intravaginal) in the child and adult. The testis is abnormally sus-

pended in a variety of forms of which the most common is described as a "bell clapper" configuration. In approximately two-thirds of cases the twist is from without inward (internal rotation). About 50% to 60% of torsion cases have similar abnormalities of suspension contralaterally. Extravaginal torsion occurs only during the neonatal period.

If torsion cannot be ruled out, expeditious scrotal exploration is performed. In the emergency room, manual detorsion can be attempted and, if successful, results in immediate relief of symptoms and converts a surgical emergency to an elective procedure. Orchiectomy is not performed unless the testis is undeniably infarcted. Orchiopexy is performed by fixing the testes directly to the dartos muscle layer with at least two opposing nonabsorbable sutures. Contralateral orchiopexy is similarly performed to prevent future torsion of that side.

Failure of the patient to seek early medical attention or misdiagnosis by the primary care physician results in orchiectomy in approximately 50% of cases. A testicular ischemia time of less than 12 hours is associated with at least a 90% salvage rate; infarction is almost certain after 24 hours of ischemia unless the torsion was intermittent. In general, the more aggressive the approach to suspected torsion, the higher is the testicular salvage rate.

Priapism

Priapism is a prolonged, involuntary, usually painful erection unrelated to sexual stimulation. Unlike a normal erection, the corpus spongiosum (i.e., glans penis and urethra) remains flaccid. With priapism, obstruction to corpus cavernosal venous outflow causes stagnation of blood, resulting in a viscous sludge that further impairs drainage. The most common conditions associated with priapism are sickle cell trait and disease and leukemia. Other causes include amyloidosis, multiple myeloma, postdialysis state, and neurologic dysfunction as seen with spinal cord tumors, spinal cord shock, and paraplegia. Several drugs, such as phenothiazines, alcohol, marijuana, antihypertensives, and heparin, have been associated with priapism.

The goal of treatment is to establish adequate venous drainage of the corpora cavernosa and prevent permanent fibrosis and associated impotence.

Treatment of the underlying cause, when known, often results in detumescence. Patients with sickle cell disease or trait are treated with oxygen, hydration, alkalinization, and transfusion. Leukemia patients require chemotherapy and splenic irradiation. Some patients respond to strong sedation. Ketamine, an anesthetic, has been successful in treating priapism and can be given in the operating room prior to definitive surgery.

Sequential intracorporal injections of dilute solutions of epinephrine or the safer phenylephrine may detumesce a shorter-lasting (6 to 8 hours) priapism, sometimes in conjunction with intracorporeal irrigation with saline. This technique is most useful and successful in patients with self-induced priapism secondary to therapeutic penile injections of papaverine with or without phentolamine for impotence.

When conservative measures fail, surgery in the form of a corpus cavernosa–spongiosa shunt (e.g., Winter procedure, formal window shunt) or corpus cavernosa–saphenous vein shunt are indicated. A Winter shunt procedure establishes bilateral fistulas between the glans penis and corpus cavernosa using a core biopsy needle. A formal cavernosa–spongiosa shunt entails approximation of opposing elliptical windows in the two structures at the level of the bulbous urethra through a perineoscrotal midline incision.

Infection

Severe acute pyelonephritis or acute focal or multifocal bacterial nephritis associated with an obstructive process requires prompt drainage by percutaneous nephrostomy or retrograde ureteral catheterization proximal to the obstruction. Simultaneous parenteral antibiotic therapy is imperative. Once the patient is afebrile and otherwise stable, the obstructing lesion can be corrected.

Scrotal gangrene is an uncommon but potentially fatal infectious process. It may be associated with urinary extravasation or other genitourinary disorder such as prostatitis, epididymitis, and traumatic scrotal or penile lacerations. Idiopathic, spontaneous scrotal gangrene, otherwise known as Fourier gangrene, accounts for approximately 50% of cases. Subcutaneous emphysema occurs in most cases. Treatment involves antibiotic coverage, colloid replacement, and prompt, aggressive débridement and drainage.

QUESTIONS

The following questions may have more than one answer.

1. The most common renal mass is a:
   a. Renal cell carcinoma.
   b. Adenoma.
   c. Cyst.
   d. Angiomyolipoma.
   e. Hemangioma.
2. During a routine right hemicolectomy, a right renal mass is noted. One should:
   a. Expose the mass and perform a wedge biopsy.
   b. Needle-aspirate the mass.
   c. Perform a nephrectomy.
   d. Expose and palpate carefully and then work up postoperatively.
   e. Excise the mass with adequate margin.
3. Which of the following modalities is not useful for maximizing early detection of prostate cancer?
   a. Prostate-specific antigen.
   b. Prostatic acid phosphatase.
   c. Transrectal ultrasonography.
   d. Digital rectal examination.
   e. Clinical symptomatology.
4. BCG bladder instillations are useful in patients with:
   a. Solitary, superficial urothelial bladder carcinoma.
   b. Squamous cell carcinoma of the bladder.
   c. Superficial, recurrent urothelial bladder carcinoma.
   d. Carcinoma *in situ*.
   e. Recurrent urothelial bladder carcinoma with superficial muscle invasion.
5. What percentage of patients with stage I testicular carcinoma eventually progress without treatment after radical orchiectomy?
   a. 10%.
   b. 20%.
   c. 30%.
   d. 40%.
   e. 50%.
6. Symptoms and signs related to benign prostatic hypertrophy can be treated pharmacologically. True or false?
   a. True.
   b. False.

7. Which testicular tumor has the worse prognosis?
   a. Seminoma.
   b. Embryonal carcinoma.
   c. Yolk sac tumor.
   d. Choriocarcinoma.
   e. Teratocarcinoma.
8. Which of the following parameters necessitate radiographic imaging of the urinary tract in the patient with blunt trauma?
   a. Adult patient.
   b. Microscopic hematuria.
   c. Systolic blood pressure higher than 90 mm Hg.
   d. Fracture of a lumbar transverse process.
   e. History of renal cysts.

9. Proper ureteral repair after trauma requires all of the following except:
   a. Tension-free anastomosis.
   b. Adequate urinary diversion.
   c. Adequate wound drainage.
   d. Watertight closure.
   e. Use of absorbable suture material.
10. Which of the following findings obviate the need for scrotal exploration in a patient with suspected testicular torsion?
   a. Positive Prehn's sign.
   b. Normal urinalysis.
   c. Unequivocally negative radionuclide testicular scan.
   d. No history of scrotal trauma.
   e. Shortened spermatic cord.

Microscopic hematuria ≡ 4+ RBC/hpf (Caused by most commonly BPH in men or prostatitis / UTI in women)

urine cytology
renal U.S. / ± IVP
cystogram / cystoscopy

urine flow normal > 15 cc/sec
(fixable) < 10 cc/sec

Fenasteride (androgen suppression) → ↓ 20% size BPH (glands ≥ 40+ gm)
Hytrin (α adrenergic blockade)
Cardura   1a
Flomax — most specific for α₁a

31

Surgical Nutrition

Steven A. Blau

Although the physicians of ancient times understood the need for a sound diet, it is only relatively recently that physicians have gained sufficient expertise in nutritional support to make nutrition a definable topic in the surgical curriculum. Its place here as a separate chapter underlines its importance, but the reader must understand that this review is concise and certainly not comprehensive.

Surgical nutrition during the 1990s has been an active area marked clinically by an increasing shift away from parenteral hyperalimentation toward enteral nutrition, a focus on some specific nutrients that have become recognized as important in clinical medicine, and an attempt to demonstrate, in large multicenter trials, the benefits of nutritional intervention.

NUTRITIONAL COMPONENTS: BASIC PRINCIPLES

It is difficult to recount the basic principles of surgical nutrition without sounding like someone's grandmother or the teacher of an elementary school science class. Physicians learned the basic principles years ago and forget them, when as medical students they filled their heads with other pertinent data. Foodstuffs, regardless of their form or the route by which they are ingested, supply the body with specific building blocks or

sources of energy. As energy substrate, protein yields approximately 4 kcal of energy per gram, carbohydrates average 4 kcal/g (intravenously administered glucose solutions provide 3.4 kcal/g glucose), and fat 9 kcal/g.

Carbohydrates

Carbohydrates include (a) simple sugars (monosaccharides), such as glucose, fructose, and mannose; (b) disaccharides and oligosaccharides, such as sucrose (ordinary table sugar) and lactose (milk sugar); and (c) complex polysaccharides, such as starch, dextrins, and glycogen. Monosaccharides in the diet are absorbed directly in the intestines. Disaccharides taken by mouth are cleaved by disaccharidases in the small intestine and then absorbed. Salivary and pancreatic amylases play a role in the breakdown of complex polysaccharides, converting them to oligosaccharides and disaccharides, which are then acted on by these same disaccharidases.

Not all saccharides can be absorbed, however. Disaccharides such as lactulose and some oligosaccharides and polysaccharides are not absorbed as carbohydrates but are fermented in the intestines to fatty acids and lactate and may then be absorbed and metabolized.

The absorbed monosaccharides may be converted to glucose and metabolized as an energy source (being converted to pyruvate and then entering the Kreb's or tricarboxylic acid cycle) or, like fructose, metabolized directly. Some tissues, such as erythrocytes, brain, and adrenal medulla, are largely dependent on glucose as their sole energy substrate. Nearly all tissues, though, can use this circulating glucose as an energy source, usually with insulin as a cofactor in its movement across the cell membrane. Excess glucose can be stored in the liver or muscle cells as glycogen. Additionally, after conversion to pyruvate and then to acetylcoenzyme A (CoA), excess glucose calories can stored as fat.

The intestinal brush border plays a crucial role in the absorption of enteral carbohydrates. This ability may be lost with prolonged periods of starvation as the brush border atrophies. Lactose intolerance is a relatively common manifestation of the loss of a specific intestinal enzyme; it exists both as a congenital defect and an acquired defect and affects a significant portion of the adult population. There are racial patterns of prevalence (it is generally more common in Blacks and Orientals) and patterns that may reflect cultural dietary practices. More importantly in clinical practice, however, is the intolerance that develops in patients who have been deprived of internal nutrition for prolonged periods and whose brush border has become atrophied.

Glycogen in the liver represents a storage depot that may be utilized by the whole body as needed in contrast to that stored in a muscle cell, which is available to meet only the needs of that cell. The liver's glycogen may be converted back to glucose in a process known as glycogenolysis (whose control is discussed below), but the liver's supply of glycogen could meet the body's needs for glucose only for about 18 to 24 hours, at best. Children, who have proportionally smaller amounts of glycogen stored in their liver, are less able to tolerate fasting partly because of this.

Fats

Lipids, by virtue of their high calorie/weight ratio, represent the body's principal form of energy storage. Triglycerides, which constitute much of the body's fat, are composed of three fatty acids (usually with an even number of carbon atoms) and glycerol. In addition to dietary triglycerides, the diet includes phospholipids and sterols, such as cholesterol. Dietary lipid may also be described according to its physical state (fat when solid at room temperature and oil when liquid, the length of the component fatty acid chains (long chains containing 16 to 24 carbons, medium chains containing 8 to 12 carbons, and short chains), the degree of saturation (zero to four double bonds), and whether the fatty acids are essential or nonessential.

When taken by mouth these triglycerides must be hydrolyzed before absorption. Bile salts and pancreatic amylases are necessary for absorption of long-chain triglycerides, yielding a mixture of fatty acids, monoacyl glycerols, and diacyl glycerols, which are taken up the intestinal cells and secreted into the small intestinal lacteals as chylomicrons (lipoprotein complexes). These compounds are rapidly cleared from the bloodstream by the action of lipoprotein lipase, which frees the fatty acids; they can be further metabolized by the liver or reesterified and stored in adipose tissue. Medium-chain triglycerides do not require the action of pancreatic lipase or bile salts, being hydrolyzed directly and then transported into the portal circulation not as chylomicrons but as albumin–fatty acid complexes.

Essential fat acids include linoleic and linolenic acids. The definition of "essential" refers not to the importance of these substances but to the fact that they cannot be synthesized from other fatty acids. This same definition applies to the essential amino acids (see below). Although technically not an essential fatty acid (because it can be synthesized from dietary linoleic acid), arachidonic acid is frequently described as such. These fatty acids are necessary precursors for prostaglandins and prostacyclins.

When stored lipid is needed to provide energy, the glycerol is cleaved and carried to the liver, where it is converted to glucose by gluconeogenesis. The fatty acids are processed via the Kreb's tricarboxylic acid cycle to produce acetyl CoA. Excess acetyl CoA is carried to the liver where it is metabolized to ketone bodies, which are released as a circulating energy substrate.

Essentially fatty acid deficiency is seen in hospitalized patients who are maintained solely on parenteral nutrition for weeks. This condition manifests most obviously as dermatitis and alopecia, the cellular defects being less obvious. The condition is preventable by administering minimal amounts of intravenous fat, which should be given to any patient who has been NPO for more than 2 weeks. Administration of fresh frozen plasma, though, may provide enough fat to obviate the need for Intralipid. Additionally, some fat may be absorbed through the skin, justifying a role for topical therapy.

There has been great interest in using ω-3 fatty acids, commonly found in fish oils, in place of ω-6 fatty acids, found in plants and, consequent to commercial feeding practices, most meats. As described above, these fatty acids participate in the synthesis of prostaglandins and cell membranes. The more common ω-6 fatty acids produce both a potent vasoconstrictor, thromboxane, and an effective vasodilator. The ω-3 pathway yields a less effective vasoconstrictor. In clinical use, the use of the ω-3 fatty acids does seem to improve some immune functions.

Protein

Ingested protein, although a source of calories, should be considered, instead, the precursor of the body's own somatic and visceral protein and not a caloric source. Proteins are hydrolyzed in the gastrointestinal tract, first by the action of gastric pepsin in an acidic environment and then by the actions of several pancreatic proteases (e.g., trypsin and chymotrypsin) and intestinal mucosal proteases in an alkaline environment. These are usually taken up as free amino acids via a number of transport systems for the acidic, basic, and neutral amino acids. Dipeptides and tripeptides may also be absorbed at the intestinal brush border, but they are further hydrolyzed to free amino acids before entering the portal circulation. Branched-chain amino acids are catabolized in muscle; the other essential amino acids are catabolized in the liver.

The body's protein exists in a dynamic state with constant synthesis, degradation, and resynthesis. The turnover of intestinal cells, for instance, supplements dietary protein intake. Adequate intake of exogenous protein provides an available pool of amino acids to decrease the body's need to catabolize its own stores. Healthy adults are in a state of nitrogen balance in that their intake of exogenous amino acids is balanced by the nitrogen losses in urine, stool, and skin.

The amino acids are preserved for this purpose only if adequate energy is provided by carbohydrate and lipid intake. If these calories are not provided in adequate amounts, the administered amino acids may be degraded as energy substrate. As such, the amino acids are stripped of their amino groups, and the carbon skeleton is metabolized to produce glucose via gluconeogenesis or acetyl CoA and ultimately lipid. The amino ($-NH_2$) groups are synthesized into urea by the liver and excreted as nitrogenous waste by the kidneys. During liver failure these nitrogenous wastes accumulate as ammonia.

The amino acids may be divided by their structure (e.g., straight-chain, branched-chain, aromatic), whether they can be synthesized by the body (and are therefore nonessential) or cannot be synthesized, or how they can be metabolized (glucogenic if the liver can generate glucose or ketogenic if fat can be synthesized) (Table 31.1).

Glutamine has become an area of intense interest in recent years. One of the major amino acids stored in muscle protein, it is released in high quantities after stress and injury where it is thought to serve as one of the body's major sources of nitrogen for growth and repair of tissues, especially to cells with rapid turnover. It seems to be a specific fuel for the enterocyte (but it is not the most important energy substrate for the colonic epithelium).

Glutamine is missing from the parenteral amino acid mixtures because of its chemical instability in acid solution and the neurologic side effects, which were reported in the early days of parenteral nutrition when the mix of amino acids was being deduced. Its absence has been suggested as part of the mechanism for the loss of

TABLE 31.1. *Structure of various amino acids*

Amino acids	Structure
Essential	
Leucine	Branched-chain amino aid; ketogenic
Isoleucine	Branched-chain amino acid; partially ketogenic
Valine	Branched-chain amino acid; glycogenic
Lysine	Ketogenic
Methionine	
Phenylalanine	Aromatic ring, partially ketogenic
Threonine	
Tryptophan	Partially gluconeogenic
Nonessential	
Cysteine-cystine	Gluconeogenic
Histidine	Semiessential
Glycine	Gluconeogenic
Alanine	Principal gluconeogenic source
Arginine	
Aspartic acid	
Glutamic acid	
Proline	
Serine	Gluconeogenic
Tyrosine	Partially ketogenic

gut microvilli when patients are fed solely by parenteral hyperalimentation and the increased loss of gut mucosal barrier function. European studies have demonstrated the value of a glutamyl dipeptide, which is stable in solution; but this dipeptide is not commercially available in the United States.

Glutamine is increasingly available in most enteral feeding mixtures and at high levels in some. Although it would be nice to demonstrate improved gut recovery with the use of the highest glutamine feeding, it has not been clinically seen. However, these elemental and simple protein diets that do contain high concentrations are clinically indicated because of the difficulties these patients commonly have absorbing more complex nitrogen sources.

The second popular amino acid currently has been arginine, which in experimental animals has been shown to increase immunologic reactivity and promote wound healing. It is available in small quantities in parenteral preparations and, especially recently, in large amounts in a variety of enteral products. Its mechanism of action may lie in its role as a secretagogue for a number of hormones, especially growth hormone.

Increases in wound healing and in T cell response have been demonstrated in humans receiving supplemental arginine in the diet. Controversy focuses on the amount of supplementation, with some investigators claiming harmful effects of excessive intake.

Vitamins

Vitamins, complex organic substances naturally occurring in plant and animal tissue, are necessary cofactors in a variety of metabolic and biochemical pathways. They are usually provided to the healthy adult by a normal diet, but hospitalized patients may have increased demands for specific vitamins they cannot obtain from a hospital diet. Patients receiving enteral or parenteral nutritional therapy therefore must have their vitamin needs met by the clinician caring for them.

Vitamins may be classified as fat-soluble (vitamins A, D, E, K), which can be stored by the body in lipid depot, and water-soluble (vitamin B complex, biotin, folic acid, vitamin C), which must be administered to meet ongoing needs. Many of the fat-soluble vitamins are now commercially available in water-soluble forms that may be administered as part of parenteral feeding regi-

mens. Commercial vitamin preparations have been extensively revised, and many preparations whose constituents were far removed from recommended dietary allowances have been removed from the marketplace. The Multi-Vitamin Infusion (MVI) currently available, approximates the recommended adult daily dietary vitamin needs except for vitamin K.

Vitamin A is absorbed with fat, and its absorption from the diet is affected by some of the same factors that affect lipid absorption, namely the presence of bile salts and pancreatic enzyme in the gut and the integrity of the brush border. After absorption, most of the body's vitamin A is stored in the liver. Transport through the body is usually via retinol-binding protein. Although its major clinical role in nonhospitalized patients is the synthesis of rhodopsin and other photopigments in the retina, in hospitalized patients it is used for its ability to promote wound healing and, at high doses, prevent stress gastritis. Although the recommended daily allowance (RDA) of vitamin A is approximately 3,000 IU (1 μg of retinyl palmitate = 3.3 IU of vitamin A), ill patients appear to tolerate daily doses as high as 50,000 IU and higher during their hospitalization, a dose previously considered toxic. Hypervitaminosis A is a real problem, however. Anecdotally reported by Arctic explorers who consumed several hundred thousand micrograms eating polar bear liver at a single meal, it is more commonly seen with the uncontrolled use of vitamin A supplements by otherwise normal people. Children are less able to tolerate either vitamin A deficiency or vitamin A excess.

Vitamin D (dihydroxycholecalciferol) may be synthesized by humans in response to sunlight, a method of providing the vitamin that is of little value for the hospitalized patient, who must rely on exogenous administration. The most important role of vitamin D is in the absorption of dietary calcium. Unlike vitamin A and the other fat-soluble vitamins, hepatic stores of vitamin D are minimal.

Vitamin E functions as an antioxidant to protect against dietary unsaturated fatty acids, and it may therefore be necessary in higher quantities when patients are on a diet high in these fatty acids. Although vitamin E deficiency may produce an anemia consequent to abnormal iron metabolism, its clinical use today is probably as a free radical scavenger. Its clinical value in this role is far from substantiated, however. Our own clinical practice is to supplement the diet with enteral vitamin E when patients require an increased Fio_2 as part of their ventilatory support. Parenteral vitamin E is not presently available in the United States. Previous experience with this parenteral agent in children has not been satisfactory.

Vitamin K is rarely a problem in the nonhospitalized patient because of its presence in a variety of foodstuffs and because intestinal bacteria can produce absorbable vitamin K analogs. The patient dependent on parenteral nutrition obviously needs vitamin K supplementation, which may not be efficiently metabolized when introduced via a central vein. Vitamin E use also requires augmentation of vitamin K intake.

Humans, other primates, and guinea pigs are unique among most vertebrates in that we cannot synthesize vitamin C. Vitamin C (ascorbic acid) deficiency produces the clinical condition scurvy with weakness, petechial hemorrhage, ecchymoses, and gingival bleeding. The exploits of Captain Cook in the South Seas in curing this condition are common knowledge. Few patients in the hospital develop this complete picture, however. Of greater concern in hospitalized patients are the defects in wound healing, which may occur because of the role of ascorbic acid in the function of the enzyme prolyl hydroxylase, which is necessary for the hydroxylation of proline and thus the structure and function of collagen. Vitamin C is also a moderately effective free radical scavenger, and hospitalized patients are regularly treated at doses of 2 g per day, or 10 to 20 times the RDA.

Trace Metals

Trace metal deficiency does not occur in patients who are on normal diets because water and foodstuffs are sufficient to meet the body's minimal need for these substances. Patients experience difficulty when they have unusual demands placed on them, or when denied access to enteral feeding. Even the weekly addition of a unit of plasma is usually sufficient to meet the body's needs. The classic signs and symptoms of trace metal deficiency states are usually seen only in patients undergoing long-term central venous hyperalimentation. "Common" deficiency states are illustrated in Table 31.2. Current clinical practice is to add commercially available trace metal supplements containing zinc, copper, manganese, and chromium to the total parenteral nutrition (TPN) regimen at least two or three times per week.

TABLE 31.2. *Trace metal deficiencies*

Element	Deficiency
Iron	Anemia, immunologic incompetence
Zinc	Alopecia, dermatitis, wound healing, loss of taste
Copper	Anemia, neutropenia
Chromium	Hyperglycemia, neuropathy, encephalopathy
Selenium	Cardiomyopathy

Fiber

Dietary fiber is composed of plant cell wall constituents such as cellulose, hemicellulose, and pectin, which are fermentable, and lignin, which is nonfermentable. Fermentable fiber is metabolized by gut bacteria to produce short-chain fatty acids, which can be used as an energy substrate by the colonic epithelium. This property of fermentable fiber makes fiber feeding relatively contraindicated in patients in hepatic failure.

The physiologic effects of fiber in the gut depend on the site. Fiber delays gastric emptying by decreasing the fluid quality of the material in the stomach. In the small bowel, bile acids are adsorbed onto fiber, which may increase the efficiency of absorption of fat-soluble substances and decrease the destruction of bile acids by bacteria. In the colon, fiber increases stool weight and, by binding cations, may effect electrolyte losses in the stool.

Whether fiber affects the absorption of nutrients significantly is a matter of controversy at present, although many manufacturers have begun to add fiber to their preparations. Their major claim is that it decreases diarrhea, a claim that is certainly not proved.

STARVATION AND STRESS

Patients in the hospital soon cease to be normal because they are alternately starved, stressed, and traumatized. As the neuroendocrine control of these states has become better understood, the clinician's ability to interact with these states has improved. Simple starvation occurs when the supply of exogenous glucose is inadequate to the patient's needs, and this commences almost as soon as he is fasted overnight. Liver glycogen, as described earlier, is converted back into glucose to provide energy and to provide glucose to the organs that require it as their sole energy source.

When this supply of glucose is exhausted, the body begins catabolizing muscle protein to produce amino acid residues, which are transported to the liver and metabolized to produce glucose by gluconeogenesis. The body's losses may average about 400 g of lean body mass per day. Continuing at this rate, however, the body would soon catabolize much of its structural protein and, to prevent this from occurring, the body "shifts" its metabolic pathways to those of "chronic" starvation. Here fat becomes the major source of energy, the glycerol becoming a principal source of the necessary glucose. Ketone bodies appear. The patient's metabolic rate falls as he conserves energy and muscle protein losses decrease.

Unfortunately, these adaptations may be interrupted by surgical "stress." This condition stems in part from specific endocrine perturbations. Catecholamines increase the metabolic rate and force the body to continue its catabolism of protein. Glucagon and cortisol secretion are increased and further stimulate hepatic gluconeogenesis from amino acid precursors. Insulin levels are inhibited early by catecholamines but recover. This relative insulin deficiency compromises the facilitated transport of glucose across the cell membranes that require it (the brain being an organ in which glucose absorption is *not* insulin-dependent).

There is accumulating evidence that not only is the neuroendocrine milieu changed but the body's intrinsic ability to handle fuels is impaired in conditions of stress and, especially, in sepsis. There is an apparent defect with enzyme pyruvate dehydrogenase that effectively limits the energy the cell can gain from circulating pyruvate through the Krebs cycle. This puts further demands on the body's muscle mass to produce more amino acids, the body being starved for energy.

Finally, the muscle cell itself seems to be under the influence of a specific mediator that causes proteolysis and hepatic protein synthesis. Originally known as leukocyte endogenous pyrogen, this mediator seems to be the lymphokine interleukin-1, or a metabolite. Because this factor continues to cause muscle protein wasting even as intravenous feeding progresses, its study seems crucial to the future of nutritional intervention. Moreover, cytokine antibodies are being developed from monoclonal research, and they may have a clinical role "turning off" the unnecessary, destructive muscle proteolysis.

Growth hormone in large quantities has become commercially available and will probably expand its role in surgical nutrition. Human studies have demonstrated that hyponitrogenous preparations can maintain nitrogen balance in human volunteers. That less nitrogen produces the same nitrogen balance is not merely a cost-saving discovery but raises the question of whether adequate amounts of nitrogen can prevent nitrogen wasting in stressed or injured patients.

NUTRITIONAL ASSESSMENT

Nutritional assessment is performed to determine the patients who are at risk because of preexisting malnutrition and who might benefit from some type of nutritional support. Numerous studies in community and university hospitals have shown that one-third to one-half of hospitalized patients fall into the category of "malnourished." Although many of these patients require little more than common sense from the kitchen in providing a diet the patient finds palatable, others may require aggressive, invasive feeding.

Assessment of the patient includes a routine history and physical examination along with a determination of the patient's current height and weight. The latter should be compared against published standards. Furthermore, a good history points out any recent unintended weight loss (usually defined as a change of more than 10 lb) and any indication of preexisting impediments to eating.

A variety of anthropomorphic tests may be performed to aid in the evaluation of the patient. Triceps skin thickness is measured with calipers and is used as an assay of fat stores. Midarm circumference, measured with a tape measure, is used as a guide to muscle mass. Wrist circumference is measured to determine the patient's stature (in order to use the proper height/weight tables). Although these determinations are usually made by a dietitian or a trained dietary aide, the physician must understand them.

The body's protein exists as somatic protein (structural elements, such as collagen, muscle protein) and visceral protein (circulating, principally albumin). Simple chemical assays provide a measure of the visceral protein mass. Serum albumin levels are the most readily available; and because albumin turnover is measured in weeks, serum albumin levels reflect chronic malnutrition. Retinol-binding protein has a half-life of 12 hours, and measurement of this protein has proved to be a good assay of current protein malnutrition. This assay, unfortunately, is not commonly available in most hospitals. Because the turnover of transferrin is somewhat more rapid (about 8 days) than albumin turnover, but longer than that of retinol-binding protein, transferrin assays are useful for assessing the patient's response to nutritional management. This level can be approximated from the readily available total iron-binding capacity (TIBC) as follows:

$$\text{Transferrin} = 0.8 \times \text{TIBC} - 43$$

Normal levels are more than 180 mg/dL. Prealbumin (another protein with a more rapid turnover than albumin) can also be measured. Its clinical use has been somewhat limited, in part because of the increased levels commonly found in patients with liver disease. Routine chemistry determinations also allow calculation of the creatinine–height index as a means of assessing the total somatic protein mass.

Adverse effects of malnutrition are frequently associated with immunologic incompetence. Two useful guides using the immunologic system as yardsticks of nutritional status include the total lymphocyte count (with severe malnutrition being associated with a count of less than 1,500 lymphocytes per cubic millimeter) and the patient's response to a battery of skin-test antigens. The latter investigation examines T lymphocyte function and number. These figures may be combined to generate a prognostic nutritional index (PNI) as follows:

$$\text{PNI } (\%) = 158 - 16.6 \times \text{ALB} - 0.78 \times \text{TSF}$$
$$- 0.20 \times \text{TFN} - 5.8 \times \text{DH}$$

where ALB is serum albumin (in grams per deciliter), TSF is triceps skinfold thickness (in millimeters), TFN is serum transferrin (in milligrams per deciliter), and DH is the rating of delayed cutaneous hypersensitivity on a three-antigen panel (0, nonreactive; 1, less than 5 mm induration; 2, 5 mm or more induration). In one study a PNI of less than 40% was associated with a minimal incidence of complications or mortality, whereas a PNI of 50% or more was associated with a mortality of 33% and a 50% incidence of complications.

The patient's basal energy expenditure may be measured or calculated. The definitive method of determining the patient's expenditure is to measure the meta-

bolic rate directly using a metabolic cart. This device directly measures oxygen consumption and carbon dioxide production and yields an energy expenditure using the following equation:

$$\text{REE} = 144 \times (3.941 \times \text{Vo}_2 + 1.106 \times \text{Vco}_2)$$

where REE is the energy expenditure (expressed in kilocalories per 24 hours), Vo_2 is oxygen consumption, and Vco_2 is carbon dioxide production.

The equipment, although increasingly available, is rather expensive and requires a qualified technician. Moreover, although the determination may be valid, it may not reflect the patient's caloric needs over a prolonged period. Anxiety, pain, or fever can alter the patient's metabolic rate acutely and can result in a falsely elevated estimate of the patient's needs. Mass spectroscopy or even bedside capnography, which continuously measures inspired and exhaled gases, would obviate this problem. Clinical utilization of the cart is more difficult when the patient is extubated and breathing room air or through a face mask in that the patient must be placed under a canopy, rather than allowing the gas lines to and from the ventilator to be accessed directly.

The metabolic cart also allows determination of the respiratory quotient (RQ), which reflects the moles of carbon dioxide produced per mole of oxygen consumed and demonstrates the relative sources of the calories (i.e., fat and carbohydrate). With addition of the patient's urine nitrogen losses, it is possible to describe the net consumption of fat, carbohydrate, and protein as energy sources. The RQ of carbohydrate is 1.0 and of fat 0.7. An elevated of RQ of 0.95, for instance, indicates that the patient was using carbohydrate as the principal metabolic fuel. Excess feeding, with the production of fat, is also detectable using the cart, as the RQ of lipogenesis is 1.3.

An alternative to direct measurements is an assessment of caloric expenditure using the Harris-Benedict equation (below), which may be used to calculate the caloric needs of the patient. The equation of basal energy expenditures (in kilocalories) is:

$$\text{Males: } 66 + (13.7 \times \text{Wt}) + (5 \times \text{Ht}) - (6.8 \times \text{Age})$$

$$\text{Females: } 655 + (9.6 \times \text{Wt}) + (1.8 \times \text{Ht})$$
$$- (4.7 \times \text{Age})$$

where Wt is weight in kilograms, Ht is height in centimeters, and Age is expressed in years. To reflect the clinical situation, this basal metabolic expenditure is augmented by both an activity factor (AF) and an injury factor (IF), so:

$$REE = BME \times AF \times IF$$

Representative injury factors are as follows:

Minor elective surgery	1.1
Major elective surgery	1.2
Skeletal trauma	1.35
Head Injury	1.6
Burn, 40%	1.4
Burn, 100%	1.9

The major failing of the Harris-Benedict equation is that it does not adequately describe caloric needs at the extremes of age, size, and illness.

Finally, the "gold standard" test of nutritional status is measurement of nitrogen balance with the patient's urine collected over 24 hours and assayed for total nitrogen; protein intake during the same period is also carefully recorded. This is not a measure of caloric balance but of the fate of protein. The nitrogen losses in the stool and skin (about 3 to 4 g /day) are approximated. Because the measurement of total nitrogen is difficult and expensive, most clinicians rely on the hospital's laboratory to report urinary urea and augment this figure by 15% to reflect the estimated nonurea nitrogen losses. All measurements of protein are reduced to grams of nitrogen by dividing the protein in grams by 6.25. It is possible to measure muscle turnover by measuring 3-methylhistidine, a fairly unique amino acid whose presence in the urine is not affected by intravenous or dietary protein intake, but this is uncommon in clinical practice.

With these determinations, the clinician is able to assign a relative assessment of the patient's degree of pre-existing malnutrition. Three clinical diagnoses may then be made: marasmus, kwashiorkor, and a combination of the two. Although these terms are associated with graphic images from studies of starvation in less developed parts of the world, the diagnoses are appropriate for hospitalized patients and are integrated into the various diagnosis-related groups (DRGs) which affect hospital reimbursement schedules.

Marasmus represents severe calorie malnutrition in which fat stores are depleted but muscle mass has been conserved. It is clinically a somewhat common consequence of malabsorption syndromes and prolonged unstressed starvation. Kwashiorkor is the classic protein

deficiency state that occurs when adequate caloric intake has been maintained but protein intake has been inadequate. These patients have markedly decreased visceral protein indices and not infrequently are encountered on trauma and burn services, where they do not receive adequate protein in their nutritional regimens. The combination condition develops, obviously, in patients who have been starved of both caloric and protein intake.

In a facility where the physician is without the appropriate ancillary personnel, the simplest approximation of the diagnosis of malnutrition may be made with just the serum albumin and the total lymphocyte count. A patient with a serum albumin level less than 3.4 g/dL is at an increase risk of surgical complications, as is a patient with a total lymphocyte count less than 1,500/mm^3. The patient with both is severely malnourished and is at a markedly increased risk of surgical morbidity and mortality. Few physicians are forced to rely solely on these determinations.

Basic to demonstrating the efficacy of nutritional intervention is a reduction in weight loss in the hospitalized patient. Although daily serum albumin and 24-hour urinary urea levels are commonly available, daily or even frequent weight determinations are difficult to obtain in most intensive care units (ICUs). The patient's weight fluctuation remains an important assessment factor, however, and every effort should be made to monitor it. Bed manufacturers are building scales directly into their more expensive models for this purpose.

On the other hand, weight gain may not always be an indicator of success, because gain in water or even in fat is not the goal of nutritional support; gain in muscle or lean body mass is. Various techniques of body component analysis have been proposed, but dunking the patient in a vat of water is certainly not a practical solution in the ICU. What has been shown to be useful and reproducible is an assessment of total body water and fat by bioimpedence, a system that relies on the different conductivities of free water and fat.

NUTRITIONAL SUPPORT

Patients who are malnourished when admitted to the hospital are obviously in need of nutritional support, but they are not the only ones. The balance between energy demand and supply is altered once a patient is hospitalized. Nutritional support must benefit the patient who came into the hospital well nourished, but who is undergoing increased stress with increased demand for energy at a time when he may not be able to increase the intake of foodstuffs sufficiently. Malnutrition develops as the balance between intake and expenditure shifts.

Support, then, is indicated to correct the damage of yesterday, the needs of today, and the anticipated demands of tomorrow. Consideration must always be made of what caloric expenditures on the part of the patient may be decreased as an aid to achieving a balance. Patients hospitalized on a burn unit, for instance, are placed in rooms with a high ambient temperature to decrease the metabolic expenditure necessary to maintain body temperature and therefore decrease the caloric needs.

One further word before pursuing the options available in today's nutritional armamentarium. The earlier discussion of discussion of protein-sparing (see Nutritional Components: Principles, above) must be observed. Most patients require 125 to 150 kcal derived from glucose or lipid to "protect" each gram of nitrogen. In septic patients, however, this amount of glucose is probably associated with severe hyperglycemia, and ratios as low as 75 : 1 or 90 : 1 may be more appropriate. This ratio breaks down again in such conditions as head trauma, when the patient requires a markedly increased nitrogen load, and renal failure, where the patient cannot tolerate the protein load but still requires the calories to maintain energy needs.

Enteral Feeding

The patient with a functional gastrointestinal (GI) tract should be fed enterally. This method of feeding is associated with fewer complications (especially sepsis) than parenteral feeding, and it is certainly less expensive. It requires less technical support both when starting and during nutritional therapy. Moreover, the delivery of nutrients via the portal blood is certainly more "physiologic" and has been shown to be more efficient. The latter point deserves some explanation. The neuroendocrine response to nutrients delivered enterally includes the appropriate insulin response from the pancreas. The insulin response to high intravenous glucose concentrations tends to lead to an accumulation of lipids (glucose moves across adipocyte cell membranes, and lipolysis is inhibited).

The major impetus to the rediscovery of enteral nutrition, though, has been concern over translocation of bacteria and endotoxin across the gut mucosal barrier. The gut barrier can be decreased in experimental animals by shock from a variety of causes, such as burns, hemorrhage, starvation, and changes in colonic microflora. The expectation is that by enteral feeding the damaged microvilli and brush border are repaired faster, a conclusion not yet documented unequivocally in clinical studies. Nutrients in the GI tract also alter the bacterial population, in both numbers and the types of microorganism.

Complications *do* occur with enteral feeding. Major complications of enteral nutritional therapy include aspiration, diarrhea, catheter or tube complications, and complications of electrolyte and water balance. These points are discussed further below.

Most enteral feeding regimens today use prepackaged products available from a number of commercial sources. This shift away from individual blenderized diets has developed because of the decreased supply of trained dietary personnel and as a consequence of the recognition of the commercial possibilities of nutritional support by a number of pharmaceutical and food manufacturers. Moreover, the canned preparations are "sterile," decreasing the risk of contamination by the staff preparing the tube feeding. Almost 100 products were listed in a recent compilation. Care must be taken to examine carefully a number of specific characteristics of the nutritional products, including the calorie/volume ratio, the osmolality of the final solution, the source of carbohydrate calories, the source and type of lipid, the source of nitrogen, and the complexity of the nitrogen source, and not to rely on the catchy "Madison Avenue" labels for the products. A brief compendium of such products may be found in Table 31.3.

Calorie/Volume Ratio

Most of the products in commercial use yield about 1.0 kcal/mL. Some manufacturers have pushed this to 2.0 kcal/mL and have advertised this increased caloric density as a "stress" or "trauma" preparation. Other manufacturers have reacted to this competition by suggesting that less water be used when preparing their solutions. The increase in caloric density is usually achieved by increasing the carbohydrate content and therefore the osmolality. Obviously, patients whose ability to maintain water balance is abnormal (patients in renal failure, for instance) are candidates for preparations of higher caloric density. So too are patients with markedly increased nutritional demands.

TABLE 31.3. *Comparison of commercial enteral feeding products*

Parameter	Vivonex T.E.N.	Criticare HN	Ensure	Nutren 1.0
Caloric density (kcal/ml)	1.00	1.06	1.06	1.00
Carbohydrate	Maltodextrin, modified starch	Maltodextrin, modified cornstarch	Corn syrup, sucrose	Maltodextrin, corn solids
% of calories	82%	83%	55%	51%
Protein	Free amino acids	Enzymatically hydrolyzed casein	Casein, soy	Casein
% of calories	15%	14%	14%	16%
Fat	Safflower oil	Safflower oil	Corn oil	Corn oil, MCT
% of calories	3%	3%	31%	33%
Osmolality (mOsm/kg)	630	650	470	300
Nonprotein calorie/nitrogen ratio	149 : 1	148 : 1	153 : 1	134 : 1
Comments and indications	Elemental diet Short bowel syndrome High glutamine	Elemental diet Short bowel syndrome	Lactose-free	Isotonic, lactose-free

OSMOLALITY

The osmolality of the solution is a major determinant of the risk of diarrhea in the patient with a normal GI tract and one with previously compromised bowel function (a long period of malnutrition, short bowel syndrome, or a malabsorption syndrome). Osmolality is increased by the use of monosaccharides and disaccharides, rather than the more complex oligosaccharides. The form of protein is also a determinant of osmolality, as elemental amino acids result in a much higher osmotic load than do di- and tripeptides and intact protein. Fats do not affect the osmolality of the solution.

CARBOHYDRATE SOURCE

The patient's lactose tolerance is a major problem that prompts making clinical decisions regarding the source of carbohydrate. Recognizing this problem, most products today are lactose-free except for those that rely heavily on casein as the nitrogen source. If the patient develops nausea and abdominal distension when using a lactose-based supplement and there is no other apparent cause for this clinical picture, the diagnosis of lactase deficiency should be entertained and a lactose-free preparation prescribed instead.

PROTEIN CONTENT

Commercial preparations differ most significantly in the form of protein provided and the amount. The supplemental nitrogen preparations usually append such alliteratives as "HN" or "high nitrogen" or "plus" to designate the enriched protein content. The clinician should not be confused by the advertising because one company's enriched product may, in fact, have less protein than the "ordinary" product of a competitor. The elemental diets designed for efficient absorption, especially in malabsorption states, use crystalline amino acids. These products are uniformly unpalatable and can almost never be given by mouth without careful adulteration. Moreover, the body's ability to absorb di- and tripeptides may be better than its ability to absorb single amino acids, and these slightly more complex diets provide the patient with more nitrogen than the diets composed of individual amino acids. Whole protein is probably contraindicated in cases of pancreatic insufficiency and should be used cautiously in patients who have not been fed for some time because of the aforementioned loss of brush border function and the lack of pancreatic proteases. In other patients, the enteral diet is commonly advanced to one with intact protein. Increasingly, and probably consequent to the interest in glutamine and arginine, combination products are available today in

TABLE 31.3. *Continued.*

Nutren 2.0	Pulmocare	Travasorb renal	Travasorb hepatic	Impact
2.00	1.50	1.35	1.10	1.00
Corn syrup solids, maltodextrin, sucrose	Sucrose, hydrolyzed cornstarch	Glucose oligosaccharides, sucrose	Glucose oligosaccharides, sucrose	Hydrolyzed cornstarch
39%	28%	81%	77%	53%
Casein	Casein	Essential L-amino acids, nonessential amino acid	L-Amino acids	Casein, L-arginine
16%	17%	7%	50%	22%
MCT, corn oil	corn oil	MCT, sunflower	MCT, sunflower	Structured lipid, menhaden oil
45%	55%	12%	12%	25%
710	520	590	600	375
134 : 1				
High calorie, high fat	High fat, low carbohydrate	Low protein, renal failure diet	High amino acid, hepatic failure diet	Arginine-enriched ω-3 fatty acids

which the nitrogen source is both whole protein, small peptides, and elemental amino acids.

LIPID

Triglycerides are the predominant lipid in the commercial preparations, and the long-chain polyunsaturated fatty acids from vegetable sources provide the body's need for essential fatty acids. Preparations differ in total lipid content, the percentage of nonprotein calories derived from lipid, and the amount of additional medium-chain triglycerides (six to ten carbon lengths) added. Medium-chain triglycerides (MCTs) are more easily absorbed from the GI tract and may be absorbed in the presence of pancreatic or biliary deficiency or short bowel syndrome. MCTs are also indicated in patients with chylothorax. Preparations with low fat content decrease the gastric emptying time, which may be an advantage in some patients.

There has been increasing emphasis on ω-3 fatty acids as already described (see Nutritional Components: Basic Principles, above), but their use has not been without difficulty. Most of the fish oil-based mixtures suffer from a generally unpleasant "fishy" odor, but because most of the products are administered via tube feeding the patient is not usually the one who complains. Recently, canola oil, a vegetable source of ω-3 fatty acids, has been incorporated into enteral products.

ROUTE OF ADMINISTRATION

Enteral nutrition diets may be taken orally or may be introduced directly into the stomach via a nasogastric tube, a cervical pharyngostomy, or a gastrostomy. They may also be introduced directly into the small bowel via a nasointestinal tube, a Moss tube (Sheridan Catheter Corporation), a combination gastrostomy and jejunostomy system (Medical Innovations Corporation), a needle catheter jejunostomy, or a formal feeding jejunostomy.

Preparations consumed by mouth must be palatable and administered to awake patients with an intact gag reflex. This route requires intermittent feeding, which probably decreases the amount that can be given and the total calories that may be consumed. This route is mostly indicated therefore in the convalescent patient with minimal increased nutritional needs. Oral feeding is plagued by the risk of aspiration.

Diets administered directly into the stomach may cause aspiration as well. A nasogastric tube effectively maintains the upper esophageal sphincter open to further increase the risk of aspiration. Feeding the supine patient has also been implicated in aspiration, as has feeding the patient whose stomach is already full. Although continuous feeding is the preferred regimen to meet caloric needs, the diet here may be administered discontinuously. A compromise is to feed continuously for 16 or 18 hours a day, allowing the patient to have an empty stomach when supine at night. The gastric residual must be frequently monitored, and gastric ileus is a definite contraindication to feeding the stomach. Therefore gastric feeding usually requires a 24- to 48-hour delay from the time of operation, rather than feeding the intestinal tract directly. Gastrostomy, whether placed surgically or endoscopically, does not *by itself* prevent aspiration. Moreover, patients who have aspirated previously are still at an increased risk even after the placement of a gastrostomy.

Feeding the small bowel directly is the technique with the least risk of aspiration, although feedings may reflux into the stomach. Rapid return of intestinal function after surgical manipulation makes feeding as early as the recovery room a possibility. Feeding is usually continuous, and there is little risk of overloading the small bowel's capacity to empty (one does not have to check for residuals). Care must be taken when administering fluid into the small bowel that the lumen of the catheter is sufficient. This problem occurs principally when administering feedings through a fine-needle catheter jejunostomy, which usually allows infusion of only elemental diets and relatively simple solutions. The volumes infused, however, are usually sufficient to overcome the problem posed by the diet's complexity in most patients.

FEEDING

The gut (regardless of route of access) must be prepared for the feeding, and therefore dilute solutions are usually instituted initially. One usually begins with half-strength elemental diets or one-quarter strength more complex diets. Initial volumes are 25 to 50 mL/hr if given continuously and about 100 to 200 mL if given by bolus infusion. As the patient tolerates the feeding, the complexity, osmolality, and volume of solution are increased.

EXOGENOUS ALBUMIN

Echoes of the colloid versus crystalloid controversy in the management of intravascular volume are heard

regarding enteral feeding. The gut becomes a secretory organ rather than functioning as an absorptive surface with a severe reduction in colloid oncotic pressure. The clinical correlate of this has been the need to increase serum albumin in patients to allow them to absorb enteral nutrients and decrease diarrhea. In children the benefits of albumin infusion for reducing diarrhea have been demonstrated, and a brief course of exogenous albumin has allowed patients to tolerate enteral feedings and to increase their own endogenous albumin production. The benefits of exogenous albumin have been more difficult to demonstrate in adults, and several studies have demonstrated that in patients with serum albumin levels as low as 2.5 g/dL supplemental albumin failed to decrease morbidity or mortality. Furthermore, the albumin is increasingly expensive, and some have suggested that exogenous albumin causes the hepatic synthesis of albumin and other proteins to *decrease.* Our enthusiasm for meeting the former goal of maintaining serum albumin at 3.0 g/dL has been tempered.

OTHER COMPLICATIONS

Diarrhea

Diarrhea in the enterally fed patient, although lacking the dramatic potential of aspiration, is the usual reason for the discontinuance of enteral feeding. It is unfortunate because the patients frequently still require the nutrition and the clinician can usually correct the problem by determining its cause. Neglecting the problem results in the nurses' ire, the patient's continuing (or worsening) malnutrition, and a call from the hospital's accountant demanding to know why you are feeding the bedsheets. Diarrhea is most commonly secondary to the osmotic load of the solution, the patient's intolerance to specific parts of the solution (e.g., lactose), or decreased GI function (e.g., loss of length, loss of villi, low serum albumin, pancreaticobiliary insufficiency). The diarrhea can usually be cured by changing the preparation, the rate of administration, or the concentration of the solution. Tincture of opium or paregoric may be added to the feeding to decrease gut motility, if necessary. Of course, for patients hospitalized in an ICU on multiple antibiotics, *Clostridium difficile* should also be considered in the differential diagnosis, especially as slowing intestinal transit time is contraindicated with this condition. The importance of contamination of the tube feeding product must also be considered, especially if the solution hangs in an open container for more than 12 hours at the bedside.

Hyperosmolar, Hyperglycemic Dehydration

The patient with diarrhea loses considerable water and is at great risk of becoming frankly dehydrated. Another form of dehydration may occur secondary to the glucose load in patients who are glucose-intolerant or diabetic. The patient's serum glucose should be kept within normal limits and fluid losses from glycosuria repleted. Management should include both changing the rate of infusion and insulin administration as indicated. Another viable alternative is to switch to a preparation with less glucose that uses fat as a source of nonprotein calories.

GOAL OF THERAPY

The goal of therapy is restoration of a positive nitrogen balance and is the same goal as with any nutritional intervention. Electrolytes must be maintained within normal limits and can be adjusted by the addition of specific elements to the diet or parenterally. Care must be taken to ensure normal water balance.

PARENTERAL FEEDING

Parenteral nutrition is indicated when the patient requires nutritional intervention and the gut is either unavailable or unsuitable as a route for feeding. The questions posed to the clinician by parenteral nutrition are technical (where to introduce what type of intravenous cannula), biochemical (the choice of caloric source between glucose and fat), and quantitative (how much of what to give for how long).

Because of their high osmolarity, hyperalimentation solutions containing significant concentrations of glucose (in excess of 10%) must be administered via a central vein. The subclavian route is preferred because the catheter is easily secured without limiting the patient's mobility. Contraindications to subclavian cannulation are obvious and include prolonged bleeding and abnormal thoracic anatomy. Positive-pressure ventilation must be considered at least a relative contraindication. Jugular venous access is associated with fewer complications (especially hemo- and pneumothoraces), but the catheter dress-

ing is difficult to maintain. Femoral venous access is usually precluded by the difficulty of keeping the area clean. Catheters that contain two or three lumens, although more expensive than the traditional single-lumen catheters, allow infusion of hyperalimentation and provide additional ports of venous access.

Permanent venous access may be provided by Broviac or Hickman catheters, which are similar to the above in that they are inserted principally into a central vein. Insertion of these catheters in a sterile environment (the operating room) and the subcutaneous tunnel that isolates the point where the catheter penetrates the skin from the point at which the catheter enters the vein serve to decrease the infectious complications and thereby allow long-term use of the same catheter. Several studies with silver-impregnated catheters or catheters with Teflon cuffs suggest a definite advantage for decreasing infectious complications. Frequent line changes (by new cannulation or exchange over a guidewire) are routine in most settings. Our practice is to change the line at least every 72 hours, with the first change generally being over a guidewire. The diagnosis of catheter-related sepsis continues to be difficult even with routine culturing of catheter tips and the intradermal portion of the catheter and semiquantitative blood cultures.

The infectious complications of parenteral nutrition cannot be overstated. In current use, the pharmacist is usually not responsible for systemic contamination, which usually results from contamination during line insertion or from lack of attention to good dressing technique. The violation of the parenteral line is an all too frequent source of subsequent sepsis. TPN lines must never be violated.

Solutions of low osmolarity include principally those in which fat calories are substituted for a portion of the calories that central TPN derived from glucose. These solutions may be introduced via a peripheral vein. The route of the catheter, though, does little to diminish the need for aseptic technique and appropriate dressing changes. Violation of these lines is also to be condemned. It is not clear how often this catheter should be replaced, but clinical experience indicates that the lines are more prone to phlebitis than other peripheral lines, and they should be changed before phlebitis occurs, probably every 48 hours.

The choice between central TPN and peripheral hyperalimentation depends on the patient's needs. The central route is obviously preferred if peripheral venous access is difficult and should be considered for all patients in whom nutritional support is likely to be maintained for long periods or in patients with markedly increased needs. Patients who require less support or for short periods are candidates for peripheral vein alimentation. Peripheral hyperalimentation can also be a useful bridge supplementing the nutrition provided by enteral nutrition early in the course of these feedings when the calories supplied are likely to be inadequate without this parenteral support. This combination of parenteral and enteral feeding has been dubbed "transitional" feeding.

Nonprotein Caloric Source

Central TPN, initially described and used on countless patients, employs a 25% dextrose solution as the source of nonprotein calories. With the commercial availability today of Intralipid (as 10% and 20% solutions), the clinician has another source of nonprotein calories available. Intralipid is a soybean-based emulsion whose principal fatty acid is linoleic acid (an essential fatty acid), with lesser amounts of oleic and palmitic acid and the other major essential fatty acid, linolenic acid. Caloric supplementation with glucose frequently requires exogenous insulin. High glucose infusions can result in lipid accumulation (because unused glucose is stored rather than utilized), especially in the liver. Lipid infusions, however, tend to result in less net lipid accumulation.

Numerous studies of the value of fat and glucose calories have failed, in the main, to illustrate anything less than their biologic equivalence. Moreover, the combination of fat and glucose produces a more "normal" hormone response (insulin and glucagon) for the patient. Studies suggesting that the body is not able to utilize fat under conditions of trauma or stress are matched by studies questioning the utilization of glucose. Fat or glucose infusions given in the amount of 125 to 150 cal/g of nitrogen seems satisfactory for producing a positive nitrogen balance in most hospitalized subjects. Burn patients may be an exception, because fat in large quantities may not adequately "protect" nitrogen. Glucose infusions may also lead to problems with sodium and water retention.

The experience with earlier lipid emulsions demonstrated extensive problems that some fear also occur with Intralipid, although current studies suggest that the complications associated with Intralipid are probably more imagined than real. There is no convincing evidence of liver, pulmonary, or renal complications with the appropriate use of Intralipid. Neither the fixed retic-

uloendothelial system nor circulating immunologic reactivity is affected. There is, though, some question of the effect of the lipid infusion on the function of platelets, especially in patients with thrombocytopenia. I do not infuse Intralipid in patients with platelet counts below 50,000/mm³ because of this. The value of fat infusions in patients who have pancreatitis with hyperamylasemia is also a concern. Although some studies have demonstrated its use in patients with pancreatitis without complications, most clinicians avoid intravenous fat and oral fat. Currently, I centrifuge a sample of the patient's blood 4 to 6 hours after the end of the Intralipid infusion. If the serum is lipemic, the patient obviously cannot clear the lipid emulsion; therefore the dosage is decreased or the fat discontinued entirely.

One specific difference between glucose and fat calories bears on the subsequent discussion of respiratory dysfunction. The two calorie sources differ significantly in their previous described respiratory quotients. Patients with borderline respiratory function may not be able to eliminate the increased CO_2 produced when glucose is oxidized, in contrast to fat. What fat emulsions do provide, and what is clearly missing in glucose-only regimens, are essential fatty acids.

Timing and Parenteral Hyperalimentation

Parenteral hyperalimentation is maintained until the patient no longer requires parenteral therapy and can be weaned to enteral feeding. Parenteral hyperalimentation needs are dictated by the patient's protein requirements and caloric needs. Patients usually cannot immediately tolerate these high glucose loads, so therapy should be adjusted with close monitoring of serum glucose and urine glucose, adding insulin as appropriate and remembering that the glucose lost in the urine clearly does not benefit the patient and may rapidly lead to nonketotic, hyperosmolar dehydration or frank diabetic ketoacidosis.

When to start TPN is also a question. Although animal studies have demonstrated defects in wound healing after only a few days without food, not all surgeons believe that these findings are germane to patients. Nearly everyone starts TPN after a week; for a patient expected to eat in a few days TPN is not implemented.

Perhaps more important is a determination of which patients benefit from TPN, especially preoperatively. The recently completed Veterans Administration study suggests that only in the most severely malnourished patients did TPN decrease surgical complications. More importantly, perhaps, the study also demonstrated that infectious complications increased in patients on TPN and that this increase outweighed any reduction in non-infectious complications in patients less severely malnourished.

Additives to TPN

The assumption by clinicians of the nutritional state of their patients forces them to be concerned not only with calories and nitrogen. Vitamins must be added to the solution, usually in the form of prepackaged supplements such as MVI. Supplemental vitamin K (which is absent from MVI) may be required along with the "supernormal" doses of vitamin A (which must be provided enterally) and vitamin C (which can provided enterally or parenterally), discussed earlier. Intravenous feeding preparations with distilled, deionized water also forces the clinician to add appropriate amounts of trace metals, which are now commercially available. Electrolytes are added as necessary with specific care to add appropriate amounts of the less common elements. Phosphate is the precursor to high-energy phosphate bonds and must be added in sufficient quantities to maintain the metabolic rate. Magnesium and potassium must be given in quantities to compensate for their roles as cofactors in protein synthesis. Calcium must be administered to compensate for the increased phosphate presented to the patient. Insulin is added to the TPN mixture if indicated, but the acutely hyperglycemic patient is probably better managed when the insulin dose is given independently until the proper dose is determined. H_2 blockers such as ranitidine or cimetidine can also be added to the TPN mixture, and there are some data to support the increased efficacy of the drug when given in a continuous infusion. Albumin is uncommonly added to the TPN solution as well.

Special Problems

There are a number of specific clinical problems that nutritional support may worsen or may cause nutritional support to lose its effectiveness. Many of the answers to questions in these areas have not been elucidated, and it is an intense field of investigation. These discussions are therefore somewhat superficial; the reader is advised to consult current journals and monographs, rather than outdated textbooks.

Hepatic Failure

Hepatic insufficiency creates two distinct problems for the physician in that liver dysfunction interferes with nitrogen processing in the liver, and the amino acids infused in parenteral or enteral nutritional therapy effect the liver and subsequently the brain.

The liver is responsible for gluconeogenesis, and patients with advanced liver dysfunction have difficulty with glucose hemostasis, requiring a continuous glucose infusion to maintain serum levels. Oxidation of medium-chain triglycerides may be inadequate, so they should be used with discretion. Nitrogen cleaved from amino acids is supposed to be recirculated as urea after it is synthesized in the liver. Because patients with advanced liver disease may not synthesize urea, determination of urea clearance may not be an adequate guide to nitrogen balance. Moreover, the liver, unable to clear these nitrogenous residues, allows formation of false neurotransmitters in the brain as the patient develops hepatic encephalopathy.

Parenteral nutrition should be effected with lower total nitrogen infusion, a shift toward more of the essential amino acids, especially of the branched-chain variety, and avoidance of aromatic amino acids. This may be achieved with products such as HepatAmine (McGaw). The same goals exist with enteral nutritional therapy. Hepatic-Aid (McGaw) and Travasorb Hepatic (Travenol) are commercial preparations that attempt to meet these goals.

Renal Failure

The same concerns of organ dysfunction compromising nutrition and the role of nutrition in recovering organ function that exist in hepatic insufficiency occur with renal insufficiency. The kidney is crucial for eliminating nitrogenous waste products. High protein loads are simply not tolerated as the patient becomes progressively azotemic and uremic. High fluid volumes are similarly unacceptable because the kidney is the primary organ for maintenance of water balance. Conservative therapy with protein and water restriction compromises the patient unnecessarily. Essential amino acids reduce the urea load because excess amino groups do not need to be cleaved. Keto- analogs of amino acids are promising but not yet commercially available. The water load may be decreased by increasing dependence on fat for nonprotein calories.

The damaged kidney in acute renal failure must be given every chance to repair itself, but this cannot be achieved during protein deprivation. Studies have shown not only increased renal recovery but increased patient survival with appropriate administration of intravenous amino acids and calories.

Commercially available parenteral renal formulations include RenAmine. Enteral preparations include AminAid (McGaw) and Travasorb Renal (Travenol), which are characterized by their decreased total nitrogen content and increased percentage of essential amino acids.

Respiratory Failure

As the body cannibalizes its own muscle protein, the muscles of respiration (actually, of ventilation) are especially affected; and patients are more likely to experience respiratory difficulty, pneumonia, and the need for mechanical ventilatory support. One of the goals of nutritional intervention is to reverse this catabolism before it has a chance to compromise the patient. After intubation the patient attached to the ventilator needs nutritional support to help the immune system overcome pneumonia and to restore muscle mass. Feeding has been demonstrated to increase the patient's ability to be weaned from the ventilator.

Feeding is a two-edged sword here because aggressive feeding with high glucose solutions results in an increased total body burden of carbon dioxide. These patients may not be able to increase minute ventilation sufficiently to compensate. One of the goals of feeding ventilated patients and patients at risk of ventilatory compromise must be to limit their glucose infusion to 4 to 5 mg/kg/min.

The exposure of the patient to oxygen tensions in excess of an FiO_2 of 0.5 may result in oxygen toxicity. Supplemental vitamin E along with large doses of ascorbic acid may be a factor in decreasing oxygen free radical injury. Vitamin E must be administered enterally.

The patient requiring ventilatory assistance is one in whom the technology is available for decreasing metabolic workload. As discussed earlier in the chapter, nutritional support is indicated when the metabolic work of the patient exceeds the caloric intake. Placing a patient on the assist/control mode of ventilation or continuous mandatory ventilation (depending on the ventilator) decreases the work the patient must perform when breathing. It also decreases the caloric needs of the patient. This maneuver is an appropriate adjunct when the caloric needs of the patient are difficult to meet. The same comments are valid regarding tracheostomy, which also decreases the work of breathing.

Pancreatitis

The goal of pancreatic rest with the absence of stimulation of the organ's secretion of bicarbonate or enzymes requires that the patient take nothing by mouth. With resolution of acute peritonitis and the return of gut function, the patient may be fed with a low-fat, elemental diet. TPN affords pancreatic rest, but there are inconclusive data to support its benefit in acute edematous pancreatitis. Some investigators have shown that these patients can tolerate intravenous lipid emulsions. Patients suffering with acute hemorrhagic pancreatitis are generally sicker, and their disease tends to run a more protracted course. They are candidates for TPN and early enteral feeding with low-fat diets.

Our preferred route for feeding patients with acute pancreatitis, especially following trauma, is via a surgically placed jejunostomy. The rationale here is that the pancreatic stimulating effect of feeding is decreased when the foodstuffs bypass the duodenum.

Stress Gastritis

Life-threatening upper GI bleeding is encountered less often in the surgical ICU because physicians have learned to control stress gastritis. Current thinking has shown a decreased incidence of stress gastritis with antacid therapy and, perhaps to a lesser extent, with cimetidine therapy and other H_2 blockers. Experimental animal models have shown that addition of food to the stomach is the most efficient means of preventing stress gastritis. Vitamin A in large quantities (25,000 to 50,000 U/day) has also been shown to decrease the severity of stress gastritis.

A comment on the control of gastric pH by antacids is necessary considering the role of aspiration as a complication of enteral feeding. Several studies have demonstrated an increase in the incidence of nosocomial pneumonia in patients managed with either antacids or H_2 blockers when these patients are compared to similar patients managed with sucralfate. The proposed explanation is that the changed gastric pH allows overgrowth of microorganisms that colonize the stomach and the hypopharynx and are then aspirated. Sucralfate provided similar protection against gastric bleeding, whether detected clinically or endoscopically. Many of these studies have methodologic flaws that have prevented widespread acceptance of their conclusions. The role of gastric alkalinization continues to be controversial.

Head Injury

Metabolically, the patient with a head injury is characterized by nitrogen losses above and beyond the increase in metabolic rate. These losses are probably due to the common treatment of high dose corticosteroids. Nitrogen losses as high as 350 mg of urea per kilogram body weight per day have been recorded. These losses increased during the early postinjury period, reaching a peak at about the tenth day after injury. The increase in metabolic activity parallels this temporal sequence, reaching a peak during the end of the first week at a mean 170% of basal metabolic activity.

Feeding the head-injured patient is compromised by the prolonged gastric ileus, which makes nasogastric feeding difficult, and by an early intolerance for glucose, which complicates parenteral nutrition. Hyperglycemia with its attendant increase in serum osmolarity must be avoided because of its effect on the water content of the brain. High glucose loads enter brain cells irrespective of the facilitated transport provided by insulin. In the presence of ischemia or hypoxia, this glucose may be metabolized anaerobically, producing lactate, which may decrease vascular tone in the cerebral circulation and thereby increase intracranial pressure.

The neurologic recovery of the patient does seem to benefit from aggressive nutritional support. Several studies have documented a significant increase in the Glasgow Coma Score in patients in whom a positive nitrogen balance could be achieved. It must be noted that a positive nitrogen balance is difficult to achieve early in the course of these patients.

Burns

Burn patients are the paradigm of the severely stressed patient with increased caloric and protein needs. With sepsis they become even more stressed, and estimated caloric needs reach 2.5 times basal requirements. Malnutrition is recognized as a preventable cofactor in the death of the burned patient and a cofactor in the loss of immunologic reactivity, which increases infectious morbidity and mortality. Burn victims represent, like patients on ventilators, a type of patient in whom the efficacy of nutritional intervention may be improved by restricting caloric waste. The ambient temperature in the burn patient's room is about 85° to 90°F, a temperature dictated by the laws of thermoneutrality. The patient's work to maintain body temperature is increased by the difference between body temperature and the temperature of the surrounding air. A cold patient shivers to generate heat, thereby burning calories that may be better used elsewhere. Occlusive dressings can decrease the evaporative water loss of the patient and thereby decrease heat and calorie losses. Even with these maneuvers, the burn patient requires aggressive nutritional intervention.

Calorie needs are not well deduced from the Harris-Benedict equation. The Curreri formula, which is appropriate only for adults, is generally accepted:

$$\text{Daily calories} = (25 \text{ kcal/kg weight}) + (40 \text{ kcal/\% body surface area burn})$$

In children, whose surface area/weight ratio is different, the following is a useful approximation of needs:

$$\text{Daily calories} = 1800 \text{ kcal/m}^2 + 2200 \text{ kcal/m}^2$$

The burn wound may be responsible early for protein losses of approximately 1 to 3 g of protein per percent body surface area burn per day. Later, skin losses may present one-fourth of the patient's total nitrogen loss. Patients require 1.5 to 3.0 g or more of protein per kilogram body weight per day. Another approach to estimating nitrogen needs is to divide the caloric needs calculated from the above equations by 100 (a nonprotein calorie/nitrogen ratio of 100 : 1). Calculations of nitrogen balance that rely solely on measured urine losses give the physician a false sense of security.

Important additional factors in burn patients include a daily recommendation of high vitamin A dosages (25,000 to 50,000 IU/day), 1 to 2 g of vitamin C, 5 mg folic acid, and supplemental zinc and vitamin B_{12}.

Rehabilitation

The relation between protein intake and increases in muscle mass is influenced by a variety of circumstances, including the age of the patient and the amount of exercise. The health club dictum of "no pain, no gain" is unfortunately valid in the ICU where the lack of exercise and prolonged periods of immobilization foster the loss of muscle mass. Without exercise, an important stimulus to the laying down of new protein in muscle has been lost. These patients should undergo passive exercise if possible and active exercise when able.

Overfeeding

Overfeeding has been increasingly recognized as a problem in surgical nutrition. It is most commonly seen in patients whose metabolic needs have decreased but who continue to receive the same high caloric diet. As discussed earlier, high glucose loads that are above the patient's current needs are metabolized to fat and stored. Fatty liver represents one such storage depot with obvious clinical significance. Demonstration of an RQ in excess of 1.0 should alert the physician to possible lipogenesis, and the caloric content of the feed is adjusted accordingly.

Pediatrics

Although all of the above concepts are valid when caring for children, the specifics and numbers may be inappropriate, especially in small children and neonates. Children have decreased metabolic reserves and immature biochemical pathways and physiologic abilities. They are more vulnerable to growth defects consequent to specific amino acid therapy. Overall, they have increased needs for essential fatty acids. They require

careful monitoring. Caring for the nutritional needs of these patients should not be taken lightly.

QUESTIONS

1. What is the caloric content of the following TPN order: 1,000 mL of D50%, 1,000 mL of 8.5% amino acids, 500 mL of 10% Intralipid. Assume that all of the substrate is used to provide calories.
   a. 1,800 kcal.
   b. 2,200 kcal.
   c. 2,500 kcal.
   d. 2,800 kcal.

2. Arginine supplementation is important because of its role in:
   a. Maintaining gut integrity.
   b. Wound healing and increased immunity.
   c. Preventing stress gastritis.
   d. Decreasing nitrogen losses.

3. Which of the following are fat-soluble vitamins?
   a. A, C, E, K.
   b. A, B, choline, D, K.
   c. B complex, C, E.
   d. A, B, C, D.

4. A 60-kg man with a 40% burn requires how many calories according to the Curreri formula?
   a. 3,100 kcal.
   b. 4,200 kcal.
   c. 2,700 kcal.
   d. 3,600 kcal.

5. The respiratory quotient of fat is:
   a. 0.5.
   b. 1.0.
   c. 0.7.
   d. 1.1.

6. Stress starvation differs from chronic starvation in that in stress starvation:
   a. Nitrogen losses are minimal.
   b. Proteolysis is extensive; fat stores are not utilized well.
   c. Fat stores are used; glycogen is stored in the liver.
   d. Fat stores are used for energy; metabolic rate falls.

7. Essential amino acids are contraindicated in:
   a. Renal failure.
   b. Head trauma.

c. Burns.

d. Never.

8. In liver failure, urea output by the liver:

   a. Increases.

   b. Decreases.

   c. Is unchanged.

   d. Depends on gastric pH.

9. Glucose has what effect on the osmolarity of an enteral feeding product?

   a. Increases osmolality.

   b. Has no effect.

   c. Decreases osmolality.

   d. Depends on the fat content.

10. Age has what effect on caloric expenditure according to the Harris-Benedict equation?

   a. Increases caloric needs.

   b. Decreases caloric needs.

   c. Has no effect; age is not a factor in the equation.

   d. Depends on the injury factor.

SELECTED REFERENCES

Deitel M, ed. *Nutritional in clinical surgery,* 2nd ed. Baltimore, Williams & Wilkins, 1985. (An excellent multiauthored text on surgical nutrition, describing both its technical and theoretical aspects.)

Lang CH, Abumrad NN. Nutrition in the critically ill patient. *Crit Care Clin* 1995;11(3).

Manual of pre-operative and post-operative care. Chicago: American College of Surgeons.

Moore FA, Moore EE. The benefits of enteral feeding. *Adv Surg* 1997;30.

Present knowledge in nutrition, 5th ed. Washington, DC: Nutrition Foundation, 1984. (Complete, inexpensive, and available directly from the publishers. Although its 900 page multiauthor text is occasionally soporific, it belongs on the surgeon's bookshelf as it is an excellent review and can be used as a continuing reference.)

Rombeau JL, Caldwell MD. *Clinical nutrition.* Vol I. *Enteral and tube feeding.* Philadelphia: WB Saunders, 1984.

Rombeau JL, Caldwell MD. *Clinical nutrition.* Vol II. *Parenteral nutrition.* Philadelphia: WB Saunders, 1986.

32

Surgical Infection

H. David Stein

This chapter is intended to present a broad overview of infection in surgical patients and the treatment of these infections with surgery or antibiotics. Specifically, the discussion covers the body's defenses against infection, factors that enable bacteria to defeat the immune mechanisms of the host, some of the causes of hospital-acquired infections, and the use of prophylactic antibiotics. Finally some specific infections including virulent soft tissue infections and antibiotics are discussed.

RELATION OF HOST TO BACTERIA

The three primary factors that determine whether a person develops an infection are systemic host factors, local host factors. and bacterial factors.

Systemic Host Factors

To protect against a bacterial infection the host has a series of mechanisms that are initiated by exposure to the bacterium. The most important immune mechanism is the ability of the circulating granulocytes to phagocytize the bacteria, with the help of humoral factors. It occurs in four steps, the first of which is chemotaxis. Within hours the neutrophil is attracted to the area of inflammation. Humeral factors that contribute to chemotaxis include complement, tissue factors released by in-

jury, vasoactive peptides released from blood clots, and lymphokines released from lymphocytes. The next step is opsonization, a process of coating the bacteria to permit the neutrophil to identify the particles that should be ingested. Immunoglobulin G complement, and perhaps fibronectin are the main circulating factors responsible. The last two steps are ingestion of the bacteria and finally degranulation, where the bacteria are killed by the lysosomes of the neutrophils. One of the most important enzyme systems used by the lysosome to kill the bacteria is myeloperoxidase, which is oxygen-dependent. Therefore the lack of available oxygen severely hampers the ability of the neutrophil to kill the invading organism and prevent the body from removing the infection.

Several factors have been demonstrated to affect the immune system adversely and should be corrected whenever possible. Starvation, age, use of medications such as steroids or chemotherapeutic agents, prolonged preoperative hospitalization, and preoperative use of antibiotics increase the ability of the bacteria to cause an infection and enhance the chance for resistant organisms to colonize the patient. The immune system may be evaluated by measuring the response to skin testing with common antigens

Evidence has suggested that in the critically ill patient, especially one who is not taking oral feedings, bacteria (especially *Enterococcus* and *Staphylococcus epidermidis*) or fungi translocate from the intestines and may cause peritonitis or systemic infections. Translocation may be diminished by early use of the oral route for alimentation. There is some evidence also that the intake of glutamine or short-chain fatty acids decreases translocation as well.

Local Host Factors

Surgical technique is important in avoiding infection. Foreign bodies, deadspace, and ischemic tissue make an infection more likely. It is also important that blood flow be maintained to the area of the wound. Not shaving the operative site until just prior to the operation (or not at all) and not operating on a patient with a distant infection have been shown to reduce the infection rate. The longer the duration of surgery, the greater is the chance of contamination and the chance of infection.

Bacterial Factors

Several bacterial factors play a role. The number of bacteria present appears to be of prime importance. Fewer than 10^5 bacteria per gram of tissue wet weight usually indicates colonization (e.g., in a burn wound or contamination in a laceration), which the body can handle. More than 10^7 bacteria usually produce an infection in a laceration or an invasive infection in a burn wound. Larger numbers of bacteria also produce the "inoculum effect" in which the minimum inhibitory concentration (MIC) of an antibiotic is increased, making the antibiotic less effective.

The virulence of bacteria may be enhanced by a number of factors. Some bacteria are able to invade intact mucosa; others are not. Some bacteria have developed protective mechanisms; for example, the pneumococcus surrounds itself with a capsule that makes it difficult for the host to destroy. Others, especially gram-negative rods, contain an endotoxin (a lipopolysaccharide in the cell wall) that leads to septic shock. Although endotoxin alone does not produce all the symptoms of classic septic shock, it does cause the release of many endogenous mediators, which are probably responsible for the symptomatology. Cytokines such as interleukin-1 (IL-1) and IL-6, and tumor necrosis factor are released by white blood cells and produce profound physiologic changes. Hageman factor may alter the coagulation system and produce disseminated intravascular coagulation. Bradykinin, histamine,

and arachidonic acid metabolites all have vasoactive properties. Complement may cause the release of toxic oxygen radicals, and myocardial depressant factor decreases cardiac function. Nitric oxide appears to be the final common pathway on a cellular level for producing smooth muscle relaxation, which is responsible for decreased systemic vascular resistance and results in hypotension.

Many bacteria, notably the anaerobes, produce exotoxins that have specific detrimental effects on the host. *Clostridium perfringens* produces an exotoxin that causes gas gangrene. *Staphylococcus aureus* or *Streptococcus* may produce TSST-1, the exotoxin responsible for producing toxic shock syndrome.

A third factor is the development of antibiotic resistance by the bacteria. Probably the least important mechanism is genetic mutation. Far more important is passage of "R" factors and selection. "R" factors are cytoplasmic factors that can be transmitted from one gram-negative bacterium to another, even if a different species. They may then render the recipient bacteria resistant to many antibiotics. Selection of resistant strains occurs commonly in the hospital setting. Placing a person on a series of antibiotics kills off the sensitive strains, leaving the resistant ones free to proliferate. Bacteria are also transmitted from one patient to another on physicians' hands or by other means when proper technique is not followed.

A fourth factor is the presence of two bacteria, usually an aerobe and an anaerobe, that develop a synergistic relationship that enables each to proliferate by producing bacterial growth factors, depressing host defenses, producing an environment conducive to bacterial growth, or suppressing antibiotic effectiveness. For example, *Escherichia coli* may cause tissue necrosis, creating a reducing, anaerobic environment that allows *Bacteroides* to propagate. The anaerobe may produce hyaluronidase, which enhances the ability of the *E. coli* to spread, or a cephalosporinase, rendering treatment of *E. coli* with a cephalosporin ineffective.

NOSOCOMIAL INFECTIONS

Nosocomial, or hospital-acquired, infections are common and occur in about 5% of all patients in the hospital. The most common infection is in the urine and can be attributed to use of indwelling catheters. If proper sterile technique is not utilized, infection is almost inevitable after 72 hours. Pneumonia is the second most common infection, and its incidence is increased by prolonged endotracheal intubation and use of respirators, especially if sterile technique is ignored. It is advisable to keep patients in the sitting rather than the supine position, as lying flat in bed increases aspiration and decreases pulmonary function. It has been shown that the routine use of antacids and H_2 blockers allows colonization of the stomach and increases the incidence of pneumonia. The use of an indwelling nasogastric tube, though preventing vomiting by keeping the stomach empty, also has the adverse effect of keeping the gastroesophageal junction open, thereby allowing reflux to occur. In addition it may cause paranasal sinusitis, which can be severe and difficult to diagnose except on computed tomography (CT).

When the use of plastic cannulas for intravenous infusions became popular, phlebitis became a major problem. Any catheter inserted under less than ideal, sterile conditions should be removed as soon as possible, and those placed under sterile conditions should be changed every 3 days. Central lines used for hyperalimentation may remain in place longer if the proper precautions are taken: sterile insertion, frequent sterile dressing and tubing changes, no medications added, and no violations of sterility. The use of transparent dressings has been associated with an increase in the incidence of infection and should be discouraged. Other central venous pressure (CVP) lines should be changed every 3 to 5 days. They can be changed over a wire if the site does not seem infected. If the patient appears septic and the line is changed over a wire, the tip should be cultured. If the tip culture is positive, and the signs of infection have not abated, the new line must be removed. Positive blood cultures from an intravenous line necessitate removal of that line immediately. Patients who are immunosuppressed may develop a suppurative phlebitis from an intravenous line. This is the equivalent of an abscess in the vein; and like any other abscess, it does not respond to antibiotics without drainage or excision. The diagnosis is suspected in an immunosuppressed patient with an unknown source of sepsis or a virulent appearing phlebitis. The diagnosis can be confirmed by aspirating or incising the vein and finding pus or a blood clot that grows out an organism. A gallium scan can be helpful for identifying septic phlebitis in one of the central veins. A blood culture positive for *Staphylococcus* must be assumed to be caused by an infected intravenous line unless there is another obvious source.

Wound infections are common nosocomial infections found in surgical patients. Although wound infections are determined by the time the patient leaves the operating room, they are usually difficult to detect until 5 to 7 days later when the classic signs of rubor, calor, tumor, and dolor (erythema, heat, swelling, and pain) are present. Early signs of a wound infection include low-grade intermittent fever, persistently elevated white blood cell (WBC) count, pain in one area of the wound, edema, erythema, and lack of a healing ridge in the fascia under the wound. Two exceptions to the usual timing of wound infections are those caused by β-streptococci or *Clostridium*. Infections by these organism may manifest within hours of the operation.

Patients who have long-standing nasogastric or nasotracheal tubes may developed a purulent sinusitis causing a serious infection. Diagnosis is best made by obtaining CT scans of the sinus to look for air–fluid levels.

SURGICAL INFECTIONS

Types

Certain infections in the soft tissues require surgical treatment and do not respond to antibiotics alone. They include abscesses, infections of closed spaces (e.g., tendon sheaths), the presence of necrotic tissue, areas with poor blood supply, and instances of synergistic gangrene.

Diagnosis

Although some of these infections are obvious and the treatment is clear, others are subtle and difficult to locate. Frequently older patients and those who are immunosuppressed exhibit signs of infection or sepsis but do not readily reveal the location of the infection. A simple cellulitis that does not respond to appropriate antibiotic therapy must be suspected of harboring a necrotizing infection. Patients may be septic and have negative blood cultures if the sepsis is caused by dead bacteria, with bacterial toxins leaking out of a closed-space infection.

The history and physical examination are still the first and most valuable sources of information. Areas of pain, swelling, edema, and erythema may be clues to an underlying infection. Crepitance in the skin may be a sign of underlying subcutaneous emphysema indicating a gas producing infection. Areas of necrosis that are not explainable by vascular lesions are frequently a sign of underlying soft tissue infection with concomitant thrombosis of the arterioles in the subcutaneous tissue.

Radiologic studies usually come next. Plain films can be helpful for demonstrating gas in soft tissues. Ultrasonography may be useful if there are specific areas that need to be explored. CT scans are more appropriate when searching a wider area. Scintiscans (with tagged WBCs or gallium) specifically looking at infections can also be helpful.

When an infection is suspected in an area, it must be identified to properly treat it. A simple cellulitis can be treated with antibiotics and must be distinguished from an abscess with surrounding cellulitis, which requires surgical intervention. To establish a diagnosis, blisters can be aspirated and Gram-stained. A needle can be inserted into the suspicious area looking for pus. A small incision can be made in the area under local anesthesia looking for pus or necrotic tissue, which would indicate the need for surgery.

Is Surgery Required for an Abscess?

Although conventional wisdom dictates that surgery is required for an abscess because of poor penetration of antibiotics, it is only partially true. The main reasons have to do with poor blood supply and high concentrations of bacteria. The presence of functioning neutrophils are required to engulf the bacteria. Each neutrophil can ingest only 30 to 50 bacteria. If there are too many bacteria, and a limited blood supply prevents more WBCs from entering the area, the body's defenses are overwhelmed. Furthermore, the bacteria produce necrotic tissue and a reducing environment with low oxygen tension. Because the neutrophils need molecular oxygen to destroy the bacteria, they are not able to complete the job and are destroyed themselves, releasing lysosomal enzymes, which inhibit other neutrophils. Aminoglycosides need an aerobic environment to function. Although the antibiotic may be present in sufficient concentration, it has no effect because the bacteria are metabolizing anaerobically in the abscess.

Treatment

The basic principle of all soft tissue infections can be summed up in the three Ds: *D*rain, *D*ébride, and *D*o it again. One must drain all loculations of pus. It is done with an incision in some cases or by needle aspiration and catheter drainage in others. In either case, all areas of pus must be drained. Second, if necrotic tissue is present it must be débrided. Necrotic tissue left in place allows the spread of infection to continue and the bacteria to proliferate. Sometimes the surgeon is afraid to remove all the necrotic tissue because of the deficit left. It must be remembered that dead tissue never revives. Large defects in the abdominal wall can be replaced with absorbable mesh, which provides a good temporary barrier, or polypropylene mesh, which is permanent in some cases. The surgeon must be willing to return the patient to the operating room until the infection is under control.

SPECIFIC INFECTIONS OR ORGANISMS

Peritonitis

Peritonitis may be primary or secondary. Primary peritonitis usually occurs in patients with preexisting conditions, especially those who develop ascites such as cirrhosis and nephrotic syndrome. The peritonitis is characterized by an infection with one organism, usually a gram-positive coccus that does not originate in the alimentary tract. It can usually be treated with systemic antibiotics. Secondary peritonitis is an entirely different condition. It represents an infection in the peritoneal cavity secondary to a separate source, such as perforated bowel, appendicitis, or a gangrenous gallbladder. The diagnosis is based on the clinical findings of peritonitis with evidence of a pneumoperitoneum or gas bubbles on abdominal radiographs. An abdominal tap may disclose enteric bacteria or more than one organism. Because secondary peritonitis is decidedly more common than primary peritonitis, its presence must be ruled out before making the diagnosis of the primary type.

Clearly the principal concern when treating primary peritonitis is the pathology. If operation is indicated it should be delayed long enough to rehydrate the patient. (Insertion of a CVP or Swan-Ganz catheter to optimize the patient's physiologic state may be indicated.) An attempt is made to correct any metabolic or electrolyte problem. With an undrained abscess, it may not be possible to completely resolve an acidosis in a patient with bowel infarction or control the glucose in a diabetic. Even if the electrolyte problem does not resolve rapidly, operation should not be delayed. Broad-spectrum or appropriate antibiotics are started as soon as the decision to operate has been made. It is not clear as to when the antibiotics may be discontinued. It seems appropriate to continue them so long as there is an active infection and to stop them only after the temperature and WBC count have been normal for at least 48 hours.

The main thrust of the operation is to treat the primary pathology. This may be done by excising the infection or repairing the defect. Once this is done, attention is turned to treating the peritonitis.

Many forms of treatment have been advocated, and the definitive remedy has not yet been determined. Irrigating of the peritoneal cavity has the advantage of removing foreign bodies (feces, old food), removing toxic fluids (small bowel contents), and diluting the number of bacteria. The early theory that irrigation spreads the bacteria has been abandoned, as bacteria spread throughout the abdomen regardless of irrigation. There is a natural flow from the center of the abdomen to the periphery, and then up to the undersurface of the diaphragm, where the lymphatics clear the peritoneal cavity of bacteria and other microscopic particles. Evidence has disclosed that extensive lavage with many liters of fluid may be harmful, as macrophages and beneficial humeral substances are washed out of the peritoneum as well. Some surgeons believe that suctioning the fluid and removing particles is all that is necessary.

Placing antibiotics in the lavage solution has not been proved to have any advantage over systemic antibiotics. The main mode of action of peritoneal antibiotics appears to be their systemic activity after rapid absorption from the peritoneal cavity. Certainly a patient on adequate doses of systemic antibiotics may eventually have toxic levels if antibiotics are added to the peritoneal irrigation. It is now accepted that the patient's own peritoneal defenses are compromised if fluid remains in the peritoneal cavity at the completion of the operation. Therefore the abdomen is suctioned as dry as possible prior to closure.

An abscess cavity can be drained, but it is impossible to drain the entire peritoneal cavity. Loculations and abscesses form regardless of the presence of drains. If drains are left in, suction drains with a closed system are preferred. The Penrose drain allows bacteria to enter the peritoneum. When necrotic tissue or foreign bodies are anticipated in the drainage fluid, large-caliber drains must be fashioned and some compromise to the closed drainage system may have to be made.

Several other modes of therapy have been described to treat severe peritonitis. Leaving in a peritoneal catheter for dialysis over several days after the operation has been tried with good results in some cases but without conclusive evidence that it is effective. Massive peritoneal débridement of all fibrin has been described, but evidence now shows that it may be more harmful than beneficial. Many modes of open drainage, treating the peritoneal cavity like an abscess, have been tried. They include frequent returns to the operating room for débridement and drainage or the use of a zipper and mesh to allow open irrigation in the surgical intensive care unit (SICU). These methods appear to offer some benefit in selected cases, but their ultimate use has yet to be determined.

Peritonitis in patients with indwelling peritoneal dialysis catheters represents a special case. If the catheter site is infected, the catheter must be removed. If the fluid appears infected, Gram stains and cultures are prepared. If more than one organism is found, bowel perforation is presumed and exploration is indicated. If only one organism is found, a trial of antibiotic installation can be started. If successful the catheter can continue to be used. If it is not successful or if fungus or *Pseudomonas* is found, the catheter must be removed.

Occult Infections

Although it would be advantageous to diagnose an infection at the earliest possible time, it is occasionally difficult. Many times the source, or even the presence, of an infection is obscure. An early diagnosis can frequently be made only by being suspicious because of one of the signs or symptoms of occult infection: unexplained tachycardia, tachypnea, pain, confusion, hypotension, ileus, organ failure, decreased platelets, hyperglycemia, or gastrointestinal (GI) bleeding. If the patient has any of these problems without a logical explanation, a source of infection is sought.

Liver Abscess

A liver abscess may be classified by the etiology (traumatic, biliary, contiguous intraabdominal infection, portal, or hematogenous) or the causative organism (amebic, echinococcal, staphylococcal, or enteric). Obviously treatment is aimed at eradicating both the source and the abscess.

Amebic abscesses may be diagnosed by a history compatible with the acquisition of an infection; stool cultures are frequently negative. Serology or aspiration may be helpful. Treatment is with metronidazole, and rarely surgery is required.

Echinococcus is suspected on the basis of the history, calcifications on radiography, and serologic tests. Treatment is initially with drugs, but surgical removal may be required. Aspiration is contraindicated.

Staphylococcal infections are usually from a hematogenous source and are frequently multiple, not responding readily to drainage. Enteric infections frequently need to be drained, either radiologically or surgically.

Emphysematous Cholecystitis

Emphysematous cholecystitis is a form of acute cholecystitis in which gas is found in the lumen or wall of the gallbladder. It occurs more often in male subjects and in patients with diabetes. The organism is often *Clostridium,* which is responsible for producing the gas. It frequently progresses to gangrene, so surgery is always indicated.

Clostridial Infections

The classic clostridial infection, or gas gangrene, is relatively uncommon. Most infections with gas-producing organisms are not caused by clostridia. Clostridial myonecrosis is characterized by severe pain, profound toxicity, foul discharge, and hemolysis. Treatment consists in penicillin and extensive débridement or ablation. Clostridial myonecrosis may be the one infection in which hyperbaric oxygen is useful.

Clostridium difficile colitis or pseudomembranous colitis is caused by overgrowth of the bacterium in the colon, usually after antibiotic therapy. Its presence is suspected when diarrhea occurs after antibiotic treat-

ment. The diagnosis is based on seeing the typical pseudomembranes on sigmoidoscopy, finding elevated *C. difficile* toxin levels in the stool, or culturing the organism from the stool. Treatment is with oral vancomycin or metronidazole. The use of antidiarrheal agents are contraindicated. Extreme cases may require surgery, especially to rule out other acute surgical conditions. If exploration is done for symptoms so severe the patient is thought to have an acute abdomen and if the only finding at surgery is an edematous colon that is thought to be pseudomembranous colitis, it is recommended that subtotal colectomy be carried out as a life-saving procedure.

Tetanus represents the systemic effect of the exotoxin produced by an infection with *Clostridium tetani*. The organism is ubiquitous in soil contaminated with feces. Susceptible wounds do not have to be large, but they are often deep, allowing the organism to grow in an environment away from oxygen. Symptoms include muscle spasms, convulsions, and trismus. Treatment of the disease, once it occurs, includes sedation, avoidance of stimuli, and intubation. Although the organism is sensitive to penicillin, antibiotic treatment has little effect once the disease has started because the symptoms are due to the exotoxin and not the organism per se. Prevention is far more effective than treatment. Immunization with tetanus toxoid is effective for 10 years. Tetanus immune globulin is used for suspicious wounds when immunization is uncertain. If a patient has a clean wound, toxoid is given if the immunization status is uncertain. If the complete series of three shots was given during the last 10 years, toxoid is not necessary. When the wounds are dirty, both tetanus toxoid and tetanus immunoglobulin are indicated if the patient is less than fully immunized.

A patient who develops septicemia with *Clostridium septicum* or *Streptococcus bovis* should be evaluated for an ulcerating carcinoma of the colon.

Staphylococcal Infections

Staphylococcus aureus is a common infecting organism in the skin. It classically produces an abscess; and if it infects a hair follicle it is called a furuncle, which is a simple abscess treated by incision and drainage. The furuncle should not be confused with a carbuncle. The latter is a necrotizing infection that usually occurs in the thick skin of the back or neck in diabetics. The carbuncle is often a mixed infection is larger than a furuncle, and is multiloculated with both pus and necrotic tissue. Treatment of the carbuncle includes excising of the necrotic tissue and being certain to incise all loculations of pus.

Staphylococcal infections may produce two systemic manifestations. Some patients develop a vasculitis with a typical purpuric rash on the extremities. The lesions are not infected and usually clear up when the staphylococcal infection is eradicated. Occasionally the vasculitis causes ischemia and necrosis. The other infection is the "toxic shock syndrome" found most often in menstruating female individuals who use superabsorbent tampons. The syndrome can be fatal as patients may rapidly develop profound shock. It is caused by certain strains of *Staphylococcus* that produce the causative toxin.

Whereas the organism used to be sensitive to penicillin, now almost all strains are resistant; therefore penicillinase-resistant penicillins (oxacillin or first-generation cephalosporins) should be used. Methicillin-resistant *Staphylococcus aureus* (MRSA) has become common, especially in hospital-acquired infections. It should be treated with vancomycin.

Streptococcal Infections

Classically, skin infections with β-streptococci cause cellulitis or lymphangitis. Treatment with penicillin is appropriate. Occasionally the toxic shock syndrome, or vasculitis, is due to streptococci as well as staphylococci. Sometimes the organism produces a spreading cellulitis or myositis (the infamous flesh-eating bacteria). The diagnosis can be established by Gram-staining the serosanguineous discharge or incising tissue. Treatment is with penicillin and physiologic support. In the absence of necrosis, débridement is not necessary. Soft tissue infections may also be caused by an anaerobic streptococcus. They are usually sensitive to penicillin. If the presence of *Bacteroides* cannot be excluded because of the source (GI or gynecologic) or the odor (*Bacteroides* infections smell like feces), metronidazole or clindamycin should be used.

A patient who develops septicemia with *Streptococcus bovis* or *Clostridium septicum* should be evaluated for ulcerating carcinoma of the colon.

Candida

Fungal infection caused by *Candida* should be thought of in a patient, especially if immunocompromised, who has an infection that is being treated but the fever or leukocytosis is not responding to antibiotics. Although the organism is frequently found as a contaminant, when it is cultured from blood, is the only organism found in infected fluid (peritonitis or abscess), or is cultured from two or more sources, it must be assumed to be a genuine infecting organism. It must be treated with systemic antifungal drugs such as fluconazole or amphotericin B.

Helicobacter pylori

Helicobacter pylori is found in the stomach of patients with gastritis, duodenitis, and duodenal ulcers. It appears to be a causative agent of peptic ulcer disease, duodenitis, and some gastritis. Diagnosis is made by mucosal biopsy and either seeing the organism on microscopic section or culturing it in a medium looking for ammonia formation. Evidence has shown that the organism can be eradicated with treatment consisting of antibiotics (metronidazole, tetracycline, or amoxicillin), bismuth salts, and a drug that lowers gastric acid. If the organism is eradicated, the recurrence or relapse rate of the ulcer is significantly reduced.

Lyme Disease

Lyme disease is an illness caused by the spirochete *Borrelia burgdorferi*. The microbe, carried by the deer tick *Ixodes dammini,* is now endemic in the Northeast. The infection is characterized by a circular rash and manifestations of a viral illness. On occasion, the acute illness is missed, and the first manifestation may be the chronic phase, involving the joints, heart, or nervous system. Diagnosis is by serologic tests, but these can be negative, especially during the chronic phase. Detection may then depend on the history of exposure and suspicion. Treatment is with a tetracycline, penicillin, or ceftriaxone.

Animal Bites

Dog or other animal bites are be treated with irrigation, débridement of ischemic tissue, and tetanus prophylaxis. Antibiotic treatment with a cephalosporin, amoxicillin-clavulanate, or ampicillin-sulbactam is used to cover the range of expected organisms including *Pasteurella multocida*. Generally, fresh dog bites, especially in the face, are closed primarily.

Human bites, on the other hand, usually become infected. They most commonly occur after a fist has come in contact with teeth. The wound is explored to determine the depths. Antibiotic treatment (similar to that for dog bites) is mandatory. Frequently *Eikenella corrodens* is cultured. It has been suggested that if the wound is recent and clean, and the joint and tendon sheaths are not involved, the patient can be sent home on oral antibiotics after débridement.

Rabies is always a threat to be considered with animal bites. This disease, caused by a virus, is fatal once contracted. It is endemic in bats and is commonly found in carnivores and omnivores such as raccoons, skunks, and foxes. In areas where the disease is endemic, domestic animals may become infected if not immunized. Any contact with the saliva of an infected animal is cause for immunization, which consists of five doses of human diploid cell vaccine (HDCV) and rabies immune globulin (RIG).

Human Immunodeficiency Virus

Infection with the human immunodeficiency virus (HIV) is spread by exchange of bodily fluid, usually blood or sexual secretions. Although spread in the United State was initially through homosexual contact and via dirty needles, spread in Africa is primarily through heterosexual contact. There is no cure, and medications merely slow the course of the disease or treat the superinfections. Surgeons may be called on to help make a diagnosis (lymph node biopsy to look for lymphoma, lung biopsy for *Pneumocystis carinii,* or drainage of an abscess looking for *Mycobacterium*). Patients with acquired immunodeficiency syndrome (AIDS) may develop an assortment of intestinal infections that can cause pain and diarrhea. An acute surgical abdomen may result from perforations of the intestines caused by cytomegalovirus, cryptosporidiosis, candidiasis, or lymphoma. Intestinal obstruction has been described with Kaposi's sarcoma and lymphoma.

ANTIBIOTICS

For an antibiotic to work, it must come in contact with the bacteria, the drug must be in an active form, the patient's defense mechanisms must be intact, and the dosage must be adequate. Prophylactic antibiotics are no exception, and the indications for use are well described. They can be used for one event, such as an operation, but are not effective over a long period. Thus one cannot use prophylactic antibiotics to prevent an infection in a burn wound or a urinary infection in a patient with an indwelling Foley catheter. The only time prophylactic antibiotics are effective over a prolonged period is if the organism being targeted is always susceptible to the antibiotic. Thus penicillin can be used to prevent postsplenectomy pneumococcal sepsis.

Prophylactic antibiotics should be used for all clean-contaminated or contaminated operations (the use of antibiotics in dirty cases is considered treatment) or if the expected infection rate will be greater than 5%. The proper antibiotic must be chosen. Usually cefazolin suffices; but when the colonic flora must be considered, as with penetrating trauma to the abdomen, the spectrum must be extended to a wide variety of gram-negative rods and also cover anaerobes such as *Bacteroides fragilis*. In this case either an aminoglycoside (or azactam), a drug against anaerobes (metronidazole) with or without ampicillin, or single-drug therapy with a second-generation cephalosporin (cefoxitin or cefotetan) should be used. The antibiotic is started about 0.5 hour before the operation commences or in the case of trauma as soon as it is decided to operate. Tissue and blood levels must be maintained throughout surgery, which in the case of cefazolin means that it should be repeated after 3 hours if the operation is still going on, but it need not be continued after the operation is completed. When a foreign body graft is to be left in place, antibiotics are routinely started before surgery and continued for 4 to 7 days. The dose of prophylactic antibiotic should be the same as is used for treatment.

Penicillin

Penicillin is still an effective antibiotic. It prevents synthesis of peptidoglycans in the bacterial cell wall. Penicillin V is the treatment of choice against β-hemolytic streptococcus, pneumococcus, and most anaerobes (excluding *Bacteroides*). The aminopenicillins (ampicillin and amoxicillin) have extended gram-negative coverage but are not effective against penicillinase resistant staphylococci. The carboxypenicillins (carbenicillin and ticarcillin) and the ureidopenicillins (mezlocillin and azlocillin) have further enhanced gram-negative coverage and can be used to treat infections with *Pseudomonas aeruginosa*. When these antibiotics are combined with β-lactamase inhibitor (e.g., clavulanate or sulbactam) they have an even broader spectrum, rivaling the third-generation cephalosporins, but the combination has no increased activity against *Pseudomonas*. The penicillinase-resistant penicillins (methicillin, oxacillin, nafcillin, dicloxacillin) are the drugs of choice against most strains of *Staphylococcus aureus*. Unfortunately, MRSA is becoming more common, especially in hospitals, and is resistant to all penicillins. Therefore a nosocomial infection with *S. aureus* should be treated with vancomycin. The most important side effect of penicillins is allergy, which may range from a rash to anaphylaxis.

Cephalosporins

Cephalosporins are related to the penicillins, and 15% of people with penicillin allergies experience an allergic reaction to the cephalosporins. Cephalosporins are generally classified as first, second, or third generation, which approximates their effectiveness against gram-negative bacteria. As a rule, first-generation cephalosporins have the best coverage against gram-positive organisms and the least against gram-negative rods. They are most useful against infections caused by gram-positive cocci. Second-generation cephalosporins (cefotetan, cefoxitin) have enhanced gram-negative coverage, are highly effective against anaerobes (including *Bacteroides*), but are less effective against staphylococci. The third-generation cephalosporins provide even more gram-negative coverage, including *Pseudomonas* coverage in some cases. They are less useful for treating infections caused by anaerobes or gram-positive organisms. They have a great advantage in that they cross the blood–brain barrier, making them useful for treating gram-negative meningitis. The side effects of the cephalosporins include allergy, hemorrhagic diathesis, thrombocytopenia, disulfiram like reaction when alcohol is ingested, nephrotoxicity when used with aminoglycosides or furosemide, and enterococcal sepsis. (None of the cephalosporins is active against *Enterococcus*.)

Carbapenems

The carbapenems are related to the cephalosporins, and people allergic to the cephalosporins may also be allergic to the carbapenems. The antibiotic imipenem would be rapidly metabolized by the renal tubular epithelium if given alone. For this reason it is combined with cilastatin, which blocks metabolism of the antibiotic. This antibiotic has one of the broadest spectra of any antibiotic covering both aerobes and anaerobes.

Monobactams

The monobactams (aztreonam) do not have cross-allergy with the cephalosporins. The spectrum is similar to that of the aminoglycosides in that there is excellent gram-negative coverage with poor coverage of anaerobes and gram-positive bacteria. They have an advantage over the aminoglycosides by not causing renal toxicity or ototoxicity.

Aminoglycosides

The aminoglycosides (gentamicin, tobramycin, amikacin) provide excellent coverage of gram-negative rods. They have no effect against anaerobes, as they require the bacteria to be metabolizing aerobically to be effective. They bind to the 30S bacterial ribosome to prevent protein synthesis. The greatest drawback to their use is their renal toxicity and ototoxicity. The nephrotoxicity may be enhanced by simultaneous administration of a cephalosporin, vancomycin, or furosemide. Hence serum levels must be determined. The trough level, obtained 30 minutes before a dose, may indicate enhanced toxicity if elevated. The peak levels, obtained at least 30 minutes after a dose, may indicate ineffective levels if too low. There is some evidence that there is significant benefit when giving aminoglycosides once a day at a dose of 4 to 7mg/kg for gentamicin or tobramycin and 12 to 15 mg/kg for amikacin. When the antibiotic is given this way the toxicity is less, the effectiveness is at least as great, and the cost is less.

Quinolones

The quinolone antibiotics have been used for urinary tract infections for a long time. Recent additions (ciprofloxacin, ofloxacin, norfloxacin) have proved useful for gram-negative and staphylococcal coverage, with poor anaerobic and streptococcal coverage. They have good soft tissue and bone penetration, making them useful for the oral antibiotic treatment of osteomyelitis. Their use may be limited by the rapid development of resistance by *Pseudomonas* and *Staphylococcus*.

Other Antibiotics

Vancomycin is the drug of choice against MRSA and is used orally for pseudomembranous colitis. It acts on bacteria by preventing synthesis of the cell wall. The main complications are renal toxicity and the "red neck" syndrome (a rash involving the upper part of the body) when the drug is infused rapidly.

Erythromycin is a macrolide that binds to the 50S ribosome preventing protein synthesis. It provides good gram-positive coverage and some anaerobic coverage. It has proved useful for enhancing gastric motility. Newly released macrolides, such as clarithromycin and azithromycin, have a longer half-life and a broader spectrum than erythromycin.

Metronidazole is effective only against anaerobes (and a few other organisms such as trichomonads and ameba). It is effective when used orally against pseudomembranous colitis caused by *Clostridium difficile*.

QUESTIONS

Select one answer.

1. The most important step in the body disposing of bacteria is:
   a. The action of interferon.
   b. The ability of the granulocyte to phagocytize the bacteria.
   c. T lymphocyte production of antibodies.
   d. The action of Tumor Necrosis Factor.
   e. Fibroblastic proliferation.
2. Which one of the following has NOT been demonstrated to increase the chance of postoperative infection?
   a. Chemotherapeutic agents.
   b. Preoperative hospitalization.
   c. Starvation.
   d. Use of steroids.
   e. Anemia.
3. Which of the following endogenous mediators has been implicated in producing symptoms of septic shock?
   a. Interleukin-1.
   b. Hageman factor.
   c. Arachidonic acid metabolites.
   d. Tumor Necrosis factor.
   e. All of the above.
4. Which of the following bacteria produces a wound infection within 48 hr of surgery?
   1. *S. aureus.*
   2. β-Streptococcus.
   3. *E. coli.*
   4. *Bacteroides.*
   5. Clostridia.
   a. 1,3.
   b. 2,3.
   c. 3,5.
   d. 2,5.
   e. 4,5.
5. All of the following are signs of soft tissue infection EXCEPT:
   a. Skin necrosis.
   b. Decreased pulses.
   c. Crepitance.
   d. Edema.
   e. Erythema.
6. Primary peritonitis differs from secondary peritonitis in that primary peritonitis:
   a. Is usually caused by one organism.
   b. Doesn't cause pain.
   c. Is associated with strangulated bowel.
   d. Frequently is associated with free air in the peritoneum.
   e. Usually is associated with foul smelling pus.
7. Which of the following statements about emphysematous cholecystitis is NOT true?
   a. Is more common in men than women.
   b. Is frequently caused by clostridia.
   c. Is more common in diabetic patients.
   d. Is characterized by gas in the lumen or the wall of the gallbladder.
   e. Can frequently be treated without surgery.

8. Complications of cephalosporin treatment include all of the following except:
   a. Allergy.
   b. Hearing loss.
   c. Renal dysfunction.
   d. Enterococcal sepsis.
   e. Hemorrhagic diathesis.
9. Clavulinic acid is added to a penicillin to:
   a. Make the drug more effective against resistant organisms.
   b. Prevent penicillin allergies.
   c. Decrease toxic side effects.
   d. Enhance oral absorption.
   e. Increase the cost.

SELECTED REFERENCES

American College of Surgeons Care of the Surgical Patient. Section IX. *Infection.* New York: Scientific American.
Howard RJ, Simmons RL. *Surgical infectious diseases,* 3rd ed. Norwalk, CT: Appleton & Lange, 1994.

33

Minimally Invasive Surgery

Sylvain Kleinhaus

HISTORY

Laparoscopy has made great strides since the first cholecystectomy was performed in 1987 in France by Mouret. We present an overview of this rapidly evolving field and highlight some of the more popular and accepted procedures in pediatric and adult surgery.

Gynecologists were the first group to use laparoscopy routinely for diagnostic purposes during the 1950s. They used open tube instruments derived from the early esophagoscopes and sigmoidoscopes. The light sources were primitive, and the field of vision was restricted to the organs in close proximity to the distal end of the open tube. Only one person at a time could view the pelvic structures, and a vivid imagination was a helpful asset when describing the pathology. The development of rod lenses by Hopkins in England and the incorporation of fiberoptic bundles into the body of the laparoscopes greatly brightened and enlarged the field of view. The unwieldy beam splitters that allowed more than one viewer and operative assistants to participate were replaced by progressively smaller television cameras, which allow all personnel involved in the operation to see and contribute and learn at the same time.

Many ingenious instruments were devised to allow one to handle and manipulate the intraabdominal structures. The most remarkable of these instruments was the multifiring clip applier, which permitted controlled cutting of vessels and ducts. Specialized catheters were developed for intraoperative cholangiography; and bipolar instruments were invented, such as scissors and forceps, making cauterization of bleeding points easier and safer. With bipolar instruments the cauterizing current does not pass through the patient but, rather, goes down one arm of the instrument, through the tissue, and then back up the second arm, thereby reducing the chance of intraabdominal injury and electrical disturbances of conduction.

One of the newest instruments developed for minimally invasive surgery (MIS) and used extensively in many procedures is the harmonic scalpel, which uses high-frequency ultrasonic energy to cut and coagulate without any need for grounding, as no electrical circuitry is employed in the patient. Small vessels (up to 2 to 3 mm in diameter) may be coagulated and cut safely without the need for clips, rendering the procedure faster and eliminating the interference by clips, which may complicate computed tomography (CT) scans done at a later date.

The resounding success of laparoscopic cholecystectomy popularized the field of MIS with the development of new and improved instruments, operations, and outcomes. All these advances, however, did not come without a price. The new technology was and is expensive to develop and market and must be fiscally reasonable. The training of the physicians is often long and difficult, and once again there must be a credentialing process to ensure proficiency of the individuals doing the surgery. As with any new process, there is a learning curve, and one must expect that early results will improve with experience.

SPECIFIC PROCEDURES

The list of procedures now performed laparoscopically essentially duplicates the list of procedures done in an open fashion. The indications for each operation should not differ from the conventional open method, and the results should at least equal those of laparotomy. The advantages of laparoscopy, such as smaller, more cosmetic incisions and in many cases shorter hospital stay, should not compromise the final results, nor should the higher costs of some laparoscopic procedures deny patients access to them.

Cholecystectomy

Cholecystectomy was the procedure that launched the modern era of MIS, and it is still one of the most commonly performed laparoscopic procedures in children and adolescents (Table 33.1). Hematologic diseases such as spherocytosis and sickle cell disease are among the more common indications for cholecystectomy in children, as well as calculous and acalculous cholecystitis of idiopathic origin. The results in children and adolescents are similar to those in adults with a low incidence of complications (7). A large experi-

TABLE 33.1. *Frequently performed MIS procedures in pediatric patients*

Laparoscopy
Cholecystectomy
Appendectomy
Antireflux procedures
Splenectomy
Abdominal exploration
Lymph node biopsy
Liver biopsy of specific lesions
Staging Laparoscopy
Exploration for intestinal obstruction
Diagnosis pelvic pathology (culture taking and surgical
    management)
Exploration for undescended testicle
Varicocele surgery

ence with laparoscopic cholecystectomy has now been accumulated for patients of all ages, and this method has definitely become the "gold standard" for biliary disease. The first series of patients undergoing laparoscopic cholecystectomy had a higher incidence of common duct injury than open cholecystectomy; but as experience has grown, the rate of injury closely approaches that of open surgery and continues to decrease (2).

Appendectomy

Appendectomy using MIS techniques is a bit more controversial (4). Many (or most) surgeons prefer the time-honored open technique through a small transverse right lower quadrant (RLQ) incision in those cases where the preoperative diagnosis clearly seems to be acute appendicitis. This is especially true in small patients where the sum of the mini-trocar incisions is no smaller than the RLQ incision. In cases where the diagnosis is equivocal and a wider, more thorough abdominal exploration might be necessary, laparoscopy certainly has many advantages. Often the absence of appendicitis can be documented, cultures prepared, and appropriate treatment initiated (e.g., primary peritonitis). In the case of adolescent and teenage girls with lower abdominal pain the diagnosis is sometimes unclear, and an exploratory laparoscopy can direct the therapy (surgical or otherwise) appropriately (6).

A perforated appendix is not a contraindication to laparoscopic exploration, as effective peritoneal toilet may be performed as well as appendectomy in those difficult cases. It is not yet clear if it will become an accepted treatment modality for this indication. Interval appendectomies may also prove to be ideal situations for the use of MIS because significant adhesions are sometimes present following a missed appendicitis, and three or four small trocar incisions are preferable to an extended McBurney or Rocky-Davis RLQ incision.

Splenectomy

Many of the same hematologic diseases that cause biliary disease also are indications for splenectomy. Idiopathic thrombocytopenic purpura (ITP) that does not respond to medical therapy can often be improved by splenectomy, and spherocytosis symptoms can be alleviated by removing the spleen. In addition, splenectomy is included when staging Hodgkin's disease and other malignancies, and the requisite biopsies may also be performed using MIS. To optimize the chances for complete remission of all these diseases, it is important to identify and remove any and all accessory spleens. This can be done effectively at the primary MIS procedure and, when necessary, as a secondary procedure regardless of which method was used during the first operation (11). In all these cases laparoscopic splenectomy, when feasible, is advantageous to the patient because of the significantly smaller incisions. The postoperative wound discomfort is less, left lower lobe atelectasis is less common, and the patient ambulates sooner. Laparoscopic splenectomy is more difficult when the patient has a large spleen, and some surgeons believe this is a relative contraindication to MIS. In cases of splenic trauma, laparoscopy is rarely employed as a treatment modality, as the presence of large amounts of intraperitoneal blood make it difficult to explore the abdomen properly for other injuries, and the splenic pedicle is more difficult to isolate laparoscopically (3).

Antireflux Procedures

One of the unfortunate consequences of our improved ability to keep severely compromised infants and children alive is that we now care for an increasing number of children who are neurologically impaired and who require gastrostomies and antireflux procedures for long-term maintenance in extended-care facilities. The antireflux procedures reduce, but do not eliminate, the incidence of reflux; and many surgeons now perform a fundoplication at the same time as the gastrostomy. The presence of a ventriculoperitoneal shunt is not a contraindication to MIS in these cases. It is important to stress that the indications for laparoscopic antireflux surgery should be identical to those for open surgery; only the approach is different. The results so far have been excellent with fewer postoperative respiratory problems and decreased needs for pain medication (12).

Many centers that treat adult patients with gastroesophageal reflux are content to do so using the newer motility-enhancing drugs and various H_2 blockers. This protocol essentially condemns the patient to long-term oral medication with the attendant expenses and side effects. Although the Nissen fundoplication (or its various modifications) is not a perfect operation, it has been used throughout the world for many years and has been performed using MIS for at least 5 years with good success.

Other Gastrointestinal Procedures

Exploratory laparoscopy and adhesiolysis for intestinal obstruction has been performed successfully for postoperative adhesions, malrotation, and other indications (5). Intestinal resection and anastomosis has also been performed, but most surgeons now do laparoscopically assisted resections (the bowel to be excised is prepared using MIS but is then brought out through a small incision; the resection and anastomosis are performed extracorporeally, and the bowel is then replaced into the peritoneal cavity under direct vision). Bleeding Meckel's diverticula have been treated in the same way, and several reports have documented the advantages of MIS for surgical treatment of Crohn's disease (8).

Liver Biopsy

The laparoscopically directed liver biopsy based on CT scan or magnetic resonance imaging (MRI) findings was one of the first widely accepted "interventional" uses of MIS and is still used today in cases where the suspected lesion is not readily accessible through a CT scan window.

Exploratory Laparoscopy

Although perforated duodenal ulcers are no longer as commonplace as they were now that *Helicobacter pylori* has been discovered and is being treated successfully by antibiotics and acid blockers, peptic ulcer disease with perforation still occurs. If one is found at exploratory laparoscopy, an omental patch may be placed over the ulcer using MIS and medical treatment initiated. In many cases, it obviates the need for an open surgical approach altogether.

Adrenalectomy

A use for MIS recently described and implemented in many centers is adrenalectomy. This method has been used successfully for both pheochromocytomas and cortical tumors, though MIS is not recommended for obvious malignancies with proved metastases or for tumors larger than 5 cm in diameter, which are more likely to be malignant.

Three approaches have been used for laparoscopic adrenalectomy: posterior, lateral, and anterior. Most surgeons now seem to be using the lateral approach. The posterior technique is preferred by some in cases where both adrenals are to be removed, and the bilateral operation can be completed without moving the patient from the prone position. The difference in the postoperative course between the open procedure, which usually requires a large laparotomy with its inherent morbidity, and the MIS procedure has been striking. Patients have been up and around the day after surgery and discharged 1 to 2 days thereafter, compared with an average of 5 to 7 days in hospital prior to MIS (13).

Hernia Repair

Although laparoscopic hernia repair has gained favor in some adult centers, many surgeons seem to be using onlay mesh with or without a plug or a variation of the Shouldice technique. The laparoscopic approach places a mesh patch on the peritoneal side of the hernial defect and tacks the mesh in place with specially developed staplers. The MIS approach seems especially appropriate in patients with bilateral hernias or in cases where previous inguinal operations have been unsuccessful.

Another use for MIS in hernia repair has been in patients with a symptomatic hernia on one side and a questionable hernia on the contralateral side. A small 30-degree scope may be placed through the open sac on the symptomatic side, and the internal ring and posterior wall of the contralateral side are visualized. The presence or absence of a hernia can be established and an unnecessary operation prevented.

Undescended Testicle

Minimally invasive surgery has also been used to explore the retroperitoneum in cases of undescended testicle. When the gonad is not palpable in the scrotum or inguinal canal, it may still be present retroperitoneally anywhere between the peritoneal aspect of the internal ring and the inferior pole of the kidney. Although ultrasound examination is useful in some cases for identifying the testicle, definitive identification can best be performed by direct visualization. The size and shape of

the testicle can be ascertained; and if there is any question as to whether the gonad is a testicle or ovary, a biopsy can be performed. Based on the results of the biopsy a gonadectomy may be indicated. If the gonad is a testicle, and it has been decided to bring it down into the scrotum, the first stage of a Fowler-Stevens repair (clipping the testicular artery, allowing the artery parallel to the vas and other small accessory vessels to perfuse the testicle) may be performed using MIS techniques (14).

Varicocele

Ligation of the venous plexus for varicocele may be performed using MIS. The veins exiting the internal ring may be clipped or ligated under direct vision, and some of the anastomotic branches to the pelvic and abdominal wall veins can be identified, separated from the arteries, and ligated. MIS is certainly advantageous in recurrent cases so one may avoid entering the scar tissue of the previous incision and dissection.

Gynecologic Indications

In the gynecologic arena, MIS has developed and grown since the early observational laparoscopies. The newer technology has allowed more exact inspection and accurately directed biopsies and cultures.

Ovarian cysts are common during infancy, but most of those visualized on prenatal or postnatal ultrasound scans are less than 5 cm in diameter. These cysts may be safely observed without intervention, and most recede and disappear. Cysts larger than 5 cm in diameter can be followed, resected or biopsied, and drained by the use of MIS. Cysts that appear during adolescence are frequently follicular cysts and eventually recede or rupture spontaneously. If they do not, laparoscopic intervention is indicated, and the contralateral ovary may be inspected as well. In the older patients there is some controversy as to whether MIS should be used for excision or aspiration of ovarian cysts, as any spillage of malignant tumor cells into the peritoneal cavity could significantly change the long-term prognosis in these patients.

Minimally invasive surgery may also be helpful for the diagnosis of ectopic pregnancies where ultrasonography is equivocal or the patient's condition calls for more immediate intervention. Definitive treatment may also be accomplished endoscopically. Laparoscopy is useful for establishing a diagnosis in cases of congenital uterine malformations such as uterus didelphys, absent uterine horns, vaginal atresia, and so on. Although these diagnoses may be suspected based on radiologic data, they are usually best substantiated by direct observation through the endoscope. Appropriate surgical treatment may also be performed using MIS.

In oncologic cases requiring irradiation along the course of the major vessels (aorta, bifurcation, iliacs), it is often recommended that the ovaries be fixed in the midline, behind the uterus, to avoid the direct effects of external beam irradiation. Oophoropexy is sometimes performed at the time of the primary procedure; but if not, it may also be accomplished laparoscopically as a second stage (9).

Minimally invasive surgery has proved useful for hysterectomy. Many if not most vaginal hysterectomies are now being performed with laparoscopic assistance. The uterine vessels can be safely ligated under direct vision, rendering the operation safer without significant abdominal scars. In addition, the field of urogynecology has flourished with the help of MIS, allowing procedures for prolapse and incontinence to be performed more easily and with greater patient acceptance.

Thoracic Procedures

Lung biopsies are being performed more often especially in urban centers where the pulmonary complications of human immunodeficiency virus (HIV) infections have been identified with greater frequency (Table 33.2). The diagnosis of *Pneumocystis carinii* infection is sometimes difficult to establish without a tissue culture and biopsy. This can be done thoracoscopically with lower morbidity and less pain than by the open method. Often bronchoscopy with washings is per-

formed under the same anesthesia. Excision of lesions identified on CT scan or MRI may be accomplished easily, especially if the masses are close to or on the pleural surfaces.

Exploration for neoplasms of the lung and chest wall may be biopsied or excised thoracoscopically. Segmental lung resection has been made much easier by the development of endoscopic stapling instruments and the harmonic scalpel.

Mediastinal masses may be biopsied or excised thoracoscopically in many cases. Duplication cysts of the esophagus, bronchogenic cysts, and small sequestrations are lesions that may be successfully excised using MIS. Pericardial windows are easily performed thoracoscopically, and this procedure has become another in the growing list of procedures that may be safely performed by MIS. Hyperhydrosis has been effectively treated by ablation of the upper sympathetic ganglia at the apex of the pleural cavity (1). In cases where vagotomy is indicated, the vagus nerves can usually be identified along the lower esophageal wall, and truncal vagotomy can be accomplished without resorting to open thoracotomy. Decortication and release of trapped lungs as well as drainage of loculated pleural effusions with precise placement of thoracostomy tubes for maximum efficiency can be done without a major thoracotomy incision. Achalasia patients are also benefiting from the progress of MIS as Heller procedures are being performed successfully. MIS has expanded into the field of spinal surgery as increasing numbers of centers are using this technique for diskectomy; thoracoscopy for thoracic disks to be removed in cases of scoliosis and laparoscopy for lumbar scoliosis and for lower back pain (10).

The scope of MIS in the care of pediatric patients is sure to expand as more surgeons are trained to perform more varied and complicated procedures safely. These advances can only encourage more patients and pediatricians to seek the benefits of progress of modern technology and innovation in providing better care for our patients.

TABLE 33.2. *Thoracoscopic procedures*

Lung biopsy and cultures
Segmental lung resections
Lymph Node Biopsy
Excision mediastinal mass
Decortication of empyema
Pleurodesis
Vagotomy and esophageal procedures
Diaphragmatic exploration
Sympathectomy for hyperhydrosis

QUESTIONS

1. For which of the following conditions is laparoscopy relatively contraindicated?
   a. Ruptured appendicitis.
   b. Ruptured spleen.

c. Ovarian cyst.

d. Acute cholecystitis.

2. Which of the following reduces the incidence of injuries during laparoscopy?

a. Three-chip camera.

b. Routine cholangiography.

c. Bipolar instrumentation.

d. Trocars of 5 mm.

3. Which of the following diagnostic modalities is most useful for locating an undescended testis?

a. Ultrasonograpy.

b. Nuclear scan.

c. Angiography.

d. Laparoscopy.

4. For which of the following is thoracoscopy indicated?

a. Repair of a tracheoesophageal fistula.

b. Repair of a congenital diaphragmatic hernia.

c. Decortication.

d. Insertion of a V-P shunt.

5. A 13-year-old girl is found to have a 2-cm ovarian cyst on ultrasound scan. The treatment of choice is:

a. Exploratory laparotomy.

b. Angiography.

c. Trial of oral contraceptives.

d. Laparoscopy.

REFERENCES

1. Cohen Z, Shinhar D, Kurzbart E, et al. Laparoscopic and thoracoscopic surgery in children & adolescents: a 3-year experience. *Pediatr Surg Int* 1997;12:356–359.

2. Deziel DJ, Millikan KW, Economou SG, et al. Complications of laparoscopic cholecystectomy: a national survey of 4,292 hospitals and an analysis of 77,604 cases. *Am J Surg* 1993;165:9–14.

3. Glasgow RE, Yee LF, Mulvihill SJ. Laparoscopic splenectomy: the emerging standard. *Surg Endosc* 1997;11:108–112.

4. Hermans B-P, Otte JB. Laparoscopic appendectomy: pros & cons—literature review of 4190 cases. *Acta Chir Belg* 1997;97:110–117.

5. Kleinhaus S. Laparoscopic lysis of adhesions for postappendectomy pain. *Gastrointest Endosc* 1985;30:304–305.

6. Kleinhaus S, Hein K, Sheran M, et al. Laparoscopy for diagnosis and treatment of abdominal pain in adolescent girls. *Arch Surg* 1977;112:1178–1180.

7. Kleinhaus S, Kaleya R, Canning R, et al. Laparoscopic cholecystectomy in teenagers. *J Adolesc Health* 1992;13:693–695.

8. Ludwig KA, Milsom JW, Church JM, et al. Preliminary experience with laparoscopic intestinal surgery for Crohn's disease. *Am J Surg* 1996;171:52–56.

9. Nagel TC, Sebastian J, Malo JW. Oophoropexy to prevent sequestrial or recurrent torsion. *J Am Assoc Gynecol Laparosc* 1997;4:495–498.

10. Olsen D, McCord D, Law M. Laparoscopic discectomy with anterior interbody fusion of L5-S1. *Surg Endosc* 1996;10:1158–1163.

11. Rogers J, Yousuf A, Kleinhaus S. Laparoscopic accessory splenectomy in recurrent chronic immune thrombocytopenic purpura. *Surg Laparosc Endosc* 1997;7:83–85.

12. Rothenberg SS. Experience with 220 consecutive laparoscopic Nissen fundoplications in infants and children. *J Pediatr Surg* 1998;33:274–278.

13. Rutherford JC, Stowasser M, Tunny TJ, et al. Laparoscopic adrenalectomy. *World J Surg* 1996;20:758–761.

14. Seibold J, Jnnetschek G, Bartsch G. Laparoscopic surgery in pediatric urology. *Eur Urol* 1996;30:394–399.

ANSWERS

Chapter 1

1. c
2. c
3. c
4. a
5. b
6. d
7. b
8. d
9. c

Chapter 2

1. e
2. c
3. a
4. b
5. b, c
6. d
7. b
8. d
9 d
10. e

Chapter 3

1. a
2. b
3. c
4. c
5. c
6. d
7. a
8. b
9. c
10. c

Chapter 4

1. a,c
2. b
3. b
4. a, c, d
5. c
6. b, d
7. a
8. b
9. b, d
10. a, d
11. b
12. d
13. c
14. b, c
15. b, d

Chapter 5

1. e d
2. d
3. d
4. c
5. d
6. e
7. c
8. d
9. e
10. c

Chapter 6

1. True
2. True
3. True
4. False
5. False
6. True
7. False
8. True
9. True
10. False

Chapter 7

1. d
2. c
3. c
4. c
5. d
6. c
7. d
8. b
9. d
10. c

Chapter 8

1. b
2. d
3. c
4. e
5. d
6. a
7. a
8. c
9. e
10. b

Chapter 9

1. e
2. c
3. a
4. b
5. b

Chapter 10

1. b
2. a
3. d
4. d
5. e
6. b
7. d
8. e
9. b
10. c

Chapter 11

1. d
2. b
3. d
4. d
5. c
6. c
7. b
8. d
9. c
10. e
11. a

Chapter 12

1. False
2. False
3. False
4. False
5. True
6. True
7. False
8. True
9. True
10. False

Chapter 13

1. False
2. False
3. False
4. True
5. True
6. True
7. False
8. False
9. False
10. True

Chapter 14

1. c
2. c
3. c
4. a
5. c
6. e
7. b
8. a
9. a
10. e

Chapter 15

1. d
2. e
3. d
4. c
5. c
6. d
7. a
8. e
9. e
10. d

Chapter 16

1. e
2. c
3. d
4. e
5. a
6. c
7. a–iii; b–i, iv; c–ii, v; d–ii, v; e–i, iv
8. a–false, b–true, c–true, d–false
9. e
10. d

Chapter 17

1. c
2. b
3. b
4. b
5. b
6. d
7. a
8. b
9. b
10. d
11. b

Chapter 18

1. d
2. a
3. b
4. a, c, e
5. d

Chapter 19

1. b
2. a, b
3. d
4. c
5. b
6. d
7. a
8. b
9. d
10. a, b, d

Chapter 20

1. b
2. d
3. d
4. c
5. a
6. b
7. c
8. c
9. c
10. c

Chapter 21

1. a, b, c, d
2. a, b, c, d, e
3. a, c, d, e
4. a, b, d, e
5. b, c, e
6. a, b, d, e
7. b, c, e
8. a, b, c, d
9. a, d
10. a, b, c, d

Chapter 22

1. b
2. a
3. b
4. d
5. a
6. a
7. c
8. b
9. c
10. c

Chapter 23

1. b
2. c
3. a
4. b
5. a
6. b
7. a
8. c
9. b
10. c

Chapter 24

1. c
2. b
3. c
4. d
5. b
6. d

Chapter 25

1. c
2. c
3. b
4. b
5. a
6. b
7. c
8. c
9. a
10. c
11. a
12. d

Chapter 26

1. b
2. d
3. d
4. b
5. c
6. b
7. c
8. c
9. False
10. False
11. True
12. False
13. False
14. False
15. True

Chapter 27

1. c
2. b
3. d
4. d
5. c
6. d
7. d
8. b
9. d
10. b
11. d

Chapter 28

1. e
2. c
3. d
4. c
5. c
6. d
7. c
8. c
9. c
10. e
11. d
12. c

Chapter 29

1. c
2. c
3. d
4. a
5. e
6. c
7. d
8. a
9. b
10. d
11. d

Chapter 30

1. c
2. d
3. b
4. c, d
5. b
6. a
7. d
8. d
9. d
10. c

Chapter 31

1. c
2. b
3. d
4. a
5. c
6. b
7. d
8. b
9. a
10. b

Chapter 32

1. b
2. e
3. e
4. d
5. b
6. a
7. e
8. b
9. a

Chapter 33

1. b
2. c
3. d
4. c
5. c

Index

Note: Page numbers in *italics* indicate figures; page numbers followed by t indicate tables.